Renal Vascular Disease

Renal Vascular Disease

SENIOR EDITOR

A C NOVICK
Chairman
The Department of Urology
The Cleveland Clinic Foundation
Cleveland, Ohio, USA

ASSOCIATE EDITORS

J SCOBLE
The Renal Unit
Dulwich Hospital
London, UK

G HAMILTON
Consultant Surgeon
University Department of Surgery
Royal Free Hospital
London, UK

WB SAUNDERS COMPANY LTD
London · Philadelphia · Toronto · Sydney · Tokyo

WB Saunders Company Ltd 24–28 Oval Road
London NW1 7DX

The Curtis Center
Independence Square West
Philadelphia, PA 19106–3399, USA

Harcourt Brace Company
55 Horner Avenue
Toronto, Ontario M8Z 4X6, Canada

Harcourt Brace Company, Australia
30–52 Smidmore Street
Marrickville, NSW 2204, Australia

Harcourt Brace Company, Japan
Ichibancho Central Building, 22–1 Ichibancho
Chiyoda-ku, Tokyo, 102, Japan

This book is printed on acid-free paper

A catalogue record for this book is available from the British Library.

ISBN 0 7020 1814 7

Editorial and Production Services by Fisher Duncan
10 Barley Mow Passage, London W4 4PH

Typeset by Phoenix Photosetting, Chatham, Kent
Printed in Great Britain by the Bath Press, Lower Bristol Road, Bath

Contents

V Treatment

Contributors

O Abud, MD
Urology Service,
Fundacion Puigvert,
Clinica de la Santa Creu, Barcelona 08025,
Spain

FJ Albers, MD
Assistant Professor of Medicine,
Duke University Medical Center,
Box 3014, Durham, NC 27710,
USA

JF Angle, MD
Division of Angiography and Interventional Radiology,
Department of Radiology,
University of Virginia Health Sciences Center,
Charlottesville, VA 22908,
USA

AG Bellucci, MD
Cornell University Medical College,
Division of Nephrology and Hypertension,
North Shore University Hospital,
300 Community Drive, Manhasset, NY 11030,
USA

SE Bergentz, MD
Professor of Surgery,
Department of Surgery,
Malmö General Hospital,
University of Lund, S-214 01, Malmö,
Sweden

MS Berkoben, MD
Division of Nephrology,
Duke University Medical Center,
Box 3014, Durham,
NC 27710,
USA

GE Chéchile, MD
Urology Service,
Fundacion Puigvert,
Clinica de la Santa Creu, Barcelona 08025,
Spain

GM Chisolm, PhD
Department of Cell Biology,
Cleveland Clinic Foundation, NC10,
9500 Euclid Avenue,
Cleveland, OH44195,
USA

JE Deal, MD, MRCP, DCH
Consultant Paediatrician and Paediatric Nephrologist,
Department of Paediatrics,
St Mary's Hospital,
London W2 1NY,
UK

RH Dean, MD
Professor and Director, Division of Surgical Sciences,
Bowman Gray School of Medicine,
Medical Center Boulevard,
Winston-Salem, NC 27157,
USA

PE DiCorleto, MD
Department of Cell Biology,
Cleveland Clinic Foundation, NC10,
9500 Euclid Avenue,
Cleveland, OH 44195,
USA

MJ Dillon, MB, FRCP, DCH
Consultant Physician and Senior Clinical Nephrologist,
Institute of Child Health,
University of London,
30 Guildford Street
London WC1N 1EH,
UK

W Gedroyc, MBBS, MRCP, FRCR
Directorate of Radiology,
St Mary's Hospital,
London W2 1NY,
UK

GG Geyskes, MD
Department of Nephrology and Hypertension,
University Hospital Utrecht,
PO Box 85500,
3508 GA Utrecht,
The Netherlands

G Hamilton, FRCS
Consultant Vascular Surgeon,
University Department of Surgery,
Royal Free Hospital,
Pond Street,
London NW3,
UK

IF Hawkins Jr, MD
Department of Radiology,
University of Florida College of Medicine,
Box 100374, Gainesville,
FL 32610-0374,
USA

BD Higgs, MD, FFARCS
Consultant Anaesthetist,
Department of Anaesthesia,
Royal Free Hospital,
Pond Street, London NW3 2QG,
UK

JL Holley, MD
Division of Nephrology,
University of Pittsburgh Medical Center,
Pittsburgh, PA 15213,
USA

KC Irwin, MD
Department of Cell Biology,
Cleveland Clinic Foundation, NC 10,
9500 Euclid Avenue,
Cleveland, OH 44195
USA

ML Jordan, MD, FACS
Division of Urologic Surgery/Renal Transplantation,
University of Pittsburgh Medical Center,
Suite 700 Liliane Kaufman Building,
3471 Fifth Avenue,
Pittsburgh, PA 15213,
USA

SR Kerns, MD
Radiology Associates of Ocala,
Medical Imaging Center of Ocala,
1490 SE Magnolia Ave Ext,
Ocala, FL 34471,
USA

NE Madias, MD
Professor of Medicine,
Tufts University School of Medicine,
New England Medical Center,
750 Washington Street, BOX 172,
Boston, MA 02111,
USA

LU Mailloux, MD, FACP
Associate Professor of Clinical Medicine,
Cornell University Medical College,
Division of Nephrology and Hypertension,
North Shore University Hospital,
300 Community Drive,
Manhasset, NY 11030,
USA

AH Matsumoto, MD
Division of Angiography and Interventional Radiology,
Department of Radiology,
University of Virginia Health Sciences Center,
Charlottesville, VA 22908,
USA

RT Mossey, MD
Cornell University Medical College,
Division of Nephrology and Hypertension,
North Shore University Hospital,
300 Community Drive, Manhasset, NY 11030,
USA

JV Nally, MD
Department of Nephrology and Hypertension
desk A-101,
Cleveland Clinic Foundation,
9500 Euclid Avenue, Cleveland, OH 44195,
USA

B Napolitano, MD
Division of Biostatistics,
Cornell University Medical College,
Department of Research,
North Shore University Hospital,
300 Community Drive, Manhasset, NY 11030,
USA

AC Novick MD
Chairman, Department of Urology,
Cleveland Clinic Foundation,
One Clinic Center,
9500 Euclid Avenue,
Cleveland, OH 44195-5041,
USA

MS Phinney, MD
Fellow, Division of Nephrology,
University Hospitals of Cleveland,
11100 Euclid Avenue,
Cleveland, OH 44106,
USA

T Pickering, MD, DPhil
Professor of Medicine,
New York Hospital, Cornell Medical Center,
520 East 70 Street,
Starr 463,
New York, NY 10021,
USA

DA Plante, MD
Associate Professor of Medicine,
University of Vermont,
College of Medicine,
Burlington, VT 05405,
USA

AD Platts, MB, BS, FRCS, FRCR
Consultant Radiologist,
Department of Radiology,
Royal Free Hospital,
Pond Street, London NW3 2QG,
UK

MA Pohl, MD
Department of Hypertension and Nephrology,
Cleveland Clinic Foundation,
9500 Euclid Avenue,
Cleveland, OH 44195,
USA

J Reidy, MB BS, MRCS, FRCP, FRCR
Department of Radiology,
Guy's Hospital, London SE1 9RT,
UK

JM Rimmer, MD
Medical Center Hospital of Vermont,
Brown II Dialysis Unit,
Burlington, VT 05401,
USA

W Sandmann, MD
Heinrich-Heine-Universitat Dusseldorf,
Mooenstrasse 5,
Postfach 10 10 07,
D-40225 Dusseldorf,
Germany

SJ Schwab, MD
Division of Nephrology,
Duke University Medical Center,
Durham, NC 27710,
USA

JE Scoble, MA, MD, MRCP
Consultant Nephrologist,
Renal Unit,
Dulwich Hospital,
East Dulwich Grove,
London SE22 8PT,
UK

Z Shapira, MD
Professor of Surgery,
Head, Department of Transplantation,
Beilinson Medical Center,
Petah-Tiqva, 49100I,
Israel

TA Sos, MD
Director of Cardiovascular and Interventional Radiology,
The New York Hospital,
Cornell Medical Center,
Department of Radiology,
525 East 68 Street,
New York, NY 10021,
USA

JC Stanley, MD
Professor of Surgery,
Head, Section of Vascular Surgery,
University Hospital,
1500 East Medical Center Drive,
Ann Arbor, MI 48109-0329,
USA

MC Smith, MD
Associate Professor of Medicine,
Case Western Reserve University School of Medicine,
Division of Nephrology,
University Hospitals of Cleveland,
11100 Euclid Avenue,
Cleveland, OH 44106,
USA

L Smith-Powell, MD
Research Associate,
City of Hope National Medical Center,
Duarte, California,
USA

F Solé-Balcells, MD
Urology Service,
Fundacion Puigvert,
Clinica de la Santa Creu,
Barcelona 08025,
Spain

DE Strandness Jr, MD
Chief, Division of Vascular Surgery,
Department of Surgery, RF-25,
University of Washington School of Medicine,
1059 NE Pacific Street,
Seattle, WA 98195,
USA

LP Svetkey, MD, MHS
Department of Medicine,
Duke University Medical Center,
Durham, NC 27710,
USA

JD Swales, Professor
Department of Medicine,
Clinical Sciences Building,
Leicester Royal Infirmary,
Leicester LE2 7LX,
UK

P Sweny, MD, FRCP
Consultant Nephrologist,
Honorary Senior Lecturer,
Royal Free Hospital,
Pond Street,
London NW3 2QG,
UK

CJ Tegtmeyer, MD
Division of Angiography and Interventional Radiology,
Department of Radiology,
University of Virginia Health Sciences Center,
Charlottesville, VA 22908,
USA

JL Terpstra, MD
Section of Vascular Surgery/Department of Surgery,
University Hospital,
2300 RC Leiden,
The Netherlands

SC Textor, MD
Associate Professor of Medicine,
Mayo Medical School,
Consultant, Division of Hypertension,
Mayo Clinic, 200 First Street SW,
Rochester, MN 55905,
USA

H Toma, MD
Department of Urology,
Tokyo Women's Medical College,
8-1 Kawadacho,
Shinjuku-ku, Tokyo,
162 Japan

G Torsello, MD PhD
Department of Vascular Surgery and Kidney Transplantation,
Heinrich-Heine-University,
Mooenstrasse 6,
Postfach 10 10 07,
40001 Dusseldorf,
Germany

D Trost, MD
Assistant Professor of Radiology,
The New York Hospital Cornell Medical Center,
Department of Radiology,
525 East 68th Street,
New York, NY 10021
USA

JH van Bockel, MD
Section of Vascular Surgery,
Department of Surgery,
University Hospital Leiden,
Leiden,
The Netherlands

MA Vernace, MD
Cornell University Medical College,
Division of Nephrology and Hypertension,
North Shore University Hospital,
300 Community Drive,
Manhasset, NY 11030,
USA

H Weibull, MD
Associate Professor of Surgery,
Department of Surgery,
Malmö General Hospital,
University of Lund,
214 01 Malmö,
Sweden

BM Wilkes, MD
Cornell University Medical College,
Division of Nephrology and Hypertension,
North Shore University Hospital,
300 Community Drive,
Manhasset, NY 11030,
USA

R Wilkinson, BSc, MD, FRCP,
Professor of Renal Medicine,
Freeman Hospital,
High Heaton,
Newcastle Upon Tyne NE7 7DN,
UK

AB Zajko, MD
Department of Radiology,
University of Pittsburgh Medical Center,
Pittsburgh, PA 15213,
USA

Preface

The past decade has witnessed important advances in the clinical approach to patients with renal artery disease. Early recognition and treatment of renovascular hypertension remain integral to obviating the lethal potential of this disease. Several recent epidemiologic studies have highlighted that atherosclerotic renal artery disease is quite common in patients with generalized atherosclerosis obliterans regardless of whether renovascular hypertension is present. The development of chronic renal failure from atherosclerotic renal artery disease, termed ischemic nephropathy, has become an important clinical issue. The exact number of patients with end-stage renal disease from ischemic nephropathy is not known, but there appear to be several thousand patients in this category. These patients usually do not respond well to renal replacement therapy, highlighting the importance of appropriately timed intervention to preserve renal function at an earlier stage of the disease.

Several non-invasive imaging and functional tests are now available for detecting renovascular hypertension and ischemic nephropathy in patients with suggestive signs and symptoms. When renal artery disease is considered to be the cause of significant hypertension or renal insufficiency, or both, several primary treatment options are available. These include: medical management, surgical revascularization, percutaneous transluminal angioplasty, and endovascular stenting. Multiple factors must be carefully weighed in determining which form of management is more appropriate for a given patient. These include the causal relationship of renal vascular disease to hypertension, the adequacy of blood pressure control with medical therapy, the natural history of untreated renal vascular disease with particular regard for the risk of sustaining impaired renal function, the medical condition of the patient, and the known results of surgical revascularization, angioplasty and stenting in specific clinical subgroups.

The pathophysiologic and pathologic features, epidemiology, clinical manifestations, screening, diagnosis and management of different types of renal artery disease in adults and children are extensively reviewed in this textbook by distinguished clinical scientists from diverse disciplines. We acknowledge with deep appreciation their efforts and expertise which blend together so well to enhance our understanding of these subjects.

We are also appreciative of the organizational efforts and secretarial assistance provided by Lenore Krell, personal secretary of the senior editor. Finally, our special thanks go to Georgina Bentliff, Tracy Breakell, and Rachael Stock of WB Saunders Co., for their patience and guidance along the road to final publication.

Our hope is that this book will serve as a comprehensive and practical reference source for physicians and surgeons managing renal vascular disease and thereby improve the care of these patients.

Andrew C Novick MD
for the Editors

PART I

Pathology and Clinical Features

1

Atherosclerosis: characterization of the disease and underlying mechanisms

GUY M CHISOLM, KIMBERLY C IRWIN, PAUL E DICORLETO

Introduction

In the following pages, atherosclerosis will be described from three perspectives, each useful in different contexts. First, descriptions of atherosclerotic lesions in humans as they are being redefined in standardized, updated terms are summarized. The Lesion Committee of the Arteriosclerosis Council of the American Heart Association has published two of three planned articles classifying human arterial lesions and the classification is briefly presented here.[1, 2] This description requires first a brief review of the normal arterial structure and the variations that exist in the artery wall sites at which atherosclerosis occurs with higher probability. The occurrence of atherosclerosis is intimately linked to the metabolism of lipoproteins due to the compelling correlations between lipoprotein levels and risk of disease. Lipoprotein metabolism is therefore briefly reviewed as background for the second perspective on atherosclerosis, which is a description of the most probable sequence of events, including the appearance of various cell populations, that occurs in the development of the atherosclerotic lesion. This sequence should be viewed as a current viewpoint and as a useful framework to evaluate new findings, rather than as an absolute description of the developmental stages of all lesions. As a final perspective, rather than evaluate each of the numerous theories that have been developed over decades to explain atherosclerosis, we have opted to describe in detail two interrelated hypotheses for atherogenesis, which are currently receiving significant attention from the atherosclerosis research community.

Atherosclerosis: general perspectives

Atherosclerosis is a complex, multifactorial disease which, with its complications, is estimated to account for over half the deaths in the US. Atherosclerosis is generally defined by the deposition of lipids within the intimal layer of large muscular and elastic arteries. It is defined by some as a subclass of arteriosclerosis, a general term used to describe disorders that result in thickening and loss of elasticity of vascular walls, or 'hardening of the arteries'. However, many use the terms atherosclerosis and arteriosclerosis interchangeably. Early atherosclerotic lesions occur most frequently in areas associated with adaptive intimal hyperplasia. This adaptation is thought to be a physiologic response to hemodynamic forces resulting from disturbed blood flow and altered shear stress. Adaptive intimal hyperplasia and atherosclerosis are more frequently associated with arterial regions where branching occurs. Adaptive hyperplasia is believed to develop into early atherosclerotic lesions under the influence of various risk factors. The major risk factors include elevated total cholesterol, elevated low density lipoprotein (LDL), untreated hypertension, smoking, diabetes and low levels of high density lipoprotein (HDL).[3] Other aggravating factors include elevated plasma levels of triglycerides (as VLDL), lipoprotein (a), homocysteine or fibrinogen, as well as the presence of hyperinsulinemia, abdominal obesity and various dietary factors. Many of these risk factors are greatly influenced by genetics.

The basic atheroslerotic lesion consists of a raised plaque. The core of this plaque, containing a mixture that includes cholesterol and cholesteryl esters, is covered by a fibrous cap. The disease begins early in life as discrete, focal lesions located primarily in the aortic arch, descending aorta and abdominal aorta. With puberty, the lesions tend to progress down the aorta until the age of 30, when the abdominal aorta is more affected than the thoracic aorta.[4, 5] As atherosclerotic lesions advance, the initial focal lesions become diffuse and circumferential with a reduction in the size of the lumen such that blood flow is compromised. Thrombosis can ultimately occlude the affected vessel or the arterial wall may become weakened with the subsequent development of an aneurysm.

Atherosclerosis frequently affects multiple organs. For example, prevalence of clinically unsuspected renal artery stenosis was discovered in patients with known atherosclerosis elsewhere, including those with abdominal aortic disease, aorto-occlusive disease and lower extremity occlusive disease.[6] Patients with pathologic conditions characterized by hyperlipidemia are more likely to have diffuse atherosclerotic lesions. These conditions include the familial dyslipidemias, diabetes mellitus, chronic renal insufficiency and prior organ transplantation.

The importance of atherosclerosis is enormous considering that its prevalence threatens the health and productivity of a high proportion of our population. In addition, the status of a patient's vascular disease is an important consideration in many procedures contemplated as therapy for other diseases. Unfortunately, the mechanisms leading to the disease are poorly understood despite considerable research toward such understanding and despite substantial progress in understanding the disease process. As a result, the therapies for prevention of lesion formation or those administered to support lesion regression are guided by reducing risk factors. As an example of the uncertainty that persists, it can be pointed out that the medical and research communities agree to a large extent that high plasma concentrations of LDL signal high risk of disease and regimens to lower LDL appear to lower risk; however, it is still not known how or why elevated LDL actually causes the disease or, for that matter, if high LDL levels alone are sufficient to cause lesion development.

Structure and composition of normal arteries

The arterial wall is made up of three distinct concentric layers, the intima, the media and the adventitia. The inner layer, the intima, is bounded by a single continuous layer of endothelial cells which lines the vessel. Underlying the endothelial cells are various numbers, but in normalcy relatively few, smooth muscle cells and occasional macrophages existing in a proteoglycan-rich matrix. The location of endothelial cells places them in direct contact with the plasma and its components making these cells regulators of permeability to large molecules which must pass through their gap and tight junctions. Molecules can be transported from plasma to intima by traversing the endothelial junctions or by vesicular transport, depending on their molecular size and charge. In addition, endothelial cells function as regulators of vascular tone. These cells are capable of producing prostacyclin and relaxing factors like nitric oxide, which are vasodilators, as well as endothelin, a potent vasoconstrictor. Endothelial cells also express under various conditions specific leukocyte adhesion molecules which in conjunction with chemoattractants serve to regulate monocyte, neutrophil and lymphocyte entry into the intima. Endothelium also represents an effective non-thrombogenic surface that separates blood from the underlying thrombogenic components, such as collagen. Endothelial cells in their normal state have a very low rate of turnover, considerably less than 1% per day.

Another cell type residing in the intima is the vascular smooth muscle cell. It is believed that intimal smooth muscle cells can express two phenotypes. One is rich in myofilaments and characterized by contractile properties, while the second is rich in rough endoplasmic reticulum (RER) and is described to be in a synthetic state. Smooth muscle cells in the latter state have been referred to as 'modified', 'modulated', 'fibroblast-like' or 'activated', as well as 'RER-rich' and synthetic.[1] In normalcy, the intima contains a greater proportion of myofilament-rich contractile smooth muscle cells than the synthetic type. The presence of smooth muscle cells in the intima of human fetuses has been observed as early as 30–33 weeks' gestation.[7] The number of intimal smooth muscle cells increases with age.

Monocyte-derived macrophages are a third cell type found in the normal intima. They are present as isolated cells and produce collagenase and elastase, which may facilitate their movement. Upon the appropriate stimulation, these resident phagocytes are capable of elaborating important growth factors for endothelial cells and smooth muscle cells, and thus may play a role in smooth muscle cell regulation, wound healing and angiogenesis. Monocyte-derived macrophages are also active in lipoprotein metabolism since they express receptors which recognize and lead to the uptake of modified forms of lipoproteins, including oxidatively modified LDL.

The intima exhibits different characteristics at different depths. The layer closest to the lumen is composed of a matrix rich in heparan sulfate and dermatan sulfate proteoglycans. The endothelium synthesizes predominantly heparan sulfate and smaller amounts of dermatan sulfate while smooth muscle cells synthesize the bulk of the dermatan sulfate. With age, the amount of dermatan sulfate and chondroitin sulfate proteoglycans surpasses that of heparan sulfate and chondroitin sulfate proteoglycans, reflecting the increased contribution of smooth muscle cells. Collagen is a major component of atherosclerotic plaques and is the most abundant extracellular protein. The regulation of collagen synthesis may influence plaque development. Smooth muscle cells produce the bulk of the collagen; Types I and III collagens dominate, although Type V and other collagens are also present.[8] Both types of smooth muscle cells, synthetic and contractile, are found in the inner intimal layer, as are a small number of macrophages.

The deepest layer of the intima has musculoelastic characteristics similar to the adjacent tunica media. This region of the intima contains abundant smooth muscle cells of the contractile phenotype arranged in layers. The elastin content is greater in children and decreases with aging. The principal proteoglycan in the musculoelastic layer is dermatan sulfate rich, consistent with its likely production by the abundant smooth muscle cells. Another important component of both layers of the intima is fibronectin, a glycoprotein that functions in cell–cell adhesion and influences cell motility.

It is important to note that all three cell types of the intima mentioned above are capable of producing a variety of growth factors and cytokines in response to particular stimuli. The capacity of intimal cells to release biological response modifiers and influence their own behavior, or that of neighboring cells, needs to be considered when theorizing on the genesis of the atherosclerotic plaque.

The second layer of the vessel wall is the tunica media. It is separated from the intima by the internal elastic lamina (IEL), which can restrict the transport of larger molecules.[9] The media of both muscular and elastic arteries is composed of circumferentially arranged, elongated layers of smooth muscle cells with intervening elastic fibers. The elastic content of this layer contributes to the resilience of the vessel. Elastic arteries contain multiple discrete lamellae of elastin, alternating with smooth muscle cell layers, in addition to, and concentrically arranged between, the internal and external elastic laminae.

The third layer of the vessel wall is the adventitia. It lies by definition outside the external elastic lamina and consists of loosely arranged connective tissue. This layer is penetrated by the vasa vasorum, the system of blood and lymphatic vessels that provides the exchange of nutrients and other substances within this outer portion of the artery. The inner layers of the vessel are largely dependent on diffusion from the luminal plasma for nutritional requirements, whereas the outer layers and adventitia depend on the vasa vasorum. In larger arteries, the vasa vasorum penetrates the outer media. The principal resident cell type of the adventitia is the fibroblast. The adventitial layer is not believed to play a role in atherosclerotic plaque development which is localized to the intimal layer.

Classification of atherosclerotic lesions

Multiple schemes for lesion classification are currently in use. In one such scheme lesion progression in both animals and humans is perceived to proceed from the early fatty streak lesion, to the fibrous plaque, then to the complicated lesion. The fatty streak is characterized by clusters of lipid-engorged monocyte-derived macrophages that accumulate in large enough numbers to create grossly visible, raised lesions. The crowded array of lipid droplets within these macrophages is predominantly composed of cholesteryl esters. These cells were referred to as foam cells by pathologists due to the characteristic foamy look of these droplets in the microscope. Fibrous plaques are characterized by a necrotic core at or near the base of the lesion; the core is comprised of extracellular lipid, rich in free (unesterified) cholesterol and cellular debris. The fibrous cap covering the necrotic core has extensive connective tissue in which smooth muscle cells reside and proliferate. Early fatty streaks and late fibrous plaques develop at similar predilection sites in the arterial system. The fatty streak is believed to be a precursor lesion that can either regress and resolve, or progress to a more advanced lesion. Complicated lesions encompass a category with a variety of manifestations, including ulceration or rupturing, which leads to thrombosis. Hemorrhaged lesions are those in which new capillaries invading the lesion are damaged, and calcified lesions are those in which apatite crystals are produced in the lesion resulting in a brittle texture.

In the second classification scheme, atherosclerotic lesion subdivisions are more precisely defined particularly for the sake of describing the human disease.[1, 2, 10] Lesions are categorized according to a series of changes believed to take place in a somewhat predictable order. They are designated Type I to Type VIII with increasing severity.[2, 10] The progression is perceived to be accelerated depending on the degree of hyperlipidemia and the presence of other risk factors. Type I lesions are present in infants, children and adults with minimal atherosclerotic disease and occur in areas of physiologic intimal hyperplasia. They are characterized by the presence of small yellow dots which may or may not be visible to the naked eye. These small dots represent focal populations of macrophages engorged with lipid droplets. These engorged macrophages are the aforementioned foam cells and are the first histologic abnormality seen in experimental animals on hypercholesterolemic diets.

Type II lesions are also observed in children. These lesions are somewhat more structurally defined and include fatty streaks. They differ from Type I lesions in that there is an increased number of cells, particularly macrophage-derived foam cells, and a greater amount of intracellular lipid in these cells. Smooth muscle cells also start to become involved in the lesion.[1, 10] Most of the lipid continues to be intracellular, but some begins to be found extracellularly. Furthermore, T-lymphocytes and mast cells can be identified in the lesion site.

Type II lesions can be divided into two groups. Type IIA lesions are located in areas of hemodynamic stress which have already undergone physiologic intimal hyperplasia. Type IIA lesions are also known as atherosclerosis prone and have a tendency to advance. Type IIB are classified as progression resistant.[1] Unlike progression-prone lesions, progression-resistant lesions have a thinner intima with fewer smooth muscle cells, suggesting less mechanical stress. With time, Type IIA lesions are believed to advance to Type III lesions. Type III lesions represent the preatheroma stage of atherosclerosis.[1, 10] They are characterized by a greater deposition of lipid intracellularly in both macrophages and smooth muscle cells, as well as extracellular lipid within the matrix between smooth muscle cells.

Type IV lesions correspond to the atheroma stage of atherosclerosis. The lesion consists of a large organized extracellular lipid core, which disrupts and deforms the intima, and a superficial fibrous cap.[10] The Type V lesion, the fibroatheroma, has the same characteristics as the atheroma, but with markedly increased layers of collagen and smooth muscle cells overlying the lipid core. These initially focal lesions can coalesce to form larger lesions that extend circumferentially around the vessel. Sites of predilection are the abdominal aorta, coronary arteries, popliteal arteries, descending aorta, internal carotid arteries and vessels of the circle of Willis. Fully developed atheromatous lesions may undergo a series of changes and result in complicated plaques, referred to as Type VI lesions.[10] These advanced lesions may calcify (Type VII), turning the aorta into a so-called 'brittle pipe'. In addition, complicated Type VI lesions may ulcerate (Type VIA) on the luminal surface and allow debris or microemboli to spill into the bloodstream. Furthermore, cracks (fissures) and ulcerations on the surface of complicated advanced lesions may result in thrombosis (Type VIC), which can acutely occlude the lumen or become incorporated into the lesion resulting in further deformation of the luminal surface. Hemorrhage may also occur inside the plaque (Type VIB) increasing the size of the lesion. These lesions ultimately affect the underlying media such that the outer wall becomes weak which may lead to aneurysmal dilatation. Type VIII lesions are advanced lesions composed predominantly of collagen and other connective tissues. These may or may not have intermediately developed as Type VI lesions.[10]

As atherosclerotic lesions progress, particular changes occur in the makeup of the matrix. For instance, certain sulfated glycosaminoglycans, particularly dermatan sulfate and chondroitin sulfate, which exist as components of high molecular weight proteoglycans, increase, while others, such as heparan sulfate-rich proteoglycans, decrease. The chondroitin sulfate/dermatan sulfate-rich proteoglycans are known to bind apo B-containing lipoproteins (VLDL, LDL). The amounts of various collagens increase. With progressive disease, there is also an increased accumulation of minor collagen types (Types IV, V and VI) and a relative decrease in elastin fibers in the late stages. However, Types I and III collagens are quantitatively dominant in both normal and diseased vessels.[1, 8, 11]

In addition to the above changes in chemical composition of the matrix, the lipid composition of the lesion changes as the lesion progresses. Initially, three-fourths of lipid in Type II lesions are composed of cholesteryl esters, primarily oleate and linoleate; the remainder is mostly free cholesterol and phospholipids. As lesions advance to Type III, the core lipids contain more free cholesterol, fatty acids, lysolecithin and triglycerides. In addition, the type of cholesteryl esters changes, such that linoleate increases relative to oleate.

Controversy still surrounds the issue of whether the fibrous lesion is a progressed form of lesion which began as a fatty streak. While the issue is unsettled, there is a dominant belief that fatty streaks can, but do not always, progress to form the more advanced lesion types. Supporting this notion and reflected in the aforementioned categorizations of fatty streaks as either Type IIA or IIB lesions depending on their respective tendencies to be progression prone or resistant, is a general finding of temporal consistency, that is, fatty streaks are typically found earlier in life in humans than fibrous plaques. In addition, the sites of predilection for fatty streaks and early atheroma overlap considerably, strengthening the contention that the latter develops from the former.

The evidence suggesting that atheroma do not develop from fatty streaks has included the discrepancies between the lipid composition of fatty streaks (Type II lesions) and that of the more advanced fibrous plaques (Type IV and V lesions). Lipid deposition in fatty streaks is predominantly cholesteryl esters, with cholesteryl oleate being the most prominent, whereas the lipid of fibrous plaques is enriched in free cholesterol, with cholesteryl linoleate dominating the cholesteryl ester pool.[12]

Recently, measurements of the composition of microscopic pools of lipids within lesions have contributed to our understanding of plaque progression. From these microanalyses and histological and electron microscope evaluations, inferences have been made as to whether the extracellular lipid pools in fibrous plaques derive from dead foam cells or from extracellular deposition of lipoproteins. A study which focused on 'fibrolipid' lesions—lesions resembling Type III in description—revealed that the lipids of the cap (luminal portion) of these lesions had lipid compositions resembling fatty streaks; whereas, the deeper core lipids had higher proportions of unesterified cholesterol and a variable content of cholesteryl ester.[12] The cholesteryl ester pool of the core had a lower oleate and higher linoleate proportion than the cap lipids.[12] These findings are important because they suggest that the cap lipids correspond to those found in fatty streaks and the newly developing core lipids are derived from extracellular deposition of lipoprotein rather than extracellular lipid remaining from foam cell death. The cholesteryl ester fraction of LDL is predominantly cholesteryl linoleate. Upon uptake by cells, the cholesteryl ester is hydrolyzed to free cholesterol. The excess cholesterol to be stored by the cell, such as that taken up as modified LDL by macrophages, is re-esterified but predominantly with oleate.[13] Thus, the cholesteryl ester pool of foam cell-rich tissue would be expected to be predominantly oleate, whereas the cholesteryl ester pool of extracellular deposits of plasma lipoprotein would be predominantly linoleate. The above findings are consistent with the concept that these fibrolipid lesions represent a transition in the development of fibrous plaques from fatty streaks.

Lipoprotein metabolism

Since deposition of lipoprotein-borne lipid in the intima appears to be the first step in the development and progression of atherosclerosis (see below), it is important to consider certain aspects of lipoprotein metabolism when reviewing this vascular disease process.[14, 15] Lipoproteins are macromolecular complexes of lipid and protein ideally suited to the transport of lipid in aqueous media such as plasma, inter stitial fluid and lymph. The larger lipoproteins consist of a hydrophobic core made up of triglycerides and cholesteryl esters in various proportions. This core is surrounded by a hydrophilic shell made up of particular apolipoproteins (apoproteins), cholesterol and phospholipids. This more polar shell allows lipids to be transported in the blood and delivered to their sites of metabolism or storage. There are four major classes of lipoproteins, namely, chylomicrons, VLDL, LDL and HDL. They can be distinguished by differences in their sizes, buoyant densities and electrophoretic mobilities, as well as by the specific apoproteins found on their surfaces.

After a meal containing lipids, pancreatic lipases in the small intestine hydrolyze the ingested triglycerides into individual fatty acids and monoglycerides. They, along with ingested cholesterol, are then absorbed into the small intestinal epithelial cells where they are re-esterified into triglycerides and cholesteryl esters, and, along with phospholipids, are packaged into the core of chylomicrons. The assembly includes one molecule of apoprotein B (apo B) per particle as the predominant apoprotein, and a minor amount of apo AI. In humans, the form of apo B made in gut, called B-48, is a truncated form of that made in liver, called B-100. B-48 is a product of the same gene as B-100, but is made after gut-specific editing of the messenger RNA coding apo B. These triglyceride-rich chylomicrons enter the mesenteric lymphatic system and are eventually emptied into the bloodstream at the vena cava via the thoracic duct. In the bloodstream, the chylomicrons immediately come into contact with endothelial cell surface-bound lipoprotein lipase. This enzyme is activated by a specific apoprotein, namely apoprotein CII, which is transferred in plasma from HDL to the surface of the chylomicron. Lipoprotein lipase catalyzes the breakdown of triglycerides into free fatty acids, glycerol and monoglycerides, while the cholesteryl esters remain intact. The free fatty acids are taken up into adipocytes for fat storage as triglyceride until they are later hydrolyzed and transported out of cells as needed for energy. The circulating chylomicron remnant becomes triglyceride poor and cholesteryl ester rich while undergoing various exchanges with HDL such that the remnant loses apo AI, apo AII and phospholipids to HDL and gains apo E. With the acquisition of apo E, the chylomicron remnant can be rapidly removed from the circulation via specific apo E receptors on hepatocytes. The end-result is the delivery of triglycerides to adipocytes and the delivery of cholesterol to the liver.

Very low density lipoprotein, which is also rich in triglyceride, is synthesized continuously in the liver. In addition to triglycerides, it also contains smaller amounts of cholesteryl esters, phospholipids, free cholesterol and proteins. Its apoproteins consist of apo Cs, AI and a single molecule of apo B (B-100). Its fate is similar to that of the chylomicron, that is, it is transported into the blood, where it encounters endothelial cell-bound lipoprotein lipase, which degrades the triglycerides and delivers free fatty acids for fat storage and later energy utilization. The remnant VLDL, which becomes intermediate in density (IDL) between VLDL and LDL, exchanges components with HDL such that the remnant acquires apo E and loses apo AI. As with chylomicron remnants, some VLDL remnants can be taken up by the liver via an apo E receptor; but VLDL remnants can also continue to lose their content of triglycerides while becoming relatively enriched with cholesteryl esters. In the latter case, all apoproteins except the single apo B molecule are lost, transforming these remnants into the lipoprotein class known as LDL.

Cholesterol is an important constituent of cell membranes as well as a precursor for adrenal and gonadal steroids and bile acids. In normal fasting human plasma cholesterol is present in the bloodstream chiefly on LDL, on which it is transported principally as cholesteryl ester. Elevated levels of both total cholesterol and LDL cholesterol have long been recognized as major risk factors for the development of atherosclerosis. In the Bogalusa Heart Study, for example, the measured area of fatty streaks found in the aorta and coronary arteries of normal children who died of non-atherosclerotic causes was proportional to premortem LDL cholesterol levels.[16]

The amount of LDL in plasma is determined largely by the presence of a specific LDL receptor (the B/E receptor) located primarily on hepatocytes, but also on peripheral cells. B/E receptors located on hepatocytes and peripheral cells recognize specific epitopes on apo B and apo E and incorporate LDL into the cell via receptor-mediated endocytosis. From there, the LDL enters endosomes that fuse with lysosomes. In lysosomes, apo B and cholesteryl esters are hydrolyzed. The receptor is returned to the surface of the hepatocyte. The resulting free cholesterol has multiple cellular effects, including downregulation of the production of new B/E receptors, decrease in HMG CoA reductase, the rate limiting enzyme in *de novo* cholesterol synthesis, and increase in the activity of the enzyme acetylcoenzyme A cholesterol acyltransferase (ACAT), which esterifies free cholesterol for intracellular storage. These mechanisms allow hepatic and other cells to regulate the supply of intracellular cholesterol by balancing the uptake from LDL particles with *de novo* synthesis from acetyl-CoA.[17]

Recent studies indicate that the size and density of LDL appear to correlate with its atherogenic properties. Low density lipoprotein has been shown to exist in two phenotypic density patterns.[18] Type A is characterized by predominantly large LDL particles, while Type B is distinguished by an increased proportion of small, dense LDL particles. In 85–90% of subjects only one phenotype is exhibited, while the remainder have both phenotypes. Type B LDL, occurring in approximately 30% of the population, is associated with a higher risk of coronary artery disease. It has been suggested that small, dense LDL may be more atherogenic by virtue of its small size, which would allow it to enter more readily the arterial intima. However, the small, dense LDL is also more susceptible *in vitro* to metal ion-mediated oxidation.[19] This phenotype is also associated with increased plasma triglycerides and apo B levels while apo AI and HDL cholesterol are typically lower.[18] It is currently uncertain whether small, dense LDL is actually more atherogenic or simply a marker of an atherogenic profile.

Unlike LDL, an elevated HDL cholesterol is believed to decrease the risk of coronary heart disease, while a low HDL cholesterol is considered a positive risk factor.[14, 15, 20] High density lipoprotein is believed to accomplish reverse cholesterol transport, the transport of cholesterol from the peripheral tissues to the liver for catabolism. It has been shown that HDL can remove cholesterol directly from foam cells in atherosclerotic lesions.[21] High density lipoprotein is made up of a variety of apoproteins, including AI, AII, AVI, Cs and E as well as phospholipids and cholesteryl esters. It is formed predominantly in the liver and modified in plasma by association of these individual components. High density lipoprotein-3 is a small, cholesterol-poor form of HDL. Initially, it interacts with free cholesterol that has been released from cell membranes of degenerating cells, then is acted on in plasma by lecithin cholesteryl acyltransferase (LCAT). This enzyme catalyzes the removal of a fatty acid from phosphatidylcholine and converts free cholesterol to the less polar cholesteryl ester, forcing the cholesteryl ester to a deeper location in the core of the lipoprotein. This conversion allows more cholesterol to be accepted by the lipoprotein. Furthermore, as the size of the HDL complex increases, more apo Cs can be accepted and the resultant complex is known as HDL-2. Other transfers are possible. For instance, cholesteryl esters can be transferred in plasma by cholesteryl ester transfer protein (CETP; also called lipid transfer protein because it transfers both cholesteryl esters and triglycerides among lipoprotein populations) from HDL to triglyceride-rich VLDL and LDL.

Early events in atherosclerotic lesion initiation and development

The following is a hypothetical sequence of events for lesion development inferred from the results of numerous studies in experimental animals and pathological and epidemiological data in humans. In reality it is likely that the disease is multifactorial and that numerous factors influence the sequence and the rapidity of lesion development. The presence of variable subsets of known risk factors, including genetic influences and the parallel presence of other diseases, could likely cause deviations in the progression of this complex disease which afflicts most people in Western societies. Despite this caveat one can nevertheless construct a 'most probable' series of steps in lesion development. As a logical starting place, one may invoke the fact that sites of predilection for lesion initiation coincide generally with regions of the arterial tree that exhibit intimal thickening in normalcy. The pattern of these sites suggests that they form in response to hemodynamic influences, such as altered shear stress, as would be expected near vascular branching points.

The most likely next step in the process is the accumulation in the interstitial space of this thickened intima of those plasma lipoproteins associated with increased risk of disease, that is, LDL and VLDL remnants. There are several factors which could influence the levels of intimal lipoprotein accumulation. First, it is important to recognize the influence of physical factors which govern lipoprotein transport to and from the intima. Molecules the size of lipoproteins traverse the normal arterial endothelium chiefly via vesicular transport and possibly via interendothelial cell junctions during the junctional interruption occurring in the course of the replacement of a dying cell by its migrating or proliferating neighboring cells. Loss of lipoproteins from the intima may occur via the reverse of the influx process, by uptake and catabolism of the particles by intimal cells or by transport across the IEL into the tunica media. While the endothelium thus regulates macromolecular transport, there is in fact a finite transport across normal endothelium and in general the entry rate into the intima from plasma is proportional to plasma lipoprotein levels.[22] Vesicular and junctional transport would both result in net movement according to the concentration gradient, that is, in the direction from plasma to intima. It has recently been demonstrated that, despite the documentation of its large pores, the IEL represents a significant barrier to macromolecular transport.[9] It follows from these considerations that elevated plasma LDL or VLDL would proportionally elevate the interstitial levels of these lipoproteins,[22] and that the IEL would help confine the entering lipoprotein to the intima by restricting its passage into the media.

The thickened intima may exhibit increased vulnerability to lipoprotein retention due to two factors. First, LDL or VLDL traversing the endothelium from plasma can diffuse further from the endothelium into an intima that has thickened, decreasing the probability that the lipoprotein would accumulate near the abluminal endothelial cell membrane and thereby decreasing the probability that a given lipoprotein molecule would leave the intima toward the plasma by endothelial vesicular transport. Secondly, LDL has a well-documented tendency to bind to dermatan sulfate and chondroitin sulfate-rich proteoglycans, collagen and other connective tissue elements. Enhanced connective tissue elaboration is a prominent property of the thickened intima. The combination of elevated LDL, LDL binding to connective tissue, expanded interstitial space and restrictions to movement across the IEL[9] act in concert to increase the residence time of LDL focally at these sites of predilection. Furthermore, endothelial cell turnover at these sites appears to be increased, which may represent an additional factor favoring enhanced accumulation, given the likely increase in permeability of the endothelium to LDL that is believed to occur during cell replication.[23]

The next series of events in the atherogenic sequence is the binding of monocytes to endothelium, the extension of processes by the monocytes toward endothelial cell junctions and the diapedesis of the bound monocytes through the endothelial cell layer and into the intima. These phenomena have been thoroughly characterized in experimental animals fed atherogenic diets. However, it has been clearly demonstrated in cultures of endothelial cells that monocyte adhesion results from the expression of certain adhesion proteins on the cell surfaces and that the expression of these adhesion molecules on endothelium *in vitro* is induced by particular cytokines or other putative ‘activating’ agents.[24] For example, oxidized LDL, interleukin-1α (IL-1α), tumor necrosis factor-α (TNF-α) and bacterial endotoxin (lipopolysaccharide, LPS) have all been shown to enhance monocyte binding to confluent endothelial cell monolayers grown in culture,[25] and, in addition, proliferating endothelial cells have been shown to express increased monocyte binding compared with confluent, quiescent cells.[26] The initiation of the series of events culminating in monocyte infiltration into the intima has been termed endothelial activation. The various currently viable theories of atherogenesis speculate as to the identity of the agent(s) responsible for endothelial cell activation in human and experimental atherosclerosis.

The monocytes gathering in the intima transform into resident macrophages and proceed to become engorged with what appear microscopically as intracellular droplets. Cells with these cholesteryl ester-rich droplets are foam cells, and as mentioned earlier, the foam cell lesion is the fatty streak (or Type II) lesion. The lipid with which these cells are engorged is derived from lipoproteins rather than from local synthesis, leading to the speculation that the macrophage presence is related to an attempt to remove an excess local accumulation of lipoprotein from the intima. An issue of considerable speculation is the mechanism by which these macrophages recognize and internalize the lipoprotein which has accumulated in the intima. Low density lipoprotein itself is not ingested by monocytes or macrophages in culture to an extent that leads to foam cell formation. In fact, the most efficient mechanism these cells have for LDL ingestion, uptake via the B/E receptor, does not lead to high levels of lipid accumulation since, as in other cells, LDL receptors are downregulated at LDL concentrations of 50 μg/ml or less, concentrations well below the likely physiological concentration of LDL in interstitial fluid. Speculations to explain macrophage engorgement of lipid have focused on modifications to the native lipoproteins that lead to their recognition and uptake by other receptors that exist on macrophages. Particular chemical modifications of LDL (acetylation and malondialdehyde association, for example) alter its structure such that LDL binds to scavenger receptors, which are expressed on macrophages and on confluent endothelium. While acetylation of LDL is unlikely to occur *in vivo*, malondialdehyde alteration is one of the chemical changes LDL undergoes upon oxidation, since malondialdehyde can be a product of oxidative breakdown of polyunsaturated fatty acids and since malondialdehyde readily binds lysyl and other amino acid residues of proteins, including apo B. Uptake of oxidized LDL by macrophages has been shown to occur *in vitro* by a number of distinct mechanisms in addition to via scavenger receptors (see below).

Lipoprotein modifications other than oxidation of LDL have also been proposed to explain foam cell formation. These include: LDL aggregation after partial enzymatic digestion, which could lead to macrophage uptake of the aggregates by phagocytosis, LDL association with proteoglycans and LDL altered by non-enzymatic glycosylation, which could lead to uptake via AGE receptors (named for their recognition of proteins modified by association with any of a series of 'advanced glycosylation end-products').[27]

Evidence exists for the modification of LDL *in vivo*.[28–31] For example, antibodies which recognize oxidized LDL, but not native LDL, bind to sites in the vascular lesions of experimental animals and humans[32–36] and with LDL-like extracts of arterial lesions.[36] The latter is an important finding since many of the above antibodies recognize not only oxidized LDL, but also other proteins modified by particular lipid peroxidation products. The evidence that oxidized LDL does in fact exist *in vivo* as early as fatty streak lesion formation adds lipoprotein modification to the sequence of events in lesion development. However, it is important to point out that it is not currently known if lipoprotein oxidation precedes or follows monocyte invasion of the intima and it has not been determined whether lipoprotein oxidation is causally involved in lesion development or whether it is an epiphenomenon (see below). Furthermore, current definitions of oxidized LDL do not discriminate between LDL oxidized by free radical interactions (such as that which occurs during LDL oxidation in the laboratory) and LDL that has incorporated lipid peroxidation products formed in nearby cells and tissues.

The next known series of events to occur in lesion progression is the migration of more smooth muscle cells from the media into the intima, which is followed by their proliferation and the potential for their development into foam cells. The presence of a population of smooth muscle cells has long been recognized as an integral component of developing atherosclerotic lesions. The cells are believed to derive from intimal smooth muscle cells and from medial smooth muscle cells after their migration through the IEL. The presumption is based in part on data which show that following mechanical vascular injury smooth muscle cells migrate from the media and proliferate to form a neointima inside the IEL at the site of injury. It is further presumed that the proliferation of these smooth muscle cells is governed by local concentrations of growth factors and cytokines. Numerous candidate agents exist that could exert such a proliferative influence and it is currently unknown what the chemoattractant and proliferative factors are that dominate in the recruitment of smooth muscle cells to a lesion. Smooth muscle cells respond by increased migration and cell division to platelet-derived growth factor (PDGF) which can be produced by endothelial cells, smooth muscle cells and macrophages and can be released by degranulating platelets. Basic Fibroblast Growth Factor (bFGF) is a potent smooth muscle cell mitogen which can be synthesized by both endothelium and smooth muscle cells. These are but two examples of many potentially important growth factors in the vessel wall.

The transformation of smooth muscle cells into foam cells is known to occur since antibodies that are smooth muscle cell-specific bind to subpopulations of foam cells in lesions. Smooth muscle cells appear to develop into foam cells as a later event than macrophage transformation into foam cells in experimental animals fed atherogenic diets; the latter event occurs within a few weeks of cholesterol feeding. While the mechanism of foam cell formation from smooth muscle is unknown, scavenger receptors have been reported to be expressed by rabbit vascular smooth muscle cells in culture[37] suggesting the possibility of unregulated uptake of modified lipoproteins by these cells.

It is important to note that large numbers of T-lymphocytes are present in atherosclerotic lesions, beginning with Type II lesions.[1] Recent efforts have focused on determining the T-cell subtypes present, the mechanisms facilitating their appearance and the potential positive or negative roles they may play in lesion development. While T-cells are especially prevalent in atherosclerotic lesions of transplanted vessels, such a transplant-related immune response does not explain the general finding of T-cells in non-transplant atherosclerosis.[38] Like monocytes, T-cells likely enter the lesion after adherence to specific glycoprotein receptors expressed on the surface of endothelial cells. It has been shown in both human and animal atherosclerotic lesions, including early fatty streaks, that T-cells are present and that Class II major histocompatibility complexes are expressed by the various cells present, including macrophages and smooth muscle cells.[39] These complexes are important in the recognition by T-lymphocytes of foreign antigens. These features suggest that the atherosclerotic lesion exhibits both inflammatory and immunologic responses.[38, 39]

The time course for T-cell adhesion to endothelium and entry into the intima appears to parallel that of monocytes in the cholesterol-fed rabbit, beginning from 1 week onward of dietary treatment and subsequently accumulating, but in lower numbers than monocytes. The influence of T-cells on lesion development is unknown. Presumably these cells recognize as yet unidentified antigens. In addition, T-cells could be producing growth factors and cytokines that influence the behaviors of other cell types in the lesion. Activation of T-cells causes them to secrete γ-interferon and lymphotoxin.[39] γ-Interferon may activate macrophages or inhibit smooth muscle cell proliferation; lymphotoxin may alter γ-interferon-induced gene expression in smooth muscle cells.[39]

Theories of atherogenesis

Numerous theories have been offered to explain how atherosclerosis develops. The viability of any theory could be evaluated by its capacity to explain the pathogenic and cellular changes occurring in atherosclerosis, including the enhanced focal intimal influx and accumulation of lipoproteins, intimal recruitment of monocytes/macrophages, foam cell formation, formation of a lipid core with necrotic debris, smooth muscle cell migration/proliferation in the fibrous cap, specific changes in matrix components, and, eventually, thrombosis and calcification. Theories of atherosclerosis typically focus, however, on defining the events leading to the early, inciting processes. Thus, it is most important that a viable theory of atherosclerosis explain the earliest events listed above in addition to being compatible with known attributes of the disease. Two examples of theories that are currently the subject of vigorous research activity are presented below.

Lipoprotein oxidation theory

A relatively new theory of atherogenesis has developed over the last 15 years that suggests that the disease process occurs subsequent to, and because of, lipoproteins becoming oxidized. The theory was initially derived from three experimental observations made in cultured cells. (1) LDL was reported to injure vascular smooth muscle and endothelial cells[40] and this injury was shown to result from lipoprotein oxidation.[41, 42] (2) Endothelial cells were reported to modify LDL such that it became a ligand for scavenger receptor uptake by macrophages,[43] and this endothelial cell modification was shown to result from oxidation.[44, 45] (3) LDL modified by malondialdehyde, a product of fatty acid oxidation, was shown to be a ligand for macrophage scavenger receptors.[46] Macrophage scavenger receptors had previously been shown to recognize certain chemically modified forms of LDL, such as acetylated LDL.[13] Uptake resulting from scavenger receptor binding to modified forms of LDL led to lipid engorgement *in vitro* resembling foam cell formation.[13]

Oxidized LDL unlike native LDL induces cell functions *in vitro* which correlate with known features of atherosclerosis. The specific features of cell behavior usually linked to lesion formation such as endothelial cell injury, endothelial cell binding of monocytes, chemoattraction of monocytes, engorgement of lipoprotein lipid by monocyte-derived macrophages and smooth muscle cell migration and proliferation, are not readily simulated in cell culture by exposing vascular cells to high levels of LDL; however, virtually all of these features can be simulated by exposure of vascular cells to oxidized LDL. Oxidized LDL injures cells, including endothelial cells, perhaps due to its high levels of oxidized sterols. Potent cytotoxins formed in LDL that has been oxidized *in vitro* include 7β-hydroperoxycholesterol, which has been shown to be present in human atherosclerotic plaques,[47] 7β-hydroxycholesterol,[48] 7-ketocholesterol[48] and 4-hydroxynonenal.[49] Oxidized LDL also contains other cytotoxins, such as 7α-hydroperoxycholesterol, cholesterol epoxides and lysophospholipids. Oxidized LDL is a monocyte chemoattractant and promotes monocyte chemoattractant protein-1 (MCP-1) production and the expression of monocyte-binding proteins on endothelial cells.[50–53] Oxidized LDL enhances smooth muscle cell movement[54] and decreases endothelial cell migration.[55] It can promote smooth muscle cell growth directly,[56] but also alters growth factor and cytokine production by vascular cells.[57–63] HDL has been shown to be capable of inhibiting some of the effects of oxidized LDL. Furthermore, vascular cells, including smooth muscle cells, endothelial cells, stimulated monocytes and macrophages have all been shown to be capable of oxidizing LDL.[44, 45, 64, 65]

A starting point for a theory of atherosclerosis consistent with these *in vitro* findings, could simply be the occurrence of high plasma levels of LDL, which have been shown to result in higher entry of LDL even into the normal intima and media,[22] and increased residence time there,[66] particularly in parts of the vasculature where the intima is thickened by hemodynamic influences. With increased residence time, the probability increases for opportunistic oxidation by intimal cells, perhaps endothelial cells or isolated monocytes. Once oxidized the LDL may cause endothelial cell injury and dysfunction and may induce the endothelium to produce MCP-1 and to express monocyte adhesion proteins. With invasion by monocytes comes the increased probability that these free radical producing cells will oxidize further the intimal pool of LDL. Macrophages have been shown in culture to express multiple receptors that recognize oxidized, but not native LDL, including both Type I and Type II scavenger receptors,[67] CD 36[68] and a subclass of macrophage Fc receptors.[69] These, however, do not constitute the only possible pathways by which foam cells could form secondary to lipoprotein oxidation. Antibodies have been found in normal human plasma which bind oxidized LDL.[70] Thus, oxidized LDL could theoretically enter macrophages as oxidized LDL–antibody complexes via Fc receptors. Aggregates of oxidized LDL, known to form *in vitro* with severe oxidation, may also form *in vivo*, and be taken up in macrophages by the phagocytic processes known to be a property of this cell type. Other attributes of oxidized LDL could further enhance the development of the lesion. The effects of oxidized LDL on cytokine and growth factor production by various vascular cells could shift the balance of influences on smooth muscle cell behavior toward favoring migration and proliferation. The injury caused by oxidized LDL could be responsible for the accumulation of dead cell debris in late stage lesions in addition to its potential role in early endothelial cell dysfunction. Oxidized LDL has also been shown to interfere with endothelium-dependent relaxation,[71] a property that could increase the probability for dangerous stenotic events. Procoagulant properties reported for oxidized LDL in cultured cells may also further jeopardize the future of a lesion site. These properties include the induction of tissue factor expression in endothelial cells.[72]

Fueling the enthusiasm for the above theory are compelling data which indicate that oxidized LDL is present in vascular lesions of both experimental animals and humans. In addition to the evidence that the characteristics of LDL isolated from lesions are similar to those of LDL oxidatively modified *in vitro* and studies showing that antibodies recognizing oxidized, but not native LDL, bind epitopes in lesions, there is further indirect evidence in favor of the oxidation theory. Studies in experimental animals and humans with an array of antioxidants have demonstrated a limiting of the disease progress by these drugs. These include vitamin E, probucol, butylated hydroxytoluene, diphenylphenylenediamine and beta carotene.[73–79] All of these agents also exert effects unrelated to their antioxidant properties, making the interpretation of the data speculative. Some, such as butylated hydroxytoluene and diphenylphenylenediamine, have known adverse contraindications for use other than experimentally. Thus, although the lipoprotein oxidation theory remains unproven, it has withstood scrutiny sufficiently well to warrant continued testing.

Response to injury hypothesis

The 'response to injury' hypothesis was proposed in the 1970s in an attempt to explain the early events of atherosclerosis, such as endothelial cell injury, the appearance of foam cells in the intima and the proliferation of smooth muscle cells.[38, 80–83] According to the earlier versions of this theory, any of a number of putative 'injury' agents were believed to damage the endothelium resulting in its denudation and the subsequent adhesion and degranulation of platelets due to exposed basement membrane. The loss of endothelium would also lead to an increased influx of lipoproteins. An example of a suspected injurious agent was homocysteine. In childhood homocystinuria a form of accelerated atherosclerosis occurs[84] that was speculated to be mediated by the injurious effect of homocysteine on the endothelium.[85, 86] Homocysteine infused into baboons gave evidence of endothelial damage followed by the development of atherosclerosis. Since its initial proposal, the response to injury theory has undergone frequent revision.[38, 80–83] It is now proposed that endothelial cell dysfunction results from a subtle form of injury, rather than a severe insult that would lead to actual endothelial denudation. The normal functions that endothelium performs as a permeability barrier, a regulator of vascular tone, a source of growth inhibitors, a regulator of intimal matrix production, a provider of a non-thrombogenic surface and a regulator of leukocyte traffic, are believed to be compromised by the injury and dysfunction. There are currently a number of proposed injurious agents, including hyperlipidemia, viral infection, homocysteine and toxins. In recent versions of the theory, oxidatively modified LDL is also considered a likely candidate, a hypothesis that blends this theory into that presented above.[38]

Central to the response to injury hypothesis is a causal connection between risk factors for atherosclerosis and endothelial dysfunction. These endothelial influences are proposed to induce, in turn, cellular changes that lead to atherosclerotic lesion formation.[24, 38] The altered endothelial function then leads to increased lipoprotein accumulation in the intima, the surface expression of adhesion molecules for monocytes and T-cells, the release of chemoattractants for these cells, the migration to the intima and proliferation of smooth muscle cells, and the elaboration by these smooth muscle cells of connective tissue.

The theory states that the effector molecules for these events are growth factors and cytokines initially secreted by endothelium, but that the effects of these agents are potentially enhanced through a chain reaction in which endothelium-derived cytokines influence other cells in the vascular site to produce other contributing cytokines and growth factors. The proposed progression of events implied by this theory might include the exposure of endothelium to an injurious agent, such as a herpes simplex virus, homocysteine or oxidized LDL, resulting in 'activation' of the endothelium.[24, 38] Growth factors and chemoattractants for smooth muscle cells, such as PDGF or bFGF, can be secreted by activated or injured endothelium.[24] Adhesion molecules for monocytes and T-cells are expressed by activated endothelium, and these cells once in the intima may be induced to produce other cytokines and growth factors. Smooth muscle cell proliferation can be affected by numerous factors that are not expressed in normal vessels but are observed in lesions, including PDGF, bFGF, insulin-like growth factor, interleukin-1, TNF-α and transforming growth factor-β1.[38] Thus, the atherosclerotic process is believed to result from a complex interplay among positive and negative factors produced by endothelial and smooth muscle cells, macrophages and T-lymphocytes, the participation of which emanates from an initial injurious influence on endothelium.

Final comments

Several other theories to explain atherogenesis, distinct from these, have been proposed, supported with data and scrutinized. It is highly likely that atherosclerosis may develop from multiple pathological influences, such that more than one single theory turns out to be true. Hemodynamic influences, prothrombotic conditions and plasma concentrations of lipoprotein (a) are among many other factors that are being explored vigorously in multiple laboratories for their potential involvement in exacerbating lesion development.

Regression of lesions also receives considerable attention from researchers. Findings from humans and animals generally support the concept that atherosclerotic lesions can diminish in size after dramatic lowering of lipids and other lifestyle changes. However, not all components of the developed lesion appear reversible. For example, data support the concept that foam cells can diminish in number, focal lipid accumulations can decrease and the smooth muscle cell number can decline in a lesion site; however, calcifications and accumulations of collagen and other connective tissue are resistant to regression and may increase as other components of the lesion are reversed.[11] Thus, regression depends to some extent on lesion severity.

Because atherosclerosis can affect the arteries of numerous organs and thereby influence local hemodynamics, the disease may also alter renal function and affect the rate of development of other disease processes in the kidney. Risk factors for atherosclerosis such as hyperlipidemia and lipoprotein oxidation may damage kidneys independent of arterial disease by evoking inflammatory and immunological responses in the kidney analogous to the sequence of events suspected in arterial walls. For example, there are similarities between atherosclerosis and glomerulosclerosis, including monocyte infiltration, smooth muscle cell proliferation and enhanced matrix formation. Both appear to be multifactorial diseases enhanced by combinations of hyperlipidemia, hypertension and coagulation abnormalities.

References

1 Stary HC, Chandler AB, Glagov S *et al.* A definition of initial, fatty streak, and intermediate lesions of atherosclerosis. *Arterioscler Thromb* 1994; **14:** 840–56.

2 Stary H, Blankenhorn D, Chandler A *et al.* A definition of the intima of human arteries and of its atherosclerosis-prone regions. A report from the Committee on Vascular Lesions of the Council on Arteriosclerosis, American Heart Association. *Circulation* 1992; **85:** 391–405.

3 Ross R. Rous-Whipple award lecture: Atherosclerosis: a defense mechanism gone awry. *Am J Pathol* 1993; **143:** 987–1002.

4 McGill HC Jr Fatty streaks in the coronary arteries and aorta. *Lab Invest* 1968; **18:** 560–64.

5 Eggen DA, Solberg LA. Variation of atherosclerosis with age. *Lab Invest* 1968; **18:** 571–9.

6 Olin JW, Melia M, Young JR *et al.* Prevalence of atherosclerotic renal artery stenosis in patients with atherosclerosis elsewhere. *Am J Med* 1990; **88:** 46N–51N.

7 Thoma R. Uber die abhangigkeit der arterienintima von den mechanischen bedingungen des blutumlaufes: erste mitteilung. *Virchows Arch Pathol Anat Physiol* 1983; **93:** 443–505.

8 Mayne R. Collagenous proteins of blood vessels. *Arteriosclerosis* 1986; **6:** 585–93.

9 Penn MS, Saide GM, Chisolm GM. Relative significance of endothelium and internal elastic lamina in regulating the entry of macromolecules into arteries *in vivo*. *Circ Res* 1993; **74(1):** 74–82.

10 Stary HC. *The Evolution of Human Atherosclerotic Lesions*. West Point, PA: Merck and Co., 1993.

11 Chisolm GM, DiCorleto PE, Ehrhart LA *et al.* Pathogenesis of atherosclerosis. In Young JR, Graor RA, Olin JW, Bartholomew JR (eds) *Peripheral Vascular Surgery*, pp. 137–60. St Louis, MO: Mosby-Year Book, 1991.

12 Guyton JR, Klemp KF. Development of the atherosclerotic core region. Chemical and ultrastructural analysis of microdissected atherosclerotic lesions from human aorta. *Arterioscler Thromb* 1994; **14:** 305–14.

13 Brown MS, Goldstein JL. Lipoprotein metabolism in the macrophage: implications for cholesterol deposition in atherosclerosis. *Ann Rev Biochem* 1983; **52:** 223.

14 Ginsberg HN. Lipoprotein metabolism and its relationship to atherosclerosis. *Med Clin North Am* 1994; **78:** 1–21.

15 Blackett PR, Kittredge D. Hyperlipidemia in children. *South Med J* 1993; **86(10):** 1083–92.

16 Berenson GS, Wattingley WA, Tracy RE *et al.* Atherosclerosis of the aorta and coronary arteries and cardiovascular risk factors in persons aged 6–30 years and studied at necropsy (The Bogalusa Heart Study). *Am J Cardiol* 1992; **70(9):** 851–8.

17 Brown MS, Goldstein JL. A receptor-mediated pathway for cholesterol homeostasis. *Science* 1986; **232:** 34.

18 Austin MA, Hokanson JE. Epidemiology of triglycerides, small dense low-density lipoprotein, and

lipoprotein(a) as risk factors for coronary heart disease. *Med Clin North Am* 1994; **78:** 99–115.

19 Chait A, Brazg RL, Tribble DL, Krauss RM. Susceptibility of small, dense, low-density lipoproteins to oxidative modification in subjects with the atherogenic lipoprotein phenotype, pattern B. *Am J Med* 1993; **94:** 350–6.

20 Ng DS, Hegele RA. High-density-lipoprotein cholesterol and atherosclerosis. *Can Med Assoc J* 1993; **149(12):** 1807–8.

21 Nakamura R, Ohta T, Ikeda Y, Matsuda I. LDL inhibits the mediation of cholesterol efflux from macrophage foam cells by apoA-I-containing lipoproteins. a putative mechanism for foam cell formation. *Arterioscler Thromb* 1993; **13:** 1307–16.

22 Bratzler RL, Chisolm GM, Colton CK *et al.* The distribution of labeled low-density lipoprotein across the rabbit thoracic aorta *in vivo. Atherosclerosis* 1977; **28:** 289–307.

23 Lin SJ, Hong CY, Chang MS *et al.* Increased aortic endothelial cell death and enhanced transendothelial macromolecular transport in streptozotocin-diabetic rats. *Diabetologia* 1993; **36:** 926–30.

24 DiCorleto PE, Soyombo AA. The role of the endothelium in atherogenesis. *Curr Opin Lipid* 1993; **4:** 364–72.

25 Faruqi RM, DiCorleto PE. Mechanisms of monocyte recruitment and accumulation. *Br Heart J* **69:** (Suppl) 1993; S19–29.

26 DiCorleto PE, de la Motte CA. Characterization of the adhesion of the human monocytic cell line U937 to cultured endothelial cells. *J Clin Invest* 1985; **75:** 1153–61.

27 Bucala R, Makita Z, Koschinsky T *et al.* Lipid advanced glycosylation: pathway for lipid oxidation *in vivo. Proc Natl Acad Sci USA* 1993; **90:** 6434–8.

28 Steinbrecher UP, Zhang H, Lougheed M. Role of oxidatively modified LDL in atherosclerosis. *Free Rad Biol Med* 1990; **9:** 155–68.

29 Steinberg D, Parthasarathy S, Carew TE *et al.* Beyond cholesterol. Modifications of low-density lipoprotein that increase its atherogenicity. *N Engl J Med* 1989; **320:** 915–24.

30 Chisolm GM. The oxidation of lipoproteins: implications for atherosclerosis. In Spate L, Bloom AD (eds) *Biological Consequences of Oxidative Stress: Implications for Cardiovascular Disease and Carcinogenesis*, pp 78–106. New York: Oxford University Press, 1992.

31 Penn MS, Chisolm GM. Oxidized lipoproteins, altered cell function and atherosclerosis. *Atherosclerosis* 1994; **108:** (Suppl.) S21–9.

32 Boyd HC, Gown AM, Wolfbauer G, Chait A. Direct evidence for a protein recognized by a monoclonal antibody against oxidatively modified LDL in atherosclerotic lesions from a Watanabe heritable hyperlipidemic rabbit. *Am J Pathol* 1989; **135:** 815–25.

33 Haberland ME, Fong D, Cheng L. Malondialdehyde-altered protein occurs in atheroma of Watanabe heritable hyperlipidemic rabbits. *Science* 1988; **241:** 215–18.

34 Mowri H, Ohkuma S, Takano T. Monoclonal DLR1a/104G antibody recognizing peroxidized lipoproteins in atherosclerotic lesions. *Biochim Biophys Acta* 1988; **963:** 239–45.

35 Palinski W, Rosenfeld ME, Ylä-Herttuala S *et al.* Low density lipoprotein undergoes oxidative modification *in vivo. Proc Natl Acad Sci USA* 1989; **86:** 1372–6.

36 Ylä-Herttuala S, Palinski W, Rosenfeld ME *et al.* Evidence for the presence of oxidatively modified low density lipoprotein in atherosclerotic lesions of rabbit and man. *J Clin Invest* **84:** 1086–95.

37 Dejager S, Mietus-Snyder M, Pitas RE. Oxidized low density lipoproteins bind to the scavenger receptor expressed by rabbit smooth muscle cells and macrophages. *Arterioscler Thromb* 1993; **13:** 371–8.

38 Ross R. The pathogenesis of atherosclerosis: a perspective for the 1990s. *Nature* 1993; **362:** 801–9.

39 Hansson GK, Seifert PS, Olsson G, Bondjers G. Immunohistochemical detection of macrophages and T lymphocytes in atherosclerotic lesions of cholesterol-fed rabbits. *Arterioscler Thromb* 1991; **11(3):** 745–50.

40 Hessler JR, Robertson AL Jr, Chisolm GM. LDL-induced cytotoxicity and its inhibition by HDL in human vascular smooth muscle and endothelial cells in culture. *Atherosclerosis* 1979; **32:** 213–29.

41 Hessler JR, Morel DW, Lewis LJ, Chisolm GM. Lipoprotein oxidation and lipoprotein-induced cytotoxicity. *Arteriosclerosis* 1983; **3:** 215–223.

42 Morel DW, Hessler JR, Chisolm GM. Low density lipoprotein cytotoxicity induced by free radical peroxidation of lipid. *J Lipid Res* 1983; **24:** 1070–6.

43 Henriksen T, Mahoney EM, Steinberg D. Enhanced macrophage degradation of low density lipoprotein previously incubated with cultured endothelial cells: recognition by receptors for acetylated low density lipoproteins. *Proc Natl Acad Sci USA* 1981; **78:** 6499–503.

44 Morel DW, DiCorleto PE, Chisolm GM. Endothelial and smooth muscle cells alter low density lipoprotein *in vitro* by free radical oxidation. *Arteriosclerosis* 1984; **4:** 357–64.

45 Steinbrecher UP, Parthasarathy S, Leake DS *et al.* Modification of low density lipoprotein by endothelial cells involves lipid peroxidation and degradation of low density lipoprotein phospholipids. *Proc Natl Acad Sci USA* 1984; **81:** 3883–7.

46 Shechter I, Fogelman AM, Haberland ME *et al.* The metabolism of native and malondialdehyde altered low density lipoproteins by human monocyte-macrophages. *J Lipid Res* 1981; **22:** 63–71.

47 Chisolm GM, Ma G, Irwin KC *et al.* Linberg *et al.* 7β-hydroperoxycholest-5-en-3b-ol, a component of human atherosclerotic lesions, is the primary cytotoxin of oxidized human low density lipoprotein. *Proc Natl Acad Sci USA* 1994; **91:** 11452–6.

48 Hughes H, Mathews B, Lenz ML, Guyton, JR. Cytotoxicity of oxidized LDL to porcine aortic smooth muscle cells is associated with the oxysterols 7-ketocholesterol and 7-hydroxycholesterol. *Arterioscler Thromb* 1994; **14:** 1177–85.

49 Hoff HF, Chisolm GM, Morel DW *et al.* Chemical and functional changes in LDL following modification by 4-hydroxynonenal. In Cerutti PA, Fredovich I, McCord JM (eds) *Oxy-radicals in Molecular Biology and Pathology*, pp. 459–72. New York: Alan R Liss, 1988.

50 Quinn MT, Parthasarathy S, Steinberg D. Lysophosphatidylcholine: a chemotactic factor for human monocytes and its potential role in atherogenesis. *Proc Natl Acad Sci USA* 1988; **85:** 2805–9.

51 Cushing SD, Berliner JA, Valente AJ *et al.* Minimally modified low density lipoprotein induces monocyte chemotactic protein 1 in human endothelial cells and smooth muscle cells. *Proc Natl Acad Sci USA* 1990; **87:** 134–8.

52 Frostegård JJ, Nilsson J, Haegerstrand A *et al.* Oxidized low density lipoprotein induces differentiation and adhesion of human monocytes and the monocytic cell line U937. *Proc Natl Acad Sci USA* 1990; **87:** 904–8.

53 Kume N, Cybulsky MI, Gimbrone MA Jr. Lysophosphatidylcholine, a component of atherogenic lipoproteins, induces mononuclear leukocyte adhesion molecules in cultured human and rabbit arterial endothelial cells. *J Clin Invest* 1992; **90:** 1138–44.

54 Autio I, Jaakkola I, Solakivi T, Nikkari T. Oxidized low-density lipoprotein is chemotactic for arterial smooth muscle cells in culture. *FEBS Lett* 1990; **277:** 247–9.

55 Murugesan G, Chisolm GM, Fox PL. Oxidized low density lipoprotein inhibits the migration of aortic endothelial cells *in vitro*. *J Cell Biol* 1993; **120:** 1011–19.

56 Blackett PR, Lee DM, Donaldson DL *et al.* Studies of lipids, lipoproteins, and apolipoproteins in Menkes' disease. *Pediatr Res* 1984; **18:** 864–70.

57 Fox PL, Chisolm GM, DiCorleto PE. Lipoprotein mediated inhibition of endothelial cell production of platelet-derived growth factor-like proteins depends on free radical lipid peroxidation. *J Biol Chem* 1987; **262:** 6046–54.

58 Malden LT, Chait A, Raines EW, Ross R. The influence of oxidatively modified low density lipoproteins on expression of platelet-derived growth factor by human monocyte-derived macrophages. *J Biol Chem* 1991; **266:** 13901–7.

59 Fong LG, Fong TAT, Cooper AD. Inhibition of lipopolysaccharide-induced interleukin-1b mRNA expression in mouse macrophages by oxidized low density lipoprotein. *J Lipid Res* 1991; **32:** 1899–910.

60 Hamilton TA, Ma GP, Chisolm GM. Oxidized low density lipoprotein suppresses the expression of tumor necrosis factor-alpha mRNA in stimulated murine peritoneal macrophages. *J Immunol* 1990; **144:** 2343–50.

61 Boulanger CM, Tanner FC, Béa M-L *et al.* Oxidized low density lipoproteins induce mRNA expression and release of endothelin from human and porcine endothelium. *Circ Res* 1992; **70:** 1191–7.

62 Jougasaki M, Kugiyama K, Saito Y *et al.* Suppression of endothelin-1 secretion by lysophosphatidylcholine in oxidized low density lipoprotein in cultured vascular endothelial cells. *Circ Res* 1992; **71:** 614–19.

63 Rajavashisth TB, Andalibi A, Territo MC *et al.* Induction of endothelial cell expression of granulocyte and macrophage colony-stimulating factors by modified low-density lipoproteins. *Nature* 1990; **344:** 254–7.

64 Cathcart MK, Morel DW, Chisolm GM. Monocytes and neutrophils oxidize low density lipoprotein making it cytotoxic. *J Leukocyte Biol* 1985; **38:** 341–50.

65 Heinecke JW, Rosen H, Chait A. Iron and copper promote modification of low density lipoprotein by human arterial smooth muscle cells in culture. *J Clin Invest* 1984; **74:** 1890–4.

66 Schwenke DC, Carew TE. Initiation of atherosclerotic lesions in cholesterol-fed rabbits. II. Selective retention of LDL vs. selective increases in LDL permeability in susceptible sites of arteries. *Arteriosclerosis* 1989; **9:** 908–18.

67 Freeman M, Ekkel Y, Rohrer L *et al.* Expression of type I and type II bovine scavenger receptors in Chinese hamster ovary cells: Lipid droplet accumulation and nonreciprocal cross competition by acetylated and oxidized low density lipoprotein. *Proc Natl Acad Sci USA* 1991; **88:** 4931–5.

68 Endemann G, Stanton LW, Madden KS *et al.* CD36 is a receptor for oxidized low density lipoprotein. *J Biol Chem* 1993; **268:** 11 811–16.

69 Stanton LW, White RT, Bryant CM *et al.* A macrophage Fc receptor for IgG is also a receptor for oxidized low density lipoprotein. *J Biol Chem* 1992; **267:** 22 446–51.

70 Salonen, JT, Ylä-Herttuala S, Yamamoto R *et al.* Autoantibody against oxidised LDL and progression of carotid atherosclerosis. *Lancet* 1992; **339:** 883–7.

71 Kugiyama K, Kerns SA, Morrisett JD *et al.* Impairment of endothelium-dependent arterial relaxation by lysolecithin in modified low-density lipoproteins. *Nature* 1990; **344:** 160–2.

72 Drake TA, Hannani K, Fei HH *et al.* Minimally

oxidized low-density lipoprotein induces tissue factor expression in cultured human endothelial cells. *Am J Pathol* 1991; **138:** 601–7.

73 Bjorkhem I, Henriksson-Freyschuss A, Breuer O *et al.* The antioxidant butylated hydroxytoluene protects against atherosclerosis. *Arterioscler Thromb* 1991; **11:** 15–22.

74 Carew TE, Schwenke DC, Steinberg D. Antiatherogenic effect of probucol unrelated to its hypocholesterolemic effect: Evidence that antioxidants *in vivo* can selectively inhibit low density lipoprotein degradation in macrophage-rich fatty streaks and slow the progression of atherosclerosis in the Watanabe heritable hyperlipidemic rabbit. *Proc Natl Acad Sci USA* 1987; **84:** 7725–9.

75 Kita T, Nagano Y, Yokode M *et al.* Probucol prevents the progression of atherosclerosis in Watanabe heritable hyperlipidemic rabbit, an animal model for familial hypercholesterolemia. *Proc Natl Acad Sci USA* 1987; **84:** 5928–31.

76 Rimm EB, Stampfer MJ, Ascherio A *et al.* Vitamin E consumption and the risk of coronary disease in men. *N Engl J Med* 1993; **328:** 1450–6.

77 Stampfer MJ, Hennekens CH, Manson JE *et al.* Vitamin E consumption and the risk of coronary disease in women. *N Engl J Med* 1993; **328:** 1444–9.

78 Sparrow CP, Doebber TW, Olszewski J *et al.* Low density lipoprotein is protected from oxidation and the progression of atherosclerosis is slowed in cholesterol-fed rabbits by the antioxidant N,N′-diphenyl-phenyenediamine. *J Clin Invest* 1990; **89:** 1885–91.

79 Gaziano JM, Manson JE, Kidker PM *et al.* Beta carotene therapy for chronic stable angina (Abstract). *Circulation* 1990; **82:** III–201.

80 Ross R. The pathogenesis of atherosclerosis: an update. *N Engl J Med* 1986; **314:** 488–500.

81 Ross R, Glomset JA. The pathogenesis of atherosclerosis (second of two parts). *N Engl J Med* 1986; **295(7):** 420–5.

82 Ross R. George Lyman Duff Memorial Lecture. Atherosclerosis: a problem of the biology of arterial wall cells and their interactions with blood components. *Arteriosclerosis* 1981; **1(5):** 293–311.

83 Ross R, Glomset JA. The pathogenesis of atherosclerosis (first of two parts). *N Engl J Med* 1976; **295(7):** 369–77.

84 Mudd SH, Skovby F, Levy HL *et al.* The natural history of homocysteinuria due to cystathionine beta synthase deficiency. *Am J Human Genet* **37(1):** 1–31.

85 Harker LA, Slichter SJ, Scott CR, Ross R. Homocysteinemia: vascular injury and arterial thrombosis. *N Engl J Med* 4; **291:** 537–43.

86 Harker LA, Ross R, Slichter SJ, Scott CR. The role of endothelial cell injury and platelet response in its genesis. *J Clin Invest* 1976; **58:** 731–41.

2

Renal artery fibrodysplasia

JAMES C STANLEY

Introduction

The term arterial fibrodysplasia refers to a heterogeneic group of non-atherosclerotic, non-inflammatory vascular occlusive diseases that have major clinical relevance in the renal circulation. Renal artery dysplastic disease occurs in less than 0.5% of the general population. The frequency is less among black and Asian hypertensives. Renal artery dysplasia, first described a half-century ago,[1] is second only to arteriosclerosis as the most common cause of surgically correctable hypertension. The three principal categories of arterial fibrodysplastic stenoses to affect the renal arteries are intimal fibroplasia, medial fibroplasia and perimedial dysplasia.[2–4] The first entity represents a distinctly different pathologic process from the latter two, which appear to represent a continuum of disease. A fourth category, less commonly encountered, includes hypoplastic dysplastic vessels that are true developmental lesions.

Occasional renal artery stenoses exhibit combinations of the commonly recognized dysplastic lesion, and others exhibit less easily categorized vessel wall derangements that are considered a variant form of arterial dysplasia. In this regard, it is important to distinguish primary from secondary fibrodysplasia. This is particularly true regarding intimal fibroplasia. Complications of the dysplastic process, namely macroaneurysms, dissections and arteriovenous fistulas, must be differentiated from the underlying fibrodysplastic lesion.

Intimal fibroplasia

Intimal fibroplasia accounts for approximately 5% of all dysplastic renal artery stenoses, being observed in pediatric patients and young adults more often than among the elderly. No gender predilection has been noted with intimal fibroplasia. Primary intimal fibroplasia affects the main renal artery, usually occurring as a smooth focal stenosis (Fig. 2.1a). Segmental renal artery intimal fibroplasia is relatively uncommon, which when present often occurs as a web-like lesion (Fig. 2.1b).

Irregularly arranged mesenchymal cells within a loose matrix of subendothelial connective tissue characterize primary intimal fibroplasia (Fig. 2.2). The internal elastic lamina may be somewhat fragmented, but is always present. This may serve to distinguish primary from secondary intimal fibroplasia, with the latter often having no demonstrable internal elastic lamina. Primary intimal proliferation is usually circumferential, whereas secondary lesions are often eccentric. The cause of primary intimal fibroplasia is unknown, but in some cases may represent vestiges of fetal arterial musculoelastic cushions, similar to the intimal cushions observed at cerebral artery bifurcations in adults.[5] Medial and adventitial tissues are usually normal in the primary form of intimal dysplasia.

Secondary intimal fibroplasia may be difficult to differentiate from primary disease. The former lesions often accompany developmental

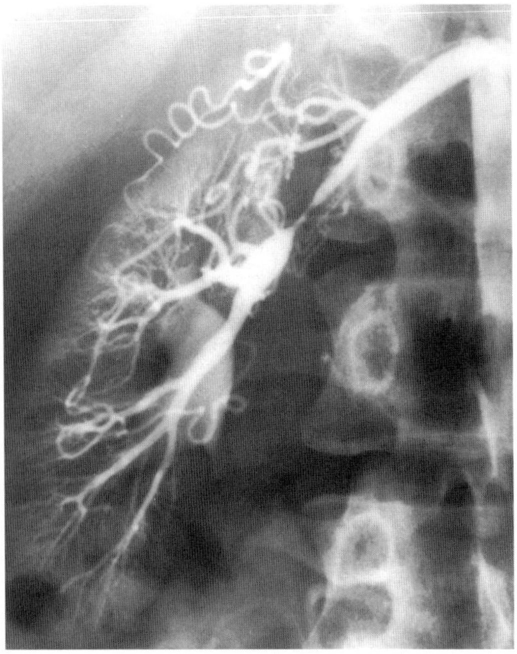

(a)

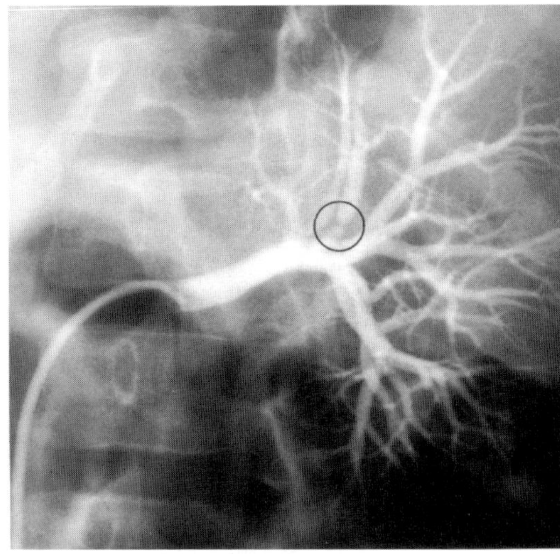

(b)

Figure 2.1. Primary intimal fibroplasia. (a) Focal stenosis of main renal artery midportion in a young adult. From ref. 12 with permission. (b) Intraparenchymal web-like stenosis of a segmental artery in a child. From ref. 38, with permission.

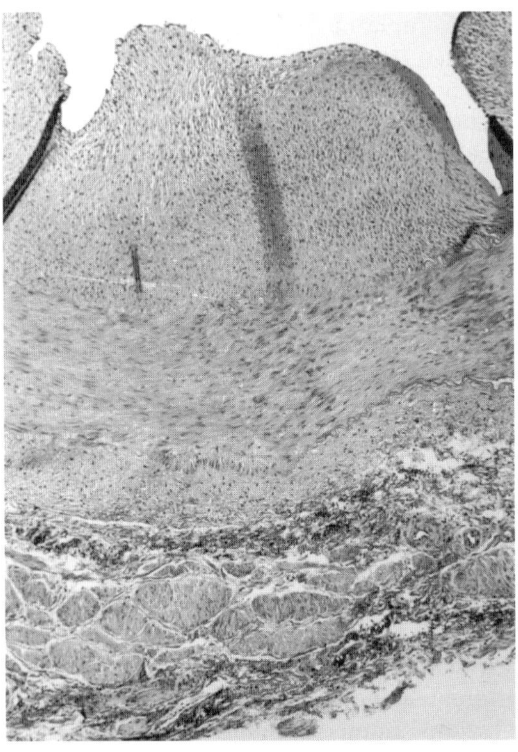

Figure 2.2. Primary intimal fibroplasia. Subendothelial mesenchymal cells within a loose fibrous connective tissue matrix are noted above an intact internal elastic lamina, normal media, and normal adventitial tissues. Hematoxylin and eosin stain, × 100. From ref. 48, with permission.

ostial narrowings or advanced medial dysplasia, perhaps as a consequence of abnormal blood flow through these stenoses. Blunt or intraluminal vascular trauma may cause an injury response and result in other secondary lesions, with medial and adventitial structures in such cases appearing relatively uninvolved. Secondary lesions may also occur following incomplete recanalization of a previously thrombosed artery. This often causes a long, tubular narrowing of the renal artery (Fig. 2.3). In this regard certain cases of intimal fibroplasia have been suggested to represent a resolved arteritis, such as might occur with rubella.[6] An infectious-immunologic etiology of certain secondary lesions receives support in immunoglobulin

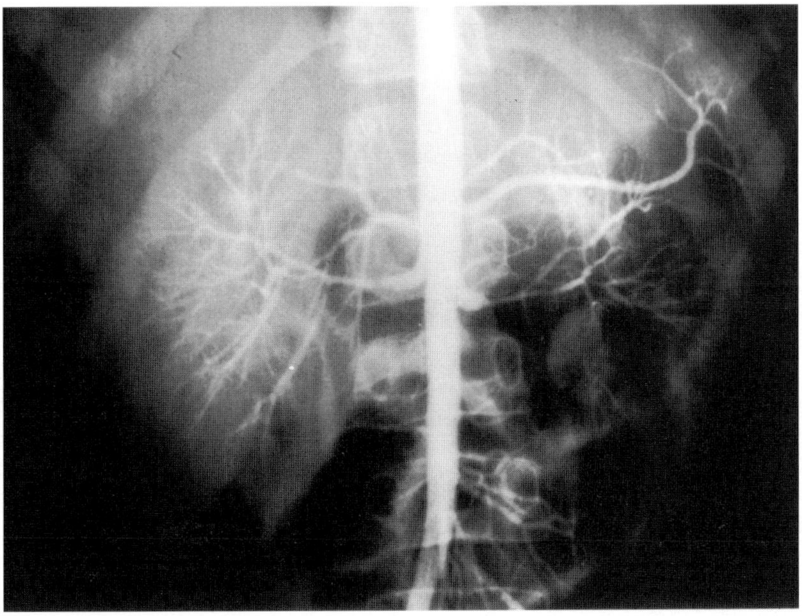

Figure 2.3. Secondary intimal fibroplasia. Long tubular stenoses in the main distal renal arteries of an infant. From ref. 49, with permission.

deposition within the stenotic vessel's intimal tissues.[7]

Progression of intimal fibrodysplasia, be it primary or secondary, once a hemodynamically important arterial stenosis develops, appears a likely consequence of abnormal surface blood flow, even if the initiating etiologic factors have resolved. The specific signals at the molecular and cellular level responsible for this tissue proliferation have not been identified. Intimal lesions appear to progress at a more rapid rate than do medial fibroplastic stenoses.[8]

Medial fibroplasia

Medial fibroplasia accounts for nearly 85% of all dysplastic renovascular stenoses. More than 90% of patients with medial fibroplasia are women, and in fact the classic 'string-of-beads' lesion has rarely been encountered in men. Medial fibrodysplasia is exceedingly uncommon among the black and Asian populations. The disease is encountered most often during the fourth decade of life. Although medial fibroplasia is considered by many to be a systemic arteriopathy, clinically overt disease is usually limited to the renal, extracranial internal carotid and external iliac arteries.

Renal artery medial fibroplasia may present as a solitary focal stenosis, but is more likely to present as multiple stenoses and intervening aneurysmal outpouchings causing a 'string of beads' appearance (Fig. 2.4). The latter has not been observed in female patients prior to menarche, with the exception of a single case report.[9] The thin-walled true mural aneurysms are usually grossly evident, and the stenoses appear as distinct webs projecting internally (Fig. 2.5). Medial fibroplasia is most often found in the distal main renal artery, with extensions into first order segmental branches affecting approximately 25% of patients.

Progression of renal artery medial fibroplasia has been reported to range from 12 to 66% in patients with main renal artery lesions.[8, 10–12] Progression is more likely to affect premenopausal women, although some investigators have noted no differences related to age.[13] Among a group of 71 potential kidney donors with angiographic evidence of renal artery fibrodysplasia, hypertension attributed to this disease developed in 26% over an average follow-up of 7.5 years compared with only 6% in

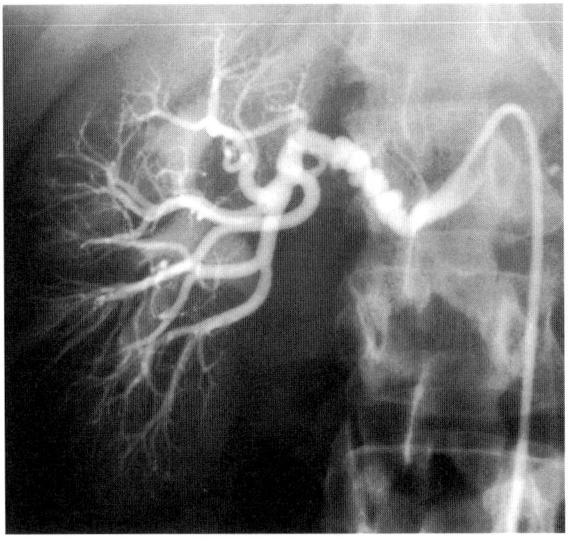

Figure 2.4. Medial fibroplasia. Serial stenoses alternating with mural aneurysms, producing a 'string of beads' appearance in the midportion and distal main renal artery. From ref. 50, with permission.

an age- and sex-matched group of control patients.[14] Fibrodysplastic renal arteries were reported to have progressed to occlusion in 18% of one series.[15] This appears to have been a unique experience, not borne out by other large series. The usual course of this disease is not one in which vessel occlusion is considered a common complication. Occasional regression of a renal artery dysplastic stenosis has been reported,[16] although the validity of such has been challenged.[17]

Two relatively distinct histologic forms of renal artery medial fibroplasia are recognized (Fig. 2.6). The first, the peripheral form, is evident by disease limited to the outer media. The second, the diffuse form, exhibits disease throughout the entire media. The latter has been observed twice as often as the former in surgical specimens. However, gradations between these extremes have been observed in the same vessel, supporting the tenet that they represent a common disease process. The peripheral form is usually encountered in younger patients. It has been speculated that with the passage of time, the peripheral disease advances to become the diffuse form. The fact that with multiple severe stenoses in series, true macroaneurysms develop in many patients who initially had a solitary lesion or a few stenoses of minimal severity, lends support to the progressive nature of this disease.

Peripheral medial fibroplasia is characterized by fibrous-appearing tissue replacing the normal smooth muscle of the outer media. Moderate accumulations of collagen and ground substances separating disorganized smooth muscle may be observed within the inner media. Intimal tissues and the internal elastic lamina are rarely affected

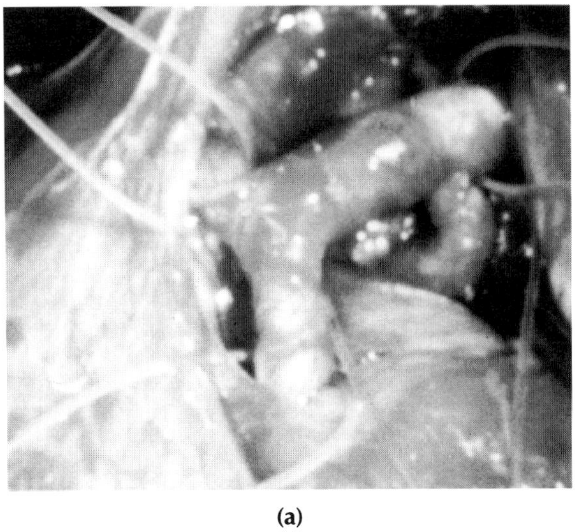

(a)

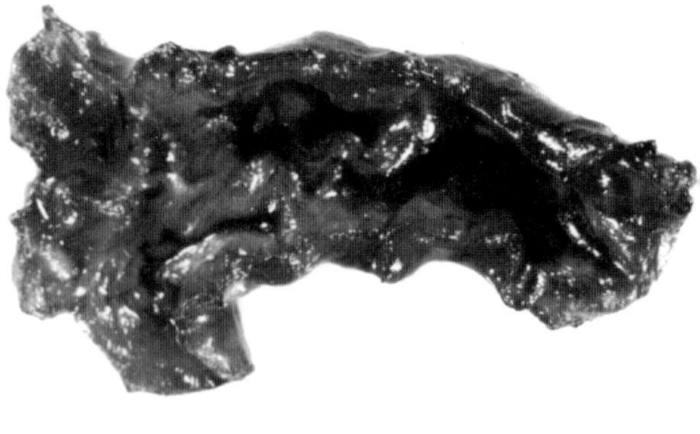

(b)

Figure 2.5. Medial fibroplasia. (a) Gross appearance of mural aneurysm (arrow) characteristic of this type renal artery dysplasia. (b) Internal appearance of webs projecting into lumen of excised main renal artery specimen. From ref. 2, with permission.

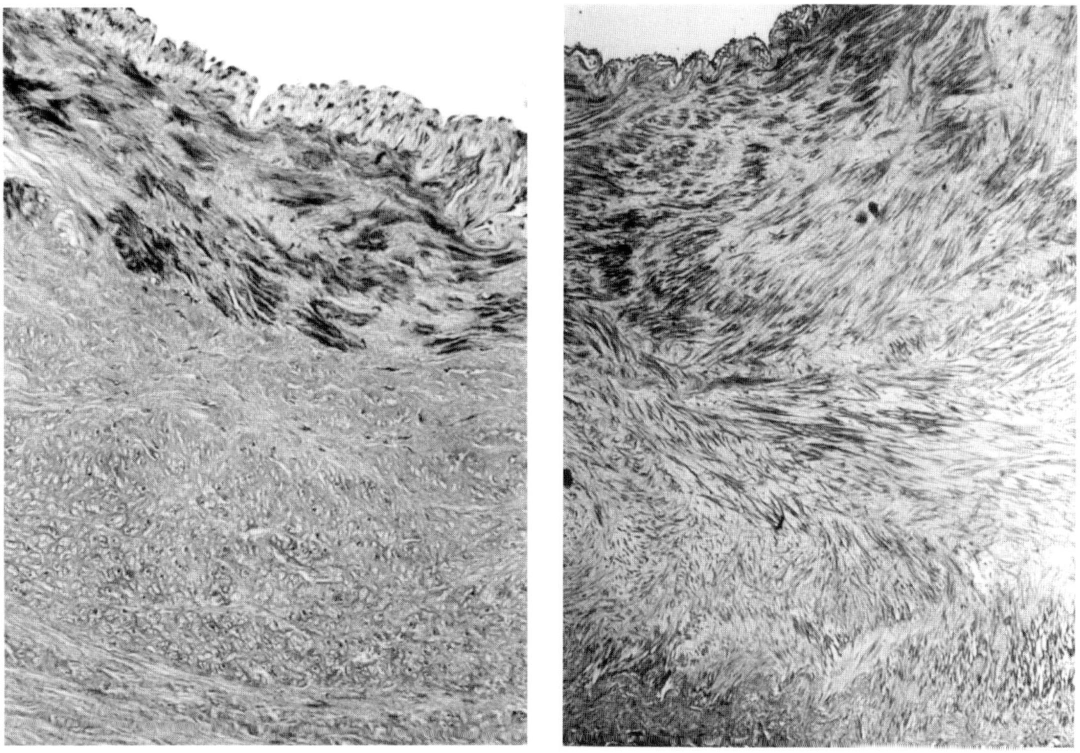

(a) (b)

Figure 2.6. (a) Peripheral form, medial fibrodysplasia: dense fibrous connective tissue in the outer media, with disordered inner medial smooth muscle, and normal intimal tissues. (b) Diffuse from medial fibroplasia: total replacement of media by disorganized cellular tissue (myofibroblasts) surrounded by fibrous connective tissue. Masson stain, × 120. From ref. 48, with permission.

in these peripheral lesions. Although the external elastic lamina may be fragmented, the adventitia is usually normal. Many of these peripheral forms of medial fibroplasia were previously classified as perimedial or subadventitial disease,[18–20] but are no longer categorized as such.

Diffuse medial fibrodysplasia is characterized by a more severe disorganization and disruption of normal medial smooth muscle architecture. This may result in an amorphous appearing media. In most vessels excessive medial accumulations of fibrous tissue alternate with areas of marked medial thinning. In some instances the media is nearly absent, and these regions account for the vessel's mural aneurysmal dilations. Internal elastic lamina fragmentation and subendothelial fibrosis may also be evident. These latter two changes are considered secondary events in instances of more advanced medial fibroplasia. Adventitial tissues are relatively uninvolved in medial fibroplasia.

Extensive fragmentation and distortion of the internal elastic lamina occur in some renal arteries exhibiting medial fibrodysplasia. Deeper dissections may extend into middle and outer medial structures as limited dissections, or they may progress as large intramural hematomas that compress the vessel lumen. Loss of vessel integrity at bifurcations with fragmentation of elastic tissue is thought to lead to development of renal artery macroaneurysms in these dysplastic arteries.[21]

Perimedial dysplasia

Perimedial dysplasia is the dominant abnormality affecting approximately 10% of dysplastic renal arteries. It may coexist with medial fibrodysplasia. Most patients exhibiting perimedial dysplasia have been female, usually in their fourth or fifth decades of life. These lesions present as either focal stenoses or multiple constrictions involving the midportion of the main renal artery without mural aneurysms (Fig. 2.7a). Excessive elastic tissue at the junction of the media and adventitia is the distinguishing feature of perimedial dysplasia (Fig. 2.7b). Minimal increases in medial ground substance surrounding intact smooth muscle cells, with little alteration of intimal tissues, characterize inner portions of the vessel wall in many of these dysplastic lesions whose dominant feature is the homogeneous collar of elastic tissue adjacent to the outer media.

Certain ultrastructural features are common to medial fibroplasia and perimedial dysplasia.[22] Both exhibit accumulations of ground substance and fibrous elements. Perimedial dysplasia is differentiated by collections of amorphous material and elastic tissue at the adventitial-medial border. Most importantly, both manifest a spectrum of change within the cellular composition of the media, ranging from near normal smooth muscle to myofibroblasts. Fibroblasts are not a usual component of the media and are infrequently observed in these diseased tissues. Similarly, macrophages and leukocytes, suggesting an inflammatory process, are not a relevant component of either medial fibroplasia or perimedial dysplasia. Normal smooth muscle cells are characterized by close apposition of cytoplasmic processes, a deeply indented and convoluted nucleus surrounded by a modest number of cellular organelles, orderly arranged thick and thin myofilaments parallel to the longitudinal cell axis with electron-dense bodies at their attachment to the plasma lamina, basal laminations, and scattered micropinocytotic vesicles.

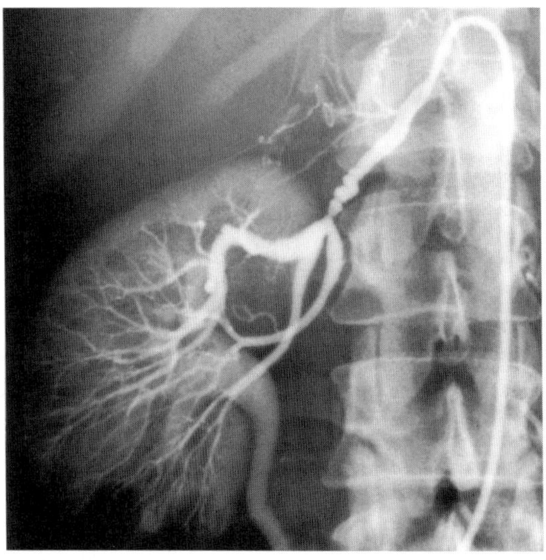

(a)

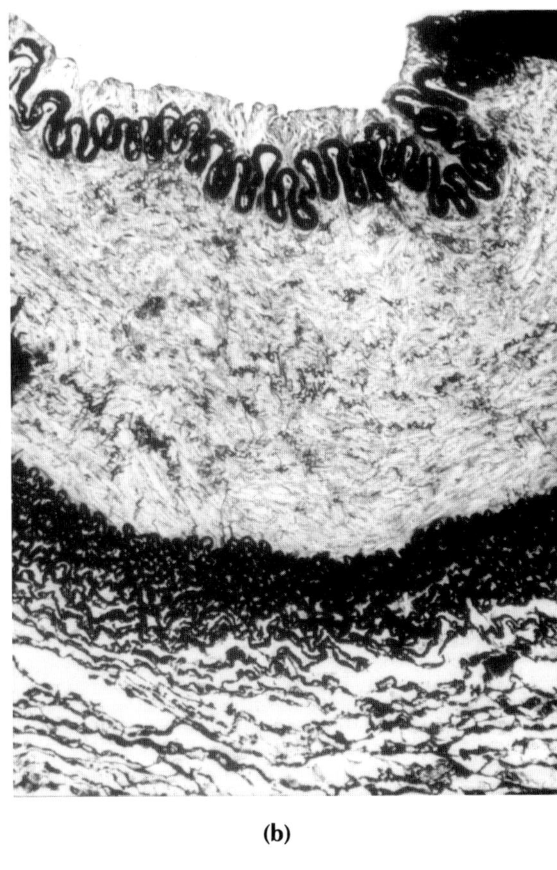

(b)

Figure 2.7. Perimedial dysplasia. (a) Multiple stenoses without mural aneurysms in the midportion of the renal artery are characteristic of these lesions. (b) These stenoses are due to excessive accumulations of elastic tissue at medial-adventitial junction. Verhoeff stain, × 120. From ref. 42, with permission.

The earliest alterations in smooth muscle ultrastructure of dysplastic vessels are focal myofilament reductions as well as perinuclear sublemmal and cytoplasmic vacuolations (Fig. 2.8). In areas of advanced dysplasia certain smooth muscle cells exhibit extreme deterioration whereas others become fibroblast-like in appearance. The former invariably are isolated from surrounding cells by excessive amounts of ground substance (Fig. 2.9a). In these tissues long slender cytoplasmic processes reflect decreased cell volumes. Cell membranes are often indistinct, and the nucleus is usually picnotic, containing dense chromatin material. Confluences of micropinocytotic vesicles are common and subcellular organelles are sparse. Myofilaments appear dense and homogeneous in these cells. Modification of medial smooth muscle cells to fibroblast-type cells represents a continuum within dysplastic tissues. Alterations in nuclear contour, loss of myofilaments, as well as increases in free ribosomes, rough endoplasmic reticulum, Golgi complexes and mitochondria, seemingly parallel altered function from one of contractility to one of secretion.

Myofibroblasts are the end product of smooth muscle transformation. Typical of these cells are a convoluted nucleus with numerous indentations and evaginations (Fig. 2.9b). Major juxtanuclear increases in subcellular organelles and the presence of peripherally located cytoplasmic filaments are characteristic of myofibroblasts. Myofilaments are scant and poorly defined. Active exopinocytotic deposition of proteinaceous matter may be evident in some cells (Fig. 2.10).

Vasa vasorum within the media of diseased arteries are usually widely separated from adjacent cellular tissue by fibrous material and homogeneous mucoid substances. The type of surrounding connective tissue appears related to the category of arterial dysplasia. Vasa vasorum within medial fibroplasia are surrounded predominantly by collagen fibrous bundles, whereas those in perimedial dysplasia are usually surrounded by amorphous mucoid substances consistent with elastic tissue.

The pathogenesis of medial fibroplasia and perimedial dysplasia has been the subject of much speculation.[2] Hormonal effects on smooth muscle, mechanical stresses on vessel walls and the peculiar distribution of vasa vasorum in arteries exhibiting these lesions are all considered contributing factors. The exact relation of these factors to each other, or their association with other unrecognized pathogenic mecha-

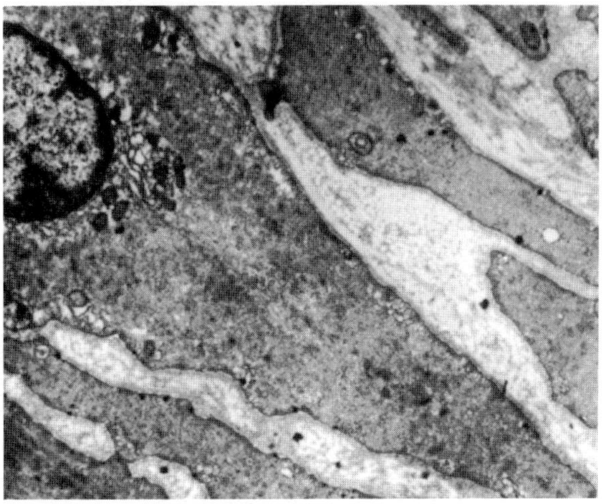

(a)

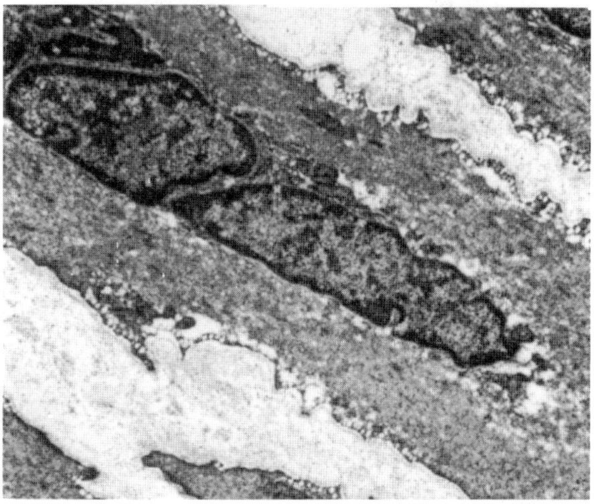

(b)

Figure 2.8. Smooth muscle cell. (a) In region of minimal fibrodysplasia. Relative normal ultrastructure except for focal reduction in myofilaments and appearance of perinuclear, sublemmal, as well as cytoplasmic vacuoles. TEM × 18 000. (b) In region of moderate fibrodysplasia. More extensive perinuclear and peripheral vacuolation is evident. Loss of organelles, basement membrane and indistinct myofilaments characterize this type cell. TEM × 12 000. From ref. 2, with permission.

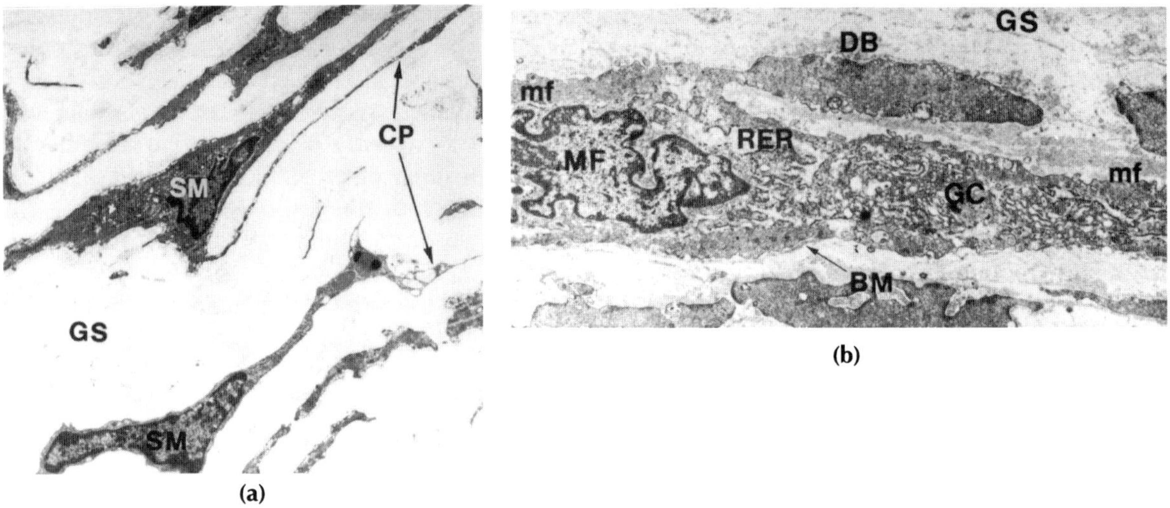

Figure 2.9. (a) Smooth muscle cell in area of advanced fibrodysplasia. Isolation of slender cytoplasmic processes by excesses in ground substances, and picnotic nuclei were typical of these markedly abnormal cells. TEM × 6000. (b) Myofibroblast associated with medial fibroplasia. Convoluted nucleus is typical of smooth muscle, but increased numbers of centrally located organelles reflect change in function from one of contractility to secretion. TEM × 8000. SM, smooth muscle; GS, ground substance; CP, cytoplasmic processes; mf, myofilament; DB, dense body; RER, rough endoplasmic reticulum. From ref. 22, with permission.

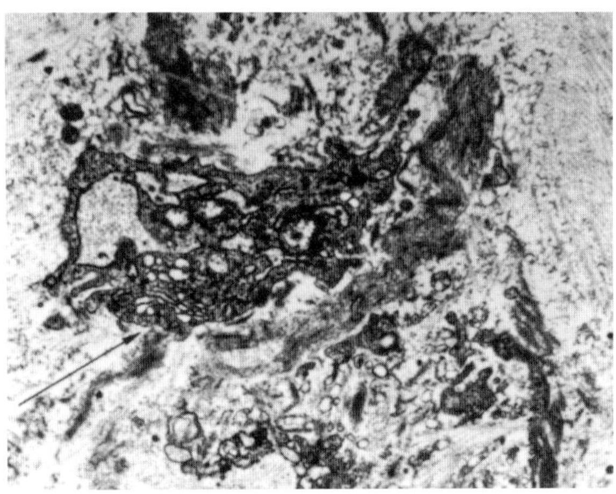

Figure 2.10. Myofibroblast in region of extensive fibroplasia, exhibiting exopinocytotic secretion of proteinaceous matter (arrow). TEM × 25 000. From ref. 2, with permission.

nisms, remains unknown. Because of the familial nature of this disease, a genetic-related autosomal dominant etiology with incomplete penetrance has been suggested. However, confirmatory arteriographic or histologic evidence to firmly establish such a contention has not been presented.[23–27] In fact, the absence of a female sex predilection in the data generated by those supporting a genetic etiology lessens the validity of their proposal.

Hormonal influences seem likely in view of arterial dysplasia's unusual female predilection. More than 95% of patients exhibiting medial and perimedial disease are women. Pregnancy, although known to cause rather profound vascular wall changes including alterations in medial structures, especially elastic tissue, is not an obvious etiologic factor in arterial fibrodysplasia. The reproductive histories of patients in a large series of patients with this arteriopathy have not revealed gravity or parity rates different from the general population.[2] Antiovulants are also known to have a significant effect on the arterial wall. However, use of such drugs by fewer than half the female patients in the Michigan series does not support any obvious cause and effect association of progesterins with arterial dysplasia.[2] A similar lack of association with oral contraceptives was reported in a case-control study.[27] Certain smooth muscle cells and fibroblasts exposed to estrogens demonstrate increased synthesis of proteinaceous substances, including collagen. It is speculated that physiologic preconditioning of vascular smooth muscle cells to a secretory state by normal circulating estrogens may account for the more frequent occurrence of medial dysplastic disease in females.

Unusual physical stresses due to ptosis of the kidneys may also be associated with fibrodysplastic changes in the renal arteries (Fig. 2.11). Comparable stretch or traction forces are less likely to occur in similar-sized vessels unaffected by this disease. Ptotic kidneys are known to be common among patients with renal artery dysplastic lesions.[28, 29] In some cases positional changes causing greater ptosis have been correlated with increases in blood pressure.[30] The fact that the right kidney is usually more ptotic than the left may account for the greater severity of right-sided disease in the majority of patients having bilateral medial fibroplasia and the fact that right-sided lesions outnumber left-sided lesions, four to one, in patients with unilateral lesions. The basis for stress-induced cellular proliferation is unknown, although cyclic stretching of smooth muscle cells in tissue culture is known to increase synthesis of collagen and certain acid mucopolysaccharides.[31] Existence of similar mechanisms *in vivo* may account for the predilection of dysplastic disease to occur in vessels subjected to mechanical stretching. In a cautionary note, one recent case-control study suggested that renal mobility was not greater in patients with renovascular fibrodysplasia.[27] This is contrary to the general experience with this disease.

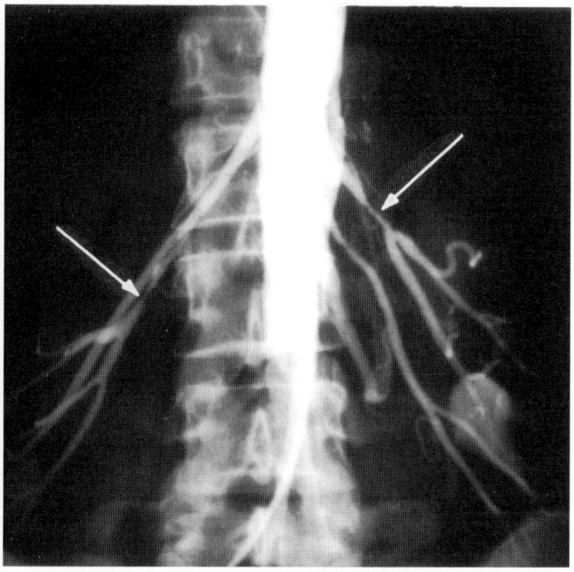

Figure 2.11. Medial fibrodysplasia manifest as irregular narrowings to ptotic kidneys (arrows) affecting midportion of main renal arteries that appear stretched during upright aortography. From ref. 4, with permission.

Mural ischemia is an additional factor that may contribute to arterial dysplasia. Vasa vasorum of muscular arteries usually arise from origins of branches of the parent artery.[32, 33] The extracranial internal carotid and external iliac arteries, in particular, have relatively few branches compared with similar-sized vessels not exhibiting this disease. Compromise of the already sparse vasa vasorum in these vessels may lead to significant mural ischemia. In addition, vasospasm may affect these arteries and contribute to vessel wall ischemia.[34, 35] The concept of mural ischemia as a causative factor receives support from the frequent involvement of the outermost media in peripheral medial fibroplasia. It is precisely this vessel wall region where ischemic changes from inadequate vasa vasorum blood flow would be expected to be greatest. In contrast, fibrodysplasia limited to the inner part of the media has not been reported. Vasa vasorum of affected vessels exhibit both dilation[36] and isolation from medial smooth muscle cells.[22] Occlusion of the vasa vasorum in dogs results in a dysplastic lesion comparable with that in humans, and lends further support to the tenet that mural ischemia contributes to arterial dysplasia.[37]

Tissue hypoxia may be a dominant factor in causing transformation of smooth muscle cells to myofibroblasts, but altered tissue pH, accumulation of metabolites, or other factors may be just as important. In this regard, cigarette smoking has been implicated as a contributing factor in this disease, although the mechanism by which this occurs has not been defined.[27] The degree of ischemia necessary to stimulate myofibroblasts are unknown, although such cells have been observed to develop in non-vascular tissues following very brief hypoxic events. Myofibroblasts are unlikely to evolve from dormant mesenchymal cells, although such could be a remote possibility. Furthermore, it is unlikely that myofibroblasts represent contractile fibroblasts, in that these cells are not normally present in the media. Myofibroblasts most likely evolve from vascular smooth muscle cells.

Developmental renal artery stenoses

Developmental renal artery stenoses are an uncommon form of renal artery dysplasia. There is no apparent gender predilection for this entity. Nearly 40% of children with renal artery stenoses are believed to have developmental lesions,[38] and among adults with intimal fibrodysplasia, approximately 20% appear to be due to growth or developmental defects. Certain adults with isolated renal arteriosclerosis may also have pre-existing developmental stenoses. Approximately 80% of patients with abdominal aortic coarctation or hypoplasia have coexisting renal artery stenotic lesions and renovascular hypertension.[39] The renal arteries in these patients usually occur at vessel origins, are hypoplastic in character, and have an 'hour-glass' appearance (Fig. 2.12).

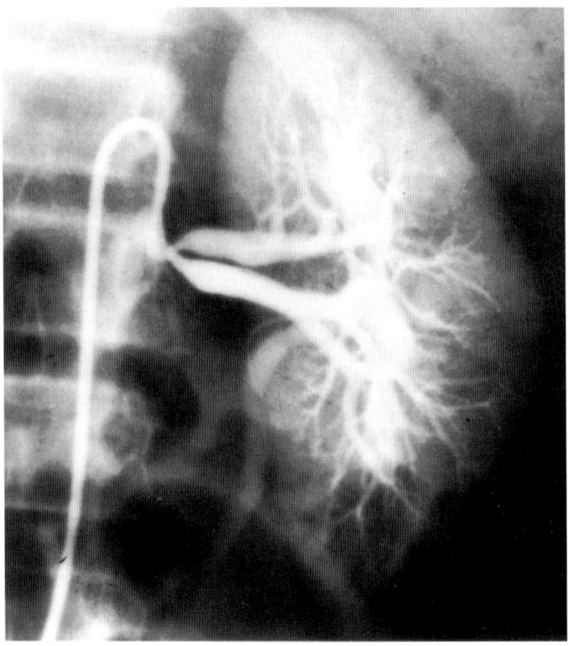

(a)

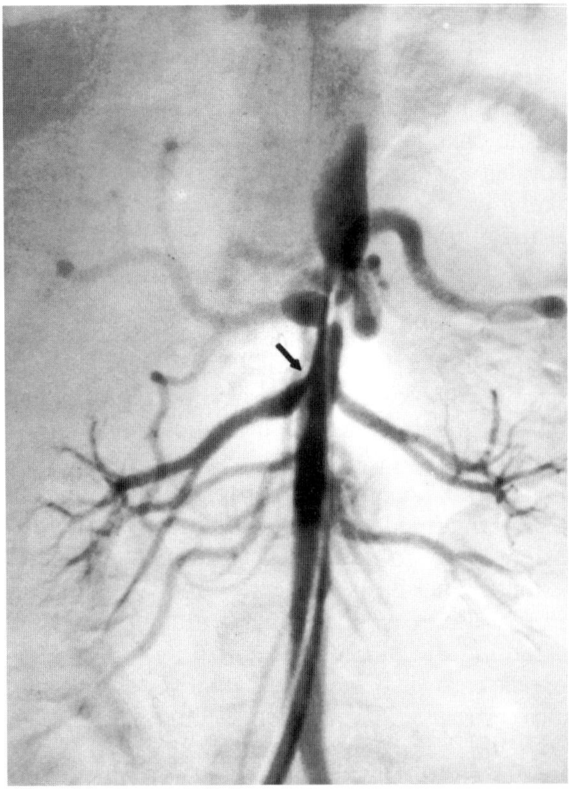

(b)

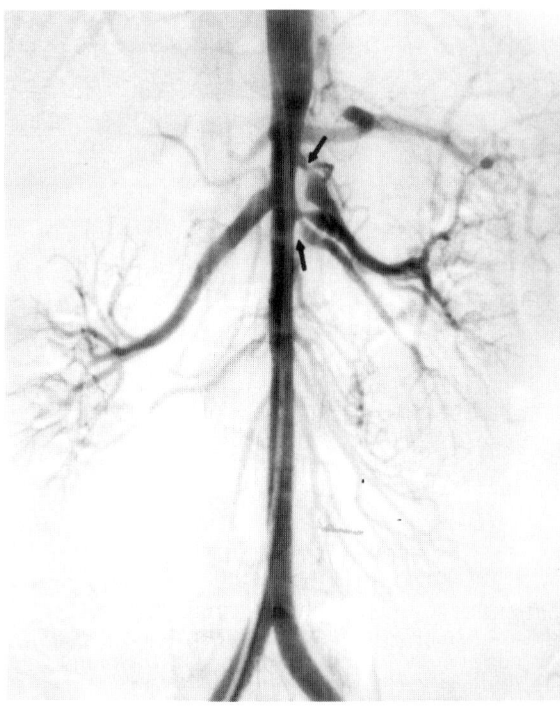

(c)

Figure 2.12. Developmental renal artery stenoses: (a) Proximal lesion in a patient with neurofibromatosis. (b) Proximal stenosis (arrow) in a patient with multiple renal arteries and midabdominal coarctation. (**c**) Multiple vessel stenoses in a patient with aortic hypoplasia. (a) From ref. 38, (b) and (c) from ref 39, with permission.

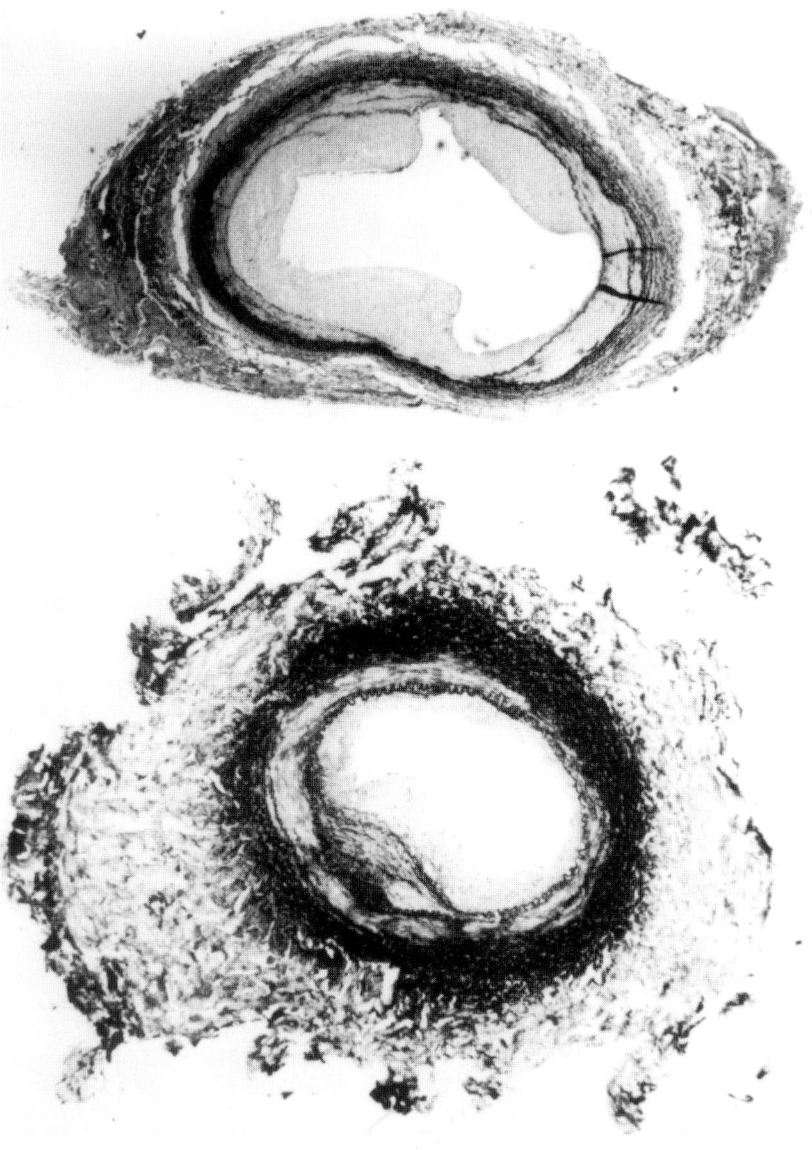

(a)

(b)

Figure 2.13. Developmental, hypoplastic renal artery: (a) Secondary intimal fibroplasia, fragmentation of the internal elastic lamina, and irregular diminutions in medial tissue are typical features of this stenotic lesion. Greatest luminal dimension is 2 mm. Movat stain, × 80. (b) Marked fragmentation and duplication of the internal elastic lamina and attenuation of medial tissues characterize this vessel. Intimal fibroplasia encroaches on the vessel lumen which is less than 1 mm in diameter. Adventitial elastic tissues appear excessive. Movat stain, × 100; (a) and (b) from ref. 41, with permission.

The histologic character of developmental lesions, especially those affecting pediatric-aged patients, usually includes abnormalities in all three vessel wall layers.[38, 40, 41] Irregular thinning of the media and intimal fibroplasia are common findings in these stenoses (Fig. 2.13a). Fragmentation and duplication of the internal elastic lamina is a frequent finding, and excess adventitial elastic tissue is often present (Fig. 2.13b).

Developmental renal artery narrowings are likely to evolve from certain *in utero* events. In normal fetal development the paired dorsal aortae fuse and in over 65% of all individuals all but one of the lateral metanephric branches of the newly formed aorta regress, resulting in a solitary renal artery to each kidney. Anything that alters the transition of the mesenchyme to medial smooth muscle tissue at this time, or its later condensation and growth, may cause both aortic and renovascular anomalies.

These renal artery constrictive lesions may follow a lack of fusion, or unequal fusion of the two dorsal aortae,[42] with subsequent obliteration of one of these channels and a narrowing of the associated renal artery. The mechanism leading to this is unknown. It appears that an acquired insult occurs *in utero* or during early life that arrests growth of the aorta and renal artery origins. This insult may be viral. Certain viruses, such as rubella, are cytocidal as well as inhibitory to cell replication, and may cause these lesions.[43, 44] In such instances inhibition of smooth muscle cell growth may preclude normal aortic development and produce accompanying renal artery ostial stenoses.

The renal arteries originate during embryonic development within mesenchymal tissue about the two dorsal aortae. They exist initially as a caudally located group of vessels to the mesonephros that are replaced with a more cephalic group of vessels to the metanephros. Development of a single renal artery apparently occurs, because of its obligate hemodynamic advantage over adjacent metanephric vessels. Abnormal flow patterns during evolution of an aortic coarctation in the region where a single renal artery would normally arise may cause coexisting polar channels to have hemodynamic advantages that allow them to persist. In support of this mechanism's existence is the fact that central abdominal aortic coarctation and hypoplasia are associated with multiple stenotic renal arteries to each kidney in nearly 80% of cases.[39, 41] Abnormalities in medial smooth muscle growth associated with neurofibromatosis in certain of these cases might also contribute to these renal artery stenoses.[45–47]

References

1 Leadbetter WF, Burkland CE. Hypertension in unilateral renal disease. *J Urol* 1933; **39:** 611–26.

2 Stanley JC. Pathologic basis of macrovascular renal artery disease. In Stanley JC, Ernst CB, Fry WJ (eds) *Renovascular Hypertension*, pp. 46–74. Philadelphia: WB Saunders, 1984.

3 Stanley JC, Gewertz BC, Bove EL *et al.* Arterial fibrodysplasia. Histopathologic character and current etiologic concepts. *Arch Surg* 1975; **110:** 561–6.

4 Stanley JC, Wakefield TW. Arterial fibrodysplasia. In Rutherford RB (ed.) *Vascular Surgery*, 4th edn, pp. 264–85. Philadelphia: WB Saunders; 1995.

5 Wright I. Age changes in the peripheral arteries in man. *Cardiovasc Anat Pathol* 1964; **11:** 157–68.

6 Stewart DR, Price RA, Nebesar R, Schuster SR. Progressing peripheral fibromuscular hyperplasia in an infant. A possible manifestation of the rubella syndrome. *Surgery* 1973; **73:** 374–80.

7 Dornfeld L, Kaufman JJ. Immunologic considerations in renovascular hypertension. *Urol Clin North Am* 1975; **2:** 285–300.

8 Meaney TF, Dustan HF, McCormack LJ. Natural history of renal arterial disease. *Radiology* 1968; **91:** 881–7.

9 Park SH, Chi JG, Choi Y. Primary intimal fibroplasia with multiple aneurysms of renal artery in childhood. *Child Nephrol Urol* 1990, **10:** 51–5.

10 Goncharenko V, Gerlock AJ, Shaff MI, Hollifield SW. Progression of renal artery fibromuscular dysplasia in 42 patients as seen on angiography. *Radiology* 1981; **139:** 45–51.

11 Sheps SG, Kincaid OW, Hunt JC. Serial renal function and angiographic observations in idiopathic fibrous and fibromuscular stenoses of the renal arteries. *Am J Cardiol* 1972; **30:** 55–60.

12 Stanley JC, Fry WJ. Renovascular hypertension secondary to arterial fibrodysplasia in adults: criteria for operation and results of surgical therapy. *Arch Surg* 1975; **110:** 922–8.

13 Schreiber MJ, Pohl MA, Novick AC. The natural history of atherosclerotic and fibrous renal artery disease. *Urol Clin North Am* 1984; **11:** 383–92.

14 Cragg AH, Smith TP, Thompson BH, *et al.* Incidental fibromuscular dysplasia in potential renal donors: long-term clinical follow-up. *Radiology* 1989; **172:** 145–7.

15 Ekelund L, Gerlock J, Molin J, Smith C. Roentgenologic appearance of fibromuscular dysplasia. *Acta Radiol Diagn (Stockh)* 1978; **19:** 433–46.

16 Nemcek AA, Holmburg CE, Reversible renal fibromuscular dysplasia. *Am J Roentgenol* 1986; **147:** 737–8.

17 McGrath TW. Fibromuscular dysplasia vs catheter-induced renal artery spasm (letter). *Am J Roentgenol* 1987; **148:** 651.

18 Harrison EG, McCormack LJ. Pathologic classification of renal artery disease in renovascular hypertension. *Mayo Clin Proc* 1971; **46:** 161–7.

19 McCormick LJ, Noto TJ Jr, Meaney TF *et al.*

Subadventitial fibroplasia of the renal artery: a disease of young women. *Am Heart J* 1967; **73:** 602–14.
20 McCormack LJ, Poutasse EF, Meaney TF *et al.* A pathologic arteriographic correlation of renal arterial disease. *Am Heart J* 1967; **72:** 188–98.
21 Stanley JC, Rhodes EL, Gewertz BL, Chang CY, Walter JF, Fry WJ. Renal artery aneurysms: significance of macroaneurysms exclusive of dissections and fibrodysplastic mural dilatations. *Arch Surg* 1975; **110:** 1327–33.
22 Sottiurai VS, Fry WJ, Stanley JC. Ultrastructure of medial smooth muscle and myofibroblasts in human arterial dysplasia. *Arch Surg* 1978; **113:** 1280–8.
23 Gladstien K, Rushton AR, Kidd KK. Penetrance estimates and recurrence risks for fibromuscular dysplasia. *Clin Gene* 1980; **17:** 115–16.
24 Major P, Genest J, Cartier P, Kuchel O. Hereditary fibromuscular dysplasia with renovascular hypertension. *Ann Int Med.* 1977; **86:** 583.
25 Morimoto S, Kuroda M, Uchida K, *et al.* Occurrence of renovascular hypertension in two sisters. *Nephron* 1976; **17:** 314–20.
26 Rushton AR. The genetics of fibromuscular dysplasia. *Arch Int Med* 1980, **140:** 233–6.
27 Sang CN, Whelton PK, Hamper UM *et al.* Etiologic factors in renovascular fibromuscular dysplasia. *Hypertension* 1979, **14:** 472–9.
28 de Zeeuw D, Donker AJM, Burema J *et al.* Nephroptosis and hypertension. *Lancet* 1977; **1:** 213–15.
29 Kaufman JJ, Maxwell MH. Upright aortography in the study of nephroptosis, stenotic lesions of the renal artery, and hypertension. *Surgery* 1963, **53:** 736–42.
30 Tsukamoto Y, Komuro Y, Akutsu F *et al.* Orthostatic hypertension due to coexistence of renal fibromuscular dysplasia and nephroptosis. *Jpn Circ J* 1988, **52:** 1408–14.
31 Leung DYM, Glagov S, Matthews MB. Cyclic stretching stimulates synthesis of matrix components by arterial smooth muscle cells in vitro. *Science* 1976; **191:** 475–7.
32 Bader H. The anatomy and physiology of the vascular wall. In Hamilton WF (ed.) *Handbook of Physiology*, Vol. 2, pp. 865–89. Washington, DC: American Physiological Society, 1963.
33 Lang J. Mikroskopische anatomie der arterien. *Angiologica* 1965; **2:** 225–84.
34 Fievez ML. Fibromuscular dysplasia of arteries: a spastic phenomenon? *Med Hypotheses* 1986; **13:** 341–9.
35 Paulson GW. Fibromuscular dysplasia, antiovulent drugs, and ergot preparations *Stroke* 1978; **9:** 172.
36 Hata J, Hosoda Y. Perimedial fibroplasia of the renal artery. A light and electron microscopy study. *Arch Pathol Lab Med* 1979; **103:** 220–3.
37 Sottiurai VS, Fry WJ, Stanley JC. Ultrastructural characteristics of experimental arterial medial fibrodysplasia induced by vasa vasorum occlusion. *J Surg Res* 1978; **24:** 169–77.
38 Stanley JC, Fry WJ. Pediatric renal artery occlusive disease and renovascular hypertension. Etiology, diagnosis and operative treatment. *Arch Surg* 1981; **116:** 669–76.
39 Graham LM, Zelenock GB, Erlandson EE *et al.* Abdominal aortic coarctation and segmental hypoplasia. *Surgery* 1979; **86:** 519–29.
40 Devaney K, Kapur SP, Patterson K, Chandra RS. Pediatric renal artery dysplasia. A morphologic study. *Pediatr Pathol* 1991; **11:** 609–21.
41 Stanley JC, Graham LM, Whitehouse WM Jr *et al.* Developmental occlusive disease of the abdominal aorta, splanchnic and renal arteries. *Am J Surg* 1981; **142:** 190–6.
42 Maycock Wd'A. Congenital stenosis of the abdominal aorta. *Am Heart J* 1937; **13:** 633–46.
43 Plotkin SA, Boue A, Boue JG. The *in vitro* growth of rubella virus in human embryo cells. *Am J Epideminol* 1965; **81:** 71–85.
44 Siassi B, Glyman G, Emmanouilides GC. Hypoplasia of the abdominal aorta associated with the rubella syndrome. *Am J Dis Child* 1970; **120:** 476–9.
45 Finley JL, Dabbs DJ. Renal vascular smooth muscle proliferation in neurofibromatosis. *Hum Path* 1988, **19:** 107–10.
46 Halperin M, Currarino G. Vascular lesions causing hypertension in neurofibromatosis. *N Engl J Med* 1965; **273:** 248–52.
47 Mena E, Bookstein JJ, Holt JF, Fry WJ. Neurofibromatosis and renovascular hypertension in children. *Am J Roentgenol* 1973; **118:** 39–45.
48 Stanley JC. Morphologic, hispathologic and clinical characteristics of renovascular fibrodysplasia and arteriosclerosis. In Bergan JJ, Yao JST (eds) *Surgery of the Aorta and Its Body Branches*, pp. 355–76. New York: Grune and Stratton, 1979.
49 Whitehouse WM Jr, Cho KJ, Coran AS, Stanley JC. Pediatric arterial disease. In Neiman HL, Yao JST (eds) *Angiography of Vascular Disease*, pp. 289–306, New York: Churchill Livingstone, 1985.
50 Stanley JC, Graham LM. Renovascular hypertension. In Miller DC, Roon AJ (eds) *Diagnosis and Management of Peripheral Vascular Disease*, pp. 231–5, Menlo Park, CA: Addison-Wesley, 1981.

3

Aneurysm and arteriovenous malformation

OSCAR ABUD, GILBERTO E CHÉCHILE, FRANCISCO SOLÉ-BALCELLS

Renal artery aneurysm

Aneurysm of the renal artery is a dilation of the main renal artery and/or its branches caused by weakening of the elastic tissue and media of the arterial wall. The increase of angiographic studies in patients with hypertension and obliterative arterial disease give us more data to know the real incidence of renal artery aneurysms. The increase in our knowledge is important in explaining the natural history of the disease, the relation with hypertension and the risk of complications such as rupture.

It is very difficult to know the true incidence of renal artery aneurysms. In necropsy studies the incidence ranges between 0.01 and 0.015%.[1] In randomized studies with injection of contrast agents into the renal artery the incidence increases to 0.7%.[2] In a series of 10 000 abdominal aortographies in patients without renal diseases the incidence of renal artery aneurysms was 0.3%.[3] In selective renal artery arteriographies the incidence increased to 0.7–1.32%.[4]

Both sexes are affected equally but some series show a slight predominance in females due to the higher frequency of fibromuscular hyperplasia. The age of presentation ranges between 20 and 75 years.[1, 5, 6]

Classification

There are four types of renal artery aneurysms: saccular, fusiform, dissecting and intrarenal.[7] Some authors classify renal artery aneurysms as displasic, acquired, dissecting and intrarenal.[5, 8]

Saccular aneurysm

This is the most common ranging between 70 and 90%.[5, 6] Usually it occurs at the bifurcation of the main renal artery or one of its branches (Fig. 3.1). Saccular aneurysms may be associated with medial fibroplasia of the renal artery. Neurofibromatosis is a disease that produces abnormalities of the media that predispose to aneurysmal development.

Unless they are calcified, differential diagnosis with arteriosclerotic aneurysms is difficult. The possibility of aneurysm rupture may depend on the degree of calcification. Aneurysms without calcification or with only partial calcification have a higher incidence of rupture.[7, 9] Saccular aneurysms may produce mural thrombosis leading to peripheral embolization with renal infarctation.[8, 10] Hydronephrosis may be the result of pelvis and/or calices being compressed by a large saccular aneurysm.[11]

Fusiform aneurysm

This is the uniform dilation of a renal artery segment (Fig. 3.2). Calcification is very rare. These aneurysms appear as poststenotic dilation in arteries with fibrotic displasia or arterosclerosis (Fig. 3.3). Progression of proximal stenosis with thrombosis is the most serious and frequent

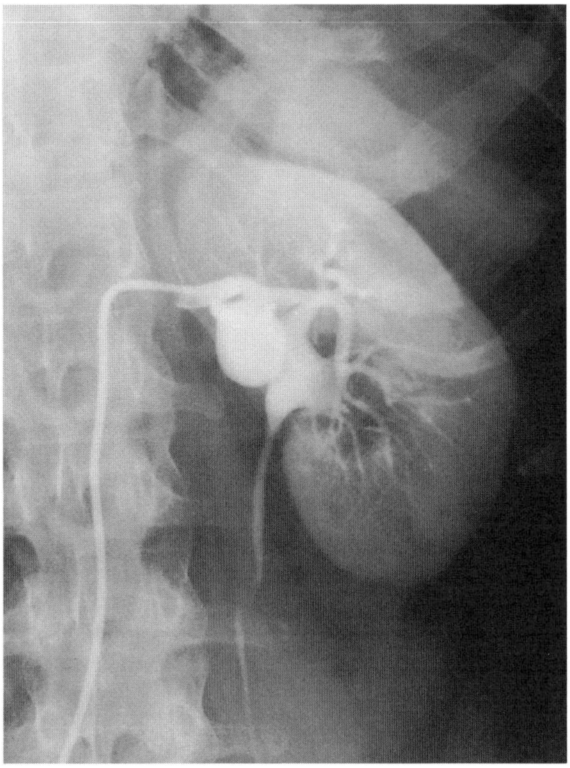

Figure 3.1. Left renal arteriogram shows a saccular aneurysm of the main artery in contact with renal pelvis.

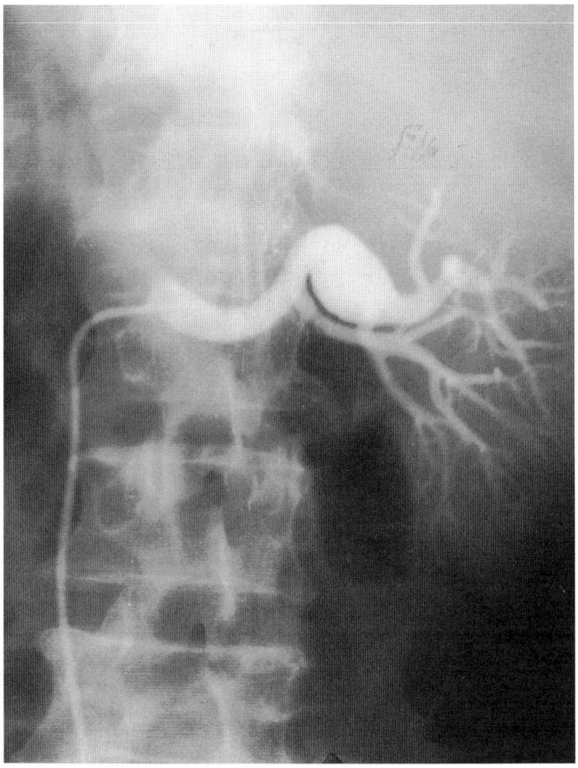

Figure 3.2. Left renal arteriogram reveals fusiform aneurysm of the main artery.

complication. Renal ischemia and hypertension in these patients demand a rapid diagnosis and surgical treatment.[12]

Dissecting aneurysm

Focal degeneration and rupture of internal elastic membrane with separation of intima from the rest of the wall is the initial lesion. Dissection may extend to secondary branches causing thrombosis and segmentary renal infarctation. Occasionally a distal repermeabilization occurs without changes in renal function. Generally, dissecting aneurysms are complications of a previous lesion in the renal artery: arteriosclerosis, intimal fibroplasia or perimedial fibroplasia. In recent years, the introduction of percutaneous angioplasty has increased the incidence of dissection by catheter. Sometimes a dissecting renal aneurysm may appear as stenosis of a dissecting aorta aneurysm. Clinical presentation as a sudden and acute flank or lumbar pain may be misdiagnosed as a lithiasic renal colic. Immediate surgical treatment is mandatory to preserve the renal unit.

Intrarenal aneurysm

Generally intrarenal aneurysms are saccular or fusiform. In a series of 250 patients with renal artery aneurysms, Smith and Hinman reported an intrarenal aneurysm incidence of 17%.[13] They found hypertension in 13% of the cases and rupture and death in 20% of the cases.

Bulbul and Farrow[6] detected intrarenal aneurysms in 8% of the patients with renal artery aneurysms. They are classified as true aneurysms or pseudo-aneurysms. The former can be fusiform, saccular or they can communicate with a venous aneurysm and the latter is caused by the rupture of the artery wall with hematoma formation and perivascular aneurysm.

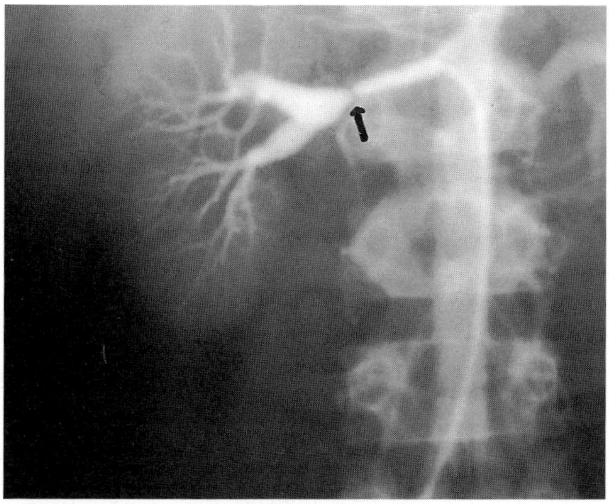

Figure 3.3. Right renal arteriogram in a 7-year-old boy shows annular stenosis (arrow) of the main artery with a poststenotic fusiform aneurysm.

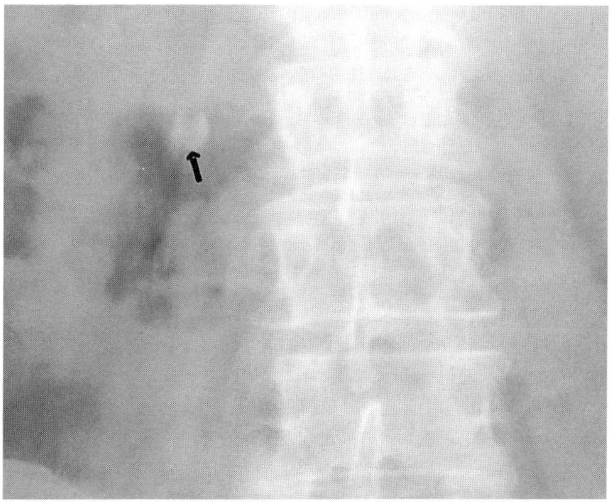

Figure 3.4. Plain abdominal radiogram reveals round calcification (arrow) over the renal hilus.

Intrarenal aneurysms can be congenital or originate from atherosclerosis, trauma, fibrous dysplasia, congenital vascular malformations, renal carcinoma or after any percutaneous procedure of the kidney. Less frequently, they can be secondary to polyarteritis nodosa, syphilis or tuberculosis.

Radiographic diagnosis

In 35–50% of patients plain abdominal radiogram may show a ring-like calcification in or near the renal hilus[14] (Fig. 3.4). The differential diagnosis should be made with splenic cyst, calcified lymph node, calcified renal cyst, renal carcinoma, renal, ureteral or biliary calculus, aneurysm of the splenic, hepatic or pancreatic artery, calcified perirenal abscess, calcification in renal tuberculosis and osteochondroma of a lumbar vertebra.

Intravenous pyelography in patients with aneurysms associated with severe renal ischemia may show decrease in renal size and/or delayed excretion of contrast. In cases with dissecting aneurysms and complete renal artery obstruction intravenous pyelography may show renal nonfunction.

If an aneurysm produces extrinsic compression of the renal pelvis, filling defects may be observed. Aneurysm expansion may appear as hydronephrosis.

Computerized tomography (CT) may diagnose retroperitoneal bleeding due to rupture of a renal artery aneurysm.[15] Large aneurysms can be diagnosed by CT with previous injection of contrast agents.[16] In cases where a renal infarction is suspected as a complication of a renal artery aneurysm, CT may show 'a thin rim of contrast agent enhancing tissue' (rim sign).[17]

New image modalities are also being used to evaluate and characterize renal artery aneurysms. Color duplex Doppler sonography is being utilized more frequently to diagnose renal pedicle diseases. It is a useful tool to diagnose and follow patients with renal artery aneurysms (Colour plate 1).

Definitive diagnosis may be established with selective renal arteriography that, moreover, gives information about configuration and size of the aneurysms and concomitant lesions such as arterial stenosis. To control the evolution of aneurysms, renal arteriography is the method of choice (Fig. 3.5),[18] however, color duplex Doppler is a very promising technique.

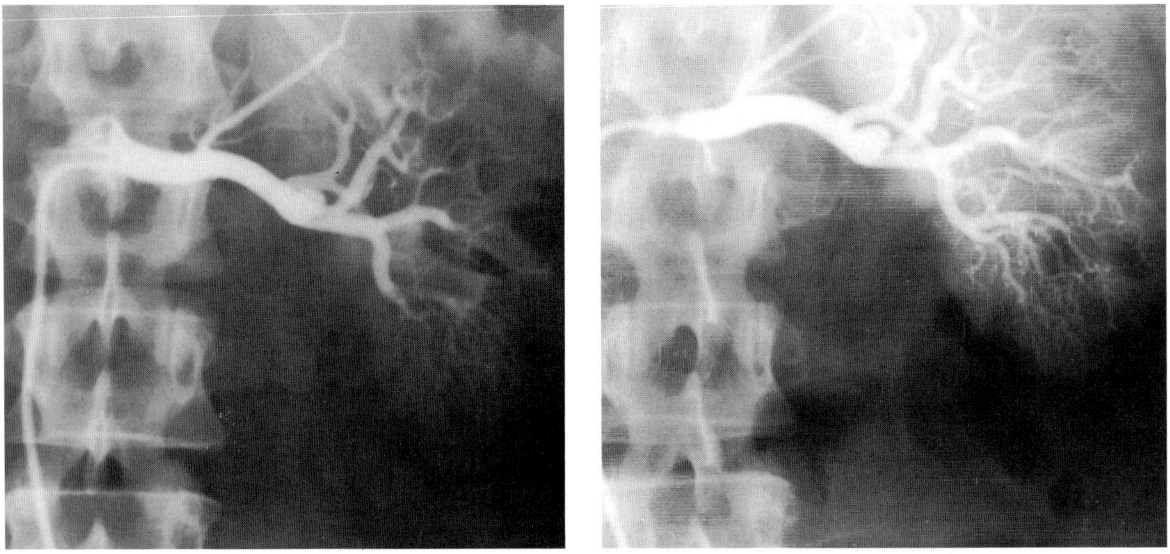

(a) (b)

Figure 3.5. Selective left renal arteriography. (a) Saccular aneurysm less than 2 cm in diameter at the bifurcation of the main artery. (b) After 6 years aneurysm does not show increase in size.

Clinical features

No pathognomic signs or symptoms accompany renal artery aneurysms. Most renal artery aneurysms are small and asymptomatic; around 35% of them are detected during evaluation of hypertension and 26% are incidentally diagnosed.[19] Renal arterial aneurysms are equally found in right or left renal arteries and both sexes are affected in the same proportion.

Thirty percent of patients have two or more lesions and 20% have bilateral lesions.[1, 18] The most common clinical manifestations are hypertension, hematuria, subcostal or flank pain, abdominal bruit and, exceptionally, a palpable pulsating mass. Hypertension continues to be the most common presentation (50–75%) presumably secondary to renal ischemia.[6, 19] Hematuria, either gross or microscopic, is attributed to be secondary to microinfarcts due to thrombosis of small vessels, to hypertension or less frequently to partial rupture into the pyelocalyceal system. Hematuria can be found in 30% of the cases.[6] Flank pain is due to aneurysmal expansion, compression of the renal pelvis or dissection, thrombosis or peripheral embolization. It may be found in a third of the patients.[20] Abdominal bruit may occur in 16% of the cases.

It is very difficult to certify if renal arterial aneurysm can produce hypertension without the presence of renal artery stenosis. In these cases, hypertension may be caused by segmental renal ischemia due to turbulent flow within the aneurysm, thromboembolism or peripheral branch compression by a large aneurysm.

Central plasma renin activity is very useful in the diagnosis and prognosis in patients with renal arterial aneurysm and hypertension. Aneurysm surgery does not cure hypertension in patients without renal ischemia.[21]

Complications

The most frequent complications of renal artery aneurysm are: arterial thrombosis with renal infarction, obstructive uropathy, erosion into a vein with formation of an arteriovenous fistula and finally spontaneous rupture. Aneurysm thrombosis without extension to the renal artery is a less serious complication (Fig. 3.6). Renal infarction is an uncommon complication and

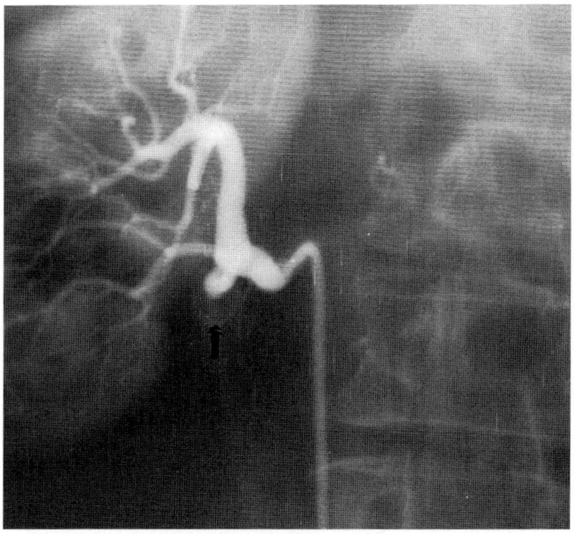

Figure 3.6. Selective right renal arteriography shows saccular aneurysm partially occupied by a thrombus (arrow).

may be caused by thrombosis, renal artery dissection or small branch embolization. Symptoms (present in 75% of cases) include diffuse abdominal pain and flank or subcostal pain with nausea and vomiting.[8]

Renal infarction may produce hypertension due to vasoactive substances liberated by ischemic areas.

Rupture of a renal artery aneurysm is a rare but very serious complication that requires an urgent operation. Novicki *et al.*[22] reported 200 cases of perirenal hematoma and 20% of them were due to aneurysm rupture. Cinman *et al.*[23] showed that in only 1 of 20 patients with perirenal hematoma, rupture of a renal artery aneurysm was the origin of the bleeding. In the series published by Stanley *et al.*,[24] the incidence of rupture was 5.6%. Smith and Hinman[13] reported that rupture was observed in 20% of intrarenal aneurysms. There is disagreement about the natural history and factors that predispose to rupture. Hageman *et al.*[3] followed 25 patients with renal artery aneurysms less than 2 cm in size for periods of 1–17 years without demonstration of rupture or increase of the size. Henriksson *et al.*[18] performed angiographic follow-up in 21 patients with 34 renal artery aneurysms finding no changes in 28 cases and a slight increase in size, thrombosis or calcification in 6 aneurysms. Poutasse[7] stated that rupture of a renal artery aneurysm tended to occur in non-calcified or incompletely calcified aneurysms larger than 1.5 cm in diameter.

Hidai *et al.*[9] reviewed 43 cases of aneurysm rupture reported in the literature showing that, except for three cases with aneurysms less than 1.5 cm in size and three cases with calcified aneurysms, the great incidence of rupture was found in non-calcified aneurysms greater than 1.5 cm in size. McCarron *et al.*[25] reported 5% of rupture in 126 cases with atherosclerotic renal artery aneurysm. Severe hypertension is an important risk factor that predisposes to rupture. Ninety percent of rupture is observed in patients with coexisting hypertension. Prognosis after the rupture of a renal artery aneurysm has improved and at the moment only 6% of patients die.[9] The risk of rupture of a renal artery aneurysm is increased during pregnancy. It has been speculated that pregnancy may predispose to rupture due to increased cardiac output and hence increased renal blood flow, hormonal influence on the vascular wall and increased intra-abdominal pressure.[6, 9] Surgery is indicated in pregnancy and in females of child-bearing age due to high incidence of rupture (around 80%).[26–29]

Recently, several authors have published their experience in performing external shock wave lithotripsy in patients with renal lithiasis and renal artery aneurysm.[30, 31] There is agreement on the safety of the treatment if it is performed with adequate preparation.

Surgical indications

Most of the authors agreed that a small (less than 1.5–2 cm), well-calcified renal aneurysm, in an asymptomatic normotensive patient does not require operative intervention. Size changes in these aneurysms can be detected with plain abdominal radiograms and color duplex sonography.

Expectant management may also be indicated in aneurysms of the same size and asymptomatic, non-calcified or only partially calcified. Follow-up of these cases may be done with serial arteriography.[3]

Absolute surgical indications accepted by most authors[25, 29, 32–34] are:

- aneurysms larger than 2 cm with or without partial calcification;
- aneurysms showing expansion (increase of size in serial radiograms);
- dissecting aneurysms;
- aneurysms associated with severe hypertension with or without renal artery stenosis;
- aneurysms associated with symptoms like flank pain or hematuria;
- aneurysms diagnosed in a woman of childbearing age who is likely to conceive;
- aneurysms occupied by thombus demonstrated in angiography that may produce peripheral branch embolization.

The most frequently used revascularization techniques are:

- aneurysmectomy followed by simple arterial repair for saccular aneurysms of the main renal artery;
- segmental resection and reanastomosis in aneurysms that affect a short segment of the main renal artery;
- extracorporeal aneurysmectomy with vascular reconstruction and autotransplantation;
- partial or total nephrectomy in patients with renal infarction or severe ischemic renal atrophy, or in patients with multiple intrarenal aneurysms.

The alternative to surgery is steel coil embolization, reserved for selected patients with small-size intrarenal aneurysms.[35] Supraselective embolization with multiple coils associated with polyvinyl alcohol may be the alternative to nephrectomy in very large aneurysms.[16]

Arteriovenous malformations

Arteriovenous malformations are uncommon lesions. Since Varela first described arteriovenous fistula, in 1928, more than 350 cases have been reported.[36] An important increase in the incidence has been observed in the last decade due to a rise in the utilization of percutaneous renal approaches for diagnosis and treatment of kidney diseases. Since most of these lesions are asymptomatic and remain undetected the real incidence of arteriovenous fistula is unknown.[37]

Classification

Arteriovenous fistula is any abnormal communication between the venous and arterial system and it may be acquired or idiopathic. Arteriovenous malformation is defined as a congenital arteriovenous fistula with multiple connections between the main renal artery or its branches and veins.[38]

Congenital arteriovenous malformations

These have a cirsoid or angiomatous configuration (Fig. 3.7) and are supplied by one or more interlobar or segmentary renal artery branches of normal caliber.[39, 40] Arteriovenous malformations comprise 14–27% of arteriovenous abnormalities, although in Yazake's series the incidence reaches 53%.[41]

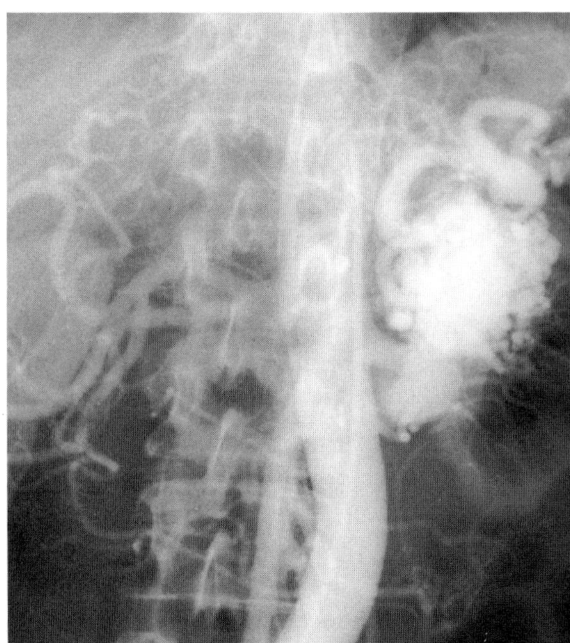

Figure 3.7. Abdominal aortogram shows a large cirsoid arteriovenous malformation in the middle part of the left kidney.

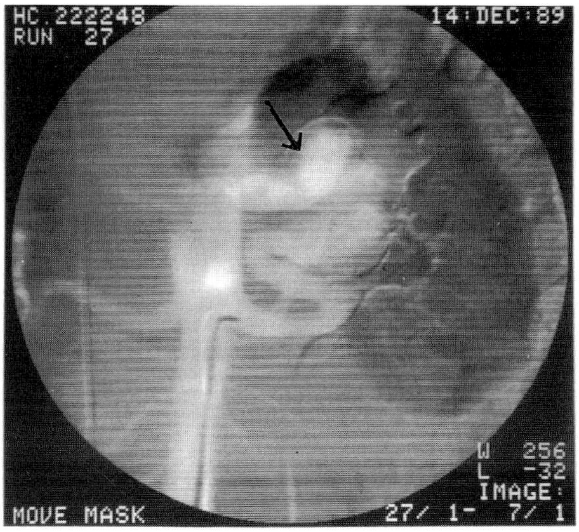

Figure 3.8. Selective digital substraction angiogram of the left renal artery demonstrating large idiopathic arteriovenous fistula; note a huge renal vein dilation (arrow).

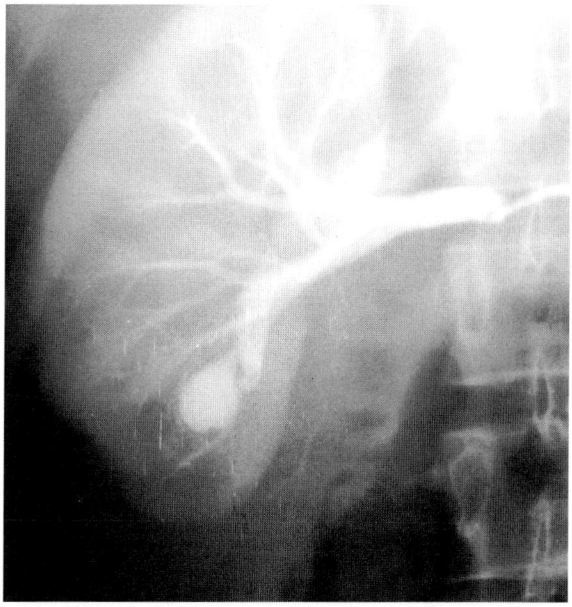

Figure 3.9. Selective right renal arteriography shows acquired arteriovenous fistula after percutaneous needle biopsy.

Idiopathic arteriovenous fistula

The term idiopathic is used to describe those fistulas in which the angiographic appearance is similar to that of the acquired variety but the exact etiology cannot be determined (Fig. 3.8). They are simple and/or cirsoid. Some authors consider that they originate as a result of venous erosion by a pre-existing arterial aneurysm associated with fibromuscular displasia.[27, 42, 43] Idiopathic arteriovenous fistula comprise between 3 and 5% of all arteriovenous fistulas.

Acquired arteriovenous fistula

This variety comprises between 70 and 75% of arteriovenous abnormalities. Selective renal angiograms show only one connection between an artery and a vein. According to the causal agent they may be classified as: spontaneous, iatrogenic, traumatic or inflammatory.

IATROGENIC ARTERIOVENOUS FISTULA

The most frequent etiology is percutaneous renal needle biopsy (Fig. 3.9). Ekelund and Lindholm[44] demonstrated that 15% of patients showed arteriovenous fistula after percutaneous needle biopsy. However, most of these fistulas closed spontaneously within a few months remaining open in only 4%. Another common cause of iatrogenic arteriovenous fistula is percutaneous biopsy of renal allograft after transplantation with an incidence of 17.5%. In 65% of the cases the fistula closed spontaneously within 6 months.[45] In the percutaneous approach for therapeutic procedures such as nephrostomy or nephrolithotomy the incidence of symptomatic arteriovenous fistula is around 1%[46–48] (Fig. 3.10). Less frequently described were arteriovenous fistula after nephrectomy, partial nephrectomy or anathropic nephrolithotomy.[49–51]

SPONTANEOUS ARTERIOVENOUS FISTULA

In this group are included fistulas associated with kidney neoplasms. They comprise between 10 and 16% of all arteriovenous fistulas. Severe cardiologic manifestations such as cardiomegaly, diastolic hypertension or systolic cardiac murmur are commonly found in arteriovenous fistulas associated with renal cancer.[52, 53] Clear cell carcinoma is the tumor that

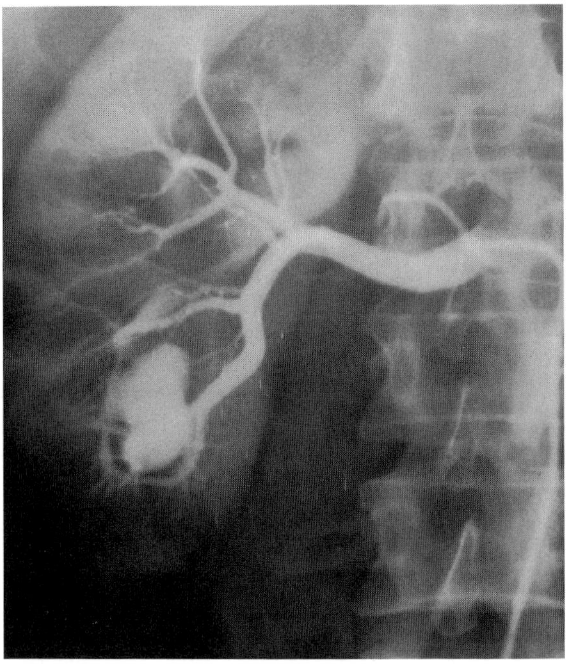

Figure 3.10. Selective right renal arteriogram shows arteriovenous fistula after percutaneous approach for nephrolithotomy.

most frequently presents arteriovenous fistula.[54, 55] Angiomyolipoma may be also associated with arteriovenous fistula.[56]

TRAUMATIC ARTERIOVENOUS FISTULA

The most common cause of traumatic fistulas are those from penetrating wounds, such as those caused by knives and gun shots. Rarely is blunt trauma a cause.[55, 57]

Inflammatory arteriovenous fistula

Inflammatory arteriovenous fistulas are least frequent. Pyelonephritis granulomatosa or chronic pylonephritis are the most common causes.[55, 58]

Clinical features

Clinical manifestations of an arteriovenous fistula depend on its size and location. The most common symptoms are: abdominal bruit, hematuria, hypertension, cardiomegaly and congestive heart failure. A bruit may be detected at the flank, lumbar or periumbilical zone.[59] Bruit is less frequent in cirsoid arteriovenous malformation.[60] Gross hematuria with clots is a common finding in congenital arteriovenous malformations. This may be explained by the fact that most cirsoid arteriovenous fistulas are frequently found beneath the caliceal or pelvic mucosa.[60] Diastolic hypertension is found in 50% of cases. Hypertension is believed to be the result of shunting of blood away from the kidney, causing relative ischemia and increased renin production. High flow arteriovenous fistulas such as postnephrectomy are associated with increase of cardiac output and decrease of peripheral resistances causing systolic hypertension with normal diastolic pressure.[58] Left ventricular hypertrophy and congestive heart failure may appear in 40% of patients.[50, 60]

Radiographic diagnosis

Intravenous pyelography is the first radiological study usually performed due to the fact that hematuria is the initial symptom in most patients. In approximately 50% of patients with arteriovenous fistula, intravenous pyelography is normal.

Common findings in excretory urography are: extrinsic compression of the renal pelvis or calices, ureteral obstruction by blood clots with resultant hydronephrosis, non-visualization of the kidney in large arteriovenous malformations or arteriovenous fistulas, and infundibular and caliceal mucosal irregularity from the dilated submucosal vascular system.[61]

Color duplex Doppler ultrasound is very effective in diagnosing and following patients with arteriovenous malformations. This non-invasive technique is particularly suitable for the detection of arteriovenous fistula following kidney allograft biopsy. Color duplex Doppler has demonstrated arteriovenous fistula in 18% of patients who underwent renal allograft biopsy.[45] The most characteristic appearence of arteriovenous fistula using color Doppler ultrasound is a mosaic of color due to combination of tissue vibration and turbulence.[62] Despite some problems detecting small lesions with this technique, it does seem potentially useful in the evaluation of renal vascular diseases. Diagnosis of arteriovenous fistula should be confirmed by angiography.[63]

Computerized tomography (CT) cannot differentiate arteriovenous abnormalities from hypervascular, solid structures such as renal cell carcinoma, benign tumors, renal abscess, complicated cystic lesions and dilated vessels (Fig. 3.11). However, dynamic CT may be useful in detecting an arteriovenous fistula associated with a huge renal vein dilation.[40] Despite the fact that magnetic resonance imaging may delineate the vascular abnormalities associated with renal cell carcinoma, without the utilization of a contrast agent,[64] definitive diagnosis of congenital arteriovenous malformations should be made with angiography. Renal arteriography confirms the lesion, and gives information about the size and the exact localization of the arteriovenous fistula. Crummy *et al.*[65] stated in 1965 two basic angiography patterns of arteriovenous fistula. Congenital vascular malformations appear as multiple small and tortuous channels supplied by multiple arterial branches. The proximal renal arterial diameter is generally normal.

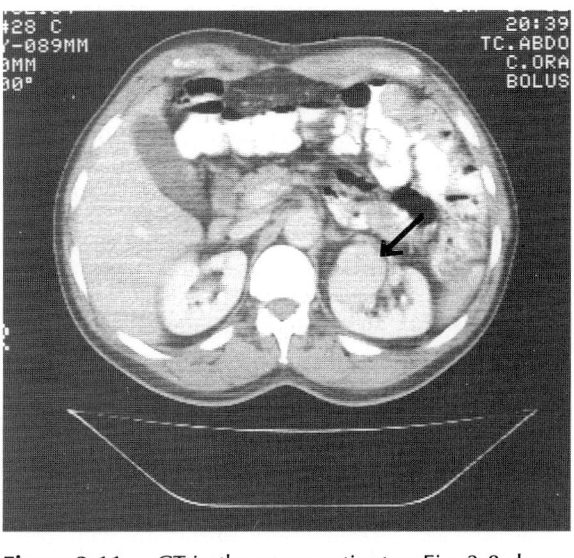

Figure 3.11. CT in the same patient as Fig. 3.8 showing that arteriovenous fistula does not differentiate from a tumoral lesion (arrow).

Idiopathic or acquired arteriovenous fistula is usually solitary with an identifiable artery and vein. The entering artery and the exiting vein are dilated with decrease of parenchyma vascularization.

Management

The management of a patient with a renal arteriovenous malformation depends on the severity of symptoms and hemodynamic effects associated with the abnormality. Expectant management is indicated in small fistulas occurring after percutaneous biopsy, because most resolve spontaneously within 18 months.[44, 55, 66, 67] Surgical treatment is necessary for patients with symptomatic disease such as recurrent hematuria, hemodynamic decompensation, hypertension, congestive cardiac failure or progressive renal failure. Although renal vein renin may be found elevated in cases with arteriovenous fistula, its measurement is not useful due to the dilutional effect that shunt has on its values. However, hypertension associated with arteriovenous malformations is cured in 62% of cases after surgical treatment.[55] Surgical success rate increases to 85% in cases with acquired post-traumatic fistula.[58]

Arteriovenous abnormalities can be managed with surgery or percutaneous embolization.

Surgery

In large arteriovenous fistulas or in cirsoid lesions, nephrectomy is the procedure most utilized.[68] Partial nephrectomy should be attempted to preserve renal parenchyma in cases with small upper or lower renal pole fistulas.[62] Simple ligation of the branch artery feeding the fistula may be performed in cases with extrarenal arteriovenous fistula.[69] In an attempt to preserve renal parenchyma in cases with large dilation of the artery and vein, closure of the fistula through a venotomy with resection of the arteriovenous aneurysm and ligation of both communicating vessels may be performed.[70, 71] Another alternative of treatment is *in situ* or extracorporeal microvascular reconstruction depending on the location of the lesion.[72]

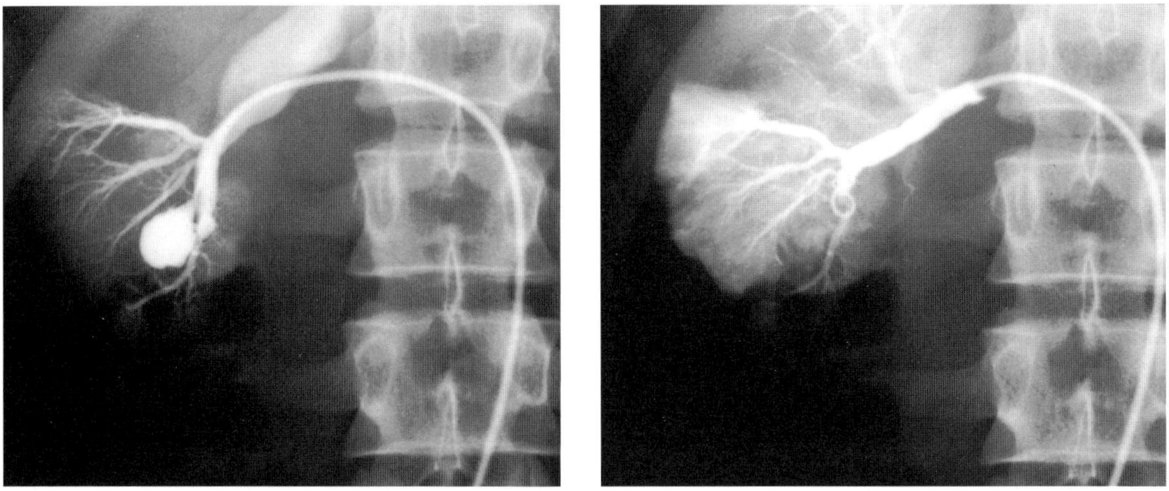

(a) (b)

Figure 3.12. Same patient as Fig. 3.9. Superselective arteriography (a) before and (b) after steel coil embolization showing occlusion of feeding artery.

Intrarenal selective embolization offers a nonsurgical therapeutic alternative for arteriovenous fistula. It can be performed as a definitive treatment or to decrease the size of the lesion in selected cases.[73] Embolization is the treatment of choice in patients with postpercutaneous procedures or post-traumatic arteriovenous fistulas. Various agents have been described for embolization: steel coils, balloons, autologous blood clot, absorbable gelatin sponge. Autologous blood clots and absorbable gelatin sponge are effective in small and peripheral arteriovenous fistulas. Nowadays non-absorbable metallic spirals (coils) are the agents most frequently utilized (Fig. 3.12).[74, 75] Balloons are more effective in large arteriovenous fistulas.[76] Before the release of obliterating agents an injection of epinephrine produces vessel spasm decreasing the risk of migration into the systemic circulation. Superselective embolization may be performed with microcoils and small coaxial catheters.[77]

Complications of embolization are: transient hypertension due to renal infarct, migration of the agent with pulmonary embolism and postembolization syndrome characterized by lumbar pain, fever and leukocytosis. This syndrome is uncommon in superselective embolizations.[74, 76]

References

1 Glass PM, Uson AC. Aneurysms of the renal artery: a study of 20 cases. *J Urol* 1967; **98:** 285–92.

2 Schwartz CJ, White TA. Aneurysms of the renal artery. *J Pathol Bacteriol* 1965; **89:** 349–56.

3 Hageman JH, Smith RF, Szilagyi DE, Elliot JP. Aneurysms of the renal artery: problems of prognosis and surgical management. *Surgery* 1978; **84:** 563–72.

4 Edsman G. Angionephrography and suprarenal angiography: a roentgenologic study of the normal kidney, expansive renal and suprarenal lesions and renal aneurysms. *Acta Radiol* 1957; **155:** (Suppl.) 104–16.

5 Lacombe M. Aneurismes de l'artere renale. Experience personnelle de 101 cas. *Chirurgie* 1989; **115:** 28–34.

6 Bulbul MA, Farrow GA. Renal artery aneyrysms. *Urology* 1992; **40:** 124–6.

7 Poutasse EF. Renal artery aneurysm. *J Urol* 1975; **113:** 443–9.

8 Frangi RS, Vermonde J, Darimont M *et al.* Aneurisme de l'artere renale et ses complications d'infarctus. *Acta Urol Belg* 1992; **60:** 131–41.

9 Hidai H, Kinoshita Y, Murayana T *et al.* Rupture of renal artery aneurysm. *Eur Urol* 1985; **11:** 249–53.

10 Martin DC. Renal artery aneurysm with peripheral embolization of kidney. *Urology* 1980; **6:** 590–1.

11 Creemers E, Van Damme H, Dusart Y, Limet R.

Hydronephrose produite par un aneurysme geat de l'artere renale. *J d'Urologie* 1990; **96:** 40–4.
12 Novick AC. Renal arterial aneurysms and arteriovenous fistulas. In Novick AC, Straffon RA (eds) *Vascular Problems in Urologic Surgery*, pp. 189–204. Philadelphia: WB Saunders, 1982.
13 Smith JN, Hinman IF Jr. Intrarenal arterial aneurysms. *J Urol* 1967; **97:** 990–6.
14 Vaughan TJ, Barry WF, Jeffords DL, Johnseude IS. Renal artery aneurysms and hypertension. *Radiology* 1971; **99:** 287–93.
15 Chen R, Novick AL. Retroperitoneal hemorrhage from a ruptured renal artery aneurysm with spontaneous resolution. *J Urol* 1994; **151:** 139–41.
16 Saltiel AA, Mantlou TAS, Patel SF. Embolization of a giant renal arterial aneurysm. *J Urol* 1990; **144:** 1227–8.
17 Frank PH, Nuttall J, Brander WL, Prosser D. The cortical rim sign of renal infarctation. *Br J Radiol* 1974; **47:** 875–8.
18 Henriksson C, Bjorkerund S, Nilson A, Pettersson S. Natural history of renal artery aneurysm elucidated by repeated angiography and pathoanatomical studies. *Eur Urol* 1985; **11:** 244–8.
19 Brekke IB, Sodal E, Jacobsen A *et al.* Fibromuscular renal artery disease treated by extracorporeal vascular reconstruction and renal autotransplantation. Short and long term results. *Eur J Vasc Surg* 1992; **6:** 471–6.
20 Lacotte B, Themelin D, Alame T *et al.* Douleur costo-lombaire, aneurysme de l'artere renale et hypertension. *J d'Urologie* 1988; **93:** 107–8.
21 Cummiles KB, Lecky JW, Kaufman JJ. Renal artery aneurysms and hypertension. *J Urol* 1973; **109:** 144–8.
22 Novicki DE, Turlington JT, Ball TP. The evaluation and management of spontaneous perirenal hemorrhage. *J Urol* 1980; **123:** 764–5.
23 Cinman AC, Farrer J, Kaufman JJ. Spontaneous perinephric hemorrhage in a 65 year old man. *J Urol* 1980; **133:** 829–32.
24 Stanley JC, Rhodes EL, Gewertz BL. Renal artery aneurysms: significance of macroaneurysms exclusive of dissection and fibrodysplastic mural dilatations. *Arch Surg* 1975; **110:** 1327–33.
25 McCarron JP, Marshall NF, Whitsell JC. Indications for surgery on renal artery aneurysms. *J Urol* 1975; **114:** 177–80.
26 Cerny JC. Renal artery aneurysm. *Arch Surg* 1968; **96:** 653–63.
27 Pliskin MJ, Dresner ML, Marrison LH *et al.* A giant renal artery aneurysm diagnosed post-partum. *J Urol* 1990; **144:** 1459–61.
28 Love WF, Robinette MA, Vernon CP. Renal artery aneurysm. Rupture in pregnancy. *J Urol* 1981; **126:** 809–11.
29 Ortenberg J, Novick AC, Straffon RA, Stewart BH. Surgical treatment of renal artery aneurysms. *Br J Urol* 1983; **55:** 341–6.
30 Carey S, Streem S. Extracorporeal shock wave lithotripsy for patients with calcified ipsilateral renal arterial or abdominal aortic aneurysms. *J Urol* 1992; **148:** 18–20.
31 Ignatoff J, Nelson J. Use of extracorporeal shock wave lithotripsy in a solitary kidney with renal artery aneurysm. *J Urol* 1993; **149:** 359–60.
32 Harrow BR, Sloane JA. Aneurysm of renal artery: report of five cases. *J Urol* 1959; **81:** 35–41.
33 Dubernad JM, Martin X, Gelet A, Mougin A. Aneurysms of the renal artery: surgical management with special reference to extracorporeal surgery and autotransplantation. *Eur Urol* 1985; **11:** 26–30.
34 Hupp T, Allemberg JR, Post K *et al.* Renal artery aneurysm: surgical indications and results. *Eur J Vas Surg* 1992; **6:** 447–86.
35 Okamoto M, Hashimoto M, Sueda T *et al.* Renal artery aneurysm: the significance of abdominal briut and use of color Doppler. *J Intern Med* 1992; **31:** 1217–19.
36 Varela MC. Aneurisma arteriovenoso de los vasos renales y asistolia consecutiva. *Rev Méd Latinoamericana* 1928; **14:** 32–44.
37 Cho KJC, Stanley JC. Non-neoplastic congenital and acquired renal arteriovenous malformations and fistula. *Radiology* 1978; **129:** 333–43.
38 Crotty KL, Orihuela E, Warren MM. Recent advances in the diagnosis and treatment of renal arteriovenous malformations and fistulas. *J Urol* 1993; **150:** 1355–9.
39 Messing E, Kessler R, Kavaney PB. Renal arteriovenous fistula. *Urology* 1976; **8:** 101.
40 Takatera H, Nakamura M, Nakano E *et al.* Renal arteriovenous fistula associated with a huge renal vein dilation. *J Urol* 1987; **137:** 722–4.
41 Yazake T, Tomita M, Akimoto M *et al.* Congenital renal arteriovenous fistula: case report, review of Japanese literature and description of non-radical treatment. *J Urol* 1976; **116:** 415–18.
42 Thomas RG, Grieve S, Lewin B. Spontaneous renal arteriovenous fistula and contralateral renal artery aneurysms. *Br J Radiol* 1962; **35:** 128.
43 Imray TJ, Cohen AJ, Hahn L. Renal arteriovenous fistula associated with fibromuscular dysplasia. *Urology* 1984; **23:** 378–80.
44 Ekelund L, Lindholm T. Arteriovenous fistulae following percutaneous renal biopsy. *Acta Radiol* 1971; **11:** 38–41.
45 Deane C, Cowan N, Giles J *et al.* Arteriovenous fistula in renal transplants: color doppler ultrasound observations. *Urol Radiol* 1992; **13:** 211–17.
46 Stables DP. Percutaneous nephrostomy: techniques, indications and results. *Urol Clin North Am* 1982; **9:** 15–29.
47 Kleist H, Pettersson S, Wikholm G. Percutaneous nephropyelostomy: a procedure not without complications. *Scand J Urol Nephrol* 1984; **18:** 71–4.

48 Fernandez I, Serrano A, Burgos J *et al.* Actitud terapéutica en el daño vascular de la endourología pielocalicial. *Arch Español Urol* 1993; **46:** 399–404.
49 Nelson BD, Brosman SA, Goodwin WE. Renal arteriovenous fistulas. *J Urol* 1973; **109:** 779–83.
50 Chew QT, Madayag MA. Post-nephrectomy arteriovenous fistula. *Urol* 1973; **109:** 546–7.
51 Snodgrass WT, Robinson MJ. Intrarenal arteriovenous fistula: a complication of partial nephrectomy. *J Urol* 1964; **91:** 135–6.
52 Wise GJ, Bosniak MA, Hudson PAB. Arteriovenous fistula associated with renal cell carcinoma of the kidney. *Br J Urol* 1967; **39:** 170–7.
53 Holmes SAV, Ball AJ. Arteriovenous fistula associated with adenocarcinoma of the kidney. *Urol Int* 1991; **47:** 81–3.
54 Bosniak MA. Radiographic manifestations of massive arteriovenous fistula in renal carcinoma. *Radiology* 1965; **85:** 454–9.
55 Morin RP, Dunnes EJ, Wright CB. Renal arteriovenous fistulas. A review of etiology, diagnosis and management. *Surgery* 1986; **99:** 114–18.
56 Barzilai IM, Braden GL, Ford LD *et al.* Renal angiomyolipoma with arteriovenous shunting. *J Urol* 1987; **137:** 483–4.
57 Cosgrove MD, Mendez R, Morrow JW. Traumatic renal arteriovenous fistula: report of 12 cases. *J Urol* 1973, **110:** 627–31.
58 McAlhany JC, Black HC Jr, Hanback CD Jr, Yarbrough DR III. Renal arteriovenous as a cause of hypertension. *Am J Surg* 1971; **122:** 117–20.
59 Tines WV, Devine CJ Jr, Devine PC, Poutasse EF. Surgical treatment of renal arteriovenous fistula: report of 5 cases. *J Urol* 1970; **103:** 692–8.
60 Takaha M, Matsumoto A, Ochi F *et al.* Intrarenal arteriovenous malformation. *J Urol* 1980; **124:** 315–18.
61 Kopchick JH, Bourne NK, Fine SW *et al.* *Urology* 1981; **17:** 13–17.
62 Renowden SA, Blethyn J, Cochlin DL. Duplex and colour flow sonography in the diagnosis of post-biopsy arteriovenous fistulae in the transplant kidney. *Clin Radiol* 1992; **45:** 233–7.
63 Sullivan RR, Johnson MB, Lee KP, Ralls PW. Color doppler sonographic findings in renal vascular lesions. *J Ultrasound Med* 1991; **10:** 161–5.
64 Selli C, Bartolozzi C, Lizzardo G, Petacchi D. Arteriovenous fistula associated with renal cell carcinoma: demonstration by magnetic resonance imaging. *Urol Radiol* 1986; **8:** 190–3.
65 Crummy AB Jr, Atkinson J, Caruthers SB Jr. Congenital renal arteriovenous fistulas. *J Urol* 1965; **93:** 24–6.
66 Morton MJ, Charboneau WJ. Arteriovenous fistula after biopsy of renal transplant: detection and monitoring with color flow and duplex ultrasonography. *Mayo Clin Proc* 1989; **64:** 531–4.
67 O'Brien DP, Parrott TS. Renal arteriovenous fistulas. *Surg Gynecol Obstet* 1974; **139:** 739–43.
68 Riba LW, Simao MP. Intrarenal arteriovenous fistula treated with partial nephrectomy. *J Urol* 1967; **98:** 293–5.
69 Cosgrove MD, Mendez R, Morrow J. Branch artery ligation for renal arteriovenous fistula. *J Urol* 1973; **110:** 632–8.
70 Merkel FK, Sako Y. Surgical treatment for traumatic renal arteriovenous fistula. *Arch Surg* 1970; **101:** 438–41.
71 Erlich RM. Renal arteriovenous fistula treated by endofistulorraphy. *Arch Surg* 1975; **110:** 1195–8.
72 Novick AC, Straffon RA, Stewart BH. Surgical management of branch renal artery disease: *in situ* versus extracorporeal methods of repair. *J Urol* 1980; **123:** 311–16.
73 Clouse ME, Levin DC, Desautels RE. Transcatheter embolotherapy for congenital renal arteriovenous malformations. Long-term follow-up. *Urology* 1983; **22:** 360–5.
74 Wallace S, Schwarten DE, Smith DC *et al.* Intrarenal arteriovenous fistulas: transcatheter steel coil occlusion. *J Urol* 1978; **120:** 282–6.
75 Bischoff W, Pohle W, Goerttler V. Treatment of arteriovenous angiomas of the kidney: surgical intervention and intra-arterial embolization. *J Urol* 1979; **122:** 825–8.
76 Corr P. Embolization in traumatic intrarenal vascular injuries. *Clin Radiol* 1991; **43:** 262–4.
77 Huppert PE, Duda SH, Erley CM *et al.* Embolization of renal vascular lesions: clinical experience with microcoils and tracker catheters. *Cardiovasc Intervent Radiol* 1993; **16:** 361–7.

4

Takayasu's arteritis

HIROSHI TOMA

Introduction

Takayasu's arteritis is a non-specific inflammatory disease affecting large arteries such as the aorta and its main branches, including the common carotid, subclavian, pulmonary, coronary and renal arteries. Most patients have obstructive symptoms due to stenosis and occlusion of the involved arteries. Involvement of the renal arteries is not uncommon in Asian and African patients, resulting in a major cause of renovascular hypertension in those countries.

In 1905, Mikito Takayasu reported a case of a 21-year-old woman who exhibited an unusual retinal arteriovenous anastomosis around the papilla, at the Annual Meeting of the Japan Ophthalmology Society.[1] At this meeting, two other ophthalmologists (K Onishi and T Kagoshima) corroborated his presentation with reports of similar cases whose radial arteries could not be palpated. In 1940 the first systematic pathological survey of a 25-year-old female suffering from Takayasu's arteritis revealed that this morbid condition was caused by vasculitis involving the aorta and its main branches.[2] The report indicated that the characteristic retinal abnormalities resulted from occlusion of the carotid artery. In 1948, Shimizu and Sano[3] described it as the 'pulseless disease', defining it in terms of the characteristic clinical features of pulselessness, coronary anastomosis in retinal vasculature and accelerated carotid sinus reflex. In 1963, Nasu[4] reviewed 21 autopsy cases and reported that the main lesions of this disease existed in the aorta and its major branches including the pulmonary artery trunk. As this disease was frequently observed in Japan, a research committee was set up by the Japanese Ministry of Health and Welfare to study it and it came to be known as 'Takayasu's arteritis'. Furthermore, there were many investigations and reviews from the point of view of pathology, clinical features, possible immunopathogenesis, diagnostic criteria, prognosis and treatment.[5–12] This chapter will focus on the more recent advances in the study of this condition.

Epidemiology

The Japanese research committee on Takayasu's arteritis performed two large nationwide epidemiological surveys.[13] The first nationwide survey on this disease was carried out from 1973 through 1975 and another was made from 1982 through 1984. Table 4.1 shows the distribution by age and sex from these two surveys in addition to data from the most recent survey in 1993. The committee reported that the number of patients was 2148 in the first survey, 2606 in the second and 1081 in the third, indicating that the number of patients with this disease was by no means decreasing. Based on these three surveys, it was evident that the peak in the age distribution was shifting to older age groups. While age distribution of patients showed a peak in the

Table 4.1. Takayasu's artertis: distribution by age and sex[a]

Age (years)	1973–5			1982–4			1993			
	Male	Female	Total	Male	Female	Total	Male	Female	Unknown	Total
<9	4	18	22		3	3	1			1
10–19	17	163	180	11	117	128	3	29		32
20–29	49	588	637	37	360	397	3	114		117
30–39	56	471	527	58	656	714	12	164		176
40–49	48	400	448	52	549	601	21	251	1	273
50–59	35	183	218	64	448	512	26	212	1	239
60–69	22	62	84	21	182	203	19	163		182
>70	7	13	20	7	39	46	4	55		59
Unknown	1	11	12	1	1	2		1	1	2
Total	239	1909	2148	251	2355	2606	89	989	3	1081

[a] From Japanese Research Committee on Takayasu Arteritis, Japanese Ministry of Health and Welfare.

twenties in the first survey, the second and third surveys disclosed a peak in the thirties and forties respectively. Male vs female ratios were 1:8.0 and 1:9.4, respectively.

Nasu[14] made a statistical investigation of 76 autopsy cases of Takayasu's arteritis between 1958 and 1973 by using the Annual Reports of Pathological Autopsy Cases in Japan published by the Japanese Society of Pathology. In 1987, Hotchi[15] also reported a similar statistical survey of 115 autopsy cases between 1975 and 1984. Comparing these two pathological surveys, the incidence of Takayasu's arteritis in all autopsy cases performed in these periods showed no difference (0.036% in Nasu's report vs 0.033% in Hotchi's survey). The sex ratio of male to female in the second survey was 1:4.5, which was the same as that of the first report. In both surveys, the disease onset peaked in the 20–40 age group whereas the peak in age distribution for death shifted from the third decade of life in Nasu's report to the forties in Hotchi's report. This shows an increase in long-term survival due to improvement of treatment of the disease.

In addition to the high prevalence in young women, many reports suggested that racial differences in the prevalence of this disease was an important characteristic. The highest incidence is in Oriental countries, such as Japan, Korea, China, India, Thailand and Singapore, in Israel, among the colored population in South Africa[16, 17] and in South America,[6] while very few cases have been reported among the Caucasian population of Europe,[18, 19] the United States[20, 21] or South Africa. Deutsch *et al.*[22] reported that 13 of 22 Israeli patients with Takayasu's arteritis were Sephardic (of Spanish or Portuguese descent), or Oriental Jews, and 9 were Arab or Bedouin. But interestingly, Ashkenazi Jews, who are of East European descent and constitute about half of the population of Israel, did not show any prevalence of this disease.

Etiology and immunopathogenesis

The etiology of this disease is still unclear. As mentioned above, an epidemiological characteristic of the disease is that the majority of the patients are young females, mainly of Asian and South American/Latin origin. These sex and racial differences suggest that genetic factors may be involved in the disease pathogenesis. Familial predisposition has been reported in 20 Japanese cases including three cases of monozygotic twin sisters.[23, 24] Isohisa and co-workers[25] first demonstrated the close association between Takayasu's arteritis and HLA-Bw52 in Japanese populations. Recently, the cooperative international survey between Japan, Korea and India also confirmed that the presence of HLA-Bw52 or B5 was closely associated with Takayasu's arteritis in all three Asian countries.[26, 27, 28] Castro *et al.*[29] reported that the haplotype Bw52 was also positively associated with this disease in Mexican populations. On the other hand, Volkman *et al.*[30] reporting on their HLA analysis in nine Caucasian and two Asian patients in North America, found a striking increase in the frequency of DR4 and MB3(DQw3) antigens among Takayasu's arteritis patients. However, Khraishi *et al.*[31] found no significant positive association of Takayasu's arteritis with DR4 and DQw3 or any of the other Class I or Class II antigens in their recent study on HLA antigens in 21 Caucasian North American patients. More recently, molecular and genetic analysis of HLA Class II polymorphism has been facilitated by using the polymerase chain reaction (PCR). Polymerase chain reaction/sequence-specific oligonucleotide (SSOP) analysis can reveal not only that two alleles are different but also how they differ, thereby allowing for a precise identification of individual alleles or polymorphic residues that are critical for disease susceptibility and resistance.[32, 33] Dong *et al.*[34, 35] investigated 64 Japanese patients and a family with Takayasu's arteritis for Class II genes by DNA typing using PCR/SSOP analysis. The results showed the frequencies of HLA-Bw52, DRB1*1502, DRB5*0102, DQA1*0103, DQB1*0601 and DPB1*0901 alleles were significantly increased in patients with Takayasu's arteritis. Therefore they concluded that the combination or haplotype of HLA-Bw52, DRB1*1502, DRB5*0102, DQA1*0103, DQB1*0601, DPA1*02, DPB1*0901 controls susceptibility to Takayasu's arteritis in Japanese populations.

Although various reports have described circulating autoantibodies such as Coomb's antibodies or anticardiolipin antibodies, as well as antiaortic antibodies, there is no evidence that these autoantibodies play a pathogenetic role in Takayasu's arteritis.[7, 36] Histological findings of inflammatory cell infiltration and necrosis of the arterial vascular cells strongly suggest that cell-mediated autoimmunity plays an important role in the immunogenesis of this disease.[36] Scott and collegues[37] showed that the infiltrating cells were CD8 positive lymphocytes and not CD4 positive cells. Studies of circulating lymphocytes showed increased numbers of activated cells and increased *in vitro* cytotoxicity against cultured human umbilical endothelial cells compared with normal lymphocytes, suggesting that cellular immunological mechanisms may play a role in the pathogenesis of Takayasu's arteritis, possibly through the direct action of cytotoxic T-cells on large elastic arteries. Talwar *et al.*[38] demonstrated inflammatory myocarditis accompanied by mononuclear cell infiltration consisting of T-lymphocytes, predominantly suppressor or cytotoxic T-cells, in patients with Takayasu's arteritis. Seko and co-workers[39] analyzed the phenotypes of the infiltrating cells and examined the expression of a cytolytic factor, perforin, in those cells of aortic tissue samples from seven patients with Takayasu's arteritis. Immunohistochemical studies showed that the infiltrating cells in the aortic tissue with Takayasu's arteritis were mainly perforin-expressing killer cells. Phenotypic analysis showed that almost 30% of infiltrating cells consisted of $\gamma\delta$ T-lymphocytes in Takayasu's arteritis, whereas there was virtually no infiltration of $\gamma\delta$ T-lymphocytes in patients with atherosclerosis. *In situ* hybridization analysis revealed expression of perforin mRNA in the infiltrating cells. They also demonstrated by immunoelectron microscope that the infiltrating cells released massive amounts of perforin directly on to the surface of arterial vascular cells. Furthermore, the authors demonstrated a marked expression of a 65-kD heat-shock protein (HSP-65), HLA Class I and II antigens and intercellular adhesion molecule-1 (ICAM-1) in the aortic tissue with Takayasu's arteritis, which might facilitate the recognition, adhesion and cytotoxicity of the infiltrating killer lymphocytes.[39] Heat-shock proteins (HSPs) are known to be synthesized by various cells in response to environmental stresses, such as temperature changes, inflammation and viral infection. There is an accumulation of evidence that $\gamma\delta$ T-lymphocytes can recognize autologous HSPs and may play an important role in autoimmunity.[40, 41] This strongly suggests that in Takayasu's arteritis the infiltrating killer cells, especially $\gamma\delta$ T-lymphocytes, may recognize HSP-65 and directly injure the vascular cells by secreting numerous perforin molecules.

In recent years, the response to injury hypothesis has been drawing attention as the most fundamental theory to explain the pathogenesis of atherosclerotic vascular lesions.[42] This hypothesis is based principally on the observation that aortic smooth muscle cell proliferation is caused by stimulation with platelet-derived and macrophage-derived growth factors. Xu *et al.*[43] reported that immunization with HSP-65 induced arteriosclerotic lesions in normocholesterolemic rabbits and recently showed that serum anti-

HSP-65 antibodies were significantly increased in patients with carotid atherosclerosis.[44] In considering the pathogenesis of Takayasu's arteritis, the infiltrating cytotoxic T-cells in the media might play, at least in part, a role in transforming the phenotype of medial smooth muscle cells, and these transformed smooth muscle cells could be a cause of fibrous thickness in intima and adventitia.[45]

Pathology

Takayasu's arteritis is a form of vasculitis characterized by stenotic and occasionally dilated lesions in the aorta, its main direct branches and the pulmonary artery trunk. According to the site of the disease, Nasu[14] classified the lesions into Type I (cranial branches), Type II (aortic arch), Type III (abdominal aorta and its main branches) and Type IV (the diffuse extensive type). Comparing the two large pathological surveys by Nasu[14] and Hotchi,[15] there has been a tendency for the lesions to extend over a broad part of such elastic arteries (Fig 4.1). There is an increase in involvement of the coronary, renal and common iliac arteries with the prolongation of the course of this disease (Table 4.2).

Histologically, Nasu[14] classified Takayasu's arteritis into the following three types; granulomatous inflammation, diffuse productive inflammation and fibrotic. The early histological changes in Takayasu's arteritis are those of granulomatous inflammation of the arterial wall and cell infiltration into the outer area of the media and a part of the adventitia through the vasa vasorum (Figs 4.2a–c). The infiltrating cells consist predominantly of lymphocytes (mainly cytotoxic T-cells), plasma cells and epithelioid cells (Fig. 4.3). The most characteristic lesion is the destruction of the elastic fibers of the media, associated with the atrophy, disarrangement and disappearance of the smooth muscle cells of the media (Fig 4.2b). Thereby, intimal and adventitial thickening with medial thining are commonly observed in Takayasu's

Table 4.2. Distribution of vascular lesions

Arteries	1958–73[14] (%)	1975–84[15] (%)
Ascending aorta	78	73
Coronary artery	11	45
Aortic arch	86	74
Brachiocephalic artery	82	57
Right subclavian artery	75	45
Right common carotid artery	82	50
Left common carotid artery	87	62
Thoracic aorta	71	81
Abdominal aorta	59	67
Celiac artery	13	9
Superior mesenteric artery	15	5
Renal artery	24	40
Inferior mesenteric artery	8	2
Common iliac artery	3	27
Pulmonary artery trunk	45	35
Intrapulmonary branches	28	17

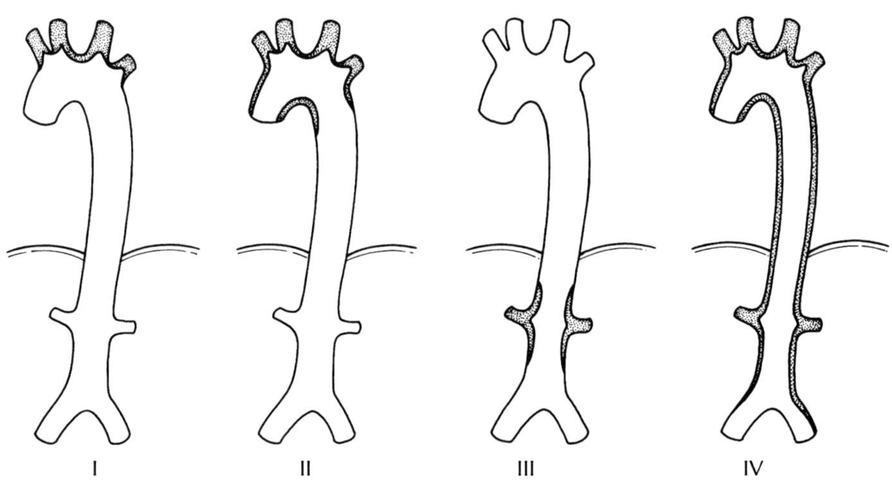

Type of lesions	I Cranial	II Aortic arch	III Abdominal aorta	IV Diffuse	Total
1958–70 14	6.9%	19.4%	4.2%	69.5%	100.0%
1975–84 115	2.0%	22.0%	0.0%	76.0%	100.0%

Figure 4.1. Incidence and type of arterial lesions in Takayasu's arteritis.[14, 15]

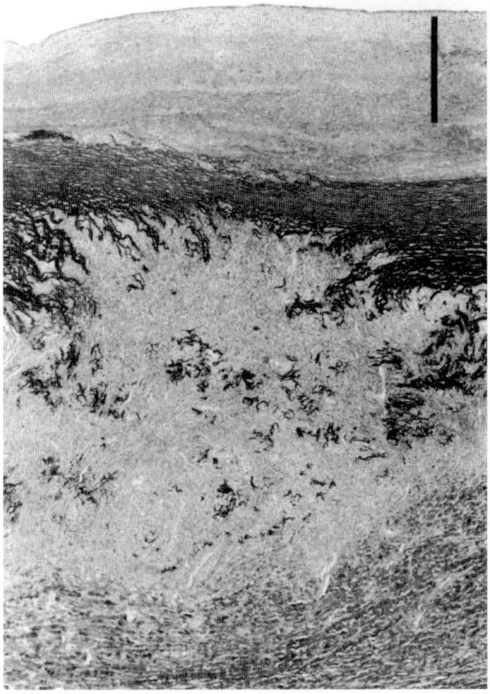

(a)

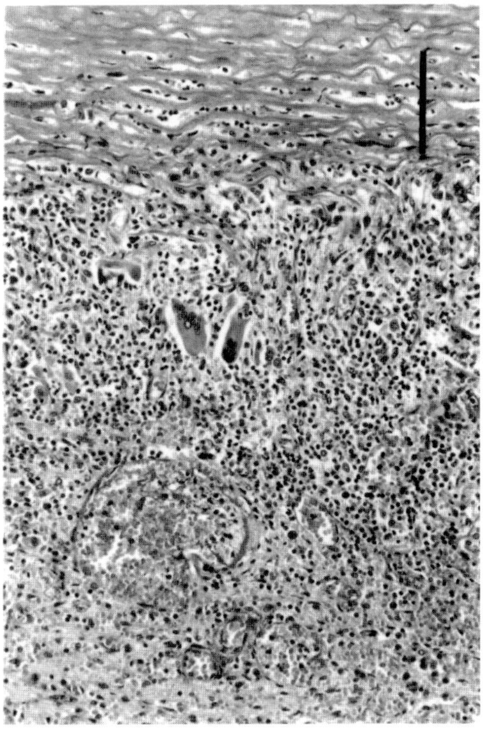

(b)

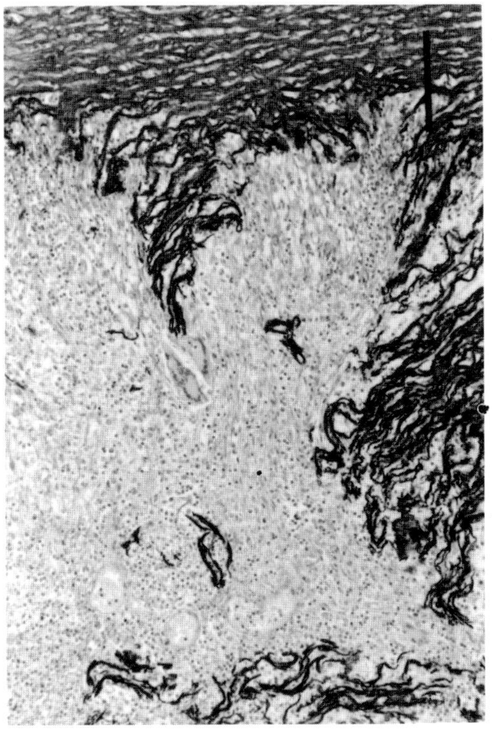

(c)

Figure 4.2. Histology of aortic wall in Takayasu's arteritis. (a) Histologic section of aorta showing marked disruption of the media associated with moderate intimal thickening. (Elastica Van Gieson's stain, a bar indicates a scale of 500 micron (μ)). (b) Massive inflammatory cell infiltration into the outer area of the media involving the vasa vasorum in the media and the adventitia. (Hematoxylin and eosin stain, a bar indicates a scale of 100 μ.) (c) Destruction of the media with elasticophagia. The elastic fibers are irregularly cut off from the adventitial side. (Elastica van Gieson's stain, the length of a bar showing 330 μ.)

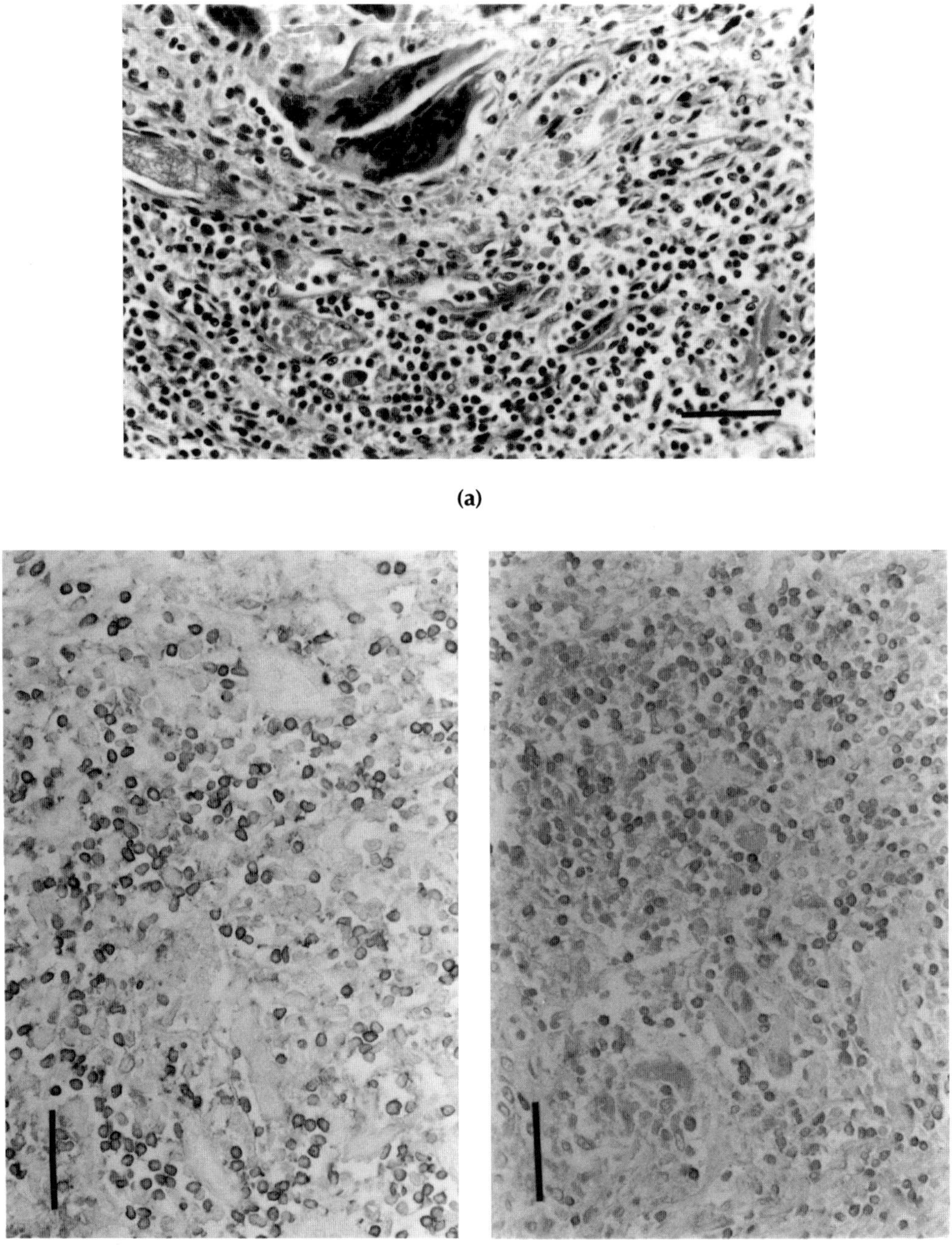

(a)

(b) (c)

Figure 4.3. The infiltrating cells mainly consist of T-lymphocytes stained with anti-CD3 monoclonal antibody associated with a small number of giant cells. CD4 positive T-lymphocytes are occupying one-third of infiltrating T-lymphocytes. (a) Hematoxylin and eosin stain; (b) avidin biotin immunoperoxidase stain with mouse anti-human CD3 mAb; (c) ABC immunoperoxidase stain with anti-human CD4 mAb; a bar indicates a scale of 50μ. By courtesy of Professor M. Kawakami, Department of Clinical Pathology, Tokyo Women's Medical College.

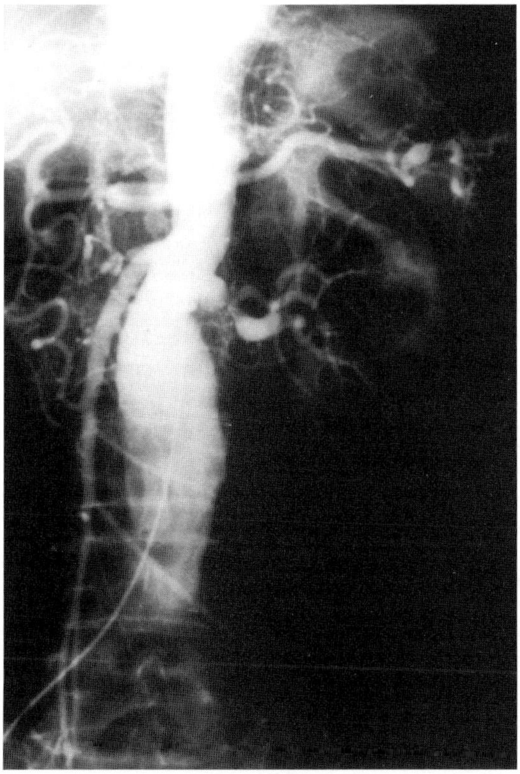

Figure 4.4. Aneurysmal dilatation of the abdominal aorta with bilateral renal artery obstruction in a 60-year-old female patient with Takayasu's arteritis.

arteritis. It is presumed to occur as a secondary phenomenon due to the impairment of the transintimal and/or transadventitial blood supply within the arterial wall itself. When the arteritis progresses rapidly, the artery becomes dilated and forms an aneurysm (Fig. 4.4) and aortic valve regurgitation occurs.

Clinical features

The clinical manifestations can be divided into the early pre-pulseless phase, characterized by a systemic inflammatory process, and the late pulseless phase, characterized by vascular occlusion.[8] Symptoms usually first appear in young adulthood (<40 years) and are variable and non-specific.[46] In the early phase of the disease, patients have non-specific systemic illness characterized by malaise, weakness, fever, night sweat, arthralgia, myalgia, vertigo and cold extremities. Therefore, it is difficult to diagnose during the early pre-pulseless phase. In the late pulseless phase the symptomatology is a direct manifestation of the location of the arterial lesions. Koide[13] reported on the incidence of clinical symptoms in a Japanese nationwide survey on Takayasu's arteritis (see Table 4.3). Vascular disorder in the extremities (with diminished or absence of pulse) is seen in 74% of patients, hypertension in 56%, symptoms of cerebral ischemia and cardiac symptoms in 40–65%, while ophthalmological symptoms are seen in 24% only. More than 60% of patients have systemic symptoms (Table 4.3).

The predominant cardiovascular symptoms were dyspnea, pulse deficit, vascular bruit and high blood pressure. Most patients have a pulse discrepancy of more than 30 mmHg between the left and right arms. An unpalpable pulse often provides the first opportunity to detect this disease. It is reported that the major sign of the disease, pulselessness, was found only in 15.8–27.3% of patients at onset but in 63.3–84.1% of patients at first diagnosis.[46, 47]

Fainting, postural dizziness or syncope is not rare and usually reflects severe occlusion of the carotid and/or vertebrobasilar systems. Uyama and Asayama[48] classified retinal vascular changes according to the disease progression: Stage 1, dilatation of small vessels; Stage 2, microaneurysm formation; Stage 3, arteriovenous anastomoses; Stage 4, ocular complications. The microaneurysm formation in the retinal vessels in Takayasu's disease did not occur until cervical arterial lesions had become extensive and severe. The stage of retinal arteriovenous anastomoses as in Takayasu's original finding corresponds to the advanced stage.

Table 4.3. Major complications in Takayasu's arteritis

	–	Yes (%)	No (%)	Unknown (%)
Aortic valve insufficiency	1475	469 (31.8)	944 (64.0)	62 (4.2)
Aortic dilated lesions	1475	349 (23.7)	957 (64.9)	169 (11.5)
Renovascular hypertension	1475	278 (18.8)	1030 (69.8)	167 (11.3)

Cardiac involvement has been increasingly recognized. Coronary arteries are involved in 45% of autopsy cases, as shown in Table 4.2.[15] Angina or myocardial infarction may be secondary to ostial stenosis or involvement of the proximal main coronary artery segment. Congestive heart failure may result from systemic arterial involvement, aortic insufficiency and hypertension. It was reported that the incidence of aortic regurgitation was significantly higher in Japanese patients than that in either Korean or Indian patients, probably as a consequence of the higher frequency of arterial lesions at the aortic arch and/or its branches in Japanese patients.[27] In addition to stenotic lesions, the incidence of aneurysmal dilatations is increasingly reported. The Japanese nationwide survey showed that 26.7% of patients had arterial dilated lesions (Table 4.4). In recent years, the rupture of aortic aneurysm is one of the main causes of death in Takayasu's arteritis.

Laboratory abnormalities in Takayasu's arteritis are shown in Table 4.4.[13] Elevated erythrocyte sedimentation rate (ESR), positive C-reactive protein (CRP), increased IgG and IgM, increased antistreptolysin O titers (ASLO), moderate leukocytosis and mild normocytic anemia are frequently present. A raised ESR is the most useful indicator to monitor the disease activity during the pre-pulseless and early pulseless stages, especially where corticosteroid treatment is indicated.[7,8,49,50,51] The ESR tends to decelerate spontaneously with time, however, a persistently elevated ESR is a reliable index of activity and disease progression.

From the standpoint of the prognosis for survival and physical activity, Ishikawa[52] classified patients with Takayasu's arteritis as a high or low risk group according to the presence and severity of the four major complications; Takayasu's retinopathy, hypertension, aortic regurgitation and aortic or arterial aneurysm. The 10-year cumulative eventless survival rate was significantly lower in patients with a severe single complication or multiple complications (a high risk group) than in the patients with no or only mild or moderate complications (a low risk group) (97.0 and 58.6%, respectively). Therefore, the presence of severe hypertension, aortic regurgitation, aneurysm and retinopathy was a useful predictor for prognosis.

Hypertension in Takayasu's arteritis

Hypertension is closely related to the prognosis of patients with Takayasu's arteritis as is the

Table 4.4. Clinical symptoms and laboratory findings in patients with Takayasu's arteritis[a]

	1973–5 Case (%) (at the initial consultation)	1982–4 Case (%) (throughout the course)
Clinical symptoms		
Cerebrovascular disorder	873/1351 (64.6)	551/1302 (42.3)
Ophthalmologic symptoms	310/1297 (23.9)	301/1276 (23.6)
Cardiac symptoms	742/1344 (55.2)	536/1296 (41.4)
Hypertension	606/1336 (45.4)	734/1318 (55.7)
Vascular disorders in the extremities	969/1341 (72.3)	930/1261 (73.8)
Acute vascular pain	492/1292 (38.1)	288/1255 (22.9)
Systemic symptoms	885/1324 (66.8)	769/1280 (60.1)
Laboratory findings		
Enhanced ESR	868/1193 (72.8)	997/1130 (88.2)
Increased white blood count	437/1249 (35.0)	506/1160 (43.6)
Anemia	563/1175 (47.9)	629/1149 (54.7)
CRP positive	666/1287 (51.7)	800/1153 (69.4)
Increase in γ-globulin	483/1008 (47.9)	502/ 972 (51.6)
Increase in ASLO	155/1067 (14.5)	142/ 920 (15.4)
RA positive	108/1185 (9.1)	119/1010 (11.8)
Positive tuberculin reaction	366/ 532 (68.8)	241/ 342 (70.5)
Aortic calcification	239/1160 (20.6)	251/1142 (22.0)
Abnormal ECG	538/1221 (44.1)	578/1169 (49.4)

[a] From Japanese Research Committee on Takayasu Arteritis, Japanese Ministry of Health and Welfare.
RA: Rheumatoid artheritis.

severity of aortoarteritis and the presence of cardiac involvement.[47] In Japan, over 50% of patients with Takayasu's arteritis have hypertension, but in Korea and India almost all the patients have hypertension (96 and 92%, respectively).[27] Hypertension in Takayasu's arteritis is secondary to marked narrowing of the aorta of renovascular origin, reduced elasticity of the arterial wall, aortic regurgitation and a combination of these.[49] Takayasu's arteritis is the most common cause of renovascular hypertension (RVH) in India and China, accounting for as many as 60% of all RVH patients, whereas fibromuscular dysplasia and atherosclerosis are the most common causes in Western countries.[9, 27, 53, 54] Chugh[53] reported that of 205 Indian patients with RVH, 125 (61%) had Takayasu's arteritis, 58 (28.3%) had fibromuscular dysplasia and 16 (7.8%) had atherosclerosis. The most recent survey on Takayasu's arteritis in Japan demonstrated that of 1475 patients with Takayasu's arteritis, 278 (21.3%) had RVH (see Table 4.3). Koide[13] reported that hypertension was observed in 118 of 135 Takayasu's arteritis patients who demonstrated decreased renal function (blood urea nigrogen >20 mg/dl and serum creatinine >2.0 mg/dl). He also showed that hypertension was noted in 79.4% of patients showing signs of proteinuria and that proteinuria was found in 13.2% of 1213 patients with Takayasu's arteritis.

There have been scattered reports of glomerular lesions associated with Takayasu's arteritis,[55, 56] including mesangial proliferative (Fig. 4.5), membranoproliferative and crescentic glomerulonephritis,[57, 58] and lupus-like membranous glomerulopathy.[59] Renal amyloidosis has also been described.[60]

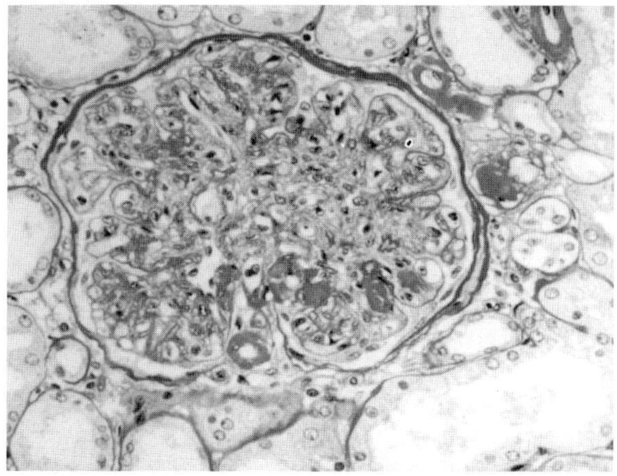

Figure 4.5. Mesangial proliferative glomerulonephritis-like glomerular lesions associating with Takayasu's arteritis showing increased mesangial matrix and thickening (reduplication) of the glomerular capillary walls in a 63-year-old female. (PAS stain, × 160). By courtesy of Professor Y. Yamaguchi, Department of Pathology, Jikei University of Medicine.

Diagnosis

Advances in imaging vascular disease in Takayasu's arteritis

Total aortography, which shows irregular vessel walls, stenosis, poststenotic dilation, aneurysm formation and occlusion and collateral circulation, has been considered mandatory for the diagnosis of Takayasu's arteritis.[6, 20, 61, 62] However, this is invasive, expensive and often requires the use of a large amount of contrast material. Moreover, there are some cases in which insertion of a catheter into the artery is impossible because of obstruction of both subclavian and iliac arteries. It would also be desirable not to have to repeat this procedure during follow-up. Recently, there have been reports concerning the diagnostic value of new imaging techniques in vascular diseases including magnetic resonance imaging (MRI)[63] and duplex ultrasound[64, 65] (Fig. 4.6).

Magnetic resonance imaging has been suggested as an ideal, non-invasive technique to evaluate various vascular diseases, and there are increasing reports suggesting its utility in aortic lesions and in the renal arteries.[66–68] Yamada *et al.*[69] described the usefulness of MRI in the diagnosis of Takayasu's arteritis. They compared MR images with those of conventional angiography in 77 patients with Takayasu's arteritis. They showed that MRI could clearly depict various aortic lesions, stenosis, dilatation, aneurysms and other abnormalities, as well as aortic wall thickening and mural thrombi, which were often difficult to detect with conventional

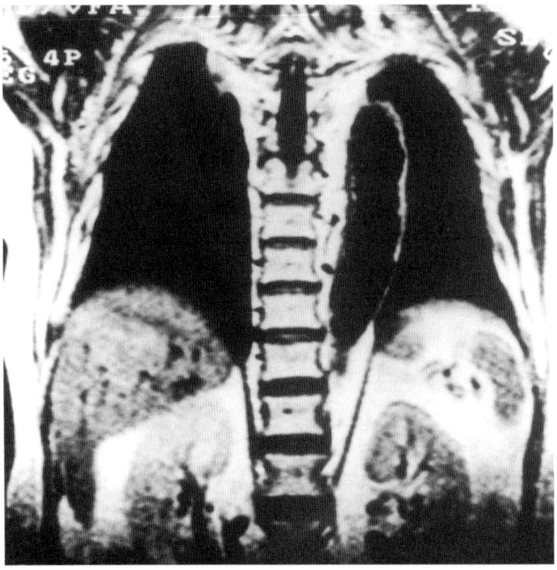

(a)

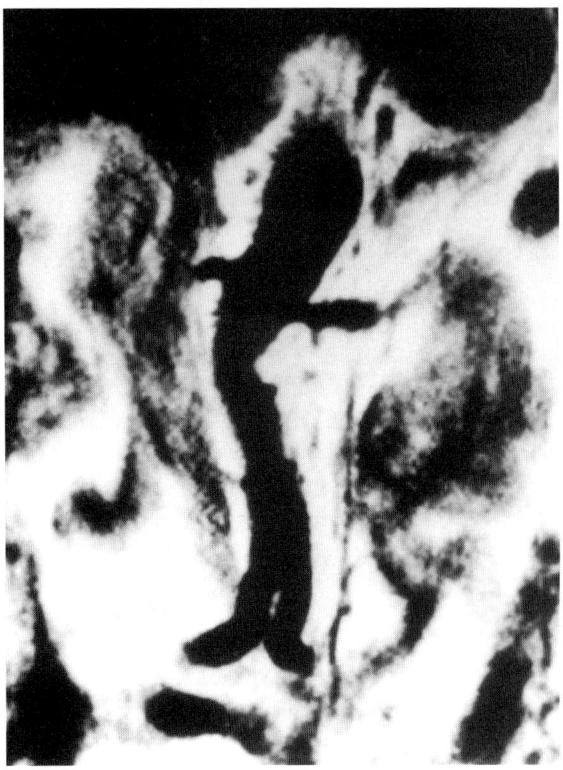

(b)

Figure 4.6. MR images in a patient with Takayasu's arteritis. The thoracic (a) and abdominal (b) aorta have irregular contours and the abdominal aorta is winding with irregular size of aortic caliber. The ostium of left renal artery is stenotic.

angiography. The authors concluded that MRI, unlike angiography, is a reliable and safe diagnostic tool for patients with Takatasu's arteritis. Tanigawa *et al.*[70] also showed that, after successful steroid therapy, decreased thickening of the arterial walls and a resolution of the pericardial effusion could be demonstrated by MRI, as well as CT scan.[71]

Duplex ultrasound is also a non-invasive method for detecting, evaluating and monitoring large vessel arteritis.[72] It combines direct visualization of large arteries (B-mode imaging) with a measurement of the velocity of blood flow (Doppler), thus providing not only an anatomic assessment of the degree of arteritis but a functional assessment as well. Maeda and his colleagues[73] recently reported that, in 19 of 23 patients with Takayasu's arteritis, B-mode ultrasonography clearly demonstrated the characteristic circumferential arterial wall thickening of carotid arteries as a 'macaroni-like', diffusely thickened intima–media complex, which was difficult to detect by conventional angiography. Buckley *et al.*[74] also described three cases of Takayasu's arteritis who could be adequately monitored with serial duplex/color flow Doppler studies. They also demonstrated that duplex analysis could play an important role in revealing hemodynamic disturbances such as aortic/mitral valve regurgitation, reduced velocity of blood flow or a high resistive flow pattern in diseased vessels that probably reflects poor arterial wall compliance secondary to inflammation and/or fibrosis in arteritis.

Diagnostic criteria

The diagnosis of this disease is often delayed for months or even years because of the variability of its natural history and the manifestation of non-specific symptoms; such as fever, myalgia, arthralgias, weight loss, general fatigue, vertigo, anemia and cold extremities. It is important to palpate both radial arteries at the time of the initial examination as an unpalpable pulse presents the first opportunity to detect this disease. The presence of hypertension in young women, the detection of vascular bruit and increased ESR

Table 4.5. Guidelines for clinical diagnosis of Takayasu's arteritis[a]

Symptoms

Cerebral ischemia: vertigo, headache, fainting, paresis, etc.
Ischemia of upper extremities: cold fingers, fatigue, pulseless
Hypertension, cardiac failure: shortness of breath, palpitation, dyspnea, angina pectoris
Visual disturbance: transient or continuous
Pain: neck pain, back pain, lumbago
General symptoms: fever, malaise, fatiguability

Important findings for diagnosis

Abnormalities of the pulse and/or blood pressure of the upper extremities (weak or diminution and/or discrepancy of the radial pulse, hypotonic pressure)
Abnormalities of the pulse and/or blood pressure of the lower extremities (accentuation or diminution of the femoral pulse, hypotension)
Vascular bruit on the neck, back or abdomen
Heart murmur (aortic regurgitation)
Ophthalmologic abnormalities (hypertensive or hypotensive fundus, visual disturbance)

Helpful laboratory findings for diagnosis

Inflammatory: increased ESR, CRP, leukocytosis, increased α-globulin
Anemia
Immunological abnormalities: increased immunoglobulin, complement (C3, C4), positive antiaortic antibody
Increased coagulability
HLA: A9-Bw52, Dw12

Imaging characteristics

Calcification: chest X-ray, CT
Stenosis, occlusion of aorta and its main branch: angiography, MRI, CT
Ectasia (ascending aortic aneurysm, aortic regurgitation): ultrasound, CT, angiography
Pulmonary arteriopathy: MRI, angiography

[a] From Japanese Research Committee on Takayasu Arteritis, Japanese Ministry of Health and Welfare.

are important checkpoints for establishing the diagnosis.

In 1984 diagnostic guidelines for Takaysu's arteritis were proposed by the Japanese Ministry of Health and Welfare's research committee and were revised in 1992 (Table 4.5).[5]

Treatment and prognosis

As the etiology of Takayasu's arteritis is not known, no specific remedy is yet available. However, it is widely accepted that corticosteroid therapy is effective for the active or acute stage of this disease.[50, 75] As the inflammatory activity is clearly indicated by a raised ESR, it should be carefully monitored throughout long-term corticosteroid therapy. To prevent frequent relapse of the disease, Ishikawa[50] advised very careful and gradual tapering of the steroid dosage. When the ESR is persistently < 10 mm/h for 3–6 months on a maintenance dose of prednisolone, a small reduction in dose is usually feasible. Moriwaki and Numano[76] suggested that HLA-Bw52-positive patients need a higher dosage of steroids for much longer periods and that there is a need to be watchful for recurrence of this disease. The recent Japanese nationwide survey in 1993 revealed that 735 of 1081 patients (68%) with Takayasu's disease underwent pharmacological treatment only, while 224 patients (20.7%) received both medical and surgical treatment. Twenty patients (1.9%) received surgery alone, and 20 patients received percutaneous transluminal renal or coronary angioplasty (PTRA or PTCA) (Table 4.6).

Table 4.6. Treatment of patients with Takayasu's arteritis in Japan (1993)

Treatment	N (%)
Medicine only	735 (68.0)
Surgery only	20 (1.9)
Medicine + surgery	224 (20.7)
PTRA or PTCA + medicine	13 (1.2)
PTRA or PTCA + medicine + surgery	7 (0.6)
Observation	82 (7.6)
Total	1081 (100)

Table 4.7. PTRA for renal artery stenosis in Takayasu's arteritis

Author	Year	*N*	Initial success rate (%)	Follow-up success rate (%)	Restenosis (%)
Hiramatsu *et al.*[77]	1983	5	100.0	40.0	60.0
Dong *et al.*[78]	1987	22	86.4		9.0
Park *et al.*[62]	1989	9	100.0		22.2
Kumar *et al.*[79]	1989	9	55.6		0.0
Zheng *et al.*[11]	1990	13	84.6	46.2	
Chugh *et al.*[53]	1992	9	77.8		
Sharma *et al.*[80]	1992	20	85.0	50.0	21.0
Fava *et al.*[81]	1993	20	83.0	33.3	
Tyagi *et al.*[82]	1993	54	89.3	84.6	13.5
Japanese survey	1993	16	43.7		

There has been an increasing number of cases successfully treated with PTRA for RVH in Takayasu's disease. Table 4.7 summarizes the reported results of renal angioplasty in this disease. In large series from India and China,[78] PTRA was highly effective in relieving renal artery stenosis in Takayasu's arteritis, while in our own experiences in Japan, the success rate of PTRA was almost 50% in patients with this disease (Table 4.7). Tyagi *et al.*[82] performed angioplasty in 54 patients with RVH caused by Takayasu's arteritis and initial angiographic success was obtained in 89.3% of lesions. Restenosis was observed in 13.5% on mean follow-up of 14.2 months, indicating that restenosis was less compared with that reported for atherosclerotic disease. When angioplasty is performed in the chronic inactive stage of the disease, RVH resulting from Takayasu's arteritis may be effectively treated by PTRA with excellent sustained, clinical results during long-term follow-up.

The major causes of death in Takayasu's disease are related to stroke, heart disease, aneurysmal rupture of aorta and RVH. There is a clear need for treatment of hypertension to minimize the risk of such disease complication. According to the recent Japanese nationwide survey on Takayasu's arteritis, 251 of 1081 patients (23.2%) were treated surgically: 84 patients for aortic valve insufficiency, 48 for carotid and vertebral artery stenosis, 38 for subclavian artery obstruction, 32 for aneurysm, 28 for renal artery stenosis and 28 for coronary artery stenosis. Of 28 patients who had renal arterial reconstruction, hypertension was cured or improved in 24 patients (85.7%) postoperatively. Surgical treatment for renal artery stenosis is currently one of the most common procedures required for Takayasu's arteritis. As shown in Table 4.8, good long-term results (approximately 90% of patients with hypertension cured or improved) with less than 5% mortality can be expected after renal revascularization. However, restenosis or late failure of renal artery reconstruction, occasionally associated with severe renal failure, may occur in some cases. It is likely that these are related to recurrence or progression of the disease. Furthermore, surgery should not be indicated until active disease has been adequately controlled with corticosteroid therapy, and steroid therapy should be continued postoperatively in case of persistence or recurrence of the disease.

Table 4.8. Reconstructive surgery of the renal artery in Takayasu's arteritis

Investigator	Year	*N*	Associated aortic surgery (%)	Postoperative deaths (%)	Follow-up (years)	Course of hypertension (%)		
						Cured	Improved	Unchanged
De Bakey *et al.*[83]	1967	16	100	0	NA	100		
Pokrovsky *et al.*[84]	1983	65	NA	12.5	1–14	63	17	10
Lagneau *et al.*[85]	1987	21	48	5	3.5	55	45	
Takagi *et al.*[86]	1989	10	10	0	10–20	70	30	
Kieffer *et al.*[87]	1990	24	89	4	5.1	63	31	6
Japanese survey	1992	28	NA	NA	1	85.7		3.6

It seems that the prognosis of this disease is favorable if adequate medical therapy is given when there are no severe complications. The 1993 Japanese survey revealed that the mortality rate was only 1.9% (20 of 1081) and 44 patients (4%) were in the progressive stage of the disease, while two-thirds of patients (720) were in the stable stage of the disease and the cure or improvement rate was 30% (227 of 1081). It is emphasized that the disease should be detected within the early phase, before any severe complications have set in, and progression into the high risk category of this disease should be prevented.

Summary

The cause of Takayasu's arteritis is still obscure. However, certain aspects of this disease have been clarified over the past decade. There is accumulated evidence that cell-mediated autoimmunity plays an important role in the immunopathogenesis of this disease. A peak in the age distribution has shifted from the twenties to the Forties over the last 20 years because of an increase in the number of long-term survivals due to improvements in treatment. Early detection of this condition is important for good prognosis before the disease has progressed to the phase of extensive, severe vascular occlusion. New non-invasive imaging techniques such as MRI and duplex ultrasound are useful for early detection and follow-up of the disease. Corticosteroid therapy is effective in ameliorating the disease condition both in the early phase and the late pulseless phase, in some cases allowing return to complete remission for a long time. Recently, percutaneous transluminal angioplasty has been reported to be successful in relieving obstructive lesions in Takayasu's arteritis. The course of the disease is unpredictable; however, in most controlled cases the disease is quiescent and the majority of lesions stable and non-progressive. Prognosis is related to the presence of severe hypertension, aortic regurgitation, aneurysm and Takayasu's retinopathy. But in patients presenting with those severe complications, medical and surgical intervention may, in some cases, effectively modify the natural progression of the disease.

References

1 Numano F. Introductory remarks for this special issue on Takayasu arteritis. *Heart Vess* 1992; **7** (Suppl.): 3–5.
2 Oota K. Ein seltener Fall von beiderseitigem Carotis-Subclaviaverschluss. Ein Beitrag zur Pathologie der Anastomosis peripapillaris des Auges mit fehlendem Radialpuls. *Trans Soc Path Jpn* 1940; **30:** 680–90.
3 Shimizu K, Sano K. Pulseless disease. *J Neuropathol Clin Neurol* 1951; **1:** 37–47.
4 Nasu T. Pathology of pulseless disease. A systematic study and critical review of twenty-one autopsy cases reported in Japan. *Angiology* 1963; **14:** 225–42.
5 Sekiguchi M, Suzuki J. An overview on Takayasu arteritis. *Heart Vess* 1992; **7** (Suppl.): 6–10.
6 Lupi-Herrera E, Sanchez-Torres G, Marcushamer J *et al.* Takayasu's arteritis. Clinical study of 107 cases. *Am Heart J* 1977; **93:** 94–103.
7 Nakao K, Ikeda M, Kimata S *et al.* Takayasu's arteritis. Clinical report of eighty-four cases and immunological studies of seven cases. *Circulation* 1967; **35:** 1141–55.
8 Fraga A, Lavalle C. Takayasu's arteritis. *Clin Rheum Dis* 1980; **6:** 405–12.
9 Chugh KS, Sakhuja V. Aortoarteritis, a common cause of renovascular hypertension in Asia. *Int J Artif Org* 1988; **11:** 319–21.
10 Hall S, Buchbinder R. Takayasu's arteritis. *Rheum Dis Clin North Am.* 1990; **16:** 411–22.
11 Zheng DY, Li LS, Fan DJ. Clinical studies in 500 patients with aortoarteritis. *Chin Med J* 1990; **103:** 536–40.
12 Virmani R, Burke AP. Pathologic features of aortitis. *Cardiovasc Pathol* 1994; **3:** 205–16.
13 Koide K. Takayasu arteritis in Japan. *Heart Vess* 1992; **7** (Suppl.): 48–54.
14 Nasu T. Takayasu's truncoarteritis in Japan. A statistical observation of 76 autopsy cases. *Pathol Microbiol* 1975; **43:** 140–6.
15 Hotchi M. Pathological studies on Takayasu arteritis. *Heart Vess* 1992; **7** (Suppl.): 11–17.
16 Essop MR, Rothlisberger C, Skoularigis J. Angioplasty for treatment of Takayasu's arteriopathy: case reports. *Angiology* 1993; **44**(10): 833–7.
17 Beale PG, Meyers KEC, Thomson PD. Management of renal hypertension in children with Takayasu's arteritis using renal autografting or allograft transplantation in selected circumstances and total lymphoid irradiation. *J Pediatr Surg* 1992; **27:** 836–9.

18 Schwarz-Eywill M, Breitbart A, Csernok E *et al.* Treatment modalities and ANCA in Takayasu's arteritis. In Gross WL (ed.) *ANCA-Associated Vasculitides: Immunological and Clinical Aspects*, pp. 497–501. New York: Plenum Press, 1993.
19 Ivarsson SA, Berqvist D, Lundstrom NR *et al.* Takayasu's aortitis with renovascular hypertension. *Acta Paediatr* 1992; **81:** 1044–8.
20 Hall S, Barr W, Lie JT *et al.* Takayasu arteritis. A study of 32 north American patients. *Medicine* 1985; **64:** 89–99.
21 Lande A, Berkmen YM. Aortitis: pathologic, clinical and arteriographic review. *Radiol Clin North Am* 1976; **14:** 219–40.
22 Deutsch V, Wexler L, Deutsch H. Takayasu's arteritis: an angiographic study with remarks on ethnic distribution in Israel. *Am J Roentgenol* 1974; **122:** 13–28.
23 Numano F, Isohisa I, Kishi Y *et al.* Takayasu's disease in twin sisters—possible genetic factors. *Circulation* 1978; **58:** 173–7.
24 Numano F. Hereditary factors of Takayasu arteritis. *Heart Vess* 1992; **7** (Suppl.): 68–72.
25 Isohisa I, Numano F, Maezawa H, Sasazuki T. HLA-Bw52 in Takayasu disease. *Tiss Antigens* 1978; **12:** 246–8.
26 Yajima M, Moriwaki R, Numano F *et al.* Comparative studies between Japanese and Korean patients (Takayasu arteritis): comparison of the findings of angiography, HLA-Bw52 and clinical manifestation. *Heart Vess* 1992; **7** (Suppl.): 102–5.
27 Yajima M, Numano F, Park YB, Sagar S. Comparative studies of patients with Takayasu arteritis in Japan, Korea and India. Comparison of clinical manifestation, angiography and HLA-B antigen. *Jpn Circ J* 1994; **58:** 9–14.
28 Park MH, Park YB. HLA typing of Takayasu arteritis in Korea. *Heart Vess* 1992; **7** (Suppl.): 81–4.
29 Castro G, Chavez-Peon F, Sanchez-Torres G. A and B antigens in Takayasu's arteritis. *Rev Invest Clin* 1982; **34:** 15–17.
30 Volkman DJ, Mann DL, Fauci AS. Association between Takayasu's arteritis and A B-cell alloantigen in north Americans. *N Engl J Med* 1982; **306:** 464–5.
31 Khraishi MM, Gladman DD, Dagenais P *et al.* HLA antigens in North American patients with Takayasu arteritis. *Arth Rheum* 1992; **35:** 573–5.
32 Sasazuki T, Nishimura Y, Muto M, Ohta N. HLA-linked genes controlling the immune response and disease susceptibility. *Immunol Rev* 1983; **70:** 51–75.
33 Yoshida M, Kimura A, Katsuragi K *et al.* DNA typing of HLA-B gene in Takayasu's arteritis. *Tiss Antigens* 1993; **42:** 87–90.
34 Dong RP, Kimura A, Numano F *et al.* HLA-DP antigen and Takayasu arteritis. *Tiss Antigens* 1992; **39:** 106–10.
35 Dong RP, Kimura A, Numano F *et al.* HLA-linked susceptibility and resistance to Takayasu arteritis. *Heart Vess* 1992; **7** (Suppl.): 73–80.
36 Sagar S, Ganguly NK, Koicha M, Sharma BK. Immunopathogenesis of Takayasu arteritis. *Heart Vess* 1992; **7** (Suppl.): 85–90.
37 Scott DGI, Salmon M, Scott DL *et al.* Takayasu's arteritis: a pathogenetic role for cytotoxic T lymphocytes? *Clin Rheumatol* 1986; **5:** 517–22.
38 Talwar KK, Chopra P, Srivastava S *et al.* Inflammatory myocarditis in Takayasu's arteritis and role of immunosuppressive therapy. *Circulation* 1988; **78** (Suppl. II): 457.
39 Seko Y, Minota S, Kawasaki A *et al.* Perforin-secreting killer cell infiltration and expression of a 65-KD heat-shock protein in aortic tissue of patients with Takayasu's arteritis. *J Clin Invest* 1994; **93:** 750–8.
40 Winfield J, Jarjour W. Do stress proteins play a role in arthritis and autoimmunity? *Immunol Rev* 1991; **121:** 193–220.
41 Born W, Hall L, Dallas A *et al.* Recognition of a peptide antigen by heat shock reactive gamma delta T lymphocytes. *Science* 1990; **249:** 67–9.
42 Ross R. The pathogenesis of atherosclerosis: a perspective for the 1990s. *Nature* 1993; **362:** 806–9.
43 Xu Q, Dietrich H, Steiner HJ *et al.* Induction of arteriosclerosis in normocholesterolemic rabbits by immunization with heat shock protein 65. *Arterioscler Thromb* 1992; **12:** 789–99.
44 Xu Q, Willeit J, Marosi M *et al.* Association of serum antibodies to heat-shock protein 65 with carotid atherosclerosis. *Lancet* 1993; **341:** 255–9.
45 Takaichi S, Yutani C, Fujita H, Yamamoto A. Ultrastructural studies on the phenotypic modulation of human intimal smooth muscle cells. *Atherosclerosis* 1993; **100:** 197–211.
46 Ishikawa K. Diagnostic approach and proposed criteria for the clinical diagnosis of Takayasu's arteriopathy. *J Am Coll Cardiol* 1988; **12:** 964–72.
47 Subramanyan R, Joy J, Balakrishnan KG. Natural history of aortoarteritis (Takayasu's disease). *Circulation* 1989; **80:** 429–37.
48 Uyama M, Asayama K. Retinal vascular changes in Takayasu's disease (pulseless disease), occurrence and evolution of the lesion. *Doc Ophthalmol Proc Series* 1976; **9:** 549–54.
49 Ishikawa K. Natural history and classification of occlusive thromboaortopathy (Takayasu's disease). *Circulation* 1978; **57:** 27–35.
50 Ishikawa K. Effects of prednisolone therapy on arterial angiographic features in Takayasu's disease. *Am J Cardiol* 1991; **68:** 410–13.
51 Mandalam KR, Subramanyan R, Joseph S *et al.* Natural history of aortoarteritis: an angiographic study in 26 survivors. *Clin Radiol* 1994; **49:** 38–44.
52 Ishikawa K. Survival and morbidity after diagno-

sis of occlusive thromboaortopathy (Takayasu's disease). *Am J Cardiol* 1981; **47:** 1026–32.

53 Chugh KS, Jain S, Sakhuja V *et al.* Renovascular hypertension due to Takayasu's arteritis among Indian patients. *Quart J Med* 1992; **85:** 833–43.

54 Chugh KS, Sakhuja V. Takayasu's arteritis as a cause of renovascular hypertension in Asian countries. *Am J Nephrol* 1992; **12:** 1–8.

55 Takagi M, Ikeda T, Kimura K *et al.* Renal histological studies in patients with Takayasu's arteritis. *Nephron* 1984; **36:** 68–73.

56 Lai KN, Chan KW, Ho CP. Glomerulonephritis associated with Takayasu's arteritis: report of three cases and review of literature. *Am J Kidney Dis* 1986; **7:** 197–204.

57 Yoshikawa Y, Truong LD, Mattioli CA, Lederer E. Membranoproliferative glomerulonephritis in Takayasu's arteritis. *Am J Nephrol* 1988; **8:** 240–4.

58 Koumi S, Endo T, Okumura H *et al.* A case of Takayasu's arteritis associated with membranoproliferative glomerulonephritis and nephrotic syndrome. *Nephron* 1990; **54:** 344–6.

59 Nakashima A, Miyazaki R, Koni I *et al.* A case of aortitis syndrome (Takayasu's arteritis) associated with glomerulonephropathy mimicking lupus membranous glomerulonephropathy. *Jpn J Nephrol* 1988; **30:** 233–8.

60 Jain S, Taraphdar A, Joshi K *et al.* Renal amyloidosis complicating Takayasu's arteritis: a rare association. *Nephrol Dial Transplant* 1992; **7:** 1133–5.

61 Matsunaga N, Hayashi K, Aikawa H *et al.* Digital subtraction angiography in Takayasu arteritis. *Acta Radiol* 1987; **28:** 247–52.

62 Park JH, Han MC, Kim SH *et al.* Takayasu arteritis: angiographic findings and results of angioplasty. *Am J Roentgenol* 1989; **153:** 1069–74.

63 Gedroyc W. Magnetic resonance angiography of renal arteries. *Urol Clin North Am* 1994; **21:** 201–14.

64 Hansen KJ, Tribble RW, Reavis SW *et al.* Renal duplex sonography: evaluation of clinical utility. *J Vasc Surg* 1990; **12:** 227–36.

65 Olin JW. Role of duplex ultrasonography in screening for significant renal artery disease. *Urol Clin North Am* 1994; **21:** 215–26.

66 Miller DL, Reinig JW, Volkman DJ. Vascular imaging with MRI: inadequacy in Takayasu's arteritis compared with angiography. *Am J Roentgenol* 1986; **146:** 949–54.

67 Oneson SR, Lewin JS, Smith AS. MR angiography of Takayasu arteritis. *J Comp Assist Tomog* 1992; **16:** 478–80.

68 Morita K, Imai H, Saito K, Miura AB, Ishikawa H. The role of gallium scintigraphy, computerized tomogram scan, and magnetic resonance imaging angiography in the diagnosis of Takayasu's disease. *J Rheumatol* 1991; **20:** 1604–7.

69 Yamada I, Numano F, Suzuki S. Takayasu arteritis: evaluation with MR imaging. *Radiology* 1993; **188:** 89–94.

70 Tanigawa K, Eguchi K, Kitamura Y *et al.* Magnetic resonance imaging detection of aortic and pulmonary artery wall thickening in the acute stage of Takayasu arteritis. *Arth Rheum* 1992; **35:** 476–80.

71 Hayashi K, Fukushima T, Matsunaga N, Hombo Z. Takayasu's arteritis: decreased in aortic wall thickening following steroid therapy, documented by CT. *Br J Radiol* 1986; **59:** 281–3.

72 Hellmann DB. Immunopathogenesis, diagnosis, and treatment of giant cell arteritis, temporal arteritis, polymyalgia rheumatica and Takayasu's arteritis. *Curr Opin Rheumato* 1993; **5:** 25–32.

73 Maeda H, Handa N, Matsumoto M *et al.* Carotid lesions detected by B-mode ultrasonography in Takayasu's arteritis: 'Macaroni sign' as an indicator of the disease. *Ultrasound Med Biol* 1991; **17:** 695–701.

74 Buckley A, Southwood T, Culham G *et al.* The role of ultrasound in evaluation of Takayasu's arteritis. *J Rheumatol* 1991; **18:** 1073–80.

75 Hoffman GS. Treatment of chronic idiopathic systemic vasculitides. In Gross WL (ed.) *ANCA-Associated Vasculitides: Immunological and Clinical Aspects*, pp. 227–34. New York: Plenum Press, 1993.

76 Moriwaki R, Numano F. Takayasu arteritis: follow-up studies for 20 years. *Heart Vess* 1992; **7** (Suppl.): 138–45.

77 Hiramatsu K, Iwata Y, Kohda E *et al.* Percutaneous transluminal renal angioplasty in Takayasu's arteritis. *Int Angiol* 1993; **2:** 69–73.

78 Dong ZJ, Li S, Lu X. Percutaneous transluminal angioplasty for renovascular hypertension in arteritis: experience in China. *Radiology* 1987; **162:** 477–9.

79 Kumar S, Mandalam KR, Rao VR *et al.* Percutaneous transluminal angioplasty in nonspecific aortoarteritis (Takayasu's disease): experience of 16 cases. *Cardiovasc Intervent Radiol* 1989; **12:** 321–5.

80 Sharma S, Rajani M, Shrivastava S *et al.* Nonspecific aorto-arteritis (Takayasu's disease) in children. *Br J Radiol* 1991; **64:** 690–8.

81 Fava MP, Foradori GB, Garcia CB *et al.* Percutaneous transluminal angioplasty in patients with Takayasu arteritis: five year experience. *J Vasc Intervent Radiol* 1993; **4:** 649–52.

82 Tyagi S, Singh B, Kaul UA *et al.* Balloon angioplasty for renovascular hypertension in Takayasu's arteritis. *Am Heart J* 1993; **125:** 1386–93.

83 De Bakey ME, Garrett HE, Howell JF *et al.* Coarctation of the abdominal aorta with renal arterial stenosis: surgical complications. *Ann Surg* 1967; **165:** 830–43.

84 Pokrovsky AV, Sultanaliev TA, Spiridonov AA. Surgical treatment of vasorenal hypertension in

nonspecific aorto-arteritis (Takayasu's disease). *J Cardiovasc Surg* 1983; **24:** 111–18.
85 Lagneau P, Michel JB, Vuong PN. Surgical treatment of Takayasu's disease. *Ann Surg* 1987; **205:** 157–66.
86 Takagi A, Tada Y, Sato O, Miyata T. Surgical treatment for Takayasu's arteritis. A long-term follow-up study. *J Cardiovasc Surg* 1989; **30:** 553–8.
87 Kieffer E, Piquois A, Bertal A *et al.* Reconstructive surgery of the renal arteries in Takayasu's disease. *Ann Vasc Surg* 1990; **4:** 156–65.

5

Atheroembolic renal disease

MELINDA S PHINNEY AND MICHAEL C SMITH

History and scope of problem

Panum described the first case of cholesterol embolism in 1862. He noted occlusion of coronary arteries by atheromatous material at autopsy.[1] Subsequently, atheroembolism was not described in the medical literature until 1945 when Flory reported autopsy findings of cholesterol emboli in multiple vascular beds. In a review of 267 autopsies, Flory found evidence of cholesterol embolism in 3.4% of patients with atherosclerotic vascular disease. However, 12.3% of patients with severe, advanced abdominal aortic atherosclerosis demonstrated significant atheroembolic disease. In contrast, in patients with mild to moderate aortic disease, only 1.3% were noted to have embolic disease, and in patients with no evidence of aortic arteriosclerosis, none had cholesterol emboli.[2] Since these early reports of cholesterol emboli diagnosed postmortem, multiple cases of cholesterol embolization have been recognized antemortem[3–6] suggesting that the entity of cholesterol embolism is more common than previously realized. It is important that physicians recognize patients at risk to develop atheroembolic disease and understand its pathogenesis, clinical manifestations and treatment.

Two forms of atheromatous embolization can occur. Dislodgement of a large portion of an atheromatous plaque can result in occlusion of a large systemic vessel. This type of embolization is usually readily apparent due to the abrupt appearance of major organ dysfunction and has been reported to cause coronary artery, cerebral artery or large peripheral artery occlusion.[1, 6–7] The second form of atheromatous embolization is a result of occlusion of multiple small vessels, generally 50–200 micron (μ) in diameter. The sequelae are often subclinical but when vascular occlusion is extensive, the clinical manifestations are protean and can mimic a picture of chronic disease with multiorgan involvement.[8] This chapter will focus on the latter, more subtle form of cholesterol embolization.

Precipitating factors

Renal cholesterol embolization occurs most commonly in hypertensive men over 60 years of age with severe abdominal aortic atherosclerosis.[2, 3, 9–13] Not surprisingly, atherosclerosis is the most strongly associated condition accompanying cholesterol emboli with 90% of patients in one series demonstrating evidence of atherosclerotic vascular disease.[9] Thurlbeck and Castleman were the first to report acute renal failure due to atheromatous emboli to the kidneys after aortic surgery. In a large autopsy series of 3000 subjects, they found that 17 of 22 patients (77%) who died after abdominal aortic aneurysmectomy demonstrated histologic evidence of renal cholesterol embolization; 14 of the 17 patients developed oliguric or anuric renal failure and 4 died from uremia. In addition, they noted renal cholesterol emboli in 31% of patients with aortic aneurysm who had not undergone surgery, and in 16% of patients with severe atherosclerosis without aortic aneurysm. Of note was the fact that cholesterol emboli were never seen in the kidneys of patients whose aorta was free from atherosclerosis.[10] Other investigators have also shown a strong similar correlation between atherosclerosis and renal cholesterol emboli.[3, 13–16]

Renal cholesterol embolization can occur spontaneously[9, 10, 17, 18] or after aortic surgery, major vessel angiography or treatment with anticoagulants or thrombolytics.[19] Inciting events have been identified in 31–90% of reported cases.[9, 10, 15] Recently, Fine and his colleagues published an extensive review of 221 cases of histologically proven cholesterol embolization. Sixty-eight patients (31%) were found to have one or more identifiable factors that contributed to cholesterol embolization, 17% of patients had undergone major vessel angiography, 13% had been treated with anticoagulants and 9% had undergone vascular surgery. The remaining 153 cases (69%) had apparently spontaneous embolization.[9] Surgical manipulation of severely diseased, atherosclerotic aortae predisposes to dislodgement of atheromatous material with subsequent distal embolization of either large portions of atheroma or showers of cholesterol crystals. Gore and Collins reviewing earlier studies of cholesterol emboli reported in 1960 that 21% of cases were consequent to aortic surgery whereas 78% of cases occurred spontaneously.[18]

Angiography involving the abdominal aorta is a well described inciting factor for the development of cholesterol embolization.[9, 15, 20–27] Harrington *et al.* reported two patients who after undergoing renal arteriography for the evaluation of hypertension, subsequently developed progressive renal failure resulting in uremia and death. At autopsy both were found to have extensive renal cholesterol embolization.[28] In a retrospective study, Ramirez and his colleagues reviewed autopsy results from 71 patients who had undergone diagnostic angiographic procedures. They found a 30% incidence of systemic cholesterol emboli after aortography and a 25.5% incidence of systemic cholesterol emboli after cardiac catheterization. This was in contrast to an incidence of 4.3% in age- and disease-matched controls who had not undergone aortic or cardiac catheterization.[29] Many other reports implicate angiography as a risk factor for cholesterol embolization.[3, 20, 23, 25, 26] The development of clinically apparent atheromatous embolization can occur within 24 h of the procedure[25] or can be delayed up to 6 weeks or more.[23, 26] Presumably, embolization of cholesterol crystals and debris from atheromatous plaques is induced when rigid angiography catheters traumatize vessel walls (Fig. 5.1). Development of newer, more flexible catheters may decrease cholesterol embolization associated with major vessel angiography.

In 1967 Moldveen-Geronimus and Merriam introduced the concept that anticoagulant therapy might precipitate cholesterol embolization.

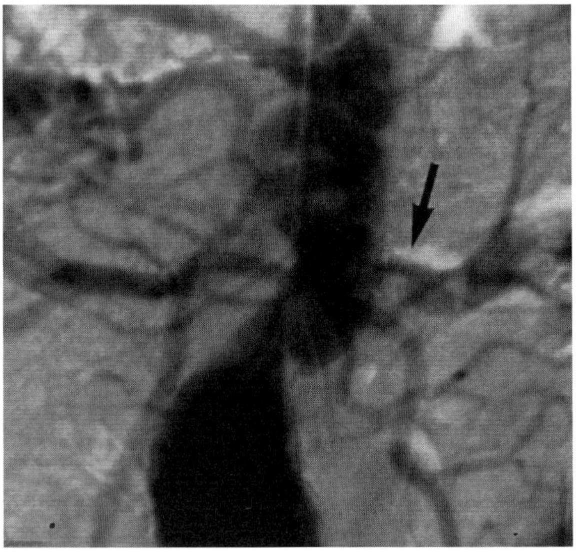

Figure 5.1. Abdominal aortic digital subtraction angiogram in a patient with diffuse atherosclerosis. The angiogram was performed to evaluate the development of resistent hypertension and demonstrates aortic atherosclerosis, a saccular infrarenal aortic aneurysm and a severe stenosis at the origin of the left renal artery (arrow) with poststenotic dilatation. The patient's baseline creatinine was 1.6 mg/dl; he developed crampy abdominal pain, lower extremity livedo reticularis and progressive renal insufficiency 2 weeks after the procedure. He then developed end-stage renal disease requiring peritoneal dialysis.

Six years earlier Feder and Auerbach reported a 'purple toe' syndrome in patients receiving oral anticoagulants, but they found no evidence of cholesterol emboli on skin biopsy.[30] However, in reviewing 121 cases of documented cholesterol embolization, Moldveen-Geronimus and Merriam noted that 16 patients demonstrated peripheral signs of livedo reticularis, purple toes and gangrene. Interestingly, in 13 of these 16 patients, histologic examination of the extremities demonstrated cholesterol emboli; 6 of these 13 patients had been receiving anticoagulants.[4] The authors speculated that a causal relationship existed between anticoagulant therapy and cholesterol embolization. Subsequently, Hyman *et al.* described four patients receiving warfarin who developed cyanosis of their toes as well as other manifestations of cholesterol embolization. In two of the four patients, biopsy of involved tissue showed cholesterol emboli.[31] Other authors have reported similar findings and emphasized a correlation between systemic anticoagulation and atheroembolic disease.[15, 32–34] Development of cholesterol embolization has also been described as a complication of thrombolytic therapy.[35–41] Glassock and colleagues reported a patient who received streptokinase therapy for a pulmonary embolus and subsequently developed livedo reticularis, cyanotic toes, hypertension and oliguric acute renal failure. Postmortem examination revealed severe atherosclerotic vascular disease of the abdominal aorta. Multiple cholesterol emboli were demonstrated in the arcuate and interlobular arteries of the kidney, in the small and medium-sized arteries of multiple other visceral organs and in the subcutaneous tissue of the legs.[38] Similar cases have been described in patients who receive recombinant tissue-type plasminogen activator for acute myocardial infarction.[37] Although the precise mechanism by which anticoagulant and thrombolytic therapy predispose to atheroembolism is unknown, some authorities theorize that these agents precipitate cholesterol embolization by preventing development of thrombi or by dissolving preformed thrombi that overlie atheromatous plaques, thus allowing the cholesterol matrix access to systemic circulation.[39] Since the abdominal aorta and its branches are the vessels most severely affected by atherosclerosis, it is logical that organs and tissues supplied by these vessels are the most commonly affected with cholesterol embolization.

Pathology

Pathologic lesions seen with renal cholesterol emboli have been well defined.[2, 8, 14, 28] On gross examination, the kidneys can demonstrate significant atrophy with depressed, wedge-shaped cortical areas of scarring that are sharply defined.[2, 4] This patchy atrophy and scarring results in a characteristic nodular, coarse surface of the kidney.[2] Typical histologic lesions involve the arcuate and interlobular arteries, vessels with diameters from 50 to 200 μm, and show biconvex clefts that remain after the cholesterol crystals dissolve during fixation (Fig. 5.2). In fresh, unfixed tissue, the cholesterol crystals can be identified by characteristic birefringence under polarized light. The crystals can be solitary, but were more often found in parallel clusters.[11]

Experimental models of cholesterol embolization have provided detailed descriptions of the histologic evolution of the lesions over time that correlate well with clinical findings on biopsy or at autopsy. In 1945 Flory produced experimental cholesterol embolization by injecting atheromatous material from human aortae into rabbit ear veins and examined the lungs 24 h and 7 days after the injection.[2] At 24 h, small arteries in the lungs were occluded by masses of red blood cells, polymorphonuclear cells and cholesterol crystals. Examination of the lungs after 7 days showed cholesterol crystals surrounded by foreign body giant cells and hyperplastic intimal tissue. In a similar experimental model, Snyder and Shapiro studied histologic specimens of lung 1, 3, 6 and 12 days after cholesterol embolization.[14] Initially, cholesterol clefts were seen in small to medium sized arteries accompanied by an acute inflammatory response comprised of leukocytes and eosinophils. At 3 days, panarteritis with more eosinophils and a few foreign body giant cells were seen along with intimal hyperplasia. By 6 days the acute inflammation had resolved and numerous for-

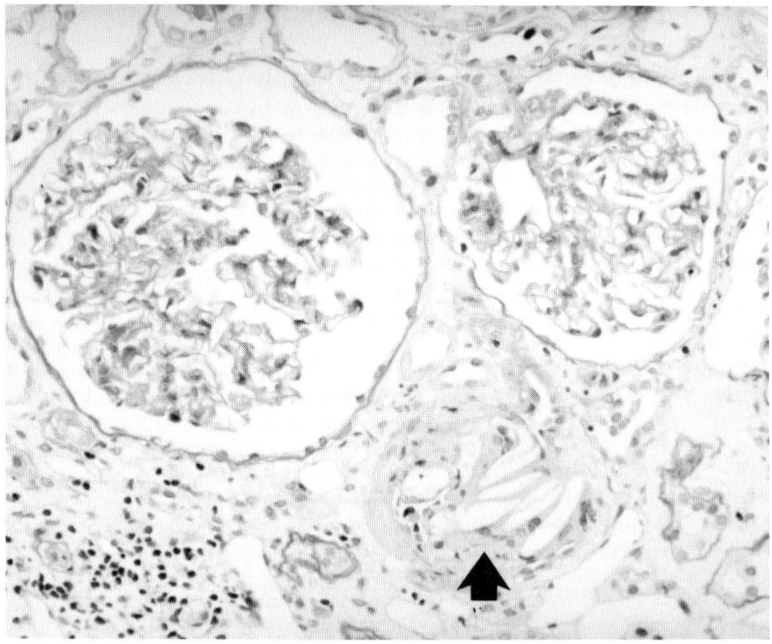

Figure 5.2. Photomicrograph of a renal biopsy specimen demonstrating the characteristic biconvex, acicular clefts of cholesterol embolization in an interlobular artery (arrow). Hematoxylin and eosin stain.

eign body giant cells were prominent. At the end of 12 days, intimal fibrosis was noted with sequestration of cholesterol crystals by foreign body giant cells. These lesions remained unchanged for 67–160 days,[14] presumably because of the resistance of cholesterol crystals to scavenger effects of macrophages.[9]

Some authors have hypothesized that significant vasospasm occurs at the time of embolization because biopsy specimens often do not show complete luminal obliteration.[10, 11, 13] Zdon and co-workers, however, infused prostacyclin, a potent vasodilator, into dogs that had experimentally induced cholesterol embolization. Vasodilation with prostacyclin failed to improve renal function, thus suggesting that reversible vasospasm does not play a major role in the renal functional deterioration caused by cholesterol embolism.[42]

Sequential histologic changes similar to those observed in experimental models can be demonstrated in the arcuate and interlobular arteries of human renal tissue as well as other vascular beds.[2] Acutely (<24 h) there is often a leukocytic infiltration with polymorphonuclear cells and eosinophils. Within 24–48 h, the cholesterol crystals are surrounded by multinucleated giant cells and fibroblasts. Endothelial proliferation and intimal fibrosis with luminal obliteration occur 2–7 days after embolization.[2, 9, 11, 14] Superimposed intravascular thrombi can occasionally be seen.[43] Immunofluorescence microscopy of renal lesions reveals no staining for immunoglobulins or complement.[26] Additional histologic manifestations that occasionally have been reported on renal biopsy include membranoproliferative glomerular changes,[5] focal necrotizing glomerulonephritis with crescent formation[21] and patchy tubular atrophy.[37]

Clinical presentation

Extrarenal manifestations

Clinical features of cholesterol embolization vary with the organs and tissues that are involved. Atheromatous embolization has been called the great mimicker because of its protean clinical manifestations. Multisystem disease is common and can be clinically evident or occult. Although embolization to the kidney is most common, autopsy studies[2, 4, 5, 9, 13, 16, 22, 23, 25, 43, 44] have demonstrated evidence of cholesterol emboli in spleen, pancreas, liver, stomach, bowel, muscle, adrenal glands, thyroid, gall bladder, myocardium, bladder, testis, skin and retinal vessels. Fine *et al.* determined the frequency of postmortem organ involvement in patients with cholesterol embolization and found that an average of 3.4 histologic sites were involved per patient autopsy.[9] Table 5.1 indicates the frequency of organ involvement according to postmortem histologic examination. The kidney (76%), spleen (56%) and pancreas (52%) were most frequently involved with cholesterol emboli. In contrast, antemortem histologic diagnosis was most frequently established by biopsy of muscle, skin or kidney or by examination of an amputated digit or limb (Table 5.2). The discrepancy between the frequency of organ involvement at postmortem examination and the frequency of histologic diagnosis antemortem reflects both the presence of subclinical disease and the suitability of tissue for biopsy.

Cutaneous involvement, demonstrated either by biopsy or at autopsy, is the most common extrarenal manifestation, occurring in 30–35% of all patients with cholesterol embolization.[9, 40] In a recent review of over 200 cases of histologically documented cholesterol embolism, Falanga and his co-workers reported a 35% overall incidence of cutaneous involvement including livedo reticularis in 49% of patients with cutaneous manifestations.[40] Gangrene (35%), digital cyanosis (28%), ulceration (17%), subcutaneous nodules (10%) and purpura (9%) occurred less frequently. Livedo reticularis, the most frequently noted cutaneous sign, is a lacy, bluish discoloration that typically affects the lower extremities and the trunk. The onset of livedo reticularis is usually abrupt and the areas of involvement are often extensive, but the appearance may wax and wane. The strong association between livedo reticularis and cholesterol embolization has led some authorities to conclude that the diagnosis of cholesterol embolization should be seriously considered in any elderly patient who develops this cutaneous finding.[40] Purple discoloration of the toes with painful dysesthesia of the affected area is not uncommon. The cyanotic areas can also wax and wane, blanch completely with pressure, and tend to fade with elevation of the involved extremity.[30] Cyanosis is believed to occur secondary to arterial obstruction with subsequent peripheral desaturation of blood.[31] Focal digital necrosis (Fig. 5.3) is common[6, 14, 16, 43] and

Table 5.1. Postmortem histologic involvement with cholesterol embolism[a]

Histologic site	Cases	%
Kidney	136	76
Spleen	101	56
Pancreas	93	52
Gastrointestinal tract	58	32
Adrenal gland	38	21
Liver	30	17

[a] Derived from refs 9 and 15; total cases = 180.

Table 5.2. Antemortem histologic diagnosis of cholesterol embolism[a]

Histologic site	Cases	%
Muscle	26	30
Skin	24	28
Kidney	18	21
Amputation	11	13

[a] Derived from refs 9 and 15; total cases = 86.

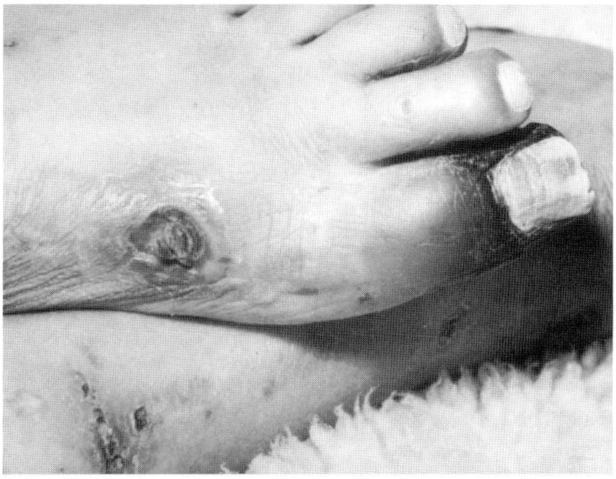

Figure 5.3. Focal digital necrosis due to cholesterol embolization after aortic angiography.

frequently occurs in the presence of normal peripheral pulses.[6, 16] However, given the high prevalence of severe atherosclerotic disease in this population, pulses are often diminished or absent due to major vessel atherosclerosis. Splinter hemorrhages have also been reported in association with atheromatous embolization.[45]

Retinal cholesterol emboli, initially described by Hollenhorst,[46] are common particularly if the source of the emboli is the aortic arch or its branches.[7] Retinal emboli were reported in 10% of patients with cholesterol emboli in one review.[25] Although retinal emboli can produce visual symptoms such as amaurosis fugax, often they are asymptomatic. Nevertheless, because of their diagnostic importance, a careful fundoscopic examination should be part of the evaluation of any patient with suspected cholesterol embolization. Hollenhorst plaques (Fig. 5.4) appear as bright-yellow crystalline plaques at bifurcations of retinal arterioles and should be distinguished from platelet fibrin thrombi that are white. This distinction is important because of the different diagnostic and therapeutic implications.[46]

Twenty to thirty percent of patients with atheroembolic disease will demonstrate clinical or histologic involvement of the gastrointestinal tract.[9, 15, 27] Symptoms of nausea, vomiting, anorexia and vague abdominal pain are common

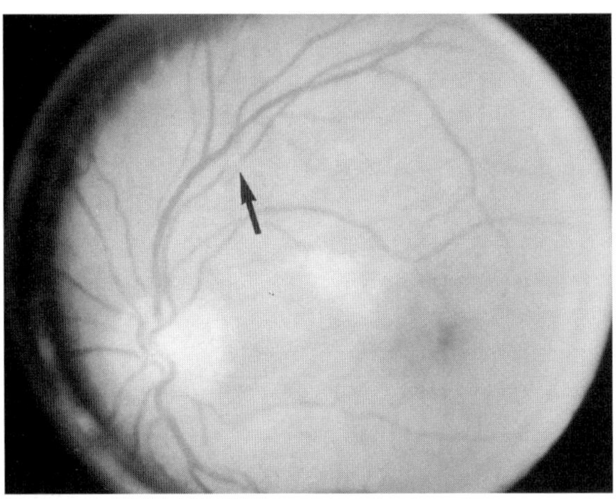

Figure 5.4 A cholesterol embolus (Hollenhorst plaque, arrow) lodged at the bifurcation of the superior temporal branch of the retinal artery.

and may be the result of pancreatitis caused by atheroemboli.[8, 43, 44] Splenic involvement with subsequent infarction can also result in abdominal pain. Embolism to small vessels in the small or large bowel can occur producing zones of bowel ischemia or infarction.[27, 41] Gastrointestinal bleeding occurs in a small percentage of patients and the manifestations range from occult blood in the stool to frank hematochezia.[16]

Renal manifestations

Cholesterol embolization most commonly affects the kidney (Table 5.1). Renal involvement occurred in 50% of cases reviewed by Fine *et al.*[9] Manifestations of renal cholesterol embolization range from mild renal insufficiency to rapidly progressive acute renal failure with uremia. Patients can have fluctuations in renal function associated with recurrent episodes of embolization.[11, 17, 18] Although flank pain with microscopic or gross hematuria has been reported, a progressive asymptomatic loss of renal function is more frequent.[43, 47] When renal function deteriorates after angiography, renal failure can be caused by cholesterol embolization or the contrast media itself. It is necessary to differentiate these entities since the course and prognosis of each is dramatically different. Typically, contrast-associated nephropathy is characterized by the abrupt onset of renal insufficiency within 12–24 h following contrast administration. The serum creatinine concentration increases over the ensuing 2–3 days, generally stabilizes by days 3–5, and usually improves over the next 7–10 days.[48] On the other hand, although oliguria and renal failure from atheromatous embolization can be evident immediately after an angiographic procedure, more often renal insufficiency develops insidiously over days to weeks following the procedure (Fig. 5.5).[3, 10, 11, 20, 23, 25, 26, 34, 49]

Hypertension is frequent with renal cholesterol embolization and can help to distinguish it from other causes of acute renal failure in which the overall prevalence of hypertension is less than 40%.[50] Handler, in 1956, was the first to report an association between hypertension and

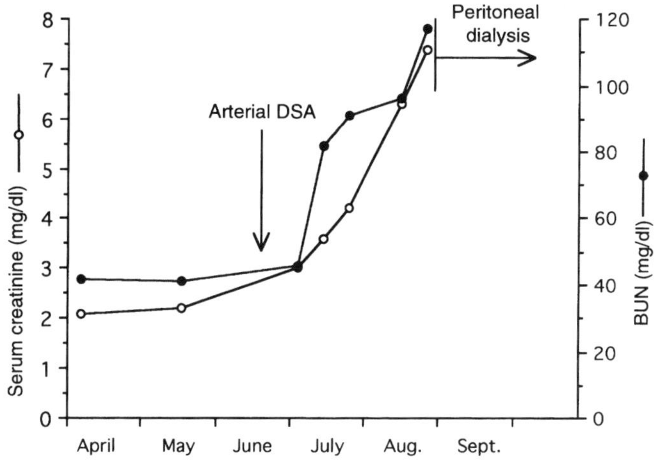

Figure 5.5. Changes in blood urea nitrogen (BUN) and serum creatinine in a patient who developed atheroembolic renal disease after renal arterial digital subtraction angiography (DSA). Renal function steadily decreased over an 8-week period.

renal cholesterol embolization.[13] In a review of 20 patients found to have atheromatous emboli at autopsy, he found that 15 of the 20 patients were hypertensive at the time of diagnosis, and in 3 of 7 recent cases the patients had an abrupt rise in blood pressure coincident with the development of renal atheroembolism. Other authors have reported onset of new hypertension or paroxysmal worsening of well-controlled or mild hypertension at the time of renal cholesterol embolization.[3–5, 11, 16] The pathogenesis of hypertension in patients with renal cholesterol embolism has not been investigated extensively, but might be the result of increased production of renin, angiotensin and aldosterone. Dalakos and his colleagues performed bilateral renal vein renin sampling in one patient who presented with malignant hypertension and papilledema.[51] They demonstrated evidence of unilateral hypersecretion of renin with a renal venous renin ratio of 2.3:1 when the left renal vein was compared with the right renal vein. At autopsy the orifice of the left renal artery was occluded by atheromatous material and evidence of cholesterol embolism was found in that kidney. These authors speculated that cholesterol embolism caused increased renin release from the involved kidney, thus causing renin-dependent hypertension.[51]

Laboratory features

Certain laboratory findings are helpful in confirming the diagnosis of cholesterol embolization. The most common laboratory abnormalities reflect embolization to the renal vascular bed. Following atheromatous emboli to the kidney, renal function deteriorates and azotemia develops. Rate of progression of azotemia is variable and is often proportional to the degree of renal parenchymal damage. In episodes of fulminant atheroembolism, azotemia occurs acutely and can progress rapidly over days to severe renal failure.[5, 10] In other cases, renal function declines more slowly and only mild to moderate renal insufficiency results.[26, 34] The erythrocyte sedimentation rate (ESR) is frequently elevated.[12, 16, 23, 31, 43, 52] In a review of 221 reported cases of cholesterol embolization, the ESR was elevated in 32 of 33 patients for whom data were available.[9] Although the pathogenesis of the increased ESR is unclear, this low false negative rate of 3% suggests that a normal ESR is strong evidence against the diagnosis of cholesterol embolization in patients with clinical findings compatible with the disease. Abnormalities in cellular elements of the blood have been noted. Thrombocytopenia has been prevalent in some, but not all studies, and might be due to platelet aggregation induced by atheromatous material.[53] Thrombocytopenia was reported in 6 of 7 patients in Cosio's review;[53] however, other investigators have failed to report a high incidence of thrombocytopenia.[9, 22] Leukocytosis has been described in up to 50% of reported cases.[9, 12, 15, 28, 43]

Eosinophilia, defined as an eosinophil count of greater than 300 eosinophils/ml or more than 3% of the total white blood count, is a characteristic finding in atheromatous embolization.[15, 49, 53–56] Its presence can help to distinguish atheroembolic renal disease from other cases of acute or subacute renal failure. The prevalence of eosinophilia ranges from 39 to 80%.[15, 49] Kasinath and his colleagues reported six patients with renal cholesterol embolism and noted eosinophilia in all. They also reviewed 36 cases of cholesterol embolization in the literature and found that 80% (29 of 36) showed peripheral blood eosinophilia.[47] The appearance of eosinophilia generally occurs within 1–3 weeks of the atheroembolic event, is variable in degree and transient in nature, lasting only for a few days.[49, 56] It appears that eosinophilia is an acute marker for episodes of atheroembolism. Pathologically, early lesions of cholesterol embolism have been noted to have significant eosinophilic infiltration that may be a histologic correlate of the peripheral eosinophilia.

Hypocomplementemia is a frequent accompaniment of cholesterol embolization. Cosio and co-workers initially described seven patients with documented cholesterol embolization in whom C3 levels were transiently decreased and temporally related to acute episodes of embolization.[53] They suggested that the complement system might amplify the inflammatory response and hence contribute to the pathogenesis of vascular damage associated with cholesterol embolization. Complement activation has been described in human atheromata and receptors for activated complement fragments have been identified within atherosclerotic lesions.[57] In addition, incubation of cholesterol crystals *in vitro* with plasma results in complement activation. Hammerschmidt *et al.* hypothesize that exposure of plasma to crystalline cholesterol *in vivo* (as a result of ulceration of, or hemorrhage into, an atheromatous plaque) can cause activation of complement, resulting in leukostasis that further potentiates ischemic injury distal to the plaque.[58] Activated C5 is known to be chemotactic for eosinophils, as well as neutrophils, possibly explaining the presence of eosinophilic infiltrates in early lesions of cholesterol embolism.

Abnormalities of urinalysis are common when renal atheroembolism occurs. Proteinuria was present in 54% (34/63) of patients reviewed by Fine *et al.*[9] Overall the degree of proteinuria reported has been variable and ranged from 1+ proteinuria by dipstick to nephrotic range proteinuria on quantitative analysis.[9, 17, 26] The urine sediment is typically bland and non-specific, but cellular elements including microscopic or macroscopic hematuria, pyuria and casts can be seen.[9, 21, 34, 47] Eosinophiluria, defined as greater than 1% of white blood cells in 15 ml of spun urine stained with Hansel's stain, was reported in 89% of patients with biopsy-proven renal cholesterol emboli in one small, preliminary study.[55] In contrast, other authors have failed to note eosinophiluria.[49] Hence, the utility of eosinophiluria in the diagnosis of cholesterol embolization remains to be determined.

Differential diagnosis

Vague and protean clinical manifestations make the syndrome of cholesterol embolization a diagnostic challenge. The symptoms and signs associated with this entity are non-specific and can suggest an underlying systemic disorder such as polyarteritis nodosa, subacute bacterial endocarditis, polymyositis or left atrial myxoma. Similarities between multiple cholesterol emboli and vasculitides such as polyarteritis nodosa are striking. Both disorders can present with non-specific symptoms of malaise, anorexia, nausea, vomiting and weight loss. Both can show evidence of renal failure, systemic inflammation (leukocytosis, elevated ESR and eosinophilia) and central nervous system abnormalities.[11, 19, 26, 43] Characteristics that often help to distinguish between cholesterol emboli and polyarteritis include a history of precipitating events such as aortic manipulation or major vessel angiography in a patient with risk factors for cholesterol embolization and the presence of disseminated atherosclerotic vascular disease. Additionally, eosinophilia occurs more commonly with multiple cholesterol emboli than with polyarteritis nodosa. On the other hand, fever, joint involvement, peripheral neuropathy and pulmonary lesions are more likely to be associated with polyarteritis and rarely reported with atheromatous embolization.[11, 23]

Certainly the most definitive means of establishing the diagnosis of cholesterol embolization is identification of characteristic lesions of intravascular cholesterol crystals in affected tissue. In early reports the diagnosis of cholesterol embolization was usually established at autopsy; however, the greater recent awareness of this entity has resulted in antemortem diagnosis by examination of resected tissue or biopsy specimens.[2, 10, 18] Diagnostic biopsy material has been obtained from skin lesions (nodules, livedo reticularis, cyanotic digits), gastrocnemius muscle, kidney and bone marrow.[5, 16, 21–23, 26, 36, 43, 59] Skin and muscle biopsy have high diagnostic yield, particularly when cutaneous findings are present. Even in the absence of cutaneous manifestations, some authors believe that skin or muscle or both should be biopsied when cholesterol embolization is suspected.[9, 16] There is a strong association between the presence of cholesterol emboli in renal biopsy specimens and clinical disease due to atheromatous embolism. In addition, the presence of renal atheroemboli is considered the best marker for other visceral involvement. The specificity of biopsy in the diagnosis of cholesterol embolization approaches 100%. On the other hand, the sensitivity for one biopsy is 75%, but increases to 94% when two biopsies from the same tissue are obtained.[19] Consequently, we believe that biopsy of skin lesions should be an initial step in establishing the diagnosis of cholesterol embolization in patients with cutaneous manifestations; renal biopsy should be strongly considered in patients with renal dysfunction who lack cutaneous findings.

Clinical course

Clinically, the course of atheroembolic renal disease is as varied as its presenting symptoms. The earliest reported cases had universally fatal outcomes. More recently, reports of extended survival and recovery of renal function have been published.[3, 5, 24, 35] This improved prognosis is probably the result of greater awareness of the syndrome which leads to earlier diagnosis. In addition, more effective supportive therapies, i.e. dialysis are available. Decline in renal function is often progressive, probably due to recurrent episodes of acute atheromatous embolization. This can result in a waxing and waning course of renal insufficiency. Occasionally, renal function deteriorates markedly and dialysis is necessary. Even with severe renal failure requiring dialysis, spontaneous recovery of renal function can occur.[3, 22, 24] Smith and colleagues reported a patient who developed end-stage renal disease that required hemodialysis for 4 months before renal function improved sufficiently to withdraw dialytic support[3] (Fig. 5.6). Siemons and associates had a similar experience with two patients who were maintained on peritoneal dialysis with eventual recovery of renal function.[24] They suggested that peritoneal dialysis is a superior mode of therapy for severe renal failure due to atheromatous renal disease because it avoids the need for vascular access, systemic anticoagulation and the potential hemodynamic instability often encountered with hemodialysis.

Despite these sporadic reports of recovery and survival after cholesterol embolism, the prognosis of this disorder remains poor. McGowan and Greenberg noted a better prognosis in patients who developed cholesterol embolization after angiography or anticoagulant therapy compared with patients with spontaneous cholesterol emboli, perhaps because of the severity of atherosclerotic disease in those in whom atheroembolism occurs spontaneously.[22] Overall, mortality ranges from 72 to 100%, and generally is the result of multiorgan involvement with cholesterol emboli, or is because of the consequences of severe atherosclerosis in multiple vascular beds (e.g. stroke, myocardial infarction.[9, 12, 25, 40]

Treatment

Prevention of its development is the most effective treatment of renal cholesterol embolization.

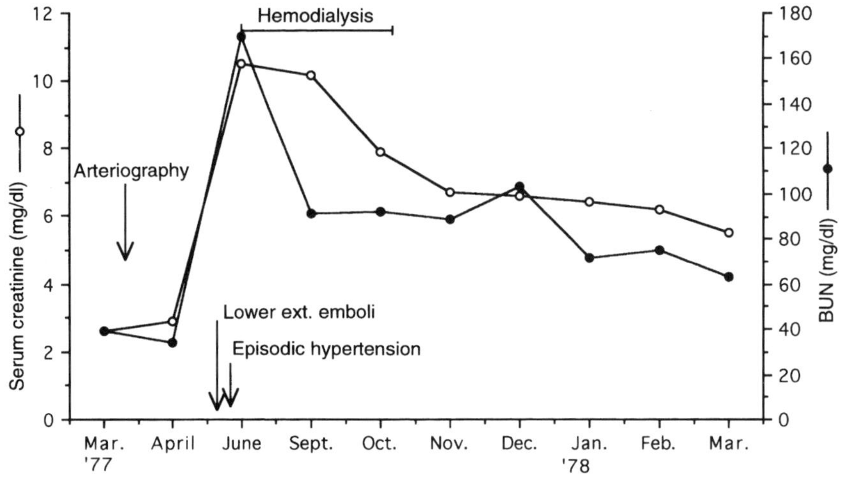

Figure 5.6. Changes in blood urea nitrogen (BUN) and serum creatinine over a 13-month period in a patient who developed atheroembolic renal disease after major vessel angiography. Arrows indicate inciting angiography, episodes of lower extremity emboli and episodic hypertension. Brackets indicate a 4-month period of hemodialysis before recovery of renal function. Modified from ref. 3, with permission.

Angiography and prolonged systemic anticoagulation should be avoided whenever possible in patients with diffuse aortic atherosclerotic disease.[3, 12] When major vessel angiography is necessary, the number of procedures should be minimized. Newer, softer, more flexible catheters should be utilized. Hopefully with increasing recognition of the potential for atheromatous embolization in patients at risk, these preventative measures will become more widely utilized.

Management of patients with cholesterol embolism is usually supportive since there is no effective therapy to treat atheroembolic renal disease. If a solitary, identifiable source of atheroemboli is found, surgical resection of the lesion can improve outcome.[6, 54] In the majority of instances, however, this is not feasible. Consequently, amelioration of factors that promote atherosclerosis (e.g. cigarette smoking, hyperlipidemia) is essential. Hypertension should be treated to prevent further deterioration in renal function as well as to minimize hypertensive cardiovascular morbidity and mortality. In patients in whom anticoagulant therapy might have been an inciting factor in the development of cholesterol embolization, recovery of renal function has been associated with discontinuation of anticoagulants.[31–33, 45] Bruns and colleagues described a patient who developed renal failure and multisystem disease associated with biopsy evidence of cholesterol emboli. Discontinuation of anticoagulant therapy resulted in prompt cessation of symptoms and dramatic improvement in renal function.[22] On the other hand, Acker described a patient taking oral anticoagulants with multiple biopsies demonstrating atheroemboli whose course improved when intermittent subcutaneous heparin therapy was substituted for oral anticoagulation.[32] Acker suggested intermittent release of heparin from subcutaneous administration provides a short anticoagulant-free period that permits some healing of eroded atheromatous plaques. Therefore, we recommend that oral anticoagulants be discontinued whenever possible. If continued anticoagulation is essential, intermittent parenteral therapy should be considered to minimize further atheroembolism.[32] If end-stage renal disease develops, institution of peritoneal or hemodialysis is indicated given reports of recovery of renal function even after prolonged periods of renal replacement therapy.

References

1 Panum PL. Experimentalle Beitrage zur Lehre Von Der emboli. *Virchows Archiv Pathol Anat Physiol Klin Med* 1863; **25:** 308–10.

2 Flory CM. Arterial occlusions produced by emboli from eroded aortic atheromatous plaques. *Am J Pathol* 1945; **21:** 549–65.

3 Smith MC, Ghose MK, Henry AR. The clinical spectrum of renal cholesterol embolization. *Am J Med* 1981; **71:** 174–80.

4 Moldveen-Geronimus M, Merriam JC. Cholesterol embolization: from pathological curiosity to clinical entity. *Circulation* 1967; **35:** 946–53.

5 Schipper H, Gordon M, Berris B. Atheromatous embolic disease. *Can Med Assoc J* 1975; **113:** 640–4.

6 Kempczinski RF. Lower extremity arterial emboli from ulcerating atherosclerotic plaques. *JAMA* 1979; **241:** 807–10.

7 Tunick PA, Culliford AT, Lamparello PI, Kronzon I. Atheromatosis of the aortic arch as an occult source of multiple systemic emboli. *Ann Int Med* 1991; **114:** 391–2.

8 Eliot RS, Kanjuh VI, Edwards JE. Atheromatous embolism. *Circulation* 1964; **30:** 611–18.

9 Fine MJ, Kapoor W, Falanga V. Cholesterol crystal embolization: a review of 221 cases in the English literature. *Angiology* 1987; **38:** 769–84.

10 Thurlbeck WM, Castleman B. Atheromatous emboli to the kidneys after aortic surgery. *N Engl J Med* 1957; **257:** 442–7.

11 Kassirer JP. Atheroembolic renal disease. *N Engl J Med* 1969; **280:** 812–18.

12 Glassock RJ. Renal arterial thrombosis and embolism. In Massry SG, Glassock RJ (eds) *Textbook of Nephrology*, pp. 916–19. Baltimore: Williams and Wilkins, 1989.

13 Handler FP. Clinical and pathologic significance of atheromatous embolization with emphasis on an etiology of renal hypertension. *Am J Med* 1956; **20:** 366–73.

14 Snyder HE, Shapiro JL. A correlative study of atheromatous embolism in human beings and experimental animals. *Surgery* 1961; **49:** 195–204.

15 Dahlberg PJ, Frecentese DF, Cogbill TH. Cholesterol embolism: experience with 22 histologically proven cases. *Surgery* 1989; **105:** 737–46.

16 Carvajal JA, Anderson WR, Weiss L *et al.* Atheroembolism: an etiologic factor in renal insufficiency, gastrointestinal hemorrhages, and peripheral vascular diseases. *Arch Int Med* 1967; **119:** 593–9.

17 Kaplan K, Millar JD, Cancilla PA. 'Spontaneous' atheroembolic renal failure. *Arch Int Med* 1962; **110:** 218–21.

18 Gore I, Collins DP. Spontaneous atheromatous embolization: review of the literature and a report of 16 additional cases. *Am J Clin Pathol* 1960; **33:** 416–26.

19 Case records of the Massachusetts General Hospital. *N Engl J Med* 1991; **325:** 563–72.

20 Ho SW-C, Thatcher GN, Matz LR. Reversible renal failure due to cholesterol embolism. *Aust NZ J M* 1982; **12:** 531–3.

21 Goldman M, Thoua Y, Dhaene M, Toussaint C. Necrotizing glomerulonephritis associated with cholesterol microemboli. *Br Med J* 1985; **290:** 205–6.

22 McGowan JA, Greenberg A. Cholesterol atheroembolic renal disease: report of 3 cases with emphasis on diagnosis by skin biopsy and extended survival. *Am J Nephrol* 1986; **6:** 135–9.

23 Young DK, Burton MF, Herman JH. Multiple cholesterol emboli syndrome simulating systemic necrotizing vasculitis. *J Rheumatol* 1986; **13:** 423–6.

24 Siemons L, van den Heuvel P, Parizel G *et al.* Peritoneal dialysis in acute renal failure due to cholesterol embolization: two cases of recovery of renal function and extended survival. *Clin Nephrol* 1987; **28:** 205–8.

25 Freund NS. Cholesterol emboli syndrome following cardiac catheterization. *Postgrad Med* 1990; **87:** 55–60.

26 Case records of the Massachusetts General Hospital. *N Engl J Med* 1991; **324:** 113–20.

27 Hendel RC, Cuenoud HF, Glansiracusa DF, Alpert JS. Multiple cholesterol emboli syndrome: bowel infarction after retrograde angiography. *Arch Int Med* 1989; **149:** 2371–4.

28 Harrington JT, Sommers SC, Kassirer JP. Atheromatous emboli with progressive renal failure: renal arteriography as the probable inciting factor. *Ann Int Med* 1968; **68:** 152–60.

29 Ramirez G, O'Neill WM, Lambert R, Blommer HA. Cholesterol embolization: a complication of angiography. *Arch Int Med* 1978; **138:** 1430–2.

30 Feder W, Auerbach R. 'Purple Toes': an uncommon sequela of oral coumarin drug therapy. *Ann Int Med* 1961; **55:** 911–17.

31 Hyman BT, Landas SK, Ashman RF *et al.* Warfarin-related purple toes syndrome and cholesterol microembolization. *Am J Med* 1987; **82:** 1233–7.

32 Acker CG. Cholesterol microembolization and stable renal function with continued anticoagulation. *South Med J* 1992; **85:** 210–12.

33 Bruns FJ, Segel DP, Adler S. Control of cholesterol embolization by discontinuation of anticoagulant therapy. *Am J Med Sci* 1978; **275:** 105–8.

34 Regester RF. Renal failure secondary to spontaneous atheromatous microembolism. *J Tennessee Med Assoc* 1980; **73:** 328–30.

35 Pirson Y, Honhon B, Cosyns JP, Van Ypersele C. Cholesterol embolism in a renal graft after

treatment with streptokinase. *Br Med J* 1988; **296:** 394–5.
36 Mendia R, Cavaliere G, Sparacio F *et al.* Does thrombolysis produce cholesterol embolisation? *Lancet* 1992; **339:** 562.
37 Gupta BK, Spinowitz BS, Charytan C, Wahl SJ. Cholesterol crystal embolization-associated renal failure after therapy with recombinant tissue-type plasminogen activator. *Am J Kidney Dis* 1993; **21:** 659–62.
38 Glassock RJ, Ritz E, Bommer J *et al.* Acute renal failure, hypertension and skin necrosis in a patient with streptokinase therapy. *Am J Nephrol* 1984; **4:** 193–200.
39 Ridker PM, Michel T. Streptokinase therapy and cholesterol embolization. *Am J Med* 1989; **87:** 357–8.
40 Falanga V, Fine MJ, Kapoor WN. The cutaneous manifestations of cholesterol crystal embolization. *Arch Dermatol* 1936; **122:** 1194–8.
41 Schwartz MW, McDonald GB. Cholesterol embolization syndrome: occurrence after intravenous streptokinase therapy for myocardial infarction. *JAMA* 1987; **258:** 1934–5.
42 Zdon MJ, Crawford B, Hermreck A. Renal function, microcirculation, and the role of PGI_2 following atheromatous embolization. *Curr Sur* 1983; **40:** 209–11.
43 Richards AM, Eliot RS, Kanjuh VI *et al.* Cholesterol embolism: a multiple-system disease masquerading as polyarteritis nodosa. *Am J Cardiol* 1965; **15:** 696–707.
44 Fisher ER, Hellstrom HR, Myers JD. Disseminated atheromatous emboli. *Am J Med* 1960; **29:** 176–80.
45 Turakhia AK, Khah MA. Splinter hemorrhages as a possible clinical manifestation of cholesterol crystal embolization. *J Rheumatol* 1990; **17:** 1083–6.
46 Hollenhorst RW. Significance of bright plaques in the retinal arterioles. *JAMA* 1961; **178:** 23–9.
47 Wellmann KF. Hematuria caused by atheromatous embolism: report of a case diagnosed intravitam. *J Urol* 1975; **114:** 299–300.
48 Alexander RD, Berkes SL, Abuelo G. Contrast media-induced oliguric renal failure. *Arch Int Med* 1978; **138:** 381–4.
49 Kasinath BS, Corwin HL, Bidani AK *et al.* Eosinophilia in the diagnosis of atheroembolic renal disease. *Am J Nephrol* 1987; **7:** 173–7.
50 Bonomini V, Campieri C, Scolari MP, Vangelista A. Hypertension in acute renal failure. *Contrib Nephrol* 1987; **54:** 152–8.
51 Dalakos TG, Streeten DHP, Jones D, Obeid A. 'Malignant' hypertension resulting from atheromatous embolization predominantly of one kidney. *Am J Med* 1974; **57:** 135–8.
52 Clinicopathologic Conference: cyanotic feet and renal failure in a 67-year-old man. *Am J Med* 1983; **75:** 509–17.
53 Cosio FG, Zager RA, Sharma HM. Athroembolic renal disease causes hypocomplementemia. *Lancet* 1985; **2:** 118–21.
54 Meyrier A, Buchet P, Simon P *et al.* Atheromatous renal disease. *Am J Med* 1988; **85:** 139–46.
55 Wilson DM, Salazer TL, Farkouh ME. Eosinophiluria in atheroembolic renal disease. *Am J Med* 1991; **91:** 186–9.
56 Kasinath BS, Lewis EJ. Eosinophilia as a clue to the diagnosis of athroembolic renal disease. *Arch Int Med* 1987; **147:** 1384–5.
57 Seifert PS, Messner M, Roth I, Bhakdi S. Analysis of complement C_3 activation products in human atherosclerosic lesions. *Atherosclerosis* 1991; **91:** 155–62.
58 Hammerschmidt DE, Greenberg CS, Yamada O *et al.* Cholesterol and atheroma lipids activate complement and stimulate granulocytes: a possible mechanism for amplification of ischemic injury in atherosclerotic states. *J Lab Clin Med* 1981; **98:** 68–77.
59 Pierce JR, Wren MV, Cousar JB. Cholesterol embolism: diagnosis antemortem by bone marrow biopsy. *Ann Int Med* 1978; **89:** 937–8.

PART II

Imaging of the Renal Artery

6

Contrast arteriography

J REIDY

Introduction

Despite the considerable developments in non-invasive imaging techniques, contrast arteriography still remains the gold standard for the investigation of renovascular disease. When in the past no effective non-invasive methods of investigation were available and the only definitive treatment was surgery, there was often a tendency among clinicians to not investigate patients aggressively for suspected renal artery stenosis (RAS). Arteriography was then a more invasive procedure with some morbidity. In addition the overall results of surgery were not especially good, particularly in the elderly where there was a significant comorbidity associated particularly with coronary artery disease.[1,2]

Developments with non-invasive imaging as well as with arteriography have considerably improved the diagnostic approach to renovascular disease. Surgical results have also improved. Additionally three other clinical developments have given impetus to the investigation and treatment of renovascular disease and particularly RAS.

Captopril therapy

This angiotensin converting enzyme (ACE) drug is now an established and very effective hypotensive agent and is also used extensively to treat cardiac failure. It is well recognized that when ACE inhibitors are given to patients with RAS, that renal perfusion may be drastically decreased with a consequent deterioration of renal function as discussed in Chapter 17. Thus, many physicians wanting to prescribe captopril for patients need to be reassured that there is no associated RAS.

Renovascular disease as an important cause of renal failure

At one time, renovascular disease was not considered to be an important cause of chronic renal failure. Recently there has been a realization that not only is it a significant cause but that it is potentially a correctable one. In one study where patients over the age of 50 were being assessed for renal replacement therapy, 14% were found to have significant RAS.[3] This is discussed in detail in Chapter 22.

Development of renal angioplasty

In the 15 years since it first became available renal angioplasty has proved to be an effective and relatively low risk method for treating RAS (Chapters 27 and 28). Recently a further and promising development has occurred with availability of intra-arterial metallic stents. As in angioplasty of the legs where risks of the procedure are felt to be very low, there has been a tendency to intervene now at an earlier stage than when surgery might usually be offered.

Incidence of renovascular disease and investigation

Renovascular disease is usually suspected in patients who present with hypertension or chronic renal failure or both. The particular problem here is that both these conditions are common and that true renovascular disease occurs in only a small percentage of the patients. Different figures can be found in the literature as to the incidence of RAS in patients with hypertension, as discussed in Chapter 22, although renovascular disease as a cause for chronic renal failure is much more common than was at one time appreciated. A further problem is that in a number of patients with generalized atheromatous disease, having arteriography for other clinical problems, significant RAS is noted often in the absence of hypertension or renal failure.[2] Several studies have also drawn attention to the common occurrence of RAS at postmortem studies in patients not known to have had hypertension or renal failure during their lifetime. If this incidental finding of RAS is well established so too is the inevitable progression of atheromatous renovascular disease.[3]

Renal artery stenoses become more severe, stenoses develop on the contralateral side and severe stenoses invariably progress to occlusion (Fig. 6.1). Occlusion is then usually associated with loss of renal function and some authors have suggested that intervention in severe RAS, whereas it may not improve renal function, if abnormal, will prevent the inevitable deterioration.[4]

The radiological screening of patients with renal failure and hypertension will vary considerably between different clinicians but will tend to be influenced by the availability and quality of non-invasive investigations that are available, as well as the results obtained with angioplasty and surgery at that center.

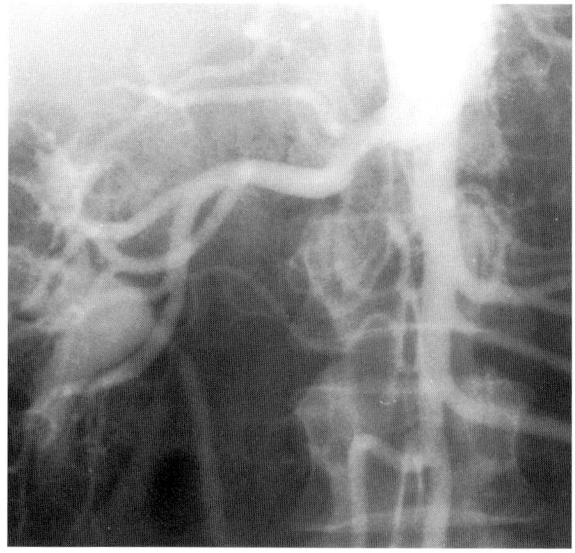

(a)

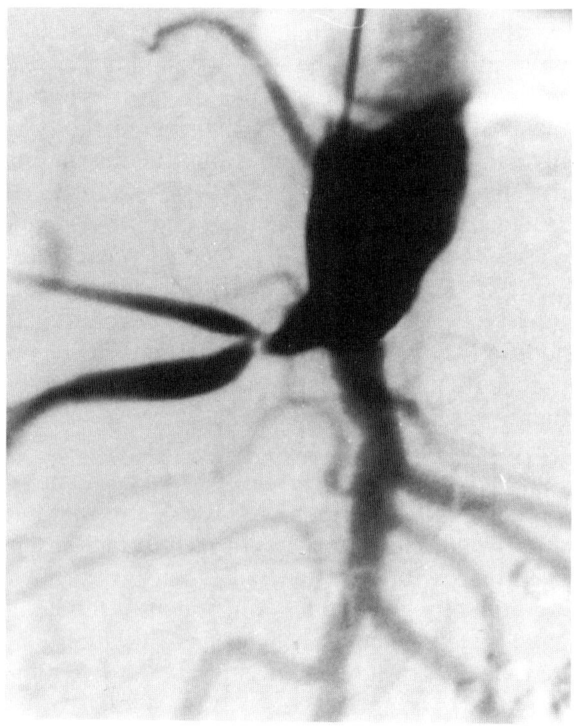

(b)

Figure 6.1. Progression of atheromatous renovascular disease. (a) Aortogram via the brachial approach. Left renal artery occlusion was an incidental finding as this patient had neither hypertension nor renal failure. (b) After 21 months the patient has renal failure. Severe stenosis of the single renal artery is now present.

Radiological screening

Generally, clinicians will screen outpatients who present with hypertension or chronic renal failure who they particularly suspect might have renovascular disease. Non-invasive radiological screening techniques are discussed separately in Chapters 7, 9 and 11. The role they play in any center will very much depend on their availability, the quality of these studies and the enthusiasm of the operators. Some general comments will be made regarding radiological screening which largely relate to our own experience and preferences.

Intravenous urography

We believe this now has no role to play in the investigation of hypertension or chronic renal failure.

Ultrasound

Ultrasound should be an essential part of the non-invasive radiological screen. Occasionally some non-vascular renal pathology may present with hypertension or be detected as an incidental finding. In the absence of any other renal abnormality, a significant difference in the size of the kidneys strongly suggests the presence of RAS. There can however be significant RAS with a normal-sized kidney and both kidneys may be normal or reduced in size in the presence of bilateral disease. Where there is renal asymmetry we believe that the patient should go straight on to arteriography as there is a high degree of suspicion.

Nuclear medicine studies

There is considerable variation in the practical role of isotope studies in different centers. Diethylenetriaminepentaacetric (DTPA) or mercaptoacetyltriglycine (MAG_3) isotope studies are fairly sensitive techniques with captopril DTPA studies giving a higher sensitivity and specificity for RAS. These techniques are discussed in detail in Chapter 15.[5]

Spiral computerized tomography and magnetic resonance imaging

Though some excellent results are being demonstrated for these relatively new techniques, they are not routinely employed. However, it is very likely that these and other non-invasive methods will improve so that intra-arterial procedures will eventually only be performed with a view to proceeding to some intra-arterial intervention. These are discussed in Chapters 7 and 11. Our current approach is to routinely carry out ultrasound and if this demonstrates clearcut asymmetry to proceed with arteriography. If the ultrasound appearances are normal, then nuclear medicine studies may be performed. If this is normal and unless there is a very high degree of suspicion, then arteriography is not requested.

Arteriographic techniques

Prior to the development of digital angiography, arteriography was performed with relatively large (6–7 F) catheters, large volumes of ionic contrast media and conventional X-ray film. This necessitated hospital admission and often before non-ionic contrast media became available, general anesthesia. When digital angiography first became available, there was a tendency to believe that intravenous studies would be adequate and would supersede the intra-arterial approach. However, since the limitations of the intravenous approach have been realized it has in most centers been superseded by intra-arterial digital angiography with small-bore catheters.

Intra-arterial digital angiography

Studies comparing intra-arterial digital angiography with conventional angiography have shown very similar results.[6]

The advantages of digital are such that it must be regarded as the investigation of choice, making it the definitive investigation for renovascular disease. When only film angiography was available, aortography with high flow rates was necessary to achieve good demonstration of the proximal renal arteries. Using 300–370 mg strength contrast media volumes of 40–50 ml with flow rates of 20–25 ml/s were usual. This necessitated larger catheters though subsequently such flow rates became possible with 5 F catheters. Digital angiography has allowed the use of smaller catheters and smaller volumes of more dilute contrast media were then found to be sufficient to obtain adequate studies. Thus using a 4 F catheter a total of 20 ml of 150/300 mg strength contrast medium injected at 10 ml/s was fairly typical.

The facility to use smaller catheters has meant that arteriography can now be satisfactorily performed as an outpatient or day-case procedure with a high degree of safety. It is now standard practice to allow patients a 2 h recovery period following a 4–5 F catheter procedure. Though the detail (spatial resolution) of digital studies will never match that achieved with conventional films, the superior contrast resolution and the subtraction of the bone and soft tissues more than compensates for this. Sometimes even well-opacified proximal renal arteries could be obscured by the presence of the spinal column with conventional film angiograms.

When several injections were needed to demonstrate adequately the renal arteries it is easy to see how the large volumes of contrast medium required led to renal arteriography having such a bad reputation. With digital angiography much smaller volumes of contrast can now be given significantly reducing the risk of postarteriography renal failure.

Even though digital angiography, non-ionic contrast media and smaller catheters have reduced the invasiveness and morbidity of renal aortography, problems related to the puncture site still can occur. This is particularly the case in patients with either hypertension or renal failure, many of whom will be elderly. We have recently changed our arteriographic technique in renovascular disease by using 3 F pigtail catheters and for the majority of patients feel that the results are very satisfactory (Fig. 6.2a).[7] The cross-sectional

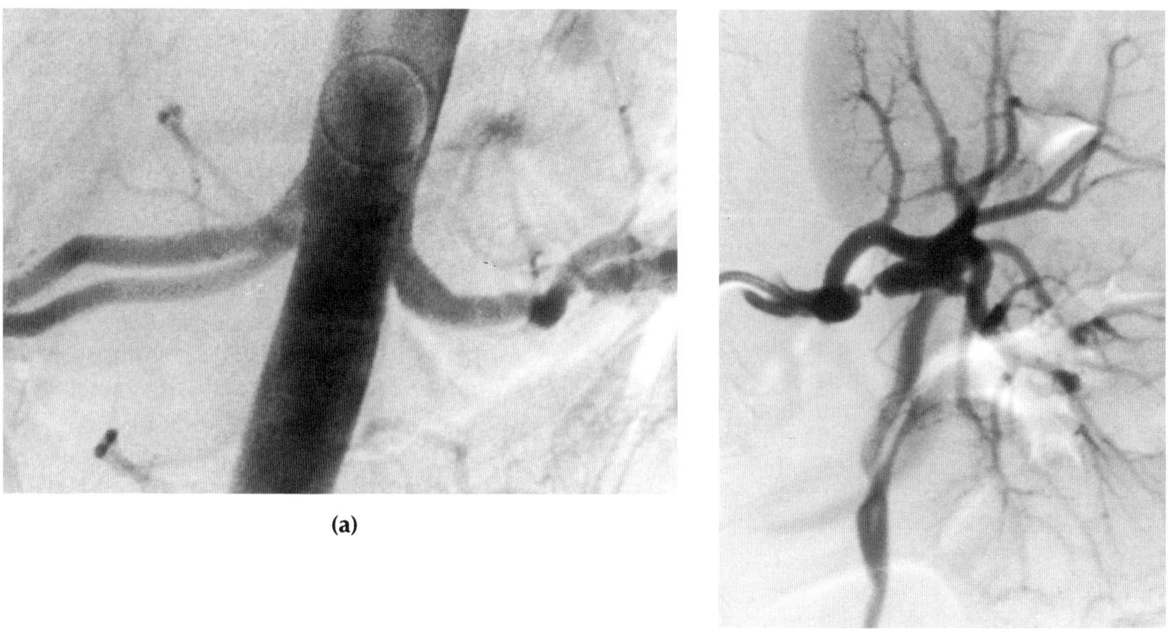

(a) (b)

Figure 6.2. A 21-year-old woman with severe hypertension. Fibromuscular dysplasia. (a) Flush aortogram with a 3 F pigtail catheter shows a good demonstration of the proximal renal arteries with no opacification of the visceral arteries. On the left side the main renal artery appears normal and there is only a suggestion of an abnormality where it bifurcates. (b) The very severe and localized branch stenosis was best demonstrated on this selective injection with 15° caudal angulation. Note the pre- and poststenotic dilatation. This lesion responded well to angioplasty.

area of a 3 F catheter is significantly smaller and only 55% that of the more commonly used 4 F catheter and just one-third that of 5 F catheters. This makes for a much smaller hole in the punctured artery and reduces the invasiveness of the procedure. The limitation of these microcatheters is the flow rate and we use a 12 ml bolus of 300 mg strength non-ionic contrast medium injected at 6 ml/s. Except in very obese patients, careful positioning of the pigtail catheter enables us to demonstrate satisfactorily the proximal renal arteries. We have shown that by using 3 F catheters for renal aortography, intra-arterial procedures have become true outpatient studies. They are simple to use and it is then only necessary to have the patient rest for 30–60 min following the procedure.

Technique of renal aortography

Except very occasionally in children when isolated branch stenoses occur, the major practical concern in patients suspected of having renovascular disease is to define the state of the main renal arteries. In the great majority of cases these are adequately shown with flush aortography.

Not only are selective injections not usually necessary, making the study more complex, but a selective injection into a diseased renal artery may cause dissection and precipitate renal artery occlusion. Sometimes even with optimal flush aortography it is not possible to be certain as to the degree of severity of an RAS, particularly when the lesion is ostial. In this situation a selective ostial injection will show the artery more clearly and will also allow measurement of the intra-arterial pressures across the lesion. Since demonstrating a significant localized stenosis will usually lead on to an angioplasty, a selective injection should only therefore be performed with a view to proceeding to renal angioplasty. A selective injection merely to demonstrate the lesion more clearly may precipitate the development of an occlusion which is a risk with a severe stenosis even without any intervention. The key to the optimal demonstration of the proximal renal arteries in renal aortography is to use a pigtail catheter and to position it properly. If this is positioned too proximally then the superior mesenteric and celiac arteries will opacify and tend to obscure the origins of the renal arteries as well as the distal branches. Alternatively, too distal a catheter placement will result in poor or no opacification of the renal arteries. The positioning of the pigtail tip and the flow rate are both critical to achieving the ideal where the aorta and the renal arteries are well opacified with minimal or no opacification or the superior mesenteric and celiac (Figs 6.2a and 6.3a). The renal arteries usually arise in the region of the lower border of L1 vertebral body and having the pigtail tip just above this level is probably a good initial guide to catheter positioning. With the small volumes of contrast injected with intra-arterial digital angiography it is better to do an injection and then adjust the position if necessary rather than making repeated hand injections and assessing with fluoroscopy. When accessory renal arteries occur they invariably occur more distally so it is extremely unlikely that any renal branches will be missed by not injecting more proximally (Fig. 6.4a). There is no place for using straight catheters with multiple side holes as a jet of contrast is produced above the level of the renal arteries.

Some form of upper abdominal compression is of value in flush renal aortography as it both reduces the bulk of the upper abdomen that is X-rayed and compresses and displaces gas-filled loops of bowel that tend to degrade the digital image. Sometimes even despite careful positioning of the pigtail catheter it is impossible to obtain good filling of the renal arteries without some superior mesenteric opacification. The tendency of the superior mesenteric artery to swing to the left or right of the midline is then likely to obscure the most proximal part of renal arteries. Slightly oblique views, e.g. 20° when the superior left anterior oblique mesenteric artery overlies the proximal left renal artery and right anterior oblique 20° when the proximal superior mesenteric overlies the right renal artery are valuable. The anatomy of the renal arteries is such that the left renal artery usually arises from the posterolateral wall of the aorta and the right renal artery is more anterior (Fig. 6.5).[8]

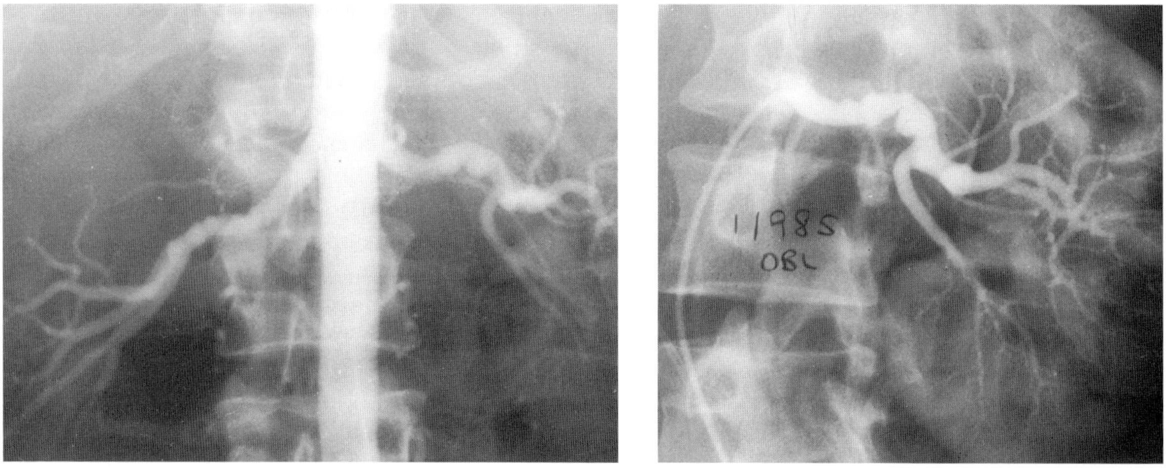

(a) (b)

Figure 6.3. Fibromuscular dysplasia in a 38-year-old woman. (a) This conventional anteroposterior aortogram demonstrates clearly renal arteries with the typical beaded appearance of fibromuscular dysplasia which spares the most proximal renal arteries. No obvious significant stenosis is seen. (b) Selective left renal arteriogram in the right posterior oblique position shows the length of the artery better and indicates clearly a severe focal stenosis involving the distal vessel. This was not evident on the earlier good quality aortogram.

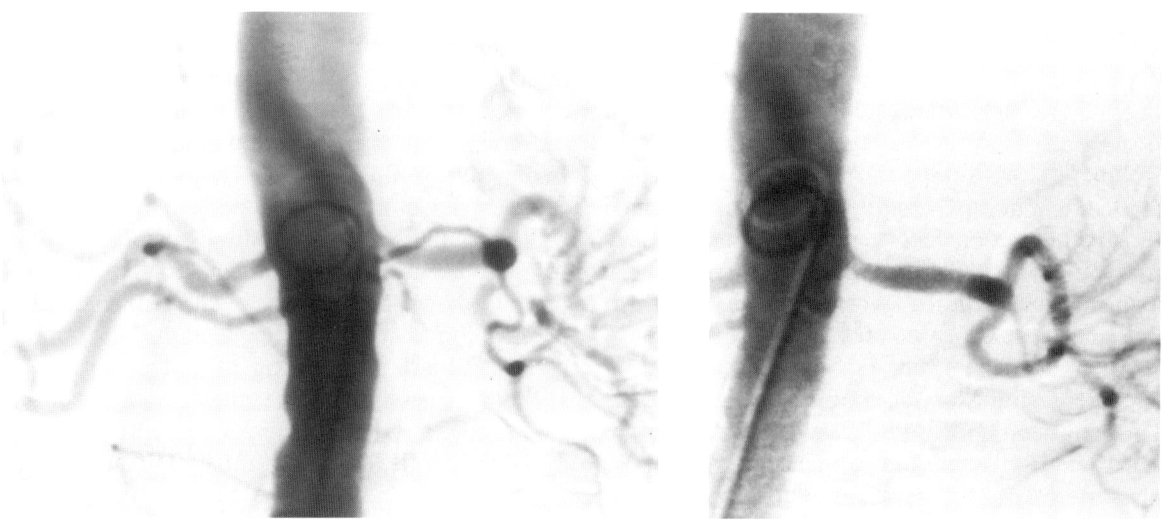

(a) (b)

Figure 6.4. (a). A 65-year-old woman with fibromuscular disease of the right two renal arteries and an atheromatous stenosis on the left. A digital aortogram clearly shows the renal arteries. On the left the proximal renal artery is not seen well and there is an intercostal crossing it. (b). Aortogram in the left anterior oblique (20°) position. The proximal renal artery is much better visualized, but it is still difficult to assess whether the stenosis is significant. The patient had further arteriography with a view to angioplasty. This was performed when a 50 mmHg gradient was demonstrated across the lesion.

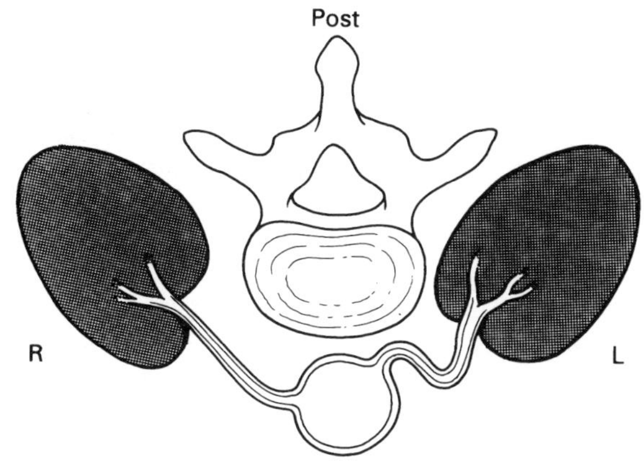

Figure 6.5. This shows the most common arrangement of the renal arteries and their relationship to the aorta. Note how the left renal artery arises posterolaterally. Thus a left anterior oblique (20°) view will profile the origin best.

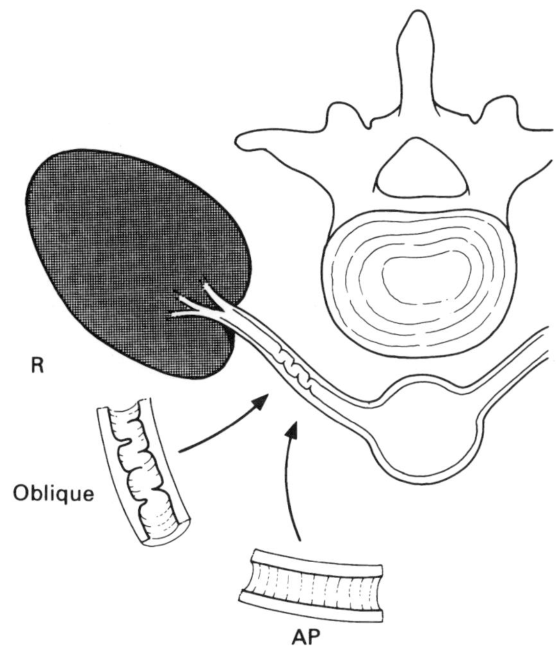

Figure 6.6. Diagramatic representation of fibromuscular dysplasia. On the anteroposterior view the dilated segments of the artery will tend to overlap the web-like stenoses. To demonstrate these to advantage a selective injection with an oblique view is necessary.

Thus a lesion at the ostium on the left or very close to it may be missed on an aortogram in the anteroposterior plane as the most proximal part of the artery is obscured by the opacified aorta (Figs 6.4 and 6.5). A left anterior oblique (usually 20°) will profile the origin of the artery and demonstrate any ostial stenosis (Fig. 6.4).[8, 9] It may be particularly difficult to demonstrate or exclude ostial disease in older patients with renal failure where there is poor opacification of the renal arteries due to poor renal perfusion. Several injections with magnification views may be necessary before optimal images are obtained. Occasionally cranial or caudal views can be valuable when a renal artery is overlapped by another renal artery or any other vessel (e.g. intercostal).[10]

Even a small angulation (e.g 10°) may separate arteries and uncover a hidden stenosis (Fig. 6.2).

A particular problem may occur in patients with fibromuscular dysplasia when the typical beaded appearances of the artery are present. This condition affects the more distal renal artery when it is coursing posteriorly as well as laterally. Thus on an anteroposterior view, the dilated segments may overlap each other and obscure the web-like stances between them (Figs 6.6 and 6.3).[8]

Such stenoses will be best seen with selective injections into the renal artery while they can be easily missed on an intravenous study.[11] Thus the best views to demonstrate the left renal artery would be a left anterior oblique and a right anterior oblique for the right renal artery (Figs 6.6 and 6.3).

Intravenous digital angiography

This has been advocated as a very safe outpatient angiographic examination that can adequately demonstrate the main renal arteries.[11]

In young patients, with good radiographic technique the renal arteries can be visualized well but there is always going to be overlying opacification of the visceral arteries. Often in older patients and those with cardiac and renal dysfunction, poor quality studies are obtained. Repeated bolus injections (25–40 ml) involve large overall volumes of contrast being given and there can never be as good an opacification of the renal arteries and kidneys as with intra-arterial studies. As has already been detailed fibromuscular dysplasia presents particular problems for intravenous digital angiography and there is a real tendency for it to underscore the severity of the disease.[5, 11]

As increasingly older patients are being evaluated for the presence of renovascular disease, many centers are now preferring the more definitive intra-arterial study. We believe that this development of small catheter outpatient arteriography has reduced intravenous angiography to a very limited role.

Problems in assessing severity of renal artery stenosis

Most often with good quality intra-arterial digital aortography it is possible to demonstrate either a severe localized stenosis or to exclude firmly the presence of a significant lesion. Occasionally, however, a stenosis is seen that despite further, more detailed views, still presents a problem regarding the assessment of its severity (Fig. 6.4). Assessing the reduction of the cross-sectional lumen of an artery, even when the stenosis is regular and concentric is difficult enough when measurements rely on a single imaging plane.[12]

Thus when a lesion is eccentric and irregular it presents far greater problems. Even in critical arteries such as the coronaries, when multiple oblique and angled views are routinely obtained, it is well established that arteriography is far from being the true gold standard.

Furthermore, attempts to improve the accuracy with digital computerized stenosis assessment and other measurements have not proved to be clinically useful.[12] With renal aortography a much more limited range of oblique and angled views are possible compared with coronary arteriography.

Our approach with moderately severe or 50% stenoses is to have the patient assessed clinically with a view to proceeding to angioplasty if further arteriography demonstrates that the stenoses is clearly significant. The patient is consented for selective arteriography with a view to proceeding to angioplasty if necessary.

Using the previous renal aortogram as a guide, the ostium of the renal artery is carefully catheterized with a 4–5 F cobra catheter (with two sideholes) or a sidewinder 1 catheter if the proximal renal artery points downwards. Initially with a catheter sitting in the ostium a selective renal arteriogram is carried out which may in itself clarify whether the stenosis is significant or not. If there is still doubt then intra-arterial pressures need to be measured (Fig. 6.4), the tip of the catheter is passed into the distal renal artery and then, while taking a continuous pressure recording, it is pulled back into the aorta. If no gradient is demonstrated then the stenosis/lesion is judged not to be significant and no angioplasty is necessary.

If a gradient greater than 15 mmHg or 10% of the systolic pressure is demonstrated then there is a good indication for proceeding to angioplasty. We do not, along with many others, believe that measurement of renal vein renins add to the decision whether to dilate a stenosis or not.[13]

Angiographic appearances in renovascular disease

Atheroma

Atheroma is a generalized disorder so that when it affects the renal arteries it is likely that other arteries will be also involved. Patients may present with hypertension or renal failure but significant renovascular disease is noted quite commonly in patients having aortography for other clinical problems.[2] Usually this occurs in peripheral vascular disease or in the assessment of abdominal aortic aneurysms. When such incidental but severe renovascular disease is discovered this presents a problem of management, as it is also well established that atheromatous renovascular disease invariably progresses.[3] When an RAS progresses and ultimately occludes, it is very likely that there will be a significant and irreversible loss of function of that kidney. Thus when a severe RAS is detected there is some urgency if a decision to treat has been made.

The association of vascular disease elsewhere may present practical problems. Major aortoiliac disease may make arterial access from either femoral artery difficult or impossible (Fig. 6.1). In this situation either intravenous digital angiography (with its inherent limitations) or an arterial approach via the brachial artery are necessary. When significant RAS that might be suitable for angioplasty has been demonstrated, views of the iliacs should be obtained, particularly in older patients and in arteriopaths, as very tortuous or diseased iliac arteries may either make one side more difficult for angioplasty access or demonstrate that the femoral approach is not really practical. Occasionally renal aortography will demonstrate an abdominal aortic aneurysm which will need treatment as a priority.

Atheromatous disease invariably affects the proximal third of the renal arteries when there is a short length of normal artery (Fig. 6.1b). Sometimes the stenosis involves the origin when it is described as ostial, but there is no clearcut distinction between an ostial lesion and a very proximal stenosis (Fig. 6.7). In ostial disease more extensive aortic disease is usually present (Fig. 6.8). The aorta shows irregularity and may be dilated (Fig. 6.9a). Assessing the severity of a stenosis is not always easy so that in doubtful cases careful selective injections and measurements of the intra-arterial pressures across the lesion are necessary. Stenoses may be smooth and symmetrical, or eccentric and asymmetric. A severe stenosis may not be so apparent when there is an irregular stenosis with endolumenal plaque (Fig. 6.4). Poststenotic dilatation may be present, but this is not a good indicator of the severity of the disease. Others have suggested that renal vein renin measurements are useful to resolve whether angioplasty is indicated when the severity of a lesion is equivocal.

In addition to optimally visualizing the main renal artery it is important to look beyond this and to assess the distal renal artery, the nephrogram and the overall size of the kidney. Usually preliminary ultrasound will have sized the kidneys. When the kidney is small (usually < 8 cm) revascularization is not felt likely to be benefi-

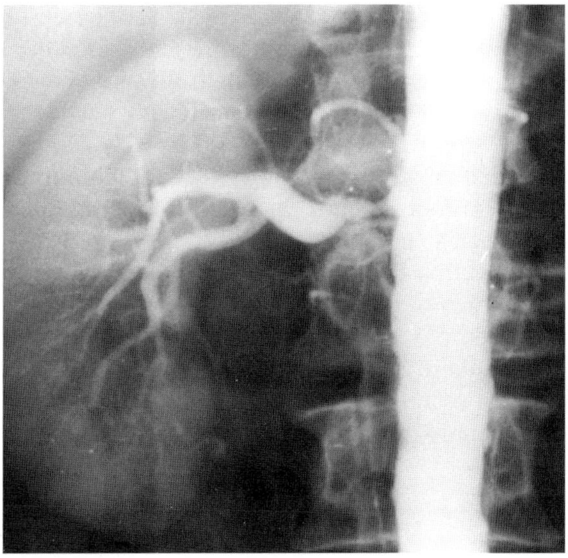

Figure 6.7. Arteriopathic 65-year-old man with renal failure. This aortogram shows occlusion of the left renal artery with no evidence of any stump. There is a very severe stenosis of a single renal artery on the right, which is very proximal and probably ostial.

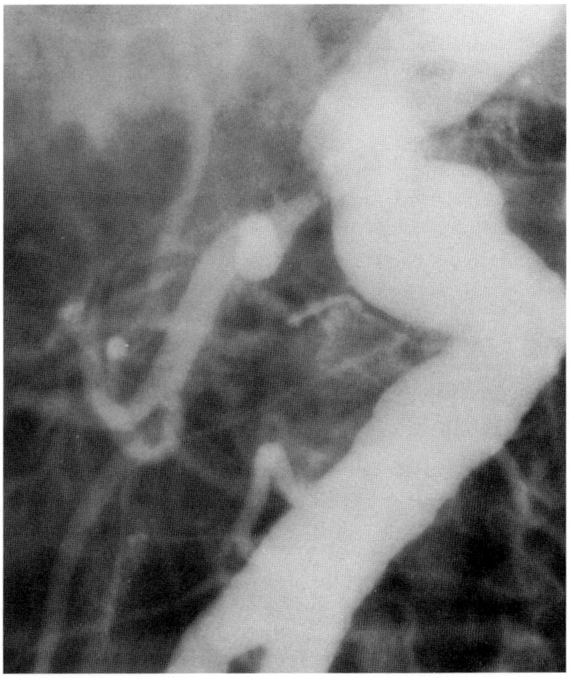

Figure 6.8. There is severe aortic disease with no sign of any left renal artery or kidney. The severe ostial stenosis on the right side proved very difficult to demonstrate and was only seen clearly on this right posterior oblique view.

cial. Thus small and tortuous distal arteries associated with a poor nephrogram are not good predictors for a successful result from angioplasty or surgery. Contrast this with an occlusion where the distal arteries are usually poorly opacified (Fig. 6.9). If, however, a nephrogram shows a good-sized kidney and other imaging (e.g. nuclear medicine) shows there is a reasonable function this then argues the case for some form of revascularization.

Sometimes in the presence of diffuse aortic disease there does not appear to be a full complement of renal branches and there an incomplete nephrogram. This may indicate that one or more accessory renal arteries (usually arising from the lower abdominal aorta) have occluded which is always more difficult to appreciate when there is no residual stump.

Fibromuscular dysplasia

This heterogeneous group of conditions has previously been classified into various types based

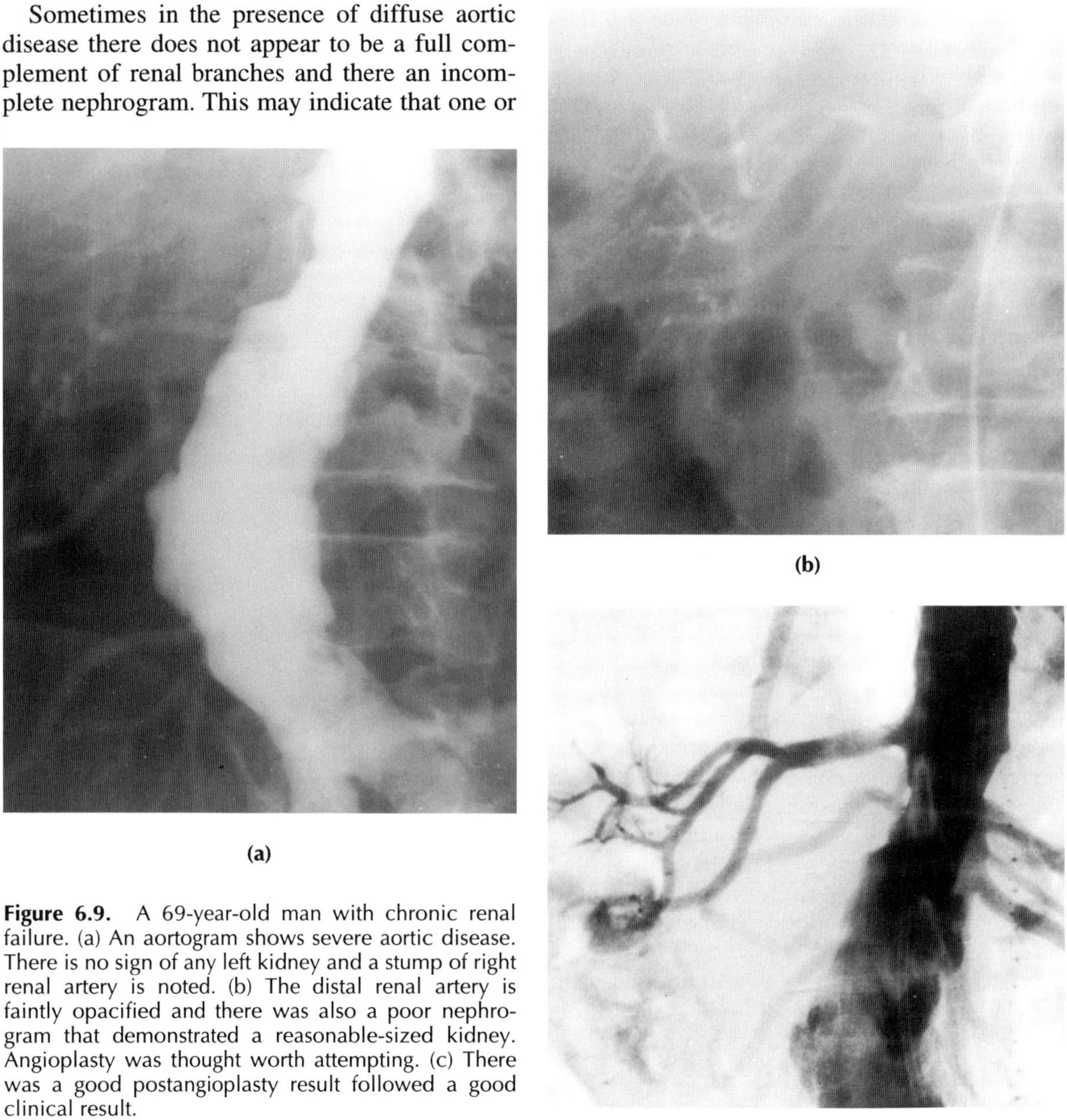

(a)

(b)

(c)

Figure 6.9. A 69-year-old man with chronic renal failure. (a) An aortogram shows severe aortic disease. There is no sign of any left kidney and a stump of right renal artery is noted. (b) The distal renal artery is faintly opacified and there was also a poor nephrogram that demonstrated a reasonable-sized kidney. Angioplasty was thought worth attempting. (c) There was a good postangioplasty result followed a good clinical result.

on the histological appearances which have been correlated with the angiographic findings as discussed in Chapter 2. In practice pathology is very rarely available so that the diagnosis is usually based on clinical and angiographic findings. Typically patients, most commonly young women, present with hypertension with no specific clinical features.

Fibromuscular disease (FMD) is occasionally seen as an incidental finding in renal donor arteriography.[14] Thus the classification of FMD is largely based on the angiographic appearances.

The most common form of FMD is medial fibroplasia when there is the typical 'string of beads' angiographic appearance (Figs. 6.3 and 6.10).

This is produced by multiple ring-like stenoses, separated by segments of dilated artery that can progress to aneurysms. The most proximal part of the renal arteries is usually spared with the distal arteries being affected and sometimes the major branches. Segmental renal artery stenosis has been described in 30–56% of patients when it is usually at the origin of major segmental branches.[15] Commonly FMD is bilateral and if there are multiple renal arteries they can all be affected. The aorta is spared but other major arteries, particularly the external iliac and carotids can be involved. In contradistinction to atheromatous RAS, non-atheromatous disease is not felt to be progressive unless seen in the early stages of disease. Others, however, have suggested that FMD can be progressive.[16, 17] As already described, the localized dilatations adjacent to the stenoses may obscure them so that the severity of the disease is underscored. Fibromuscular dysplasia can be easily missed with intravenous digital angiography and on poor quality arterial studies.[11]

The characteristic appearances in medial fibroplasia must be distinguished from the other types of FMD – intimal fibroplasia, fibromuscular hyperplasia and subadventitial fibroplasia. Here the angiographic appearances are similar with smooth segmental stenoses (Figs. 6.2 and 11). These lesions are more commonly unilateral and can involve the more proximal renal artery (Fig. 6.11). They are often symmetrical and associated with poststenotic dilatation.

There is some practical importance in distinguishing the more common medial fibroplasia from the other types of FMD. Medial fibroplasia with the typical beaded appearance dilates easily at lower pressures and excellent long-term results are obtained with angioplasty. This is in contrast to the other types where the smooth segmental stenoses do not always dilate satisfactorily, where they may be resistant to even high pressure balloon dilatation and when the clinical results are not so good.

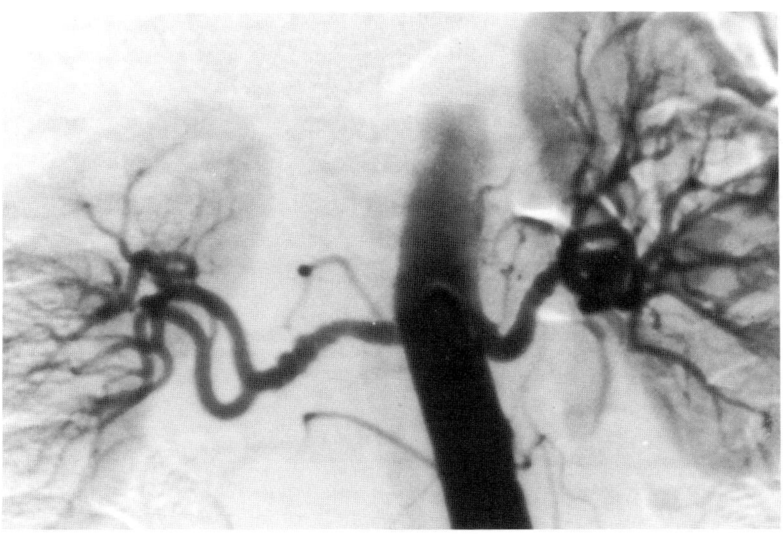

Figure 6.10. Typical appearances of fibromuscular dysplasia. The most proximal renal artery spared and the 'string of beads' sign is seen affecting both renal arteries.

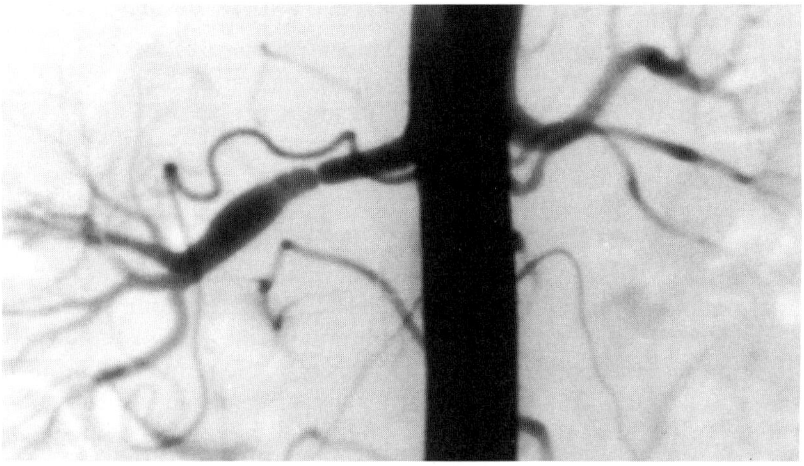

Figure 6.11. A 25-year-old woman with severe hypertension. The digital flush aortogram shows a severe and focal stenosis of the right renal artery. This was associated with poststenotic dilatation. This dilated satisfactorily with a good clinical result.

Takayasu's disease

Most commonly this occurs in younger patients from South-East Asia and India.[18] Classically it occurs with associated clinical features but it may present with no obvious antecedent illness. As its other name of aortoarteritis suggests, aortic disease is essential to the diagnosis and may consist of diffuse or focal stenotic disease, occlusion or a fusiform abdominal aortic aneurysm most commonly infrarenal (Fig. 6.12). All the major abdominal arteries may be involved but the renal arteries are most commonly affected with severe ostial stenoses being typical. In a recent angiographic survey of 110 patients with aortoarteritis the renal arteries were involved in 68, being bilateral in 37.[18] The abdominal aneurysms present can involve the renal origins and rarely the renal arteries are involved directly. Sometimes these appearances are seen in patients from outside the Indian subcontinent and South-East Asia, with no history of any systemic illness and the angiographic appearances may be identical.

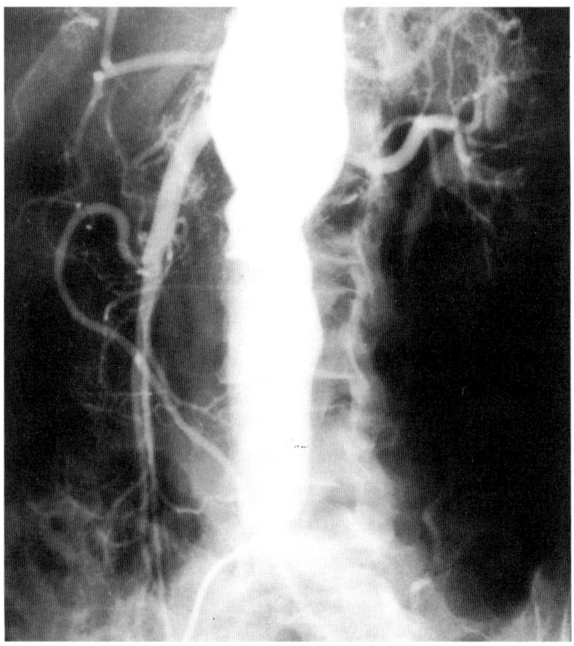

Figure 6.12. A 48-year-old Indian woman with burnt-out Takayasu's disease. This aortogram shows aneurysmal dilatation of the abdominal aorta in the region of and above the renal arteries. The distal abdominal aorta is grossly abnormal. The right renal artery is occluded and there is a severe stenosis involving the left renal artery.

Renal artery stenosis in children

Renal artery stenosis is uncommon in children although a relatively high incidence (4–20%) is found in children being investigated in hospital practice.[19, 20] A greater range of causes is found in children compared with adults. Whereas some authors have classified RAS histologically,[19] others have used the location and length of the stenosis.[21] Our approach has been to use a clinicoangiographic approach. This accepts that there are no sharp divisions between the different causes. Fibromuscular dysplasia with typical angiographic appearances occurs and very rarely isolated focal RAS is seen with appearances of the less common forms of fibromuscular dysplasia. Branch renal artery stenosis is more common in children, usually associated with RAS of the main artery.[15] Occasionally it may cause difficulties when it is present in isolation and will only then be detected by a good selective renal arteriogram. Usually then a nuclear medicine study will suggest the presence of focal renovascular disease. When severe aortic stenosis presents in children, invariably with severe proximal RAS and often visceral artery stenoses, the condition has been called middle aortic syndrome[22] (Fig. 6.13). A lateral aortogram is important to demonstrate the most proximal part of the celiac and superior mesenteric arteries. There is no clearcut separation of this condition from non-active Takayasu's disease associated with severe stenosis. However, in middle aortic syndrome, the patients are younger, there is no evidence of an acute arteritis and the disease appears to arrest at puberty.[22] The middle aortic syndrome abnormality is sometimes seen when it is associated with Williams' syndrome.[19] Finally there is a clear association with neurofibromatosis and RAS which may be bilateral and may also be associated with some aortic disease.[23]

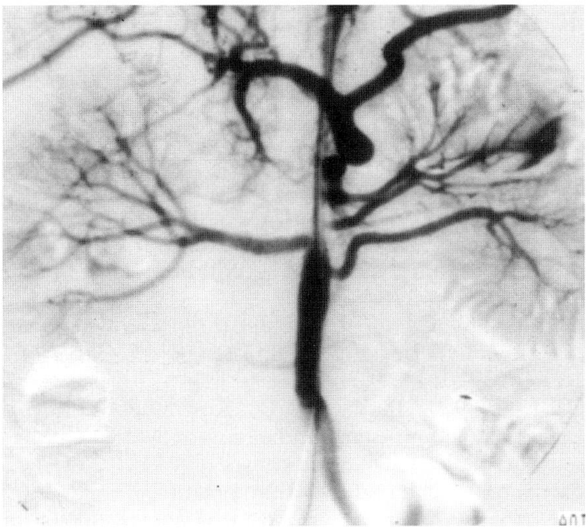

Figure 6.13. Middle aortic syndrome. Note the tubular stenosis involving most of the abdominal aorta. There are multiple renal arteries that are stenosed. The superior mesenteric artery is also severely stenosed.

Renal artery aneurysm

These are rare and usually affect the distal renal artery and at the hilum of the kidney. They are often asymptomatic and may be first detected on a plain film of the abdomen that has demonstrated curvilinear calcification. Multiple views with selective injections may be necessary to show the detailed arterial anatomy that is required before surgery can be considered. Assessment of the aneurysm size is important when indications for treatment are assessed and the neck of the aneurysm is important if new treatments such as transcatheter embolization are to be considered.

Renal artery embolism

This is rarely seen and investigated in the acute phase. When the whole of the renal artery is occluded, it may not be possible to distinguish this from occlusion of a severely diseased renal artery. Usually there will be a short proximal stump of renal artery but this may not be present. There may be very poor demonstration of the distal renal arteries with only a faint nephrogram. The clinical circumstances should then suggest the diagnosis. It is more likely that clearcut embolism will be detected when embolus affects a smaller branch of the renal artery rather than the main stem when an occlusion with a sharp cut-off will be seen (Fig. 6.14).

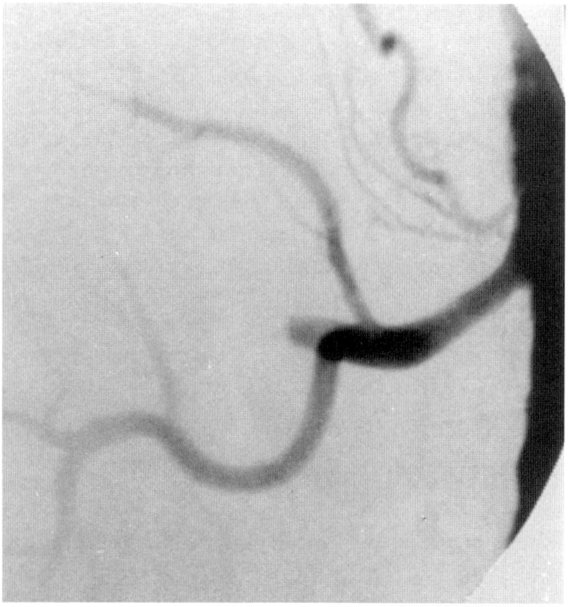

Figure 6.14. Renal artery embolism. On an earlier aortogram the whole of the right renal artery was demonstrated. On this subsequent study the middle branch is occluded with a sharp cut-off. These appearances are typical of embolism.

References

1 Scoble JE, Maher ER, Hamilton G. Atherosclerotic renovascular disease causing renal impairment—a case for treatment. *Clin Nephrol* 1989; **31:** 119–22.

2 Wilms GE, Marchal G, Peene P, Baert AL. The angiographic incidence of renal artery stenosis in the arteriosclerotic population. *Eur J Radiol* 1990; **10:**195–7.

3 Zierler RE, Bergelin RO, Issalson JA *et al.* Natural history of atherosclerotic renal artery stenosis: a prospective study with duplex ultrasonography. *J Vasc Surg* 1993; **19:** 250–8.

4 Pattynama PM, Becker GJ, Brown J *et al.* Percutaneous angioplasty for atherosclerotic renal artery disease: effect on renal function in Azotaemic patients. *Cardiovasc Intervent Radiol* 1994; **17:** 143–6.

5 Mann SJ, Pickering G. Detection of renovascular hypertension. State of the art. *Ann Int Med* 1992; **117:** 845–53.

6 Kim D, Porter DH, Brown R *et al.* Renal artery imaging: a prospective comparison of intra-arterial digital. *Angiology* 1991; **42:** 345–57.

7 Reidy JF, Ludman C. Technical note: the safety of outpatient arteriography using 3F catheters. *Br J Radiol* 1993; **66:** 1048–9.

8 Dean RH, Burko H, Wilson JP *et al.* Deceptive patterns of renal artery stenosis. *Surgery* 1974; **76:** 872–81.

9 Gerlock AJ, Goncharenko V, Oplis M, Sloan RT. Right posterior oblique: the projection of choice in aortography of hypertensive patients. *Radiology* 1978; **127:** 45–8.

10 Harrington DP, Levin DC, Garnic JC *et al.* Compound angulation for the angiographic evaluation of renal artery stenosis. *Radiology* 1983; **146:** 829–31.

11 Wilms GE, Baert AL, Staesson JA, Amery AK. Renal artery stenosis: evaluation with intravenous digital subtraction angiography. *Radiology* 1986; **160:** 713–15.

12 Chong WK, Raphael MJ. The significance of haemodynamic significance: I General considerations. *J Intervent Radiol* 1972; **7:** 55–63.

13 Roubidoux MA, Dunnick NR, Klotman PE *et al.* Renal vein renins: inability to predict response to revascularisation in patients with hypertension. *Radiology* 1991; **178:** 819–22.

14 Cragg AH, Smith TP, Thompson BH *et al.* Incidental fibromuscular dysplasia in potential renal donors: long-term clinical follow-up. *Radiology* 1989; **172:** 145–7.

15 Cluzel P, Raynaud A, Beyssen B *et al.* Stenoses of renal branch arteries in fibromuscular dysplasia: results of percutaneous transluminal angioplasty. *Radiology* 1994; **193:** 227–32.

16 Lorelius LE, Hemmingson A, Hagg A *et al.* Progressive fibromuscular dysplasia of the renal artery. Angiographic and clinical follow up. *Acta Radiol* 1985; **26:** 705–8.

17 Goncharenko V, Gerlock AJ, Shaff MI, Hollifield JW. Progression of renal artery artery fibromuscular dysplasia in 42 patients as seen on angiography. *Radiology* 1981; **139:** 45–51.

18 Mandalam KR, Joseph S, Rao VR *et al.* Aortoarteritis of abdominal aorta: an angiographic profile in 110 patients. *Clin Radiol* 1993; **48:** 29–34.

19 Robinson L, Gedroyc W, Reidy J, Saxton H. Renal artery stenosis in children. *Clin Radiol* 1991; **44:** 376–82.

20 Stanley JC. Renal vascular disease and renovascular hypertension in children. *Urol Clin North Am* 1984; **11:** 451–63.

21 Mali WP, Puijlaert CB, Kowenberg J *et al.* Percutaneous transluminal angioplasty in children and adolescents. *Radiology* 1987; **165:** 391–4.

22 Sumboonnanonda A, Robinson BL, Gedroyc WM *et al.* Middle aortic syndrome: clinical and radiological findings. *Arch Dis Child* 1992; **67:** 501–5.

23 Greene JF, Fitzwater J, Burgess J. Arterial lesions associated with neurofibromatosis. *Am J Clin Pathol* 1924; **62:** 481–7.

7

Magnetic resonance angiography of the renal arteries

W GEDROYC

Introduction

Renal arterial disease is increasingly recognized as an important cause of renal dysfunction.[1] The association between renal artery stenosis and hypertension has been documented for many years but the importance of renal artery stenosis as a cause of renal failure has been underemphasized in the literature until the last few years. The capability of minimally invasive therapeutic maneuvers such as angioplasty, percutaneous metallic stent placement coupled with improving surgical techniques, allow substantial improvement and preservation of renal function,[2, 3] so that patients who would in the past have required renal replacement/dialysis at a relatively earlier stage may now be successfully maintained in many instances by their native function alone.

Intra-arterial angiography (digital subtraction angiography [DSA] or conventional cut-film) remains the currently accepted gold standard for the diagnosis of renal artery stenosis (RAS). All other methods are currently compared against this so-called gold standard despite the fact that this technique is relatively invasive and requires an inpatient stay. Alternative methods for the diagnosis of RAS all have major drawbacks. High levels of operator skill, bowel gas interference, etc. in ultrasound Doppler studies and poor reproducibility between institutions have been major hindrances in the development of viable alternative techniques to intra-arterial DSA. In view of this, there is a clear need for a sensitive and specific test for the diagnosis of RAS to reduce the amount of negative conventional angiograms that are performed.

Magnetic resonance angiography (MRA) has the potential to fill this need. It is entirely non-invasive and operator independent, and in comparison with the various ultrasound and nuclear medicine techniques, produces images of renal arteries that are immediately recognizable to all physicians as familiar anatomic structures allowing a substantial amount of ready acceptance of this technique.

Principles of magnetic resonance angiography (simplified)

The details of the physics of MRA are complex and difficult. A comprehensive grasp of these principles is not necessary for standard clinical practice, but a knowledge of the available options and how these options can be utilized to provide the best image possible is desirable. In addition, a more detailed knowledge of the strong points and disadvantages of the individual techniques, plus an ability to interpret the artifacts that each technique produces, is important.

The following section attempts to cover these points in a simplified fashion.

The two main conventional MRA bright blood techniques are time of flight (TOF) sequences and phase contrast sequences. Each of these sequences may require either a two-dimensional (2D) acquisition, exciting one slice at a time, or a three-dimensional (3D) volume where a whole volumetric slab of tissue is excited at the same time. A further dynamic gadolinium-enhanced technique has recently been described and this will be described in brief detail at the end of this section.

Time of flight

All MRA sequences are based on gradient echo, low flip angle scans. In these scan sequences flowing blood produces a high signal as it enters the imaging volume. This effect is called flow-related enhancement. A high signal, however, is only produced by the flowing blood if the spins are fully unmagnetized and unsaturated as regards radio frequency pulses. Saturation pulses in fact can be used in conjunction with these sequences to null the signal from inflowing blood in a particular direction allowing selective venous or arterial studies to be obtained, as required. The areas of high signal on individual axial slices in a 2D acquisition are conformed into a volume covering the imaged area. The background which does not image brightly in these sequences is subtracted and the resultant high signal areas are reformatted into angiographic-like structures using a reconstructive algorithm which is usually the maximum intensity projection (MIP). Maximum intensity projection techniques pass rays through the stack of images and pick out the bright areas and conform them into a 3D representation of the vasculature within that area. These rays are usually projected at 10° increments so that 18 views give a full 180° of rotation. The resultant projections can either be viewed as still images with 10° increments between each image, or as a cine loop to give a 3D impression with apparent movement of the vasculature as if one were looking around the arterial structures from one extreme lateral to the other. The MIP algorithm is used in most MRA sequences.

Flow-related enhancement and therefore brightness of signal is maximized by using thin axial sections at right angles to the direction of blood flow. One of the main drawbacks of TOF angiography is the loss of signal encountered in 'in plane' flow situations. An example of this is a tortuous kinked artery which may show signal loss in portions of the artery that are parallel to the axis of the slice.

Three-dimensional TOF sequences have much better spatial resolution than 2D TOF sequences but can usually only cover a relatively small volume of tissue at any one site thus restricting the area imaged, making this a difficult technique to apply to the abdomen.

Time of flight sequences have been used to image renal arteries but results are very mixed and reports directly comparing TOF and 3D phase contrast studies (see below) have shown that the latter are much more sensitive for diagnosing RAS.

Phase contrast

This technique is based on the phenomenon that moving spins such as flowing blood develop a phase shift as they pass through the imaging volume and are bombarded by radio frequency pulses in the magnetic field. Stationary tissues do not undergo any phase shift and therefore flowing blood can be easily differentiated from stationary tissue. A further refinement of this technique is that the brightness of the signal produced is proportional to the velocity of the blood because the faster the blood flows within the imaging volume, the greater the phase shift developed and the amount of phase shift is directly proportional to the brightness of signal. The amount of phase shift produced by flowing blood in this sequence can be used quantitatively to measure velocity and also flow, if vessel cross-sectional area is known.[4]

Every phase contrast study that is carried out must have a calibration or velocity encoding rate (VENC) set prior to starting the examination. The value of this should approximately be equal to the mean peak average flow of the blood being imaged. If the blood velocity in the area imaged is significantly greater or less than the VENC rate set, artifactual signal loss may be seen confusing interpretation. The main difficulty with setting an appropriate VENC rate is that the flow velocity is obviously changed by the underlying pathological conditions. When the investigator sets the VENC rate the true extent or presence of an underlying pathological condition is usually not entirely clear and as a result an inappropriate value may be used causing slightly more confusion. Fortunately, the latitude within this area seems to be rather more than was initially anticipated and this rarely causes a substantial diagnostic problem. An example of an area in which this may cause some difficulty in interpretation is a near occlusion. The flow beyond this may be extremely turbulent and variable, some of it quite slow and a relatively high VENC rate may preclude any of the signal being properly imaged, falsely giving the impression of complete occlusion rather than a severe stenosis.

Phase contrast studies provide excellent background suppression and a very high vascular signal. They do not suffer from problems of loss of signal due to 'in plane' flow as is seen with 2D TOF in particular. In our experience 3D phase contrast provides substantially superior images of both native and transplant renal arteries than TOF sequences. Usually the very best TOF sequences can only image the origins of the renal arteries plus their proximal 1–2 cm. The 3D phase contrast studies consistently image all of the renal artery, at least to the hilum and often beyond in normal patients (Figs 7.1, 7.2 and 7.3). Renal arteries are often tortuous both at their origins and more peripherally and the experience of the group at our hospital is that phase contrast MRA copes with imaging these tortuous relatively small vessels much more successfully and consistently than does TOF. As a result we have abandoned using TOF in this area.

Technique

The technical factors that are set for a routine MRA study using phase contrast arteriography by either native or transplant arteries are as follows.

1 3D phase contrast study.
2 TR33, TE 7.3.
3 Flip angle 20°.
4 Saturation bands placed immediately below the imaging volume. The saturation bands are used to null the signal within the imaging volume from the inferior vena cava and portal vein. Often this is not completely successful in the portal vein because venous return from within the imaging volume will provide some portal vein signal causing some confusion since the portal vein is projected in front of the renal arteries and may obscure them. The 3D nature of the study, however, usually allows one largely to separate the portal vein from the arterial structures. Occasionally, very fast renal vein flow may cause problems and some investigators recommend placing the saturation bands over the peripheral margins of the kidneys laterally to try and diminish this flow. The disadvantage of this is that if the saturation bands are not placed absolutely correctly they may null some arterial flow and also increase the length of the study acquisition. We have not routinely used this approach.
5 Abdominal compression is applied to try and diminish the amount of respiration movement.
6 256×128 matrix is used.

Using the above parameters, a standard study takes 18 min to acquire. The time taken to reconstruct such a study varies depending on the computer power available but on the most modern systems will take 2 min of console down time for the images to be reconstructed.

The 3D phase contrast volume is centered over the expected sites of the renal artery origins. These are usually at the level of approximately L1/2 intervertebral disk native kidneys. When transplant kidneys are examined, the exact position of the transplant artery is much more variable, and depends on the exact site the surgeon has carried out the anastomosis. This is often not known precisely before the patient is examined in the MRI unit, so it is not uncommon for a few studies to be repeated because the renal artery has been partially missed if it has an unusually low or high anasatomosis. Similarly, native artery studies are occasionally repeated because renal arteries may be missed if they are unusually placed. Multiple arteries within the

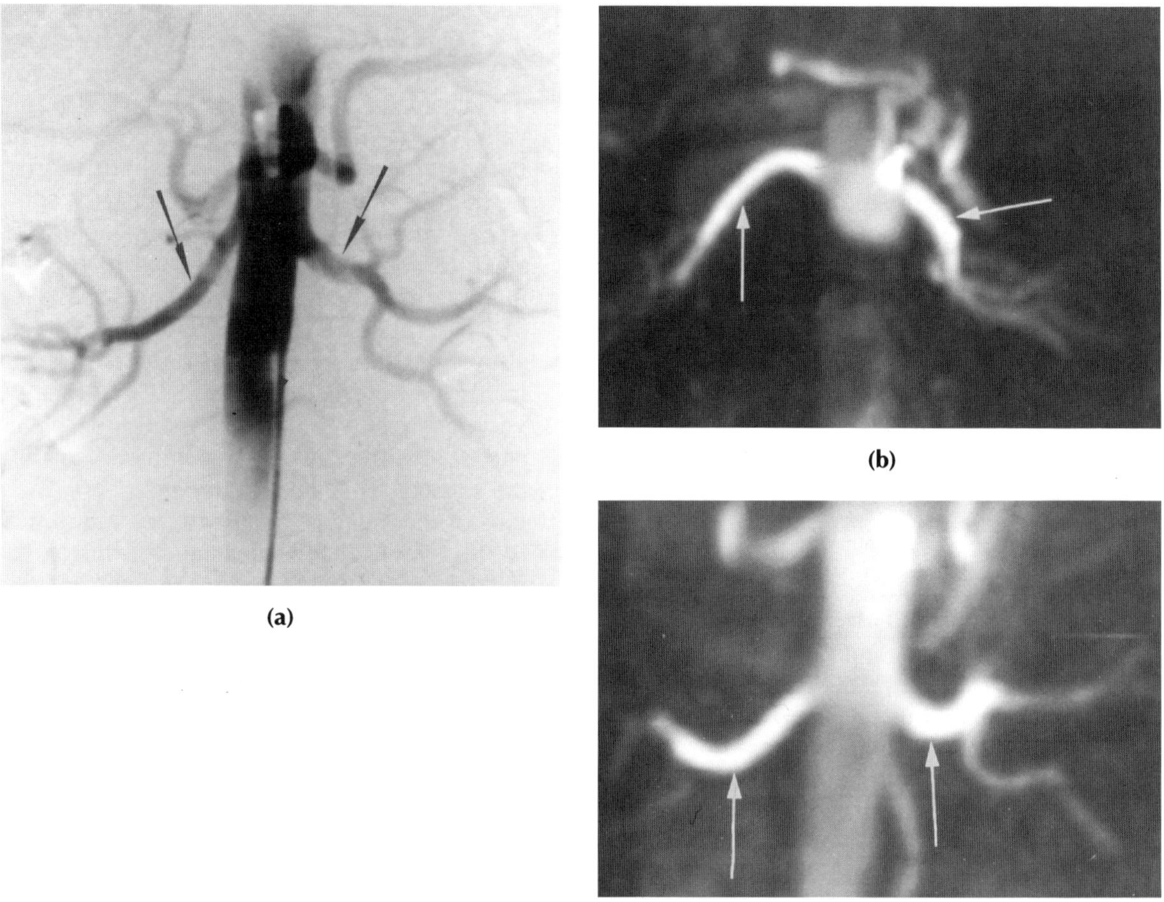

(a) (b) (c)

Figure 7.1. Normal renal arteries. (a) Intra-arterial DSA showing normal renal arteries (black arrows). (b, c) Axial and coronal projections from the MRA study showing normal renal arteries. Note normal signal throughout the length of renal arteries to and beyond the renal hila indicating normal study.

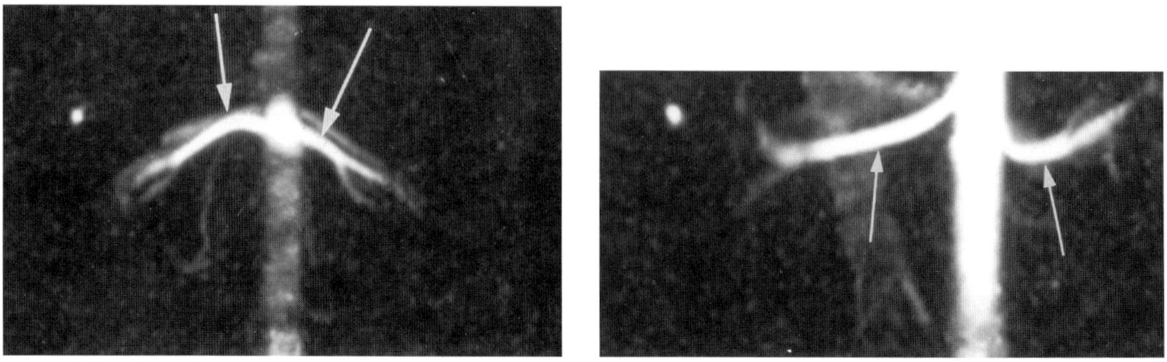

(a) (b)

Figure 7.2. Normal renal arteries. (a) An axial collapsed projection showing uniform homogeneous signal in both renal arteries (white arrows). (b) Coronal projection from MRA study showing homogeneous signal in both renal arteries (white arrows) indicating normal renal arteries.

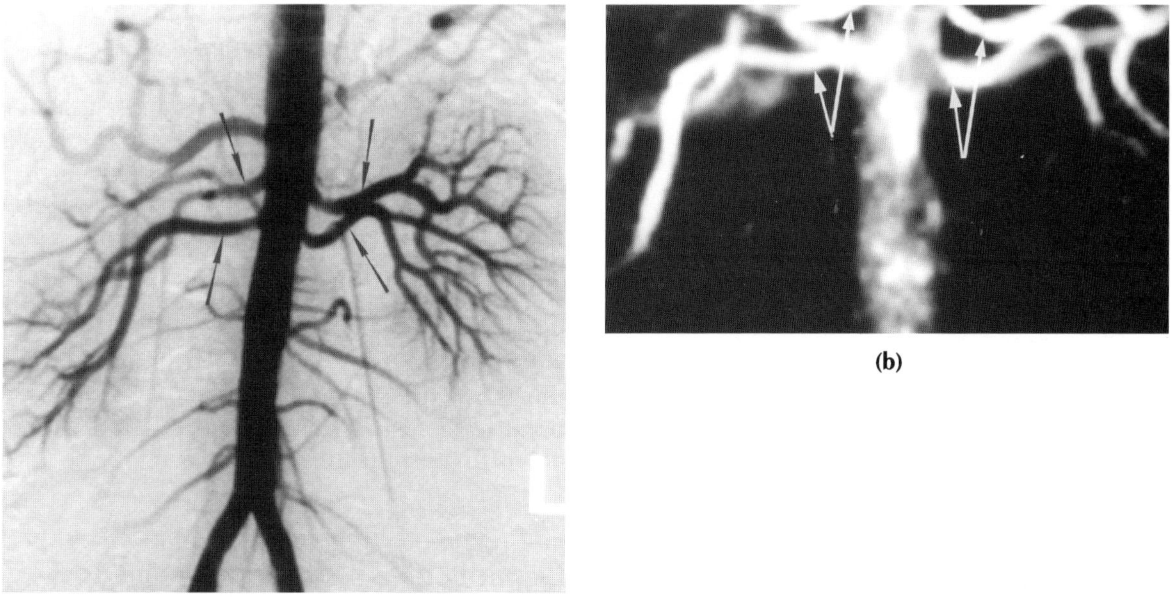

(b)

(a)

Figure 7.3. Multiple renal arteries. (a) Intra-arterial DSA showing two renal arteries on each side (black arrows). The irregularity of the proximal part of the upper left artery was not seen on further oblique projections of the angiogram. (b) Coronal MRA projection of the same patient as (a). Two renal arteries on each side are noted (white arrows). Origins of the accessory arteries arising well above or below the image volume, however, would not be seen.

imaging volume are usually easily visualized but accessory arteries that arise significantly below or above the volume will not be visualized adequately because the length of the volume is only 9 cm and will not cover a wide enough area in this situation.

Interpretation of images

The origins and main parts of the renal arteries of normal patients are easily visualized using the above technique. Figures 7.1 and 7.2 show normal native renal arteries. Turbulence may cause a small amount of signal loss at vessel origins (Fig. 7.4) and this is a factor in all conventional MRA techniques currently. The ability to interpret correctly the presence of turbulence-associated signal fallout has to be developed if MRA studies are to be consistently interpreted. In particular, one of the most difficult aspects of renal MRA interpretation is learning where the cutoff between signal loss due to turbulence alone and that due to a mild RAS lies. As the stenosis becomes more severe it is usually easily visualized with signal loss across the full width of the vascular structure. The large amount of signal loss seen in a true stenosis is partly due to the stenosis itself and partly due to associated turbulence beyond the stenosis. As a result, it is possible to overestimate the severity of lesions seen on MRA if criteria learned from conventional angiography alone are applied (Figs 7.5, 7.6, 7.7 and 7.8). It is necessary to develop new criteria for the estimation of the severity of stenoses with MRA.

A mild but significant stenosis causes enough signal loss in a renal artery for the vessel outline to be almost completely lost over a short segment of artery. As the severity of the RAS worsens, proportionally more signal is lost over longer lengths of the renal artery so that a moderate stenosis may show almost complete signal loss over a centimetre or so of artery on MRA,

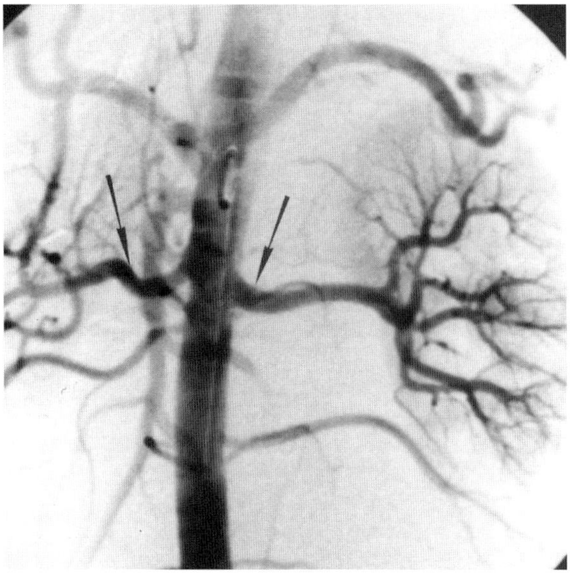

(a)

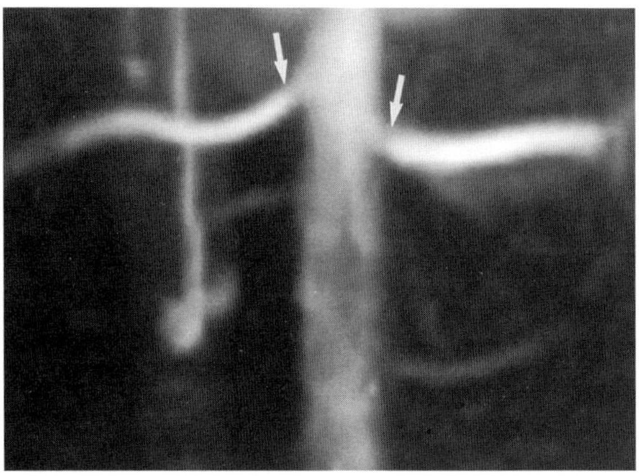

(b)

Figure 7.4. Normal renal arteriogram with some turbulence of vessel origins. (a) Intra-arterial DSA flush injection showing normal single renal arteries (black arrows). (b) Coronal projection MRA. Normal unstenosed arteries (white arrows) are visualized to the renal hilum. Note slight signal loss at renal artery origins which is due to turbulence and does not signify stenosis.

whereas a severe stenosis (>90%) with rather poor distal flow may show almost no appreciable signal within the main renal artery and only a little signal more peripherally. It is often difficult in such a severe situation to distinguish between complete occlusion with distal reconstitution and a very severe stenosis with low distal flow (Fig. 7.10). Under these circumstances a search has to be carried out for any evidence of peripheral signal to try and help with assessment (Figs 7.9 and 7.10). All of the above factors concerning interpretation apply equally to renal transplant arteries. Stenoses are seen as areas of signal loss along the length of the artery with the more severe stenoses having longer segments of signal loss (Figs 7.9 and 7.10). In addition, transplant arteries are more clearly visualized because there is little respiratory motion in the pelvis to blurr the images produced.

Dynamic enhanced gadolinium aortography and studies of renal arteries

Prince[5] described a technique using a continuous infusion of gadolinium which allowed a clear depiction of arterial structures. The major drawback of many MRA techniques is that substantial turbulence causes much signal loss. As a result, patients who have abdominal aortic aneurysms in which there is massive swirling turbulence, often show little signal on conventional MRA sequences in either aorta or renal arteries. The above technique, however, uses a continuous infusion of gadolinium during a spoiled GRASS volume acquisition (T1 weighted gradient echo scan) lasting 5 min. Whereas conventional MRA techniques use flow-related enhancement or phase shift developed by flowing blood to provide the signal for MRA, this technique utilizes the shortening of the T1 value that is produced by the circulating gadolinium diethylenetriamine-pentaacetic (DTPA) contrast agent. As a result, this technique is not significantly sensitive to turbulence and signal fallout is not seen in aneurysms. Therefore, the full extent of abdominal aneurysms and ectatic aortae can be easily and clearly visualized. Similarly, the renal arteries can be clearly seen. Such a study is acquired as a coronal volume acquisition and is then reconstructed using standard post-processing facilities (Fig. 7.14). Extremely

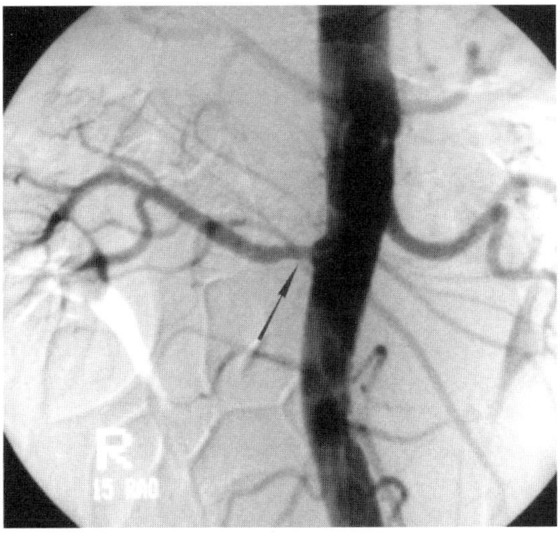

(a)

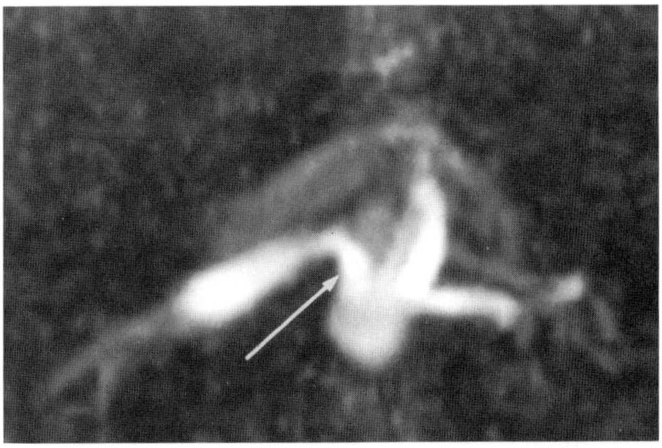

(b)

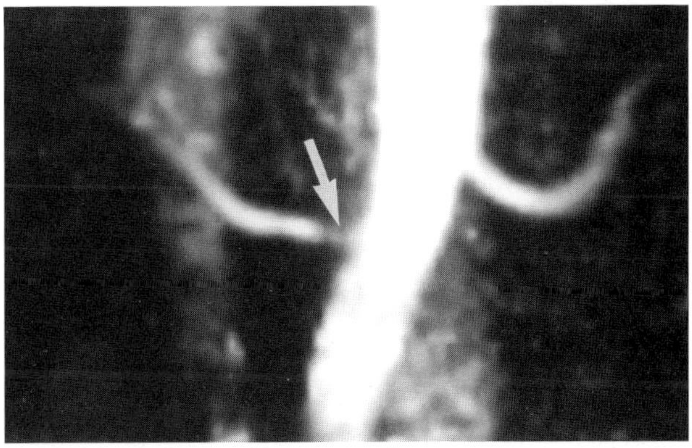

(c)

Figure 7.5. Mild right RAS. (a) Intra-arterial DSA showing normal left renal artery. Right renal artery shows a moderate stenosis (black arrow) in the first part of the renal artery. Note that the origin of the right renal artery is not completely profiled and this remained the case despite multiple oblique projections. (b) Axial MRA projection shows the origin of the right renal artery very clearly. The right renal artery origin (white arrow) can be seen to run in an anterior direction for its first portion explaining why intra-arterial DSA cannot adequately profile a renal artery origin away from the aorta in such cases. (c) Coronal MRA projection showing area of signal loss in the proximal part of the right renal artery (white arrow) suggesting a moderate stenosis.

promising images are being obtained using this technique which allows a study of the full length of the abdominal aorta from diaphragms to mid iliac arteries with depiction of the main vessels and renal arteries. The particular strength of this technique over conventional MRA studies is that aneurysms will be easily distinguished and depicted allowing their relationship to the renal arteries to be seen. More detailed results of the performance of this technique compared with conventional arteriography are still awaited.

MRA evaluation

Several series have been published examining the performance of MRA in the renal arterial territory. A relatively early paper by Kim *et al.*[6] used 2D TOF studies alone and reported a sensitivity of 100% and a specificity of 92%. No other group has been able to reproduce such high figures. Debatin *et al.*[7] compared the use of 3D phase contrast arteriography and 2D TOF in a series of 39 patients with angiographic confirmation in all patients. The sensitivity and

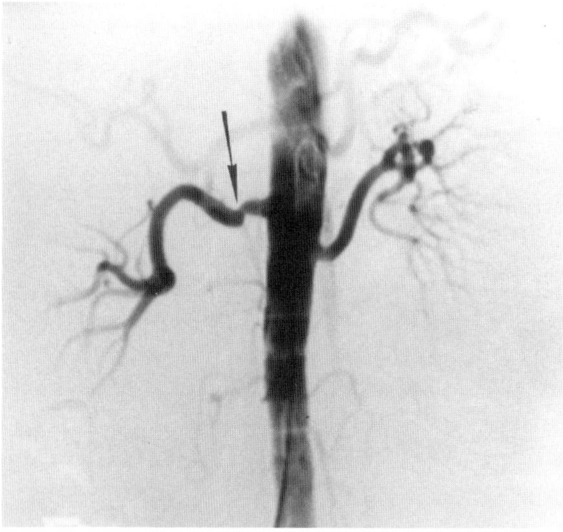

(a)

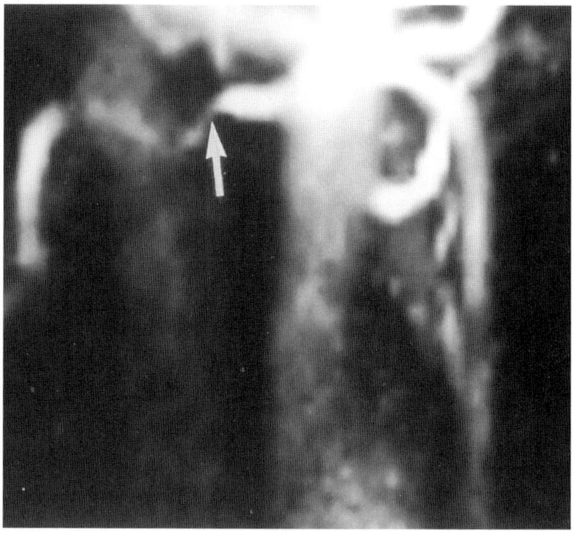

(b)

Figure 7.6. Moderate right RAS. (a) Intra-arterial DSA of renal arteries showing a stenosis of the right renal artery (black arrow). (b) Coronal projection MRA showing substantial signal loss in the right renal artery (white arrow) indicating a moderate stenosis over apparently a rather longer segment than was appreciated on the intra-arterial DSA. The increased length of the abnormality on the MRA is due to turbulence beyond the stenosis causing further signal fallout.

specificity results for this series are as shown below:

	Sensitivity %	Specificity %
3D phase contrast	84	97
2D TOF	53	97
3D phase contrast + 2D TOF	87	97

The overall conclusions of this series were that 3D phase contrast techniques were significantly superior to 2D TOF in this application and that MRA shows substantial promise in this area.

The above results are very much in keeping with the findings of our own group at St Mary's. We have studied 74 consecutive patients with conventional arteriography and 3D phase contrast MRA. The sensitivity from our series was 86% with a specificity value of 94%.

Three-dimensional phase contrast MRA is also a very sensitive and specific technique for examining renal transplant arteries. The prevalence of transplant artery stenosis varies between reports but is approximately between 8 and 25%.[8, 9] Although rates differ from unit to unit and between surgeons, the overall prevalence of transplant artery stenosis is probably rather near the 20% mark than the lower figure depending on how energetically the observer looks for it. We have used the same techniques as above in the pelvis to examine renal transplant arteries. In a similar fashion to native arteries 2D TOF studies did not appear to give adequate images of the pelvic vasculature in comparison with 3D phase contrast studies which show renal transplant arteries clearly and consistently (Figs 7.11 and 7.12).

We have studied 72 completed renal transplant cases with all patients having both conventional arteriography and 3D phase contrast MRA. Sensitivity rates of 84% and specificity rates of 90% were described for this group of patients[10] and we have subsequently carried out receiver operating characteristic curve analyses of intra-arterial DSA compared with 3D phase contrast MRA. These curves do not show any significant difference between intra-arterial DSA and MRA confirming that in this area 3D phase

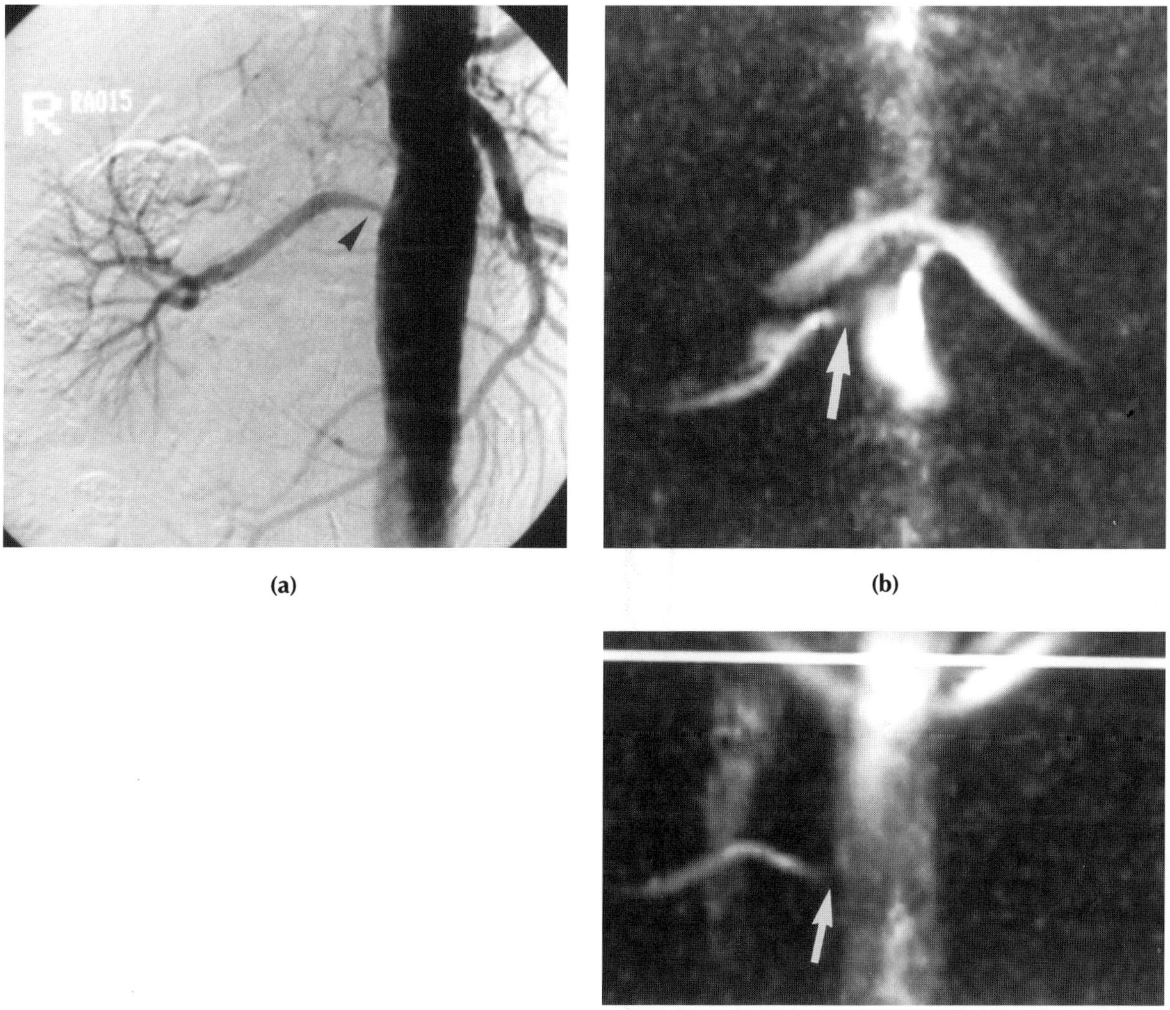

(a) (b)

(c)

Figure 7.7. Moderate right RAS. (a) Intra-arterial DSA of renal arteries. Occluded left renal artery. Moderately stenosed first part of right renal artery (black arrow). (b, c) Axial and coronal projections from the MRA study respectively. These show occluded left renal artery and signal loss in proximal part of right renal artery (white arrow) confirming the stenosis shown on intra-arterial DSA. Note signal loss across the full width of vessel.

contrast MRA is comparable with intra-arterial DSA in terms of sensitivity and specificity.

Discussion

The increasing recognition of RAS as an important cause of impaired renal function together with its well-known role in hypertension has resulted in much greater awareness of this condition. In addition, the possibility of a significant deterioration in renal function in patients who are prescribed angiotensin converting enzyme inhibitors who have bilateral RAS or RAS in a single kidney[11, 12] (which is often unsuspected) has accelerated further efforts to detect reliably the presence of occult RAS to try and prevent this occasionally permanent deterioration of renal function.

Despite the use of other techniques such as nuclear medicine and ultrasonography, conventional arteriography is still the key investigation

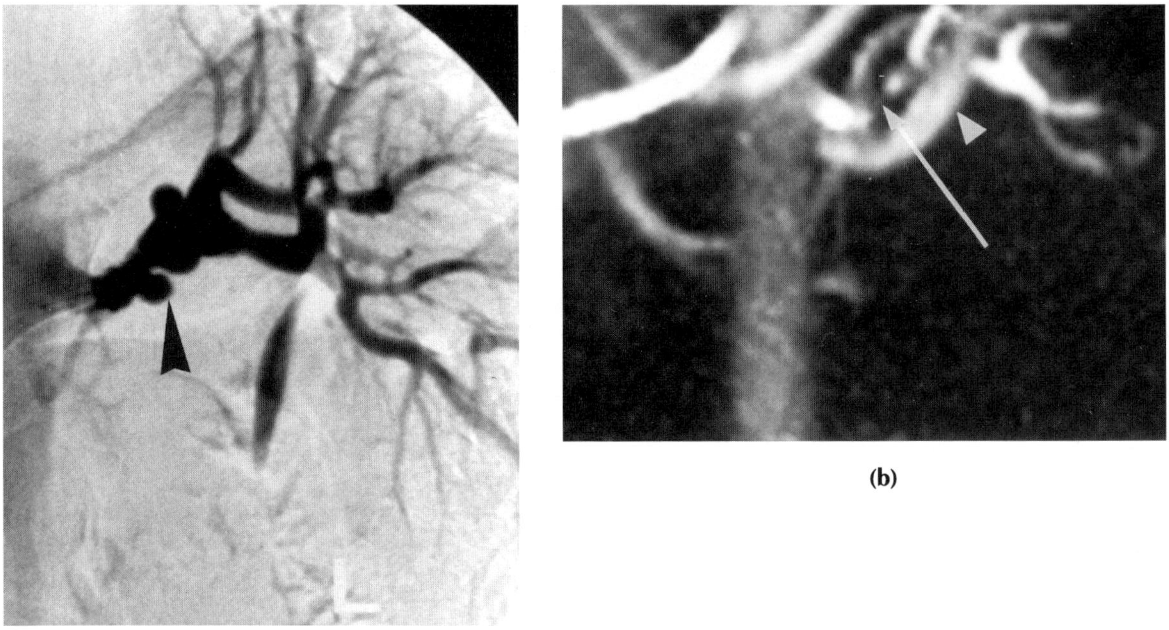

(b)

(a)

Figure 7.8. Left RAS due to fibromuscular hyperplasia. (a) Selective intra-arterial DSA study of right renal artery showing beading and aneurysm formation typical of fibromuscular hyperplasia (black arrow). (b) Coronal MRA projection. Note area of signal loss in left renal artery (white arrow) corresponding to the stenosis caused by fibromuscular hyperplasia. Right renal artery is normal and visible to well beyond the renal hilum. There is prominent renal vein signal (white arrow) in this young patient.

in this condition. Arteriography, however, has many well-known complications related to both its invasive nature and to the contrast load used. In addition, it requires ionizing radiation and is usually associated with a period of inpatient hospital stay, thus elevating the cost of the examination substantially.

Conventional arteriography, despite its relatively high spatial resolution, is also significantly limited by its planar nature. Multiple oblique views are often required in patients with tortuous or ectatic arteries and even after this the origins of the renal arteries may prove impossible to profile adequately away from a distended tortuous aorta or iliac artery (for transplants) (Fig. 7.5). The 3D representation provided by MRA in this situation is a major advantage of this technique. Not only can vessels be viewed in a full 180° rotation but the whole acquired stack can be collapsed and viewed in an axial format which often provides additional information that cannot be obtained (Figs. 7.1 and 7.2) by conventional angiographic techniques. The origins of vessels are often only adequately visualized in this projection and new insights may be gained about the path and angulation of the renal arteries.

Renal transplant arteries are often surprisingly tortuous and the 3D capabilities of MRA in this area have added greatly to our ability to diagnose transplant RAS and assess the transplant artery fully. We have recently seen three patients in our practice where, despite multiple projections using conventional angiography, the stenoses could not be definitely identified. MRA, however, easily depicted the stenoses because of its 3D abilities (Fig. 7.13). Furthermore, the sensitivity of MRA to turbulence and flow may allow it to provide some hemodynamic information about the significance of an arterial stenosis particularly in cases where the conventional angiogram shows minor or equivocal changes.

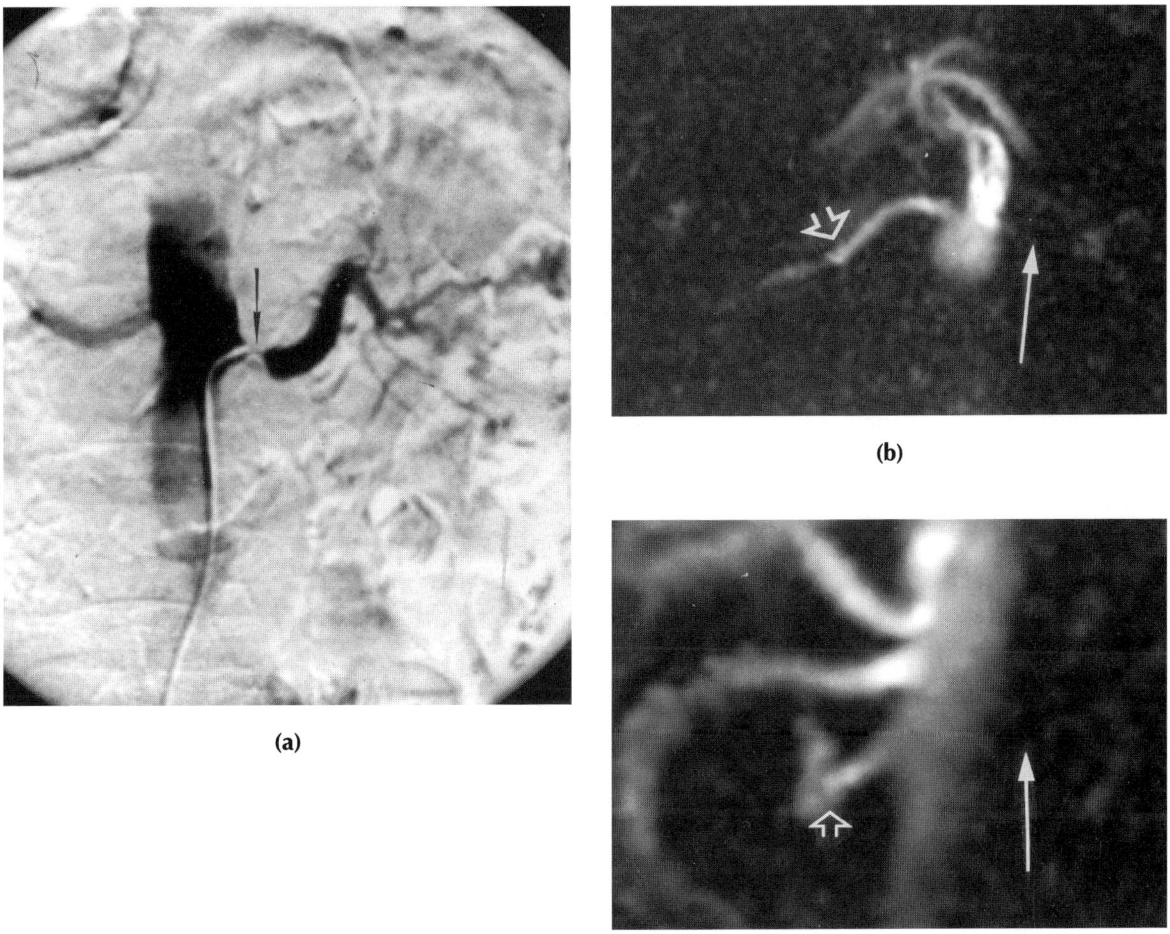

(a) (b) (c)

Figure 7.9. Severe left RAS. (a) Selective intra-arterial DSA study showing extremely severe left RAS (black arrow). (b, c) Axial and coronal MRA projections respectively showing normal right renal artery (open white arrow). The left renal artery shows almost complete signal loss from its origin to the renal hilum (white arrow). Some signal can be seen within the renal vasculature itself, particularly on the axial image in (b). This could be due to either a severe stenosis with substantial signal fallout along the length of the main artery, or due to complete occlusion of the main artery with distal reconstitution.

With the increasing interest in the diagnosis and treatment of RAS we clearly need a suitable screening technique for this condition. It is important that patients with normal renal arteries do not have to consistently undergo conventional arteriography for full assessment of the renal arteries. Conventional angiography is unsuitable for a proper screening role and it seems likely that MRA, particularly using 3D phase contrast techniques, may be able to fill this important role in future. The current published results using the above techniques strongly support the view that a normal MRA of the renal arteries is a very strong indicator that no further investigation for RAS needs to be carried out. The results outlined above suggest that MRA is a sensitive and specific technique for imaging native and renal transplant arteries. The overwhelming advantage of this technique over other non-angiographic procedures is that it produces images that are instantly recognizable as arteries. Multiple renal arteries in normal patients are

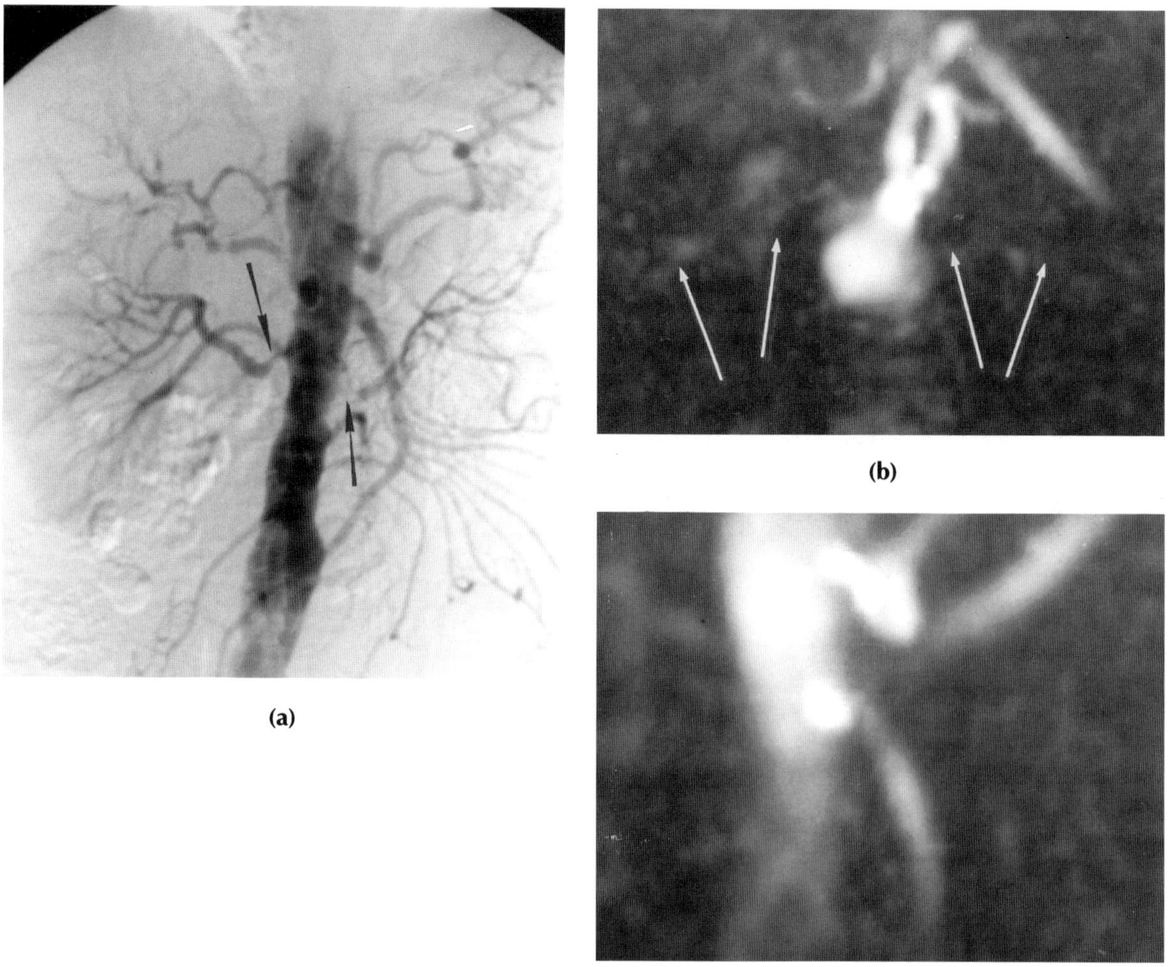

(a)

(b)

(c)

Figure 7.10. Bilateral RAS stenosis. (a) Intra-arterial DSA showing bilateral renal artery stenosis (black arrows). Note very atheromatous aorta. (b, c) Axial and coronal projections of same patient as (a) Note very low signal in both renal arteries (white arrows) with an interruption in the signal in proximal part of the left renal artery.

reliably imaged unless their origin is outside of the imaging volume. This pitfall can be overcome by using thick coronal 2D phase contrast single slices which can cover a wider field of view[13] or alternatively using the previously described dynamic gadolinium infusion technique which allows a larger field of view. It is difficult because of time constraints to image a larger area than 9 cm with the 3D phase contrast technique alone. The presence of multiple renal arteries, however, arising outside the volume imaged is realistically rarely a clinical problem except in the workup of live related renal transplant donors.

Inevitably, future developments will lead to substantial improvements in the quality of images obtained with MRA. An increase in matrix sizes to 512 × 512 will shortly be available which will allow improved spatial resolution plus a lessening in the amount of signal loss

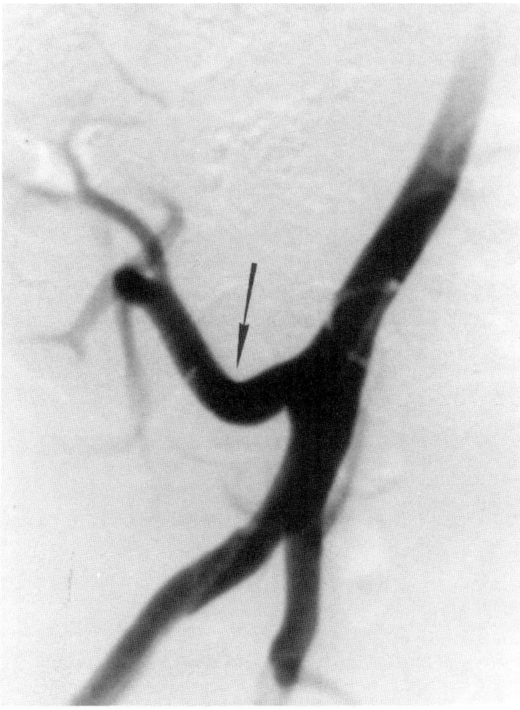

(a)

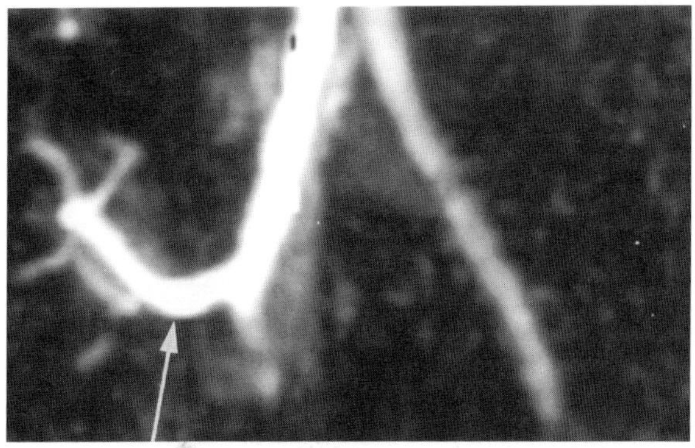

(b)

Figure 7.11. Normal renal transplant arteriogram. (a) Intra-arterial DSA injection in common iliac artery showing normal transplant artery (black arrow). (b) Coronal MRA projection showing normal renal transplant artery (white arrow) in the same patient as (a).

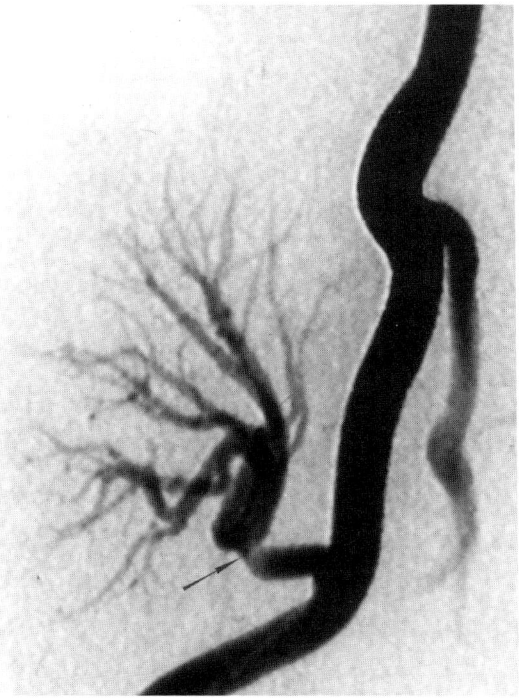

(a)

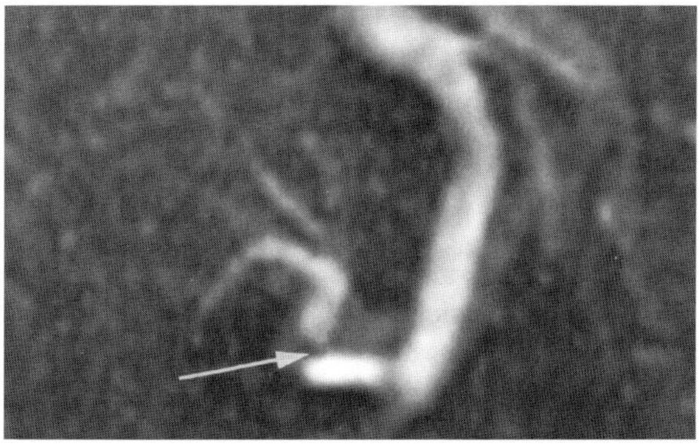

(b)

Figure 7.12. Real transplant artery stenosis. (a) Intra-arterial DSA showing unusual transplant artery stenosis at renal hilum (black arrow). (b) MRA of same patient as in (a) Coronal projection shows significant loss of signal in area of renal hilum corresponding to the abnormality in (a) (white arrow).

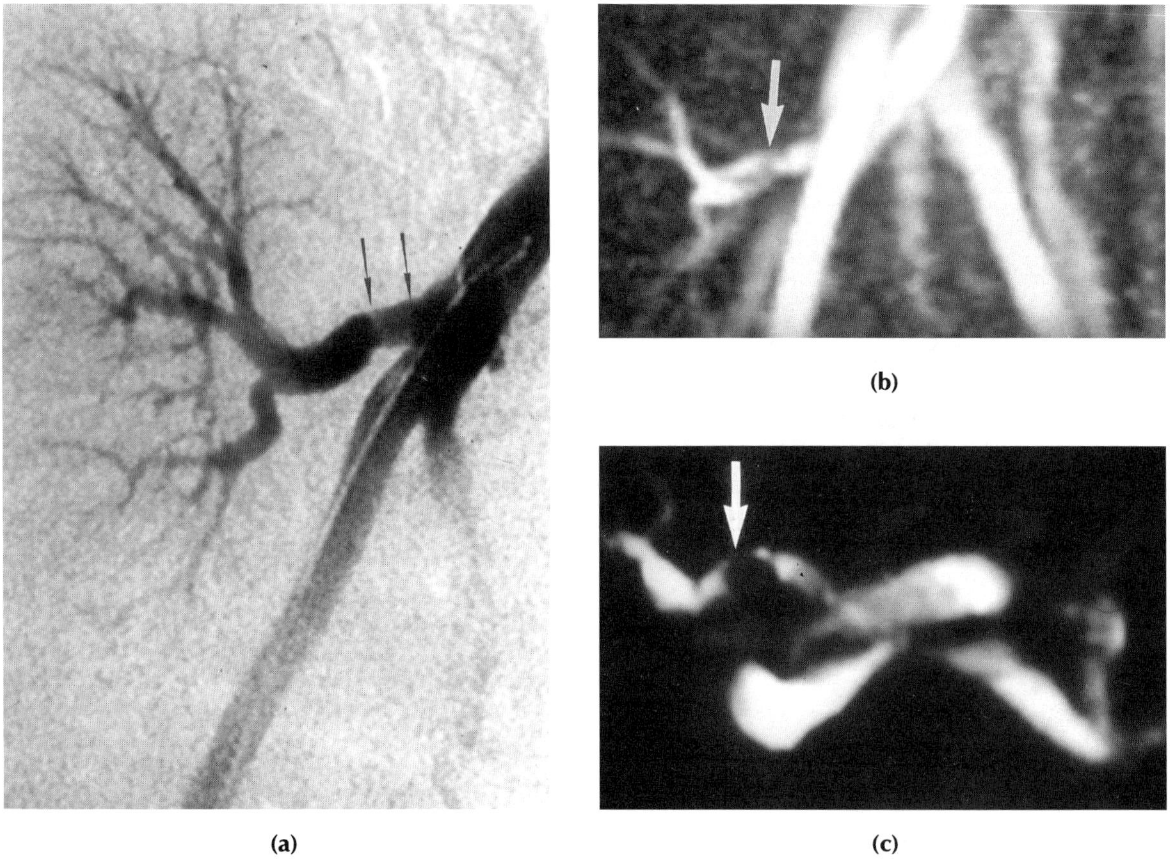

Figure 7.13. Transplant artery stenosis which was difficult to visualize on intra-arterial DSA. (a) Intra-arterial DSA of right renal transplant artery shows a questionable abnormality in the midpart of the transplant artery (black arrows). This area could not be adequately visualized despite multiple oblique projections. (b) Coronal MRA projection. (c) Collapsed axial view, clearly show a significant stenosis in the apex of an S-bend in the transplant artery (white arrows).

secondary to turbulence. The use of dynamic infusion gadolinium techniques will allow renal arteries to be visualized when they are associated with abdominal aortic aneurysms which has been a major problem using 3D phase contrast techniques alone. Further, software developments should also allow a lessening of the movement artifacts currently seen in MRA plus further improved resolution.

Another important aspect that has only been touched on so far is the ability of phase contrast arteriography to provide velocity and flow information. The phase shift seen in an MRA study of this nature is proportionate to the velocity of the blood flow. The blood flow velocity is proportionate to the intensity of the signal produced and therefore velocity can be relatively easily calculated. If vessel cross-sectional area is known, then flow in a vessel may be easily calculated. Commercial software packages already exist that allow flow rates to be measured using the above techniques. A variety of groups[14] are exploring the applications of this technique although studies are still at a relatively early stage. One of the difficulties in the renal vasculature, however, is that a reliable alternative technique for measuring total and individual renal blood flow to allow comparisons with MRA results is not available. No real work has yet emerged on the use of this technique in renal artery stenosis.

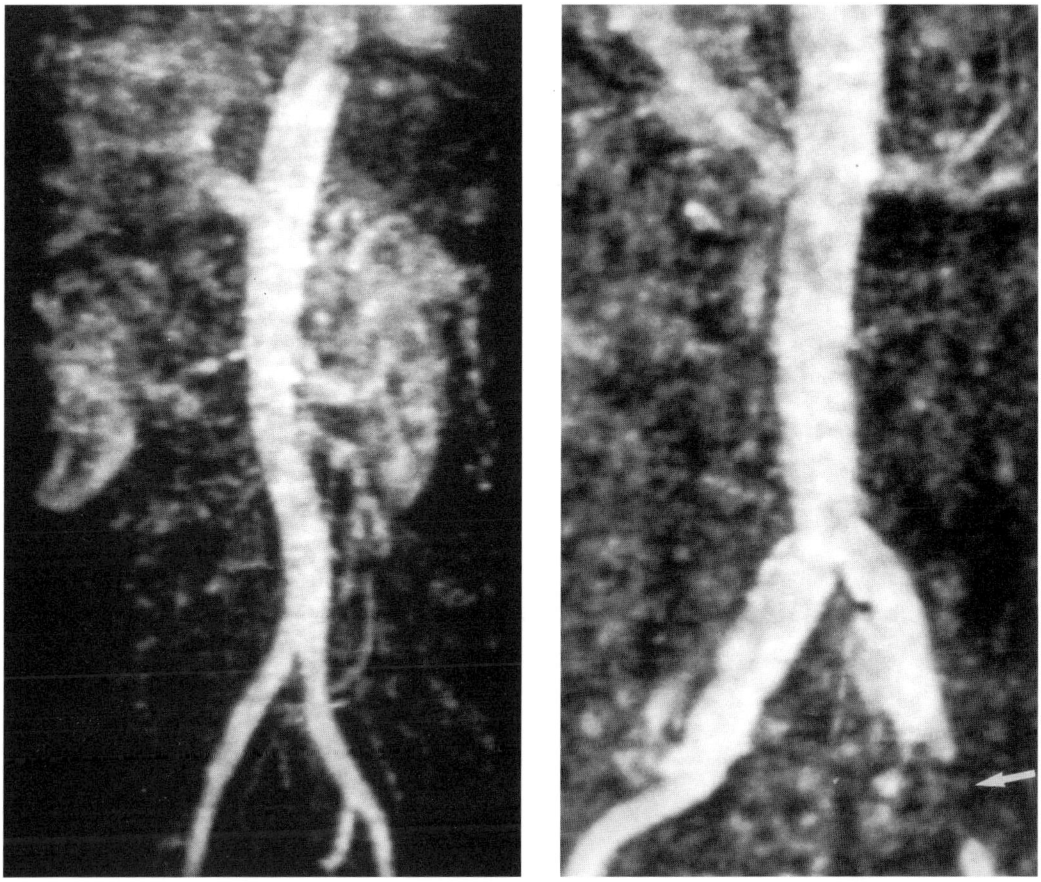

(a) (b)

Figure 7.14. Early images from gadolinium infusion aortograms. (a) Coronal infusion image clearly demonstrates the length of the aorta from diaphragm down to mid iliac arteries. Possible renal artery stenosis on right. (b) Different patient from (a) using the same technique showing iliac artery occlusion on the left (white arrow).

References

1 European Dialysis and Transplantation Association (EDTA) Conference Proceedings, 1992.

2 Kremer Hovinga TK, de Jong PE, Vander Hem GK *et al.* Relief of renal artery stenosis: a tool to improve or preserve renal function in renovascular disease. *Nephrol Dial Transplant* 1990; **5:** 481–8.

3 O'Donovan RM, Gutierrez ON, Izzo JL. Preservation of renal function by percutaneous renal angioplasty in high-risk elderly patients: short term outcome. *Nephron* 1992; **60:** 187–92.

4 Pelc NJ, Herfkem RS, Shimakawa A *et al.* Phase contrast cine magnetic resonance imaging. *Magn Reson Imaging* 1991; **4**(7): 229–54.

5 Prince MR. Gadolinium enhanced MR aortography. *Radiology* 1994; **191:** 155–64.

6 Kim D, Edelman R, Kent KC *et al.* Abdominal aortic and renal artery stenosis: evaluation with MRA. *Radiology* 1990; **174:** 727–31.

7 Debatin SF, Spritzer CE, Crist TM *et al.* Imaging of renal arteries: value of MR angiography. *Am J Roentgenol* 1991; **157:** 981–90.

8 Gedroyc WMW, Reidy JF, Saxton HM. Arteriography of renal transplantation. *Clin Radiol* 1987; **38:** 239–43.

9 Lacombe M. Arterial stenosis complicating renal allo-transplantation in man. *Ann Surg* 1975; **181:** 283–8.

10 Gedroyc W, Negus R *et al.* Magnetic resonance angiography of renal transplants. *Lancet* 1992; **339:** 789–91.

11 Blyth WB. Captopril and renal auto-regulation. *N Engl J Med* 1983, **308:** 390–1.

12 Hrickik DE, Browning PJ, Kopelman R *et al.* Captopril-induced functional renal insufficiency in patients with bilateral renal artery stenosis on RAS in a solitary kidney. *N Engl J Med* 1983; **38:** 373–6.

13 Debatin SF, Spritzer CE, Sontman HD. Evaluation of MR angiography in preoperative renovascular assessment for potential living-related donors. *Proc Radiol Soc North Am* 1992; **363:** 162.

14 Wolf RL, King BF, Torres VE *et al.* Cine phase contrast flow volumetry of the renal arteries. *Proc Radiol Soc North Am* 1992; **366:** 162.

8

Carbon dioxide angiography

SCOTT R KERNS, IRVIN F HAWKINS JR

Introduction

Several different modalities currently exist for imaging the renal vasculature including magnetic resonance imaging, three-dimensional (3D) helical computed tomography and Doppler ultrasound. However, the cornerstone modality is catheter-injected contrast angiography utilizing either cut-film or digital subtraction imaging. This invasive procedure entails risks including anaphylactoid reactions and contrast-induced nephropathy. Anaphylactoid reactions remain a problem despite the use of low osmolar contrast agents, premedication regimens and patient selection.[1, 2] Contrast-induced nephropathy is the third leading cause of hospital-acquired renal dysfunction.[3] Although the renal changes are usually transient, dialysis may be required in some patients.[4–6] Major risk factors primarily include pre-existing renal insufficiency and insulin-dependent diabetes mellitus.[7–9] It had been hoped that the development of low osmolality contrast media (LOCM) would reduce the incidence of contrast-induced nephropathy, but early reports failed to show this.[5, 10] More recent studies have suggested a reduced incidence of contrast-induced nephropathy in high risk patients with LOCM.[7, 11–13] However, the risk is not eliminated, and the risk to normal patients may not be affected.[12] Universal use of LOCM would add at least US $1.1 billion/year to the estimated cost of health care, while selective use in the high risk groups would add up to US $350 million/year.[14] The debate as to whether or not such a large part of the health care budget should be assigned to reducing risk in a relatively small percentage of the patient population will certainly continue.

At the University of Florida this problem has been addressed in a novel fashion by developing an entirely different class of intravascular contrast, carbon dioxide gas.[15, 16] Carbon dioxide (CO_2) is now being used not only for diagnostic imaging but also to guide percutaneous interventional vascular procedures. Special equipment and imaging techniques have been developed to overcome the particular problems posed by using gas as an intravascular contrast agent. This chapter will present the historical background of this technique, nature of intravascular gas behavior, principles of successful imaging using CO_2, issues of safety and clinical uses and limitations of CO_2 angiography.

Historical background

The use of gas as a negative contrast agent in radiology is not new. In the 1950s CO_2 was first used as an intravascular contrast agent to help detect the presence of pericardial effusions.[17–19] The physiological effects of intravascularly injected CO_2 have been studied and no significant changes in blood gas parameters or hemodynamics seem to occur even with relatively large injection volumes.[20, 21] The use of CO_2 to image the abdominal aorta, its branches and the peripheral circulation was later pioneered by Hawkins.[15] He originally used cut-film subtraction techniques and hand-injected the gas. Subsequently, digital subtraction imaging, dedicated gas injectors, smaller catheter delivery systems, modified examination tables, use of intra-arterial vasodilators and special postprocessing software have made CO_2 angiography a safe, reliable and accurate method of vascular imaging. However, optimal use of this technique requires a thorough understanding of the behavior of intravascular gas and how this can affect imaging.

Behavior of intravascular carbon dioxide

Intravascular bubbles of CO_2 behave in a much different manner than a bolus of conventional iodinated contrast. When liquid iodinated contrast is injected into flowing blood the contrast mixes with the blood and is carried diluted downstream. The rate at which the contrast mixes with radiolucent blood, and the rate at which the blood is flowing into the region of contrast injection, will determine how fast the contrast is diluted. Therefore, the overall positive density at any given point in a vessel will depend upon how much contrast has been injected per unit time, how fast the blood is flowing and to what degree mixing has occurred proximal to that point.

When CO_2 gas is injected into flowing blood the initial gas–liquid interface is maintained for a period of time. Carbon dioxide displaces blood rather than mixing with it. The composite negative density at given point will therefore depend on how much of the radiolucent blood has been displaced by the low density gas. To what degree this affects imaging greatly depends on how fast the gas is injected relative to the underlying blood flow in the region of interest. If the gas is injected at a slow rate the buoyant gas will literally float on the stream of flowing blood and is carried downstream out of the area being imaged. In this case only non-dependent branch vessels will be filled by the buoyant gas, and their luminal diameters may be underestimated because only the top portion of the vessel may be filled. Conversely, if a proper volume of gas is injected, at a high enough rate, all of the blood can be temporarily displaced out of the area being imaged. In this case a more accurate account of the patency and diameter of vessels in the area imaged is achieved. However, we and others have found that there is an upper limit to the injection volume after which no further improvement in imaging occurs.[22] Increasing the injection volume simply increases the amount of blood displaced on the periphery of the area imaged without affecting the density difference between the vessel and the surrounding soft tissues. We have found that the injection rate appears to have more of an advantageous effect on imaging than injection volume. Unlike with iodinated contrast in which high volumes are needed to overcome dilution due to mixing with blood, high injection rates in CO_2 angiography appear to displace blood more effectively than slower injections of larger volumes. A quick 'burst' of gas temporarily displaces blood more effectively than a slow 'dribble' which provides only a stream of bubbles. Of course, larger volumes will necessarily be needed in larger vessels, but increasing injection rates can decrease the total amount of gas needed for successful imaging.

The buoyancy of CO_2 must be taken into account when attempting to image structures or vessels that are dependent. Although higher injection rates may be able to overcome this by displacing the entire blood volume within the portion of the vessel being imaged, one can enhance this effect by simply rotating or elevating the body part in such a manner that it is less dependent. Only a 15 or 20° change in position can make a dramatic difference.

When iodinated contrast is injected it will circulate through the bloodstream, and eventually be excreted by the kidneys in large part. Conversely, CO_2 immediately begins to undergo dissolution in the blood and is expired by the lungs on the first pass. Carbon dioxide is quite soluble in serum, approximately 20 times that of oxygen.[21] If too small a volume is injected the gas begins to break up into bubbles which dissolve within the area of interest.[22] This causes the vessel to appear as a series of discontinuous bubbles on any given image. This would seriously degrade the study, but postprocessing software is available which allows the summation of images to provide an accurate and useful composite image. This allows diagnostic information to be obtained with somewhat smaller injection volumes.

An early concern with CO_2 angiography was whether or not the gas bubbles would become trapped in the capillary bed essentially causing a gas embolus situation with resulting ischemia. Experiences in both animal and human studies at our institution have shown that this is not the case. In fact, in most arterial studies much of the gas injected is dissolved by the time it reaches the capillary level. The dissolved CO_2 is then carried to the lungs where it is expired. One caveat is that in low flow situations the gas that has not dissolved could potentially become trapped in any inverted U-shaped structure or vessel. In this instance the kinetic energy of the flowing blood may not be enough to 'push' the trapped, buoyant gas through the distal arteriolar and capillary beds to be released into the venous circulation. In addition, continuing exposure to saturated blood may slow dissolution of the trapped gas. In the patient with renal vascular disease this situation is most likely to occur in patients with renal transplants, or bypasses to native renal arteries, since the arteries involved tend to originate off the non-dependent aspect of the native feeding vessel. Keeping the total volume of CO_2 as low as possible while still obtaining diagnostic information, and spacing sequential injections by 1–2 min, is a prudent practice to avoid potential trapping.

The viscosity of gas is approximately 0.25% that of iodinated contrast. This can be easily demonstrated by comparing the amount of effort needed to hand-inject a given volume of gas through a very small gauge needle with that needed for the same volume of iodinated contrast. Carbon dioxide arteriography can therefore be performed with much smaller catheters (3 French) which reduces procedural complications.[23] Bleeding vessels and arteriovenous fistulas are well demonstrated with CO_2,[24] and collateral reconstitution of vessels distal to a total occlusion may be seen only during CO_2 arteriography, due to the low viscosity of the gas which allows it to pass much more readily through small collaterals, direct arteriovenous connections or breaches in vessel walls.

Imaging principles

The use of CO_2 as an intravascular contrast agent involves many theoretical and practical concepts which are foreign to many radiologists. Carbon dioxide is a colorless, odorless, compressible gas. We use highly pure gas available in disposable cylinders (AngioDynamics, Glens Falls, NY) since we have discovered that reusable cylinders accumulate water vapor resulting in corrosion of their interior. Purity of the gas, and prevention of room air contamination, are extremely important to avoid the known adverse effects of air embolization.

Several different methods for injecting CO_2 have evolved over the years. Originally hand-injection was used, and this remains the most simple method. However, because of the compressibility of the gas, the delivery is difficult and unpredictable. The gas typically compresses in the syringe and is then injected suddenly in a rather explosive manner. This problem can be alleviated somewhat by clearing the injection line and catheter of fluid with a 3 ml syringe of gas followed by the main bolus.[23, 25] However, this is somewhat cumbersome since several stopcocks need to be opened and closed quickly in the correct sequence for successful imaging. Standard contrast injectors can be used, but since they are not closed systems the risk of air contamination is high. Since pure CO_2 is heavier than room air the injector nozzle should be kept in the upright position during filling. The injector should also be opened briefly to atmosphere when the desired injection volume is loaded. If it is not, more than the intended volume may be injected inadvertently due to the compressibility of the gas.[16]

Many of these problems specific to CO_2 angiography have been solved with the development of a dedicated injector system which is undergoing clinical trials (AngioDynamics, Glens Falls, NY). This injector delivers pure, dry CO_2 through a closed system reducing the

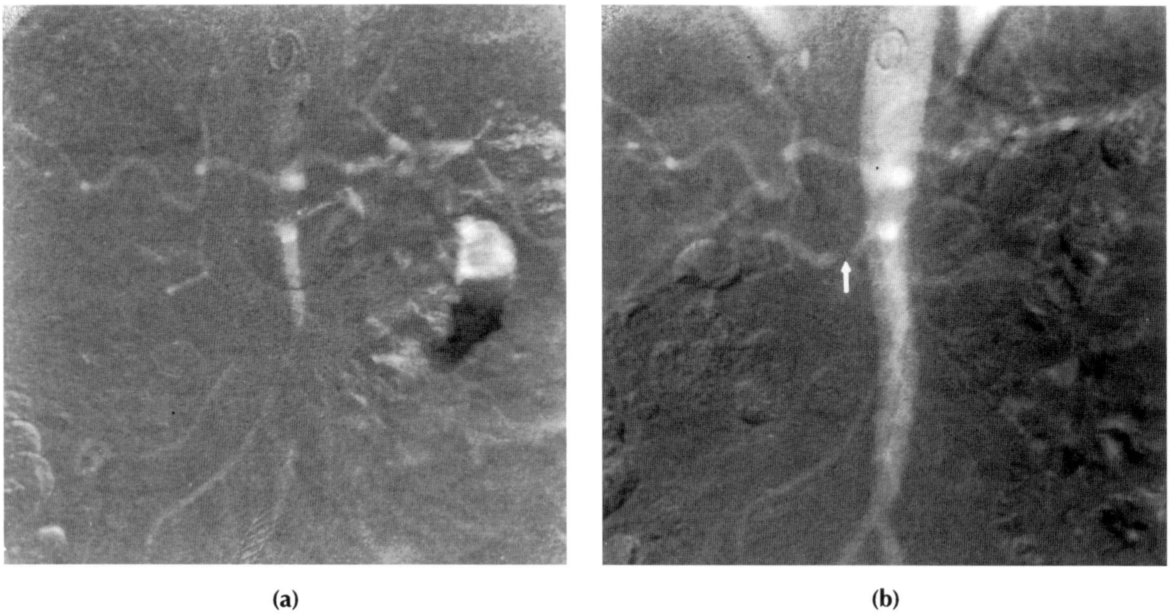

Figure 8.1. (a) Small volume injection (10 ml) fills primarily celiac axis and superior mesenteric artery. (b) Larger injection (140 ml) fills entire aorta and branch vessels demonstrating right renal artery stenosis (arrow).

possibility of room air contamination. Multiple transducers and high speed valves guard against inadvertent high injection volumes. The catheter size and length, injection rate and injection volume are entered by the operator. The injector delivers this specific bolus much more accurately than any other method. Between injections a constant saline flush keeps the catheter clear. A hand-held mini-injector has also been described,[22] but it lacks the safeguards mentioned above.

Although CO_2 imaging was originally performed using cut-film subtraction techniques,[15] the advent and continuing development of digital subtraction angiography (DSA) and more powerful postprocessing capabilities have increased the accuracy and usefulness of CO_2 angiography. Similar to all techniques utilizing DSA, image quality is maximized if all motion during accumulation of images is kept to a minimum. We sedate our CO_2 angiography patients as little as possible so they may halt respiration during image acquisition. Since bowel peristalsis can significantly degrade images in the abdomen and pelvis 0.5 mg glucagon may be given intravenously though this is not always necessary. Any motion artifact that remains can usually be reduced or eliminated by using post-processing software available on most current systems such as pixel shifting, remasking and edge enhancement.

Injection volumes and rates for renal vascular imaging depend on whether native vessels are being studied, or if transplants, reimplanted native renal arteries or renal artery bypasses are the subject of the study. As mentioned previously, the buoyancy of CO_2 must be considered during imaging..Native renal arteries course posteriorly and therefore will not fill with gas if an inadequate amount and/or rate is used (Figs 8.1a and 8.1b). In order to completely clear all blood from the aorta, and thus fill the posteriorly oriented native renal arteries, we have found that an injection of the order of 75–100 ml delivered in 0.5 s is usually adequate. Smaller volumes may be adequate depending on the size of the aorta and the runoff. Similarly, renal arteries may fill preferentially during systole. Postprocessing image summation allows accurate assessment of the renal artery anatomy (Figs 8.2a and 8.2b). If this does not result in visualization of the renal arteries, the patient may be obliqued on the table

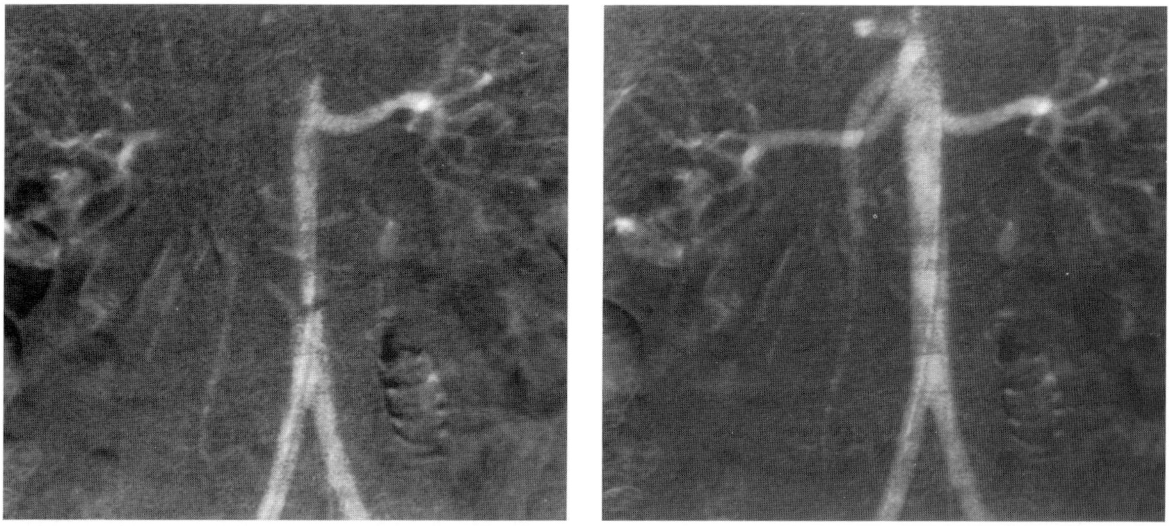

Figure 8.2. (a) Single image suggests non-filling of right renal artery. (b) Composite image using postprocessing summation software shows normal renal arteries and aorta.

with the side of interest elevated approximately 15–20° to take advantage of gas buoyancy. We are currently investigating the possibility of interfacing a mobile examination table that can cant side-to-side with the C-arm. Selective injection of 100 µg nitroglycerine immediately prior to imaging may transiently increase renal blood flow and improve visualization though results are highly variable.

Reimplanted native renal arteries (e.g. after aortic aneurysm repair), renal artery bypass grafts and renal transplants tend to image very well since these vessels originate off the non-dependent aspect of the supplying vessel. Smaller injection volumes may be used (e.g. 40–50 ml) since only the non-dependent portion of the supplying artery needs to be filled with gas. As with native renal arteries, these vessels can be selectively catheterized and selective angiography may be performed with improved image quality.

Safety

At the University of Florida, CO_2 angiography has primarily been used in high risk patients who have renal insufficiency, diabetes mellitus or other risk factors for iodinated contrast, or have had a suspected or documented reaction to conventional contrast. Since CO_2 is a normal constituent of the body there is no chance of a reaction to it. In our large clinical experience we have noticed neither intravascular nor catheter-related thrombosis during CO_2 angiography. Iodinated contrast, on the other hand, may induce thrombosis, especially with LOCM and a finite reaction rate remains despite pre-treatment.[2, 26–28] In our experience all commonly used medications may be injected through the same catheter used for CO_2 angiography unlike with some iodinated contrast agents.[29–31]

If CO_2 is injected distal to the renal arteries there is no chance that it will come in contact with the renal parenchyma since it is eliminated by the lungs in one pass. This is not the case with iodinated contrast which is distributed throughout the intravascular and extravascular space and is eliminated eventually by the kidneys. However, to use CO_2 to image the renal arteries one must necessarily expose the kidneys directly to the gas. The effect on function and histology of CO_2 directly injected into the renal artery was evaluated in the dog model.[32] Renal blood flow and function was measured with ^{131}I iodohippurate sodium in 14 dogs given CO_2 either in the prone position or with the kidney directly over the catheter to maximize possible effects of gas trapping. There appeared to be no significant difference in renal blood flow or function, though in all groups renal blood flow decreased immediately after the study but returned within 24 h. No significant histological changes were seen with the exception of one dog in which the kidney was positioned directly above the catheter. Acute tubular necrosis developed which was thought to be due to ischemia from frequent injections and gas trapping rather than a toxic effect of CO_2 itself.

The safety of CO_2 as an intravascular contrast agent has been demonstrated in clinical use as well. Several small series have noted no significant change in renal function, usually as reflected in the serum creatinine level, when patients who also received iodinated contrast are excluded.[33–36] In our large clinical experience we have noted no definite effect of CO_2 on renal function, though large-scale controlled studies have yet to be completed. The only definite complication directly attributable to CO_2 occurred in a patient with an abdominal aortic aneurysm and renal insufficiency (serum creatinine 3.5 mg/dl) who developed profuse watery diarrhea after receiving approximately 2000 ml of CO_2 over a 30-min period. This was temporary and thought to be due to transient ischemic colitis. Typical volumes used are far lower than this, and no other cases of mesenteric, renal or extremity ischemia have occurred. A thorough understanding and adherence to the principles delineated above should allow adequate diagnostic information in most cases with avoidance of complications.

Care should be taken to ensure the catheter is below the diaphragm before injection of CO_2 since there is a question of neurotoxicity. Studies performed on rats in which CO_2 was injected directly into the carotid artery showed damage to the endothelial cell membrane on microscopic examination with multifocal ischemic infarction.[37] Conversely, selective injections have been performed on canines without detectable changes on neurological examination, EEG monitoring or at gross pathology.[38] Until the exact direct effect of CO_2 on the intracranial circulation is clarified we recommend no injections of CO_2 within the thorax.

Clinical uses and limitations

Carbon dioxide angiography is useful in almost all situations in which vascular imaging is needed in patients with a history of reaction to iodinated contrast and/or at risk for contrast-induced nephropathy. This technique is useful for not only diagnostic arteriography and venography, but can also be used to guide percutaneous interventional vascular procedures.[39, 40] Focusing on the patient with renal vascular disease, this technique is advantageous not only in those who need arteriographic evaluation of the renal arterial system prior to possible revascularization, but also those with other vascular diseases such as abdominal aortic aneurysms, mesenteric ischemia and peripheral vascular disease (Fig. 8.3). These patients frequently have concurrent renal vascular disease and may benefit from CO_2 arteriography even though they are not presenting with azotemia or hypertension.

The most frequent indication for CO_2 arteriography in this patient population is the evaluation of possible renovascular hypertension (Figs 8.4a and 8.4b). The main renal artery and its second and third order branches are usually well seen.[33, 35] Frequently, several injections must be made to obtain adequate diagnostic information adjusting patient position as needed. As many injections as necessary can be made since CO_2 appears not to be nephrotoxic. In those cases in which CO_2 arteriography is non-diagnostic, or where the results are discordant with non-invasive tests, repeat confirmatory arteriography can be performed with a small amount of low osmolar iodinated contrast. Since there is some evidence that the incidence of contrast-induced nephropathy is directly related to the total volume of contrast used,[4, 6] CO_2 arteriography can

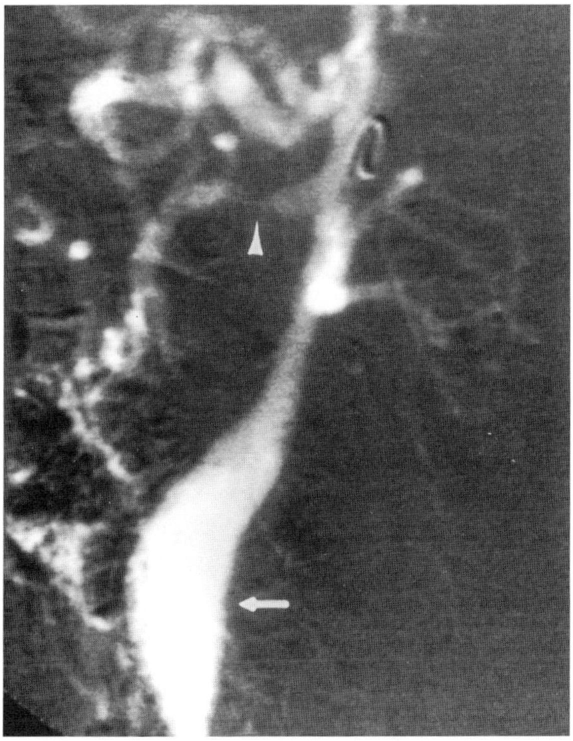

Figure 8.3. Cross-table aortogram shows stenosis of superior mesenteric artery (arrow), and gas floating on slowly flowing blood within an intrarenal aortic aneurysm (arrow).

thus significantly lessen the chance of postprocedure renal failure.

We and others have noticed that intraparenchymal branches are in many cases poorly imaged.[22, 33] For this reason entities that primarily affect intraparenchymal branches such as polyarteritis nodosa or renal infarcts are not well evaluated with CO_2. Similarly, no nephrogram phase occurs and therefore contour defects, such as infarcts, are not seen (Figs 8.5a and 8.5b). However, CO_2 aortography can determine the location, number and size of renal arteries prior to selective iodinated contrast injections.

Aortorenal bypass grafts have a substantially high rate of early postoperative problems including suture line stenosis and graft thrombosis.[41] Intraoperative ultrasound has been advocated as a means to detect these problems early and surgically correct them before renal function is affected.[42–44] Alternatively, CO_2 arteriography has been used successfully to insure wide patency of aortorenal grafts prior to discharge.[36] The procedure is accurate, safe and fast, usually requiring only a 3 French catheter and a single injection (Fig. 8.6).

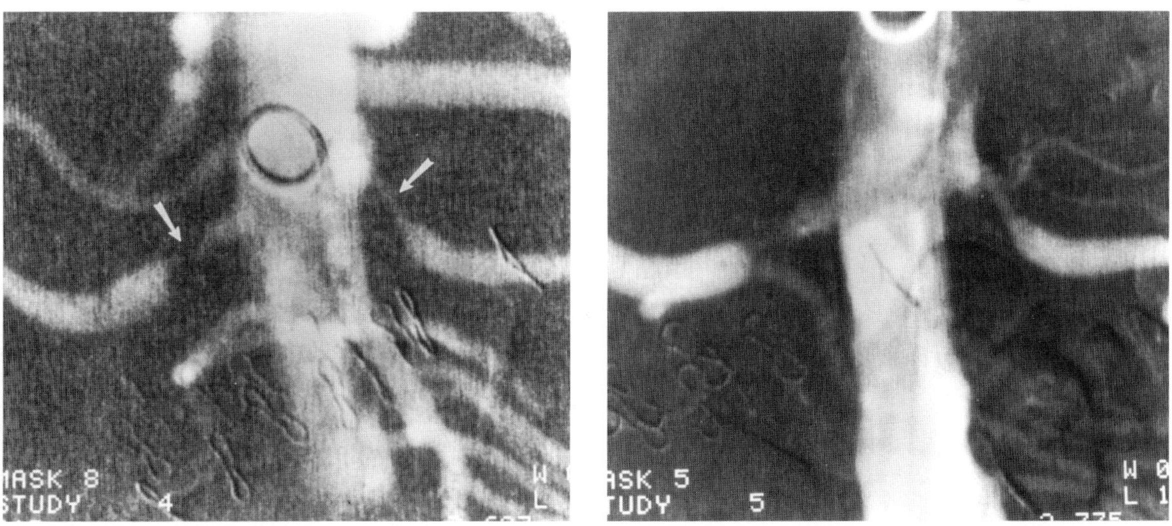

(a) (b)

Figure 8.4. (a) CO_2 aortogram demonstrates bilateral ostial renal artery stenosis (arrows). (b) Comparison image using iodinated contrast confirms findings.

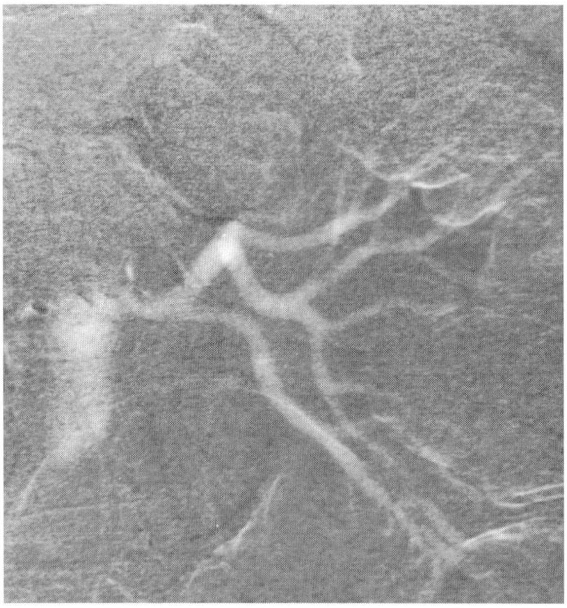

(a)

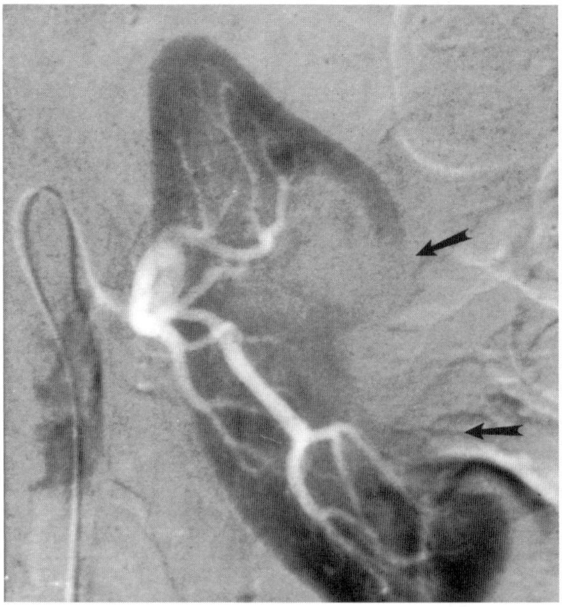

(b)

Figure 8.5. (a) Anteroposterior selective CO_2 left renal arteriogram shows paucity of vessels to midportion of kidney. (b) Renal arteriogram (RAO) selective iodinated contrast image better demonstrates loss of intrarenal branches and nephrogram consistent with a focal infarct (arrows).

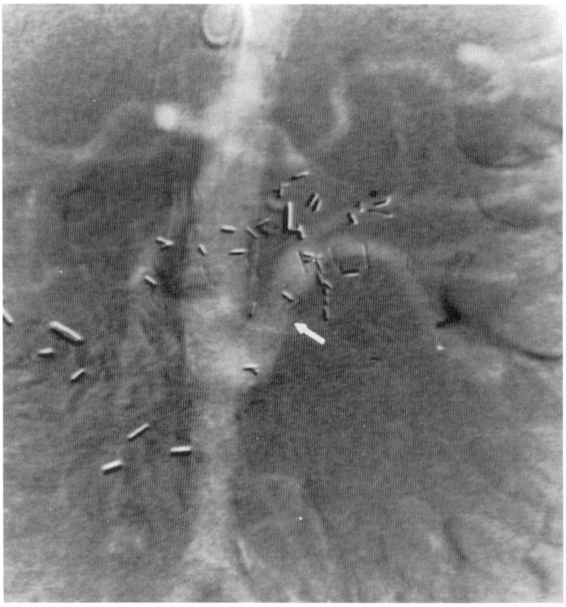

Figure 8.6. Widely patent aortorenal bypass graft (arrow).

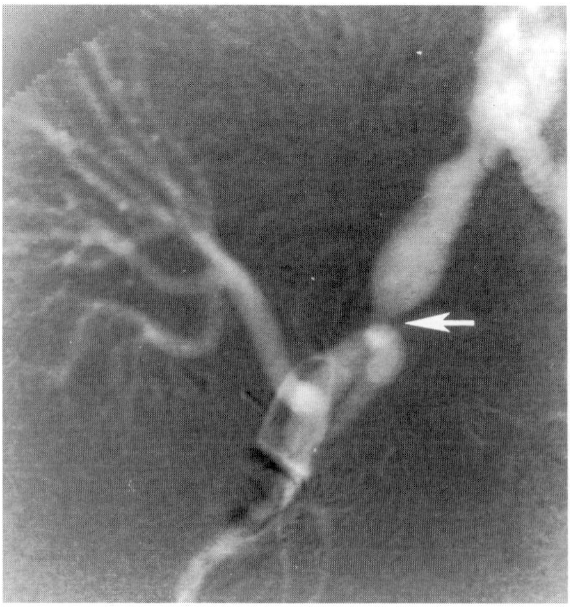

Figure 8.7. Atherosclerotic common iliac artery stenosis (arrow) causing reduction of inflow to iliac fossa renal transplant.

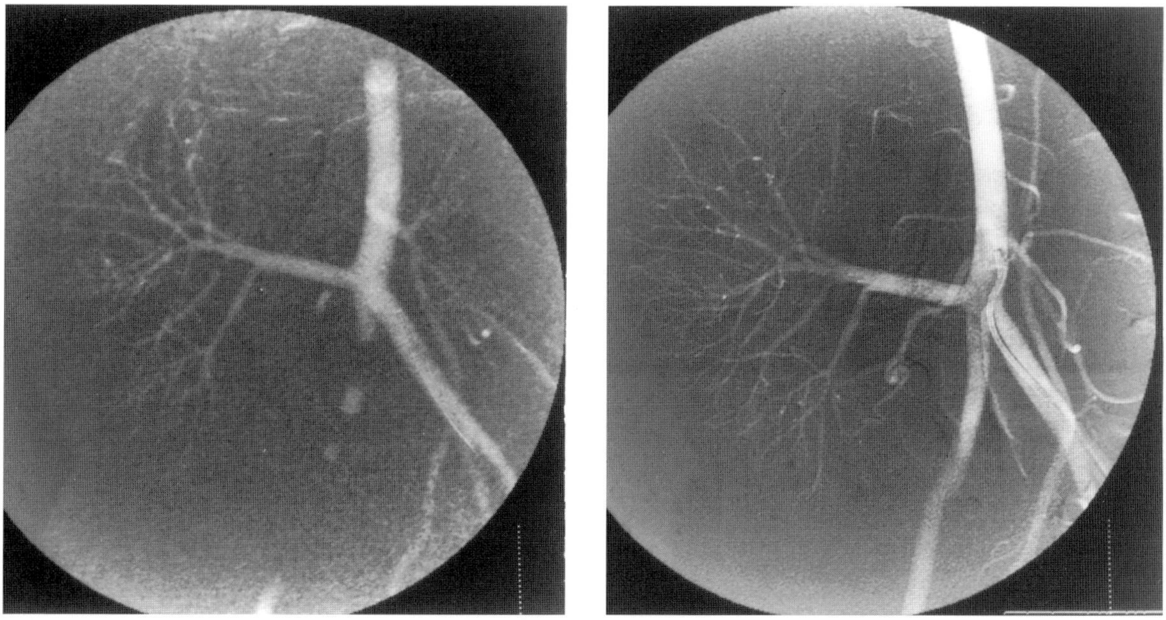

(a) (b)

Figure 8.8. (a) CO_2 aortogram shows good visualization of main renal artery and intrarenal branches in a pediatric renal transplant patient. (b) Comparison iodinated contrast image.

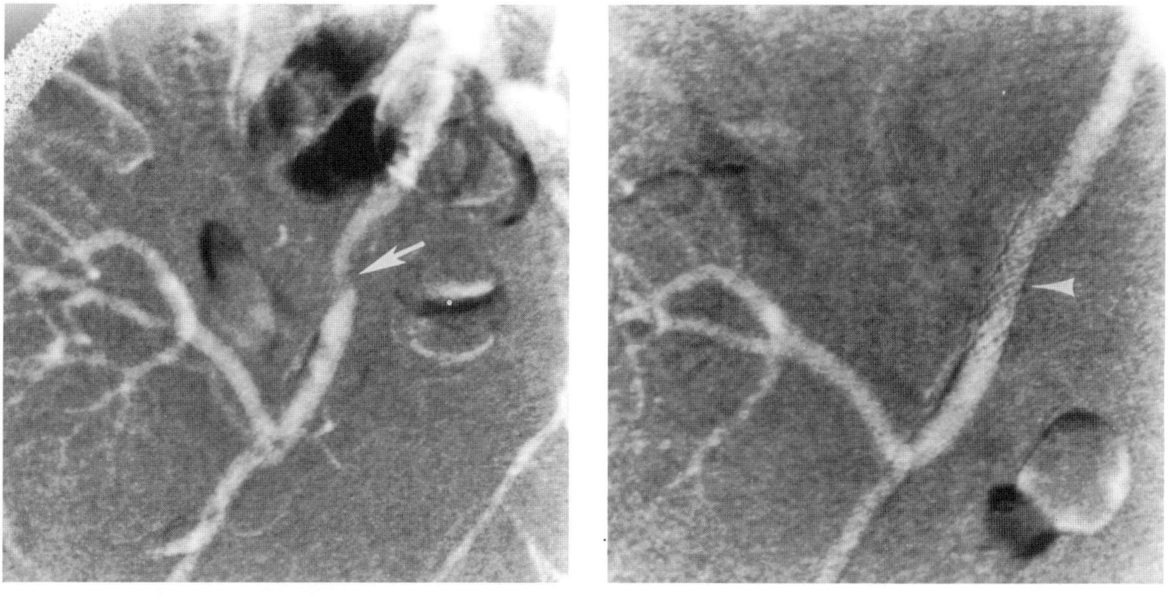

(a) (b)

Figure 8.9. (a) Renal transplant patient with right leg claudication and stenosis of common iliac artery (arrow). (b) Repeat angiography after placement of a Palmaz stent (arrow) across the iliac stenosis.

Onset of hypertension and/or azotemia in patients with renal transplants suggests the possibility of renal artery stenosis or stenosis of the inflow vessel. Transplant renal artery stenosis may present at any time after transplantation, and may be due to surgical technique or may have an immunologic origin. In older patients feeding iliac arteries may narrow due to concomitant atherosclerotic disease (Fig. 8.7). Carbon dioxide arteriography is ideally suited for the angiographic evaluation of these patients since the gas rises into the non-dependently positioned graft filling not only the main vessels but also the intraparenchymal to a degree not seen in native kidneys (Figs 8.8a and 8.8b). Accurate information prior to possible revascularization is obtained with little or no risk to the graft provided proper precautions are taken including waiting 2–3 min between injections to allow the gas to dissolve and reduce the chance of ischemia. Evaluation of the lower extremities in renal transplant patients with concurrent peripheral vascular disease allows accurate preoperative imaging and intervention without risk to the graft (Figs 8.9a and 8.9b).

Summary

Digital subtraction angiography using CO_2 as an intravascular contrast agent has proven to be both safe and clinically useful in the evaluation of both the patient who presents with renal vascular disease, and the patient who has other vascular abnormalities with concomitant renal insufficiency or history of iodinated contrast reaction. A thorough understanding of the nature of intravascular CO_2 behavior is necessary to perform this technique safely and to optimize imaging studies. The main native renal arterial vasculature is accurately imaged, though iodinated contrast at this time remains superior in depicting small vessel and parenchymal disease. Renal transplants and aortorenal bypass grafts are exceptionally well visualized by this method. Further research continues utilizing CO_2 for diagnostic arterial and venous imaging, and as a guide to percutaneous vascular interventional procedures.

References

1 Katayama H, Yamaguchi K, Kozuka T *et al.* Adverse reactions to ionic and nonionic contrast media. *Radiology* 1990; **175:** 621–8.

2 Greenberger PA, Patterson R. The prevention of immediate generalized reactions to radiocontrast media in high-risk patients. *J Allergy Clin Immunol* 1991; **87:** 867–72.

3 Hou SM, Bushinsky DA, Wish JB. Hospital acquired renal insufficiency: a prospective study. *Am J Med* 1983; **74:** 243–8.

4 Manske CL, Sprafka JM, Strony JT, Wang Y. Contrast nephropathy in azotemic diabetic patients undergoing coronary angiography. *Am J Med* 1990; **89:** 615–20.

5 Gomes AS, Lois JF, Baker JD *et al.* Acute renal dysfunction in high-risk patients after angiography: comparison of ionic and nonionic contrast media. *Radiology* 1989; **70:** 65–8.

6 Martin-Paredero V, Dixon SM, Baker JD *et al.* Risk of renal failure after major angiography. *Arch Surg* 1983; **118:** 1417–20.

7. Moore RD, Steinberg EP, Powe NR *et al* Nephrotoxicity of high-osmolality versus low-osmolality contrast media: randomized clinical trial. *Radiology* 1992; **182:** 649–55.

8 Porter GA. Contrast-associated nephropathy. *Am J Cardiol* 1989; **64:** 22E–26E.

9 Lautin EM, Freeman NJ, Schoenfeld AH *et al.* Radiocontrast-associated renal dysfunction: incidence and risk factors. *Am J Roentgenol* 1991; **157:** 49–58.

10 Schwab SJ, Hlatky MA, Pieper KS *et al.* Contrast nephrotoxicity: a randomized controlled trial of a nonionic and an ionic radiographic contrast agent. *N Engl J Med* 1989; **320:** 149–53.

11 Harris KG, Smith TP, Cragg AH, Lemke JH. Nephrotoxicity form contrast material in renal insufficiency: ionic versus nonionic agents. *Radiology* 1991; **179:** 849–52.

12 Barrett BJ, Carlisle EJ. Metaanalysis of the relative nephrotoxicity of high- and low-osmolality iodinated contrast media. *Radiology* 1993; **188:** 171–8.

13 Katholi RE, Taylor GJ, Woods WT *et al.* Nephrotoxicity of nonionic low-osmolality versus ionic high-osmolality contrast media: a prospective double-blind randomized comparison in human beings. *Radiology* 1993; **186:** 183–7.

14 Evens RG. Economic impact of low-osmolality contrast agents on radiology procedures and departments. *Radiology* 1987; **162:** 267–8.

15 Hawkins IF. Carbon dioxide digital subtraction arteriography. *Am J Roentgenol* 1982; **139:** 19–24.

16 Hawkins IF, Herrera MA. Carbon dioxide has promise as arterial contrast agent. *Diagn Imaging* 1985; **7:** 82–4.

17 Stauffer HM, Durant TM, Oppenheimer MJ. Gas embolism: roentgenologic considerations including the experimental use of carbon dioxide as an intracardiac contrast material. *Radiology* 1956; **166:** 686–92.

18 Paul RE, Durant TM, Oppenheimer MJ, Stauffer HM. Intravenous carbon dioxide for intracardiac gas contrast in the roentgen diagnosis of pericardial effusion and thickening. *Am J Roentgenol* 1957; **78:** 224–5.

19 Scatliff JH, Kummer AJ, Janzen AH. The diagnosis of pericardial effusion with intracardiac carbon dioxide. *Radiology* 1959; **73:** 871–82.

20 Moore RM, Braselton CW. Injections of air and of carbon dioxide into a pulmonary vein. *Ann Surg* 1940; **112:** 212–18.

21 Oppenheimer MJ, Durant TM, Stauffer HM *et al.* *In vivo* visualization of intracardiac structures with gaseous carbon dioxide: cardiovascular-respiratory effects and associated changes in blood chemistry. *Am J Physiol* 1956; **186:** 325–34.

22 Schmitz-Rode T, Alzen G, Gunther RW, Pott H. CO_2 spray mini-injector for digital subtraction angiography versus PC-controlled injection system: experiments in dogs. *Cardiovasc Intervent Radiol* 1993; **16:** 297–302.

23 Hawkins IF, Kerns SR. Carbon dioxide digital subtraction angiography. In Cope C (ed.) *Current Techniques in Interventional Radiology*, pp. 11.1–11.17. Philadelphia: Current Medicine, 1994.

24 Takeda T, Iko K, Yuasa Y *et al.* Intraarterial digital subtraction angiography with carbon dioxide: superior detectability of arteriovenous shunting. *Cardiovasc Intervent Radiol* 1988; **11:** 101–7.

25 Hawkins IF, Akins EW, Seeger JM. Carbon dioxide (CO_2) as a contrast agent for angiography and angioscopy. In Ahn SS, Moore WS (eds) *Endovascular Surgery*, pp. 473–80. Philadelphia: WB Saunders, 1992.

26 Hwang MH, Piao ZE, Murdock DK *et al.* Risk of thromboembolism during diagnostic and interventional cardiac procedures with nonionic contrast media. *Radiology* 1990; **174:** 453–7.

27 Kopko PM, Smith DC, Bull BS. Thrombin generation in nonclottable mixtures of blood and nonionic contrast agents. *Radiology* 1990; **174:** 459–61.

28 Robertson HJF. Blood clot formation in angiographic syringes containing nonionic contrast media. *Radiology* 1987; **163:** 621–2.

29 Irving HD, Burbridge BE. Incompatibility of contrast agents with intravascular medications. *Radiology* 1989; **173:** 91–2.

30 Pallan TM, Wulkan IA, Abadir AR *et al.* Incompatibility of Isovue 370 and papaverine in peripheral arteriography. *Radiology* 1993; **187:** 257–9.

31 Shah SJ, Gerlock AJ. Incompatibility of Hexabrix and papaverine in peripheral arteriography. *Radiology* 1987; **162:** 619–20.

32 Hawkins IF, Mladinich CRJ, Storm B *et al.* Short-term effects of selective renal arterial carbon dioxide administration on the dog kidney. *J Vasc Intervent Radiol* 1994; **5:** 149–54.

33 Weaver FA, Pentecost MJ, Yellin AE *et al.* Clinical applications of carbon dioxide/digital subtraction arteriography. *J Vasc Surg* 1991; **13:** 266–73.

34 Miller FJ, Mineau DE, Koehler PR *et al.* Clinical intra-arterial digital subtraction imaging. *Radiology* 1983; **148:** 273–8.

35 Seeger JM, Self S, Harward TRS *et al.* Carbon dioxide gas as an arterial contrast agent. *Ann Surg* 1993; **217:** 688–98.

36 Harward TRS, Smith S, Hawkins IF, Seeger JM. Follow-up evaluation after renal artery bypass surgery with use of carbon dioxide arteriography and color-flow duplex scanning. *J Vasc Surg* 1993; **18:** 23–30.

37 Coffey R, Quisling RG, Mickle JP *et al.* The cerebrovascular effects of intraarterial CO_2 in quantities required for diagnostic imaging. *Radiology* 1986, **151:** 405–10.

38 Shifrin EG, Plich MB, Verstandig AG, Gomori M. Cerebral angiography with gaseous carbon dioxide CO_2. *J Cardiovasc Surg* 1990; **31:** 603–6.

39 Kerns SR, Hawkins IF, Sabatelli FW. Current status of carbon dioxide angiography. In Katzen BT (ed.) *Radiologic Clinics of North America*, pp. 15–29 Philadelphia: WB Saunders, 1995.

40 Rees CR, Niblett RL, Lee SP *et al.* Use of carbon dioxide as a contrast medium for transjugular intrahepatic portosystemic shunt procedures. *J Vasc Intervent Radiol* 1994; **5:** 383–6.

41 Dean RH, Wilson JP, Burko H, Foster JH. Saphenous aortorenal bypass grafts: serial arteriographic study. *Ann Surg* 1974; **180:** 469–78.

42 Hansen KJ, O'Neil EA, Reavis SW *et al.* Intraoperative duplex sonography during renal artery reconstruction. *J Vasc Surg* 1991; **14:** 364–74.

43 Dougherty MJ, Hallett JW, Naessens JM *et al.* Optimizing technical success of renal revascularization: the impact of intraoperative color flow duplex ultrasonography. *J Vasc Surg* 1993; **17:** 849–57.

44 Lantz EJ, Charboneau JW, Hallett JW *et al.* Intraoperative color Doppler sonography during renal artery revascularization. *Am J Roentgenol* 1994; **162:** 859–63.

9

Duplex ultrasound scanning

D EUGENE STRANDNESS JR

Introduction

The search for a suitable screening test for patients suspected of having renal artery stenosis has had a long and difficult history. Since the incidence of renal artery disease amongst the large number of patients with hypertension is very low (estimated to be in the 1–3% range),[1] it is imperative that any screening test be very specific and have a very high negative predictive value. This is necessary to avoid the overuse of arteriography which remains the gold standard for the detection of the problem. Such arteriographic studies are very expensive and potentially dangerous, making its widespread use as a screening test impossible. In addition, there are other concerns that have emerged which must be taken into account with regard to the diagnostic tests that can and should be employed.

With the availability of better antihypertensive agents as well as direct methods for treating renal artery lesions, there is a need for methods that can be used both for screening and follow-up studies. In this regard it is important that the method provide objective information that can be used for comparison from one visit to another. This permits an accurate assessment of any changes that might have occurred in the interim.

Ultrasonic duplex scanning when first developed was applied only to the carotid arteries.[2] This was due to the fact that the technology at that time did not have the versatility to permit its use for other areas in the body. However, as transducer design improved and lower transmitting frequencies became available, it was possible to explore the application of the method for the visceral vessels.[3–5] The renal arteries pose special problems that must be appreciated if the method is to be used successfully. The greatest barriers to ultrasound in the abdomen are the distances to the vessels of interest and the presence of gas in the bowel which is a barrier to the transmission of ultrasound. The distance of the artery from the transducer is less of a problem with the availability of lower transmitting frequencies and the use of different access ports to the kidneys. The problem with bowel gas can be minimized by having patients studied after an overnight fast.

Early experience

As the technology improved and early studies were being performed, the technique of scanning and the interpretation of the findings became the central concerns. For all arteries in the body, the methods employed to detect and grade the degree of narrowing have involved the use of the Doppler method to estimate the velocity changes that are observed. The earliest observation was made by Satomura in 1959 who showed that continuous wave ultrasound could be transmitted through the skin as long as appropriate acoustical coupling was used.[6] It was also noted that the frequency shift provided by flowing blood could be recorded from the back scattered ultrasonic signal. This type of information became the basis for nearly all future developments and applications of Doppler to the study of vascular disease.

There were two major problems and hurdles that had to be overcome with the use of continuous wave Doppler. The first was the method of signal analysis that was used; the second was that when used alone the method was essentially 'blind' to the structures being interrogated.[7] For example, with a continuous wave Doppler system, it is possible to detect blood flow signals in the abdomen but there is no way of knowing from which vessels the signals are arising nor can one determine the velocity in absolute terms due to a lack of information relative to the angle of incidence of the sound beam with the vessels. The solution to detecting flow at all points along the sound beam was achieved by the development of the pulsed Doppler.[8] This method sends out packets of ultrasound whose position in tissue can be determined by noting the time required for the back scattered ultrasound signal to return to the transducer.[9] This is possible since the speed of sound in tissue is known.

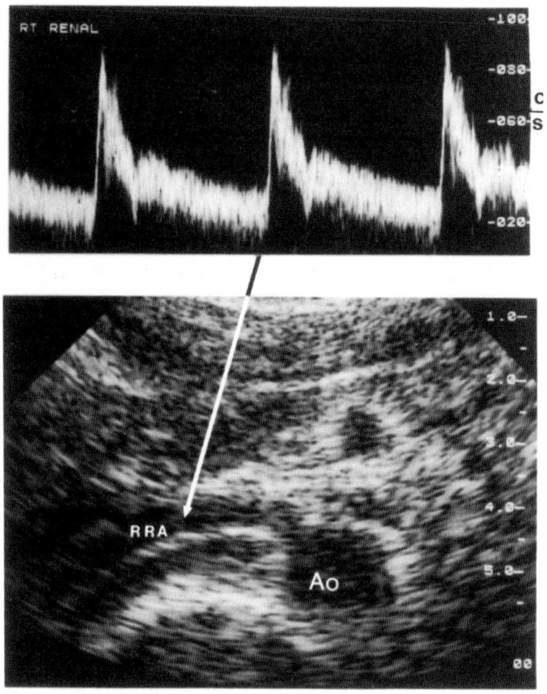

Figure 9.1. The normal velocity patterns in the renal artery are characterized by a peak systolic velocity in the range of 100 cm/s. The end-diastolic velocity is always above the zero flow point. All velocity signals must be taken at an angle close to 60°. From ref. 10, with permission.

Once the back scattered Doppler signal is obtained, it must be analyzed to determine the frequency shift that occurred, which, in turn, is a reflection of the velocity of the target, which, in the case of blood flow, is the red blood cell. The development of the Fast Fourier Transform spectrum analyzer (FFT) solved many of these problems.[9] The FFT permits a display of the frequency and intensity of the back scattered signal (Fig. 9.1). However, even with the use of the pulsed system and the FFT, the true value of the frequency shift (velocity) requires information relative to the angle of the sound beam with the vessel being studied. In order to make maximal use of the pulsed Doppler, associated imaging is vital since the user would then have all the necessary parameters to make estimates of velocity changes as related to location along and within the artery of interest.

The combination of pulsed Doppler and B-mode imaging became known as duplex imaging.[10, 11] While the resolution of the imaging component of these systems has improved dramatically over the past several years, it is not yet possible to use the imaging component alone to detect and quantify the degree of arterial narrowing. While there is no doubt that some of the changes associated with diseases such as atherosclerosis can be appreciated from the imaging, the extent of diameter and cross-sectional area reduction depends entirely upon the detected velocity changes along the course of the artery and within suspected areas of narrowing.[2]

From a clinical standpoint the two diseases that we are asked to evaluate are fibromuscular dysplasia and atherosclerosis. Fibromuscular disease is primarily a disease of young to middle-aged females. From an anatomic standpoint, it comes in three separate forms – medial, intimal and adventitial. The medial is the most common with multiple fibrous rings interspersed with areas of arterial wall thinning (string of beads). With the intimal variety, the fibrous bands are confined to the intima. The adventitial form of the disease is the most uncommon. Regardless of the type, these lesions can narrow the artery and be a cause of hypertension.

By far the most common renal artery lesions are secondary to atherosclerosis.[12] The lesions that involve the renal artery are no different than those found elsewhere in the arterial circulation. In contrast to the fibromuscular lesions which typically involve the mid to distal renal arteries, atherosclerosis commonly is an aortic lesion which extends into the proximal one-third of the renal artery. The fact that it is an orificial lesion and frequently heavily calcified can make it a difficult lesion to treat by balloon angioplasty.

For a renal artery lesion to be a causative factor in the pathogenesis of hypertension, it must reduce the pressure distal to the stenosis to the point where the renin–angiotensin system is activated. The level of diameter reduction sufficient to do this is in the 50–60% range.[13] In the case of atherosclerosis, the lesions are usually discrete and it is uncommon to have more than one stenosis in a renal artery. However, with fibromuscular disease, the lesions are often multiple which makes it very difficult from a radiographic standpoint to assess the actual extent of diameter reduction that is present (Fig. 9.2). The lesions responsible for the development of hypertension can also be bilateral. With atherosclerosis, the bilateral lesions can in the long term be responsible for the development of ischemic renal failure.[14]

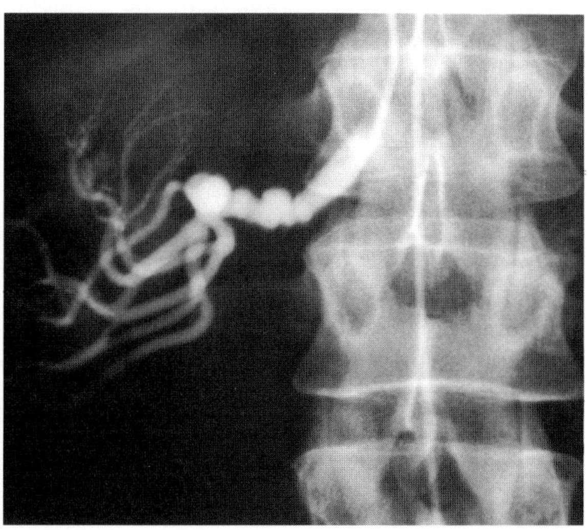

Figure 9.2. The lesion shown in the distal renal artery is typical of fibromuscular dysplasia. Due to the multiple lesions, it is difficult to assess the degree of diameter reduction by arteiography.

Physiology of arterial flow

The organs and tissues of the body from a hemodynamic standpoint can be considered in three major categories which are useful both in understanding their function and how ultrasound can be of assistance in detecting the presence of disease.[15] The categorization that I find most helpful relates to the resistance to flow. There are three organs of low resistance that need high levels of blood flow at all times during the day and night. These include the brain, liver and kidney. With these organs, the end-diastolic flow is always above the zero flow point. The other two patterns noted are dependent upon the level of activity at the time they are studied. Under resting conditions, the gut and extremities can be considered high resistance which is characterized by a brief period of reverse flow in late systole and early diastole with the end-diastolic flow going to zero.[15] However, with even minimal activity, the reverse flow component will disappear and the end-diastolic velocity will be above zero during the period of excess metabolic demand.

One of the confounding factors that complicates the issues involved in studying patients with or suspected renovascular disease is the development of parenchymal vascular disease (arteriolonephrosclerosis). This small vessel disease will lead to an increase in resistance to blood flow.

One of the first to study this issue was Rittenhouse *et al.*, who in a dog model noted that as the resistance to flow increased the end-diastolic velocity decreased.[16] This was further confirmed by Norris *et al.*, who performed similar experiments using a canine renal model.[17] From an ultrasonic standpoint, it is possible to quantitate the peripheral resistance by relating the end-diastolic velocity or frequency to the peak systolic velocity (the end-diastolic ratio, EDR). We evaluated this in 42 normal persons (16 men, 26 women) with a mean age of 54 years. All were normotensive. The EDR in this group of normal subjects was in the 0.33–5 ± 0.06 range.[18] However, when we examined the effects of aging alone on this parameter, we found that there was a trend toward it decreasing.[3] Since we do not have tissue from these kidneys of 'normal aging' controls, we cannot be certain as to the basis for this change. As will be noted there are changes in the resistance as estimated by the EDR which may be of use in the clinical evaluation of patients with suspected renovascular disease.

Role of duplex scanning in screening

Since the prevalence of renovascular hypertension is so low, it is not feasible to screen all hypertensive patients. Even today the patients who are sent for screening have to satisfy certain clinical criteria, which are as follows:[19]

1 malignant hypertension;
2 young patients with hypertension;
3 the presence of an abdominal bruit in a patient with hypertension;
4 decreased serum potassium;
5 azotemia
6 patients whose blood pressure is difficult to control.

In our institution, when patients who fall into the above categories are screened by duplex scanning the diagnostic yield is in the range of 25%. This is acceptable since once identified, the treatment provided may be altered. This is particularly true of those patients with fibromuscular dysplasia where balloon angioplasty may be curative.

An important variable that needs to be known is the degree of narrowing of the renal artery that is required to activate the renin–angiotensin system. For the peripheral arteries, the 'critical stenosis' is defined as that which reduces the diameter of the artery by 50% which is equal to a 75% reduction in the cross-sectional area. For the renal artery, in a dog model, it has been shown that a 60% diameter reduction will be required to produce a pressure drop.[13] In our validation of duplex scanning against arteriography, we chose the 60% diameter lesion as the one most likely to be associated with the development of hypertension.

Once it became apparent that the renal arteries could be studied by ultrasound, it became necessary to develop criteria for grading the degree of narrowing.[3,5] For some areas of the arterial circulation, it is possible to use absolute velocity criteria for the grading of the degree of narrowing but in most cases, this does present a problem. This is due to several facts which are as follows:

1 The range of normal velocities for any particular artery is large. For example in the normal renal arteries that we examined, the peak systolic velocity was in the range of 100 ± 20 cm/s (1 SD).[18]
2 Instead of trying to use an absolute velocity for predicting the degree of narrowing, we chose to use the ratio of the peak systolic velocity in the abdominal aorta to that recorded from the area of narrowing (the RAR ratio).[5] The aortic velocity serves as the reference value against which that recorded from the renal artery can be compared.

As our studies progressed, it became apparent that while the RAR ratio was useful for detecting a clinically significant renal artery stenosis, this alone would miss many patients who had renal artery lesions of lesser magnitude. This could leave the impression with the referring physician that no renal artery lesions were found. To permit detection of lesser lesions, we selected a cutoff value for peak systolic velocity that would have a very high negative predictive value thus avoiding unnecessary arteriograms. To this end, we chose a cutoff value for the peak systolic velocity that would be 2.5 SDs above our normal range. This was found to be 180 cm/s.[20]

Given these considerations, we arrived at the following velocity criteria for the evaluation of renal arteries:

1 normal–peak systolic velocity less than 180 cm/s;
2 renal artery stenosis present–peak systolic velocity greater than 180 cm/s;
3 renal artery stenosis <60% diameter reduction, peak systolic velocity >180 cm/s, RAR less than 3.5;

4 renal artery stenosis >60%, peak systolic velocity >180 cm/s, RAR >3.5;
5 total occlusion–no signals from the renal artery; it was also noted that a renal artery occlusion was commonly associated with a renal length of <9cm.

In our early studies, which were somewhat limited by numbers, we noted that in patients with a >60% diameter reducing stenosis, renal length (which we assumed reflected renal mass) tended to decrease over time.[21] In order to establish the repeatability of this measurement, we conducted a study to determine the range of lengths that a single technologist could achieve by ultrasound. A total of ten subjects were scanned on two separate occasions 5–13 days apart.[22] The same instrument was used for all studies and ten separate images of each kidney were taken for measurement. An horizontal image of the kidney was used for each measurement.

The mean difference in length between the first and second study was 3 mm (p>0.05). The average standard deviation was 2.6 mm. The standard deviation of the difference between the first and second studies was 4.3 mm resulting in one-tailed 95% confidence interval for a change in renal length of 7.1 mm. Based upon these data we considered any change of 1 cm in length as being significant. As will be shown this type of measurement became very important when we examined the changes that occurred over time when a high grade renal artery lesion was found.

Scanning method

Because of the problems of bowel gas, we prefer to carry out the studies in the morning after an overnight fast. This makes the likelihood of success much greater. By instituting this procedure our success rate has remained in the 90% range for completing the study.

The procedure is started with the patient in the supine position with the head of the examining table elevated 30°. A low frequency scanhead (2.5–3.0 MrHz) is used to image the abdominal aorta in the longitudinal plane. It should be noted that the availability of color Doppler in the system assists the technologist in identifying the key landmarks for the study which include the aorta, left renal vein and the origin of the renal arteries. The renal arteries do not follow a straight path to the kidneys from their origin.

Once the abdominal aorta at the level of the renal and superior mesenteric arteries is identified, a center stream signal from the aorta is obtained. The scanhead is then rotated 90° to permit the identification of the origin of the renal arteries. The left renal vein is a useful landmark since the renal arteries lie immediately beneath this vessel. Once identified, the entire renal artery is scanned out to the hilum of the kidney to be sure that no lesions are missed. If at all points along the renal artery, the peak systolic velocity is <180 cm/s, the patient is classified as normal.

The presence of a stenosis is recognized by the sudden increase in peak systolic velocity. There are two other findings that are helpful. The first is the presence of turbulence which is recognized in color by the random admixing of colors distal to the site of narrowing. The other is the presence of a bruit, represented by flashes of color at systole and found outside the boundaries of the renal artery. This when seen is associated with the presence of high grade lesions. Once the peak systolic velocity is recorded, the RAR can be calculated. If >3.5, the patient is classified as having a >60% diameter reduction. The occluded artery is suspected by failure to identify a signal from the renal artery.[20]

To further assess the kidney itself, the patient is turned on their side with the kidney now approached from the flank. From this position, it is possible to measure renal length as well as the flow patterns within the parenchyma of the kidney. All measurements of renal length are made from the same position at the time of each follow-up visit.

Results of duplex vs arteriography

The arteriographic approach used at our institution for renal arterial studies is the intra-arterial digital subtraction method (DSA). With this method there are both advantages and disadvantages. It is possible to limit the dye load which is important since many of these patients have some degree of renal insufficiency. A potential disadvantage is that multiple views of the renal arteries may not be obtained. For classification purposes, the renal arteries were classified into four categories:[20]

1 normal;
2 less than 60% stenosis;
3 greater than 60% stenosis;
4 occluded.

For the comparison of duplex scanning against arteriography we considered only that population of patients who had atherosclerotic involvement. It is difficult if not impossible to estimate the degree of diameter reduction in patients with fibromuscular disease of the renal artery. This is due to the presence of multiple lesions (string of beads) that are frequently found. The role of duplex for patients with fibromuscular dysplasia will be covered later.

For the latest validation study there were 41 patients (27 males and 14 females) with a mean age of 63 ± 10.9 years.[20] Hypertension was present in all 41 patients with diabetes being a comorbid condition in nine cases (22%). Twenty-seven patients (66%) had some element of renal insufficiency (creatinine > 115 µm/l–1.3 mg/dl). The mean systolic and diastolic blood pressures were 175 ± 27 mmHg and 94 ± 19 mmHg. The mean creatinine level was 202 ± 153 µm/l (2.28 ± 1.7 mg/dl: range 80–887 µm/l).

Results of screening

For the analysis of duplex against arteriography, 38 of the 41 patients included for comparison had atherosclerosis as the basis for the renal artery narrowing. One patient had a dissection and another patient presented with multiple emboli to both kidneys. The results as compared with arteriography for the detection of renal artery stenosis are shown in Table 9.1. The comparison resulted in a sensitivity of 95% (95% confidence interval [CI] 90–100%) and a specificity of 90% (95% CI 71–100%).

For the detection of a >60% diameter reducing stenosis, the comparison is as shown in Table 9.2. As noted there were 26 arteries that had a <60% stenosis or were normal by arteriography. In 16 of these cases the RAR was <3.5 giving a specificity of 62% (95% CI 43–80%). Since there were differences in the classification in the ten cases where the RAR and arteriography were employed, we reviewed these cases in more detail:

1 only one of the ten renal arteries was in fact normal;
2 in the remaining nine cases, both studies revealed a stenosis with the difference being on the degree of narrowing;
3 in four of the cases where a stenosis of <60% was noted by arteriography, three went on to have an angioplasty while the fourth underwent direct surgical repair.

Ten of the eleven occluded renal arteries were correctly identified by duplex scanning. Seven kidneys had accessory renal arteries which were not identified by duplex scanning. However, none of these accessory renal arteries had stenotic lesions which were the cause of their hypertension. However, there are certainly instances when accessory renal arteries can be involved and be the source of problems.

Another important factor in utilizing a combined imaging/Doppler method, is its ability to not only identify the presence of renal artery stenosis but also localize the site(s) of involvement in the renal artery. As one might expect, the best and most accurate method of identifying the location is arteriography. In this regard, we did carry out an evaluation of this in 61 arteries

Table 9.1. Comparison of duplex scanning vs arteriography for the detection of renal artery stenosis

	Arteriography		
Duplex	Normal	Abnormal	Total
Velocity <180cm/s	9	3	12
Velocity >180cm/s	1	61	62
Total	10	64	74

Table 9.2. Duplex scanning vs arteriography for the detection of a >60% diameter reducing stenosis

	Arteriography		
Duplex	<60%	>60%	Total
RAR <3.5 normal	16	4	20
RAR>3.5 abnormal	10	44	54
Total	26	48	74

where disease was found by both methods. In 58 of the arteries, there was agreement as to location. In two renal arteries, duplex identified lesions in the mid and distal renal artery, whereas arteriography found them to be located at the origin and proximal renal artery.[20]

If duplex is going to play a role when compared with arteriography, it is important to know how well arteriographers do when they are compared against each other in reading films. The results in simply classifying the presence or absence of disease is shown in Table 9.3.

Given these results, it would appear that duplex scanning has sufficient accuracy to permit its use for screening purposes with some provisos which are as follows:

1 the laboratory has sufficient experience and workload to maintain proficiency;
2 the technologists involved have done sufficient cases under supervision to provide the necessary expertise to carry out the studies;
3 the referral population is large enough to provide a constant flow of patients for study. At present we have referred 30–40 patients per month for screening. The diagnostic yield for this screening has been in the 25% range which seems to be adequate given the low prevalence of renal vascular hypertension.

Renal hilar scanning

Because of the difficulties associated with renal duplex scanning, attempts have been made to simplify the procedure by examining the arterial signals from the renal hilum. The first to describe this was Handa *et al.*[23] The parameters used for the diagnosis were the acceleration time and acceleration index (Fig. 9.3). The normal values for these parameters were <100 ms for acceleration time (AT) and <3.78 kHz/s/MHz for the acceleration index (AI). These authors found that these were 100% sensitive for the detection of siginficant stenoses in the main renal arteries. Martin *et al.*[24] performed a similar study and found that acceleration times ≥100 ms had a sensitivity of 93%.

Stavros *et al.*[25] used pattern recognition to assess renal hilar arterial patterns. The principle is simple. If there is a hemodynamically significant stenosis proximal to the recording site, there will be loss of the early systolic peak (ESP) with blunting of the arterial waveform (tardus parvus; TP) (Fig. 9.4). By the simple

Table 9.3. Interobserver variability of two radiologists reading the same films

	Radiologist 1		
	Normal	Abnormal	Total
Radiologist 2			
Normal	9	3	12
Abnormal	1	61	62
Total	10	64	74

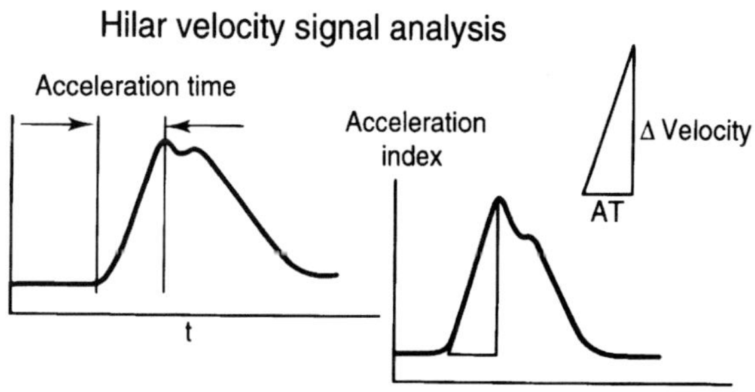

Figure 9.3. Hilar velocity signal analysis. The methods by which the accleration time and acceleration index are measured are shown. These waveforms are recorded from the hilum of the kidney. From ref. 10, with permission.

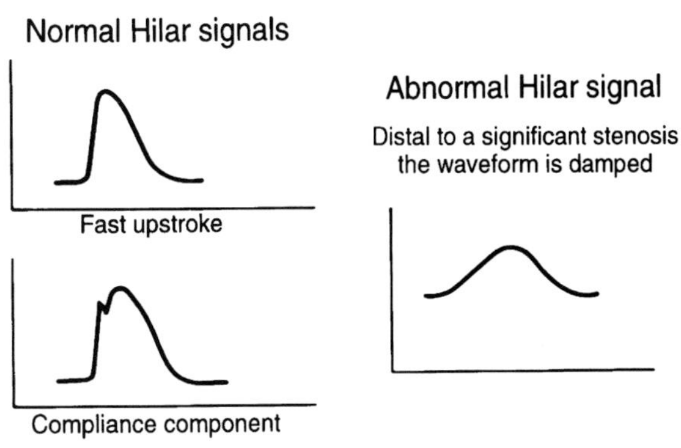

Figure 9.4. The normal hilar velocity patterns consist of a very rapid upstroke and systolic peak. In some normals, a notch near the peak is often found. When there is a hemodynamically significant stenosis proximal to the recording site, the waveform loses its rapid upstroke and becomes damped (tardus parvus).

observation of loss of the ESP, the sensitivity was found to be 95%. In those cases where the findings were positive, a complete duplex examination would be performed. If it was negative, no further examination was performed. If this were as good as it appears, it might serve as a very simple and fast method of screening making it nearly ideal for the detection of renal artery disease.

To investigate this in our own patient population, we carried out a prospective study.[26] There were 44 patients who were screened by separate technologists. These were randomized to the standard approach and the hilar method. The technologists who did the studies were unaware of the findings of the other. The mean examination time for the standard study was 69 min and 14 min for the hilar scan. In the 86 renal arteries that were scanned, 15 (17%) were found to have a renal artery stenosis that exceeded 60% diameter reduction. For AT and AI, the sensitivity for both was 67%. The sensitivity for ESP/TP was 72%. The specificity was 89% for AT, 79% for AI and 99% for ESP/TP waveforms. While the specificity of the hilar studies was satisfactory, its sensitivity was low.

There are several problems with the hilar alone approach. As noted the sensitivity is not good enough for detection of high grade lesions. In addition, the hilar studies will never permit detection of lesions that are not yet significant from a hemodynamic standpoint. Thus, this approach would underestimate the prevalence of renal artery stenosis.

Patient management

It is impossible to draw any firm conclusions about the impact of a positive and negative screening test on patient management but certain trends are beginning to emerge. These have to be considered under the basis for the disease and the reason for referral for study. The population where a positive scan appears to have the most immediate impact are those women with fibromuscular disease. When renal artery stenosis is found, there has been a trend to having an arteriogram done with the prospect of performing transluminal angioplasty which can be curative. The problem with renovascular disease secondary to atherosclerosis is much more complex. These patients are older, have more generalized disease in the circulation and do not do as well with endovascular methods as do the patients with fibromuscular disease. In addition, surgical results while satisfactory do carry a substantial risk to the patient which must be taken into account. When invasive studies are done in this group, they are done because of the failure of treatment for the hypertension or the patient is showing evidence of early renal failure. In the past few years, the issue of ischemic renal failure has been raised. While exact figures are not available, it has been estimated that up to 150 000 patients in the United States may be on renal dialysis due to this problem.[14] If that is the case, then the detection of bilateral renal artery lesions becomes more important since they will be the ones that are most likely to lead to such an outcome.

Natural history and outcome studies

While there is no doubt that atherosclerosis is a chronic progressive disease, the time course over which it develops or progresses when established has remained largely a mystery. Until the availability of duplex scanning, the only information available on the natural history of renal artery lesions was by repeat arteriographic studies which were not prospective so the population is undoubtedly skewed. Four studies done in this manner have given us some clues as to the rate at which this occurs.

1 Meaney *et al.* reviewed 39 patients with atherosclerotic disease who underwent serial arteriograms at intervals ranging from 6 months to 10 years. In ten of these patients, there appeared to be an increase in stenosis severity, with four progressing to a total occlusion giving an overall progression rate of 36%.[27]
2 Wollenweber *et al.*, in a similar arteriographic study carried out over a 42-month period, found progression of the lesions in 50%.[28]

3 Schreiber *et al.*, in the largest study to be done, found that 44% of the 85 patients developed progressive lesions over a mean follow-up period of 52 months. In the 37 patients who showed progression of their lesions, 14 of these went on to total occlusion. The progression to total occlusion was highest in those patients who had a stenosis that exceeded the 75% level.[29]
4 In Tollefson and Ernst's more recent study, 48 patients with a minimum of two arteriograms at least 1 year apart were followed up for a mean of 7.3 years. Of the 79 renal artery lesions, stenosis progression was found in 42 or 53% with seven progressing to total occlusion.[30]

Our interest in the natural history of renal artery stenosis as documented by duplex ultrasound was stimulated by an early and rather limited study. Taylor *et al.* showed that the status of the renal artery could be monitored over time but, most importantly, there was a decrease in renal length that appeared to be related to the degree of narrowing. There were 15 patients (19 renal arteries with a >60% stenosis) that had a mean follow-up of 13 months. While all of the renal arteries remained patent, there was a significant decrease in renal length noted (mean difference: 1 cm; $p<0.01$).[21]

After these initial observations, we elected to start a natural history study of patients found to have atherosclerotic narrowing of one or both renal arteries at the time of screening. These patients were identified as having atherosclerosis by age, sex and location of their lesions. All patients with fibromuscular disease were excluded from follow-up. There were two analyses that were performed on the patients with the first addressing the relationship between the degree of narrowing and changes in renal length with the second examining the changes in the renal artery lesions themselves.

Before considering the outcome data, it is important to review some of the factors and difficulties in documenting disease progression. By the time patients with renal artery stenosis are first seen, the disease has already reached an advanced stage. While the disease at this stage will have activated the renin–angiotensin system, its effects on the renal parenchyma will remain an uncertainty. For example, if renal mass does decrease distal to a high grade renal artery stenosis, we do not understand why or how it occurs. It might represent a loss of functional nephrons in combination with loss of the interstitium. We do know that the results of renal revascularization are in part dependent on the size of the kidney.

Ideally, we would like to be able to observe the progression of a renal artery stenosis in a step-wise manner along with the rate at which it occurs. This is not possible by almost any means including arteriography. Nonetheless, it is possible to use categories with which one may be able to state with some certainty that a change has occurred. In this regard and based upon our validation studies, we can use the same categories to document changes over time. These are:

1 normal;
2 <60% narrowing;
3 >60% stenosis;
4 renal artery occlusion.

The first part of our study examined the changes in renal length that occurred over time. There were 54 patients (22 males, 32 females with a mean age of 65.8 years) who were followed an average of 14.4 months (range 4–24 months). These patients were followed every 6 months with a repeat ultrasonic duplex scan. None of patients with normal renal arteries or <60% stenosis showed a decrease in length of >1 cm during follow-up. On the other hand, 26% (13/49 sides) with a >60% stenosis were found to have a >1 cm loss of renal length. The average decrease in length was 1.9 cm (range 1.2–3.4 cm). The estimated risk for a 1 cm decrease in length was 19% at 1 year. After the first year, the patients with bilateral high grade lesions were three times more likely to have one or both kidneys decrease by >1 cm (Fig. 9.5).[31]

In order to document progression of disease by categories of narrowing, we studied 80 patients (36 males, 44 females with a mean age of 66 years). These patients were studied every 6 months for a mean interval of 12.7 months. There were a total of 139 arteries included in the target group. The status of the renal arteries and their cumulative incidence of progression to a higher degree of narrowing is shown in Table 9.4.[32]

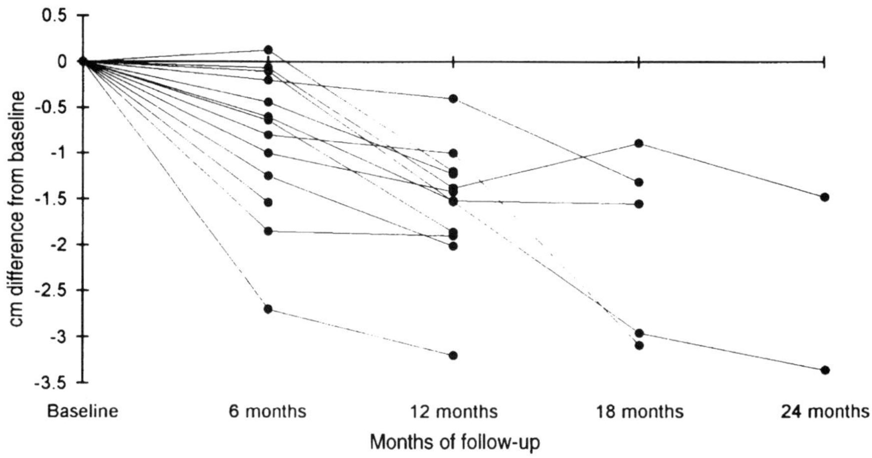

Figure 9.5. The changes in renal length that occurred over time in patients with a >60% diameter reducing lesion are shown. From ref. 31, with permission.

Table 9.4. Cumulative incidence of renal artery disease progression

Baseline duplex[a]	Follow-up interval 0 months	6 months	12 months	18 months	24 months
Normal arteries					
No. entering interval	36	27	24	18	7
CI	0	0	0	0	0
<60% stenosis					
No. entering interval	35	22	14	8	2
CI	0	3±3	23±9	29±10	42±14
≥60% stenosis					
No. entering interval	63	46	32	22	10
CI	0	0	5±3	5±3	11±6

CI: cumulative incidence (%).
age ± SEM.
[a]5 baseline occlusions omitted.

The renal artery disease progression was assessed by life-table analysis in 95 arteries followed for 6 months, 70 arteries followed for 24 months, 48 arteries followed for 18 months and 19 arteries followed for 24 months. None of the arteries classified as normal at the time of entrance into the study showed progression to a >60% stenosis or total occlusion. Seven of the 35 renal arteries having a <60% stenosis at the baseline progressed to a >60% stenosis resulting in a cumulative incidence of progression of 23 ± 9% at 12 months and 42 ± 4% at 24 months. All four renal arteries that progressed to a total occlusion had a >60% stenosis at the baseline visit. The cumulative incidence of progression to occlusion was 5 ± 3% at 12 months and 11 ± 6% at 24 months.

Discussion

The role of a screening test is to establish the underlying basis for a patient's presenting problem. In the case of patients with hypertension, we are attempting to determine if renal artery stenosis is present and is the cause for the hypertension. The problem is compounded by the fact that renal artery lesions constitute a very small percentage of the patients in this very large population (1–3%). However, with more experience and a better understanding of the patients with hypertension, it is now known that the yield for finding renal artery lesions will increase dramatically if screening is limited to particular subsets of patients with hypertension. If screening is limited to those patients whose hypertension acutely worsens, in patients with malignant hypertension and those referred to specialty centers for hypertension difficult to control the yield will be as high as 30%. This will increase to 45% in patients whose hypertension is accelerated and associated with renal failure.[33, 34]

Like most other diagnostic tests, the technique and application of duplex scanning has evolved and improved both from a technological standpoint and our understanding of how the test should be performed and the results interpreted. In some of the early studies done by Greene *et al.*[35] and Avasthi *et al.*,[36] the sensitivity and specificity for detecting a renal artery stenosis of >50% was 83 and 73% respectively. The criteria employed were a peak renal artery velocity >100 cm/s, absence of flow in diastole and detection of turbulent flow as noted by the audible character of the Doppler signal. Other criteria have been suggested and include peak frequency, the presence of a bruit, spectral broadening and an abrupt decrease in the peak systolic velocity from one segment of artery to the next.

When we began our studies we were aware of the various parameters that might be used but each of them had problems which were difficult to standardize and implement into daily practice. The major problems associated with detection of renal artery lesions can be summarized as follows:

1 The arteries are deeply placed.
2 They do not follow a straight course to the kidney making it difficult to obtain a constant angle of incidence of the ultrasound with the renal artery. This becomes critical when one is attempting to derive absolute values for the detected velocities.
3 The range of normal values for velocity is such that it is difficult in any single patient to use a cutoff value for the detection of relatively minor degrees of stenosis. In addition, if the upper limit of normal is set too low, unnecessary arteriographic studies are likely to be more common which defeats the purpose of the screening procedure.
4 The study itself is very difficult to do unless one has considerable experience and ongoing exposure to a sizable population of patients with this problem.

Fortunately, during the evolutionary period of development of the method there were parallel improvements in the technology which have made the method much easier to use. For example, the incorporation of color into the Doppler portion of the duplex scanner has made several aspects of the scans simpler. With color one is able to see the origin and course of the renal arteries thus in many cases avoiding the relatively blind search that one had to do with black and white alone. However, one must realize that color is a 'pathfinder' and should not be used to quantitate the degree of stenosis that may be present. Another indirect but useful application of color is its ability to detect the presence of a bruit generated by the vibration of the arterial wall. The arterial wall vibration is transmitted to the soft tissues and appears as bright flashes seen during peak systole. The appearance of a bruit is strongly suggestive of the presence of a high-grade stenosis in the renal artery. Finally, with color it is possible to see flow within the kidney itself which is useful as a landmark for placement of the sample volume of the pulsed Doppler.

Given the uncertainties of the method, we have developed the criteria that are currently in place and work well for us. In our experience, there are factors not included in the standard protocol which can introduce some uncertainty. The first is the presence of an aortic aneurysm which will by virtue of the increase in diameter result in a lower peak systolic velocity which is used as the reference value in calculating the renal aortic ratio. If we find the peak systolic velocity from the aorta to be less than 40 cm/s, we do not use this as the reference value but depend on the extent of the velocity increase in the renal artery at sites of narrowing, the appearance of bruits and the presence of poststenotic turbulence.

A continuing problem not unique to the renal circulation is the variability associated with the estimation of the degree of stenosis. If we accept arteriography as the gold standard, any disagreements with regard to the degree of stenosis predicted by duplex will be assigned as an error for duplex scanning. While we know the intra- and interobserver variability for arteriography in other areas of the arterial circulation, we do not have a similar appreciation for it in the renal artery. In our own studies of this problem the greatest uncertainty when two radiologists read the same films is for the presence or absence of minimal lesions which is not unexpected.

As a concrete example of the problem, let us examine the consequences of the 'apparent errors' for the detection of a >60% stenosis in our own studies. As noted earlier there were ten cases where we found the RAR to be >3.5 predicting the presence of a high grade stenosis. The arteriographic studies detected one clear error, but in the remainder of the cases the disagreement was on the degree of narrowing not on the presence or absence of disease. If one were to use very rigid criteria for the cutoff point in this setting, the nine patients would be denied further consideration and therapy for renal artery stenosis. In fact, in four of the ten, where there was disagreement, three were treated by angioplasty and one by direct surgical repair.

An example where some dispute arose over the diagnosis and future therapy is shown in Fig. 9.6. This middle-aged woman with severe hypertension was found by duplex to have a stenosis in the distal right renal artery giving an RAR of 3.6. When the arteriogram was performed, the interventionist felt the lesion was not sufficiently abnormal to proceed with angioplasty. Is this correct? One way to settle this issue would be to do renins and if there was lateralization to the right, I would argue that an angioplasty should be done. While this was recommended, further testing was not carried out.

Another great advantage of duplex scanning is for follow-up purposes. Since we have quantitative criteria for the initial detection of stenoses, these can be used during follow-up to document the results of therapy, be it endovascular or surgery. We studied this in nine patients with fibromuscular dysplasia (14 arteries) that under-

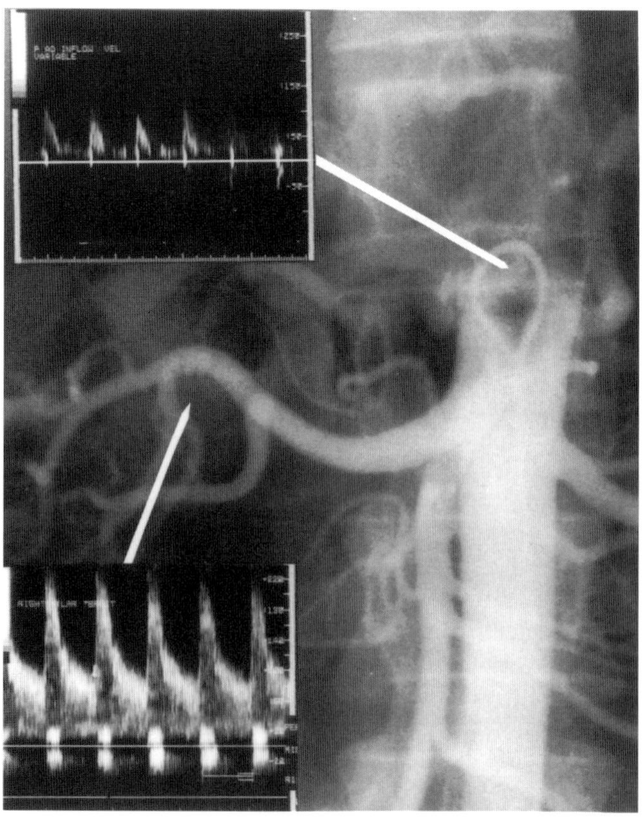

Figure 9.6. This middle-aged female with hypertension was found to have a velocity pattern in the distal renal artery consistent with a >60% stenosis. The arteriogram while demonstrating a lesion of fibromuscular dysplasia was not thought to appear significant enough to warrant angioplasty. See text for details.

went transluminal angioplasty for the treatment of their hypertension. There were a total of 18 treatments of which 14 were considered successful by a fall in the blood pressure and a decrease in the RAR to 3.5 or lower.[37] We have found that both angioplasty and arterial surgery for the treatment of atherosclerotic lesions can be evaluated in an identical manner. There are no other diagnostic tests which provide this degree of flexibility and quantitation of results.

Since the duplex scanning can be repeated to examine the same lesions and arteries over time, it is an ideal method of monitoring disease progression and its effects on renal mass. In most other arterial beds, progression of disease is followed by changes in the clinical picture which are quite simple to recognize and relate to the change in the status of the disease. This is not necessarily true for the kidneys for the following reasons:

1. Since there are two kidneys disease progression in one renal artery may be manifest only as increased need for antihypertensive medication.
2. With bilateral lesions, progression to the level of renal failure may be subtle and not recognized until it is too late from a therapeutic standpoint.
3. It has been recognized for a long time that one of the consequences of long-standing renovascular stenosis is loss of renal mass. In fact one of the considerations that must be taken into account when contemplating arterial reconstruction is the size of the affected kidney. At present there are no firm guidelines that would indicate at what renal size arterial reconstruction should *not be done*. Our studies clearly show that once a lesion in the renal artery becomes >60%, there is progressive loss of renal mass which is quite rapid. This raises several questions which will have to be answered by future studies. These are as follows:
   a. is the quantitation of renal length decrease an indication for intervention?
   b. if the process is bilateral, should intervention be done before loss of renal mass occurs?

These are not trivial questions because intervention particularly surgical, carries considerable risk particularly if it is done for patients who are in some degree of renal failure. It would be ideal to repair these arteries at a stage where the revascularized kidney is able to restore function to a normal level. The problem is compounded by the fact that angioplasty which appears to work quite well in patients with fibromuscular dysplasia, is not as successful in patients with atherosclerotic disease due to the very high and early recurrence rate that follows due the development of myointimal hyperplasia. Thus, at present, the patient with atherosclerosis who needs some form of intervention is left with very few options.

Another advantage of duplex scanning is that it can also be used to scan other arterial beds that can be involved by atherosclerosis. In a cohort of 60 patients who were documented to have renal artery stenosis by duplex scanning, a similar study was done of the carotid arteries and peripheral circulation monitored by the measurement of the ankle/brachial index (ABI).[38] For those patients with a <60% diameter stenosis of the renal artery, the prevalence of a 50–100% diameter reducing lesion in the carotid artery was 25%. For those patients with a >60% diameter reducing lesion, the prevalence of a high grade carotid lesion was 46%. In the leg arteries the prevalence of ABIs of less than 0.95 (upper limit of normal) was 50% in the patients with a <60% renal artery stenosis. This increased to 73% in that subset with the high grade renal artery lesions.

These findings show that the presence of severe atherosclerosis in one major arterial bed is very likely to be associated with disease in other areas. The finding of a high prevalence of carotid arterial disease in patients with renal artery stenosis suggests that a scan of this area should also be done. Evidence is emerging that the presence of high grade stenoses (>80% diameter reduction) in the carotid artery is associated with a high incidence of stroke. In addition, the concomitant presence of hypertension makes it likely that it will contribute to the progression of the carotid lesion and a poor outcome.

Finally, as an adjunct to screening for lesions in the renal arteries, there are suggestions that the degree of resistance in the kidney might also be studied and perhaps be of some clinical value. As noted earlier, an increase in resistance is reflected in the end-diastolic velocity and its relationship to the zero flow point. The higher the resistance to flow, the lower the end-diastolic velocity. Of what value might this be? It is of interest that patients with fibromuscular dysplasia all have uniformly low resistance patterns even in the non-involved kidney. This is in contrast to those patients with atherosclerosis who show lower values which may reflect parenchymal changes at the microcirculatory level.

Some of the problems associated with the use of resistance changes from a clinical standpoint are that they are non-specific and also appear to be affected by age alone in the absence of hypertension. The one area where continued work needs to be done is to study the effect of parenchymal resistance changes on the outcome after angioplasty and direct arterial surgery. Our evidence for this as a factor is incomplete at present but is certainly something we shall be studying in more detail as time passes.

References

1 Gifford RW. Epidemiology and clinical manifestations of renovascular hypertension. In Stanley J, Ernst CB, (eds) *Renovascular Hypertension*, pp. 77–99. Philadelphia: WB Saunders, 1984.
2 Phillips DJ, Powers JE, Eyer MK *et al.* Detection of peripheral vascular disease using duplex scanner III. *Ultrasound Med Biol* 1980; **6:** 205–18.
3 Kohler TR, Zierler RE, Martin RL *et al.* Noninvasive diagnosis of renal artery stenosis by ultrasonic duplex scanning. *J Vasc Surg* 1986; **4:** 450–6.
4 Taylor DC, Moneta GL. Duplex scanning of the renal and mesenteric circulation. In Rutherford RB (ed.) *Seminars in Vascular Surgery*, pp. 23–31. Philadelphia: WB Saunders, 1988.
5 Taylor DC, Kettler MD, Moneta GL *et al.* Duplex ultrasound in the diagnosis of renal artery stenosis: a prospective evaluation. *J Vasc Surg* 1988; **7:** 363–9.
6 Satomura S. Study of flow patterns in peripheral arteries by ultrasonics. *J Acoust Soc Jpn* 1959; **15:** 151–8.
7 Strandness DE Jr, Schultz RA, Sumner DS, Rushmer RF. Ultrasonic flow detection: a useful technique in the evaluation of peripheral vascular disease. *Am J Surg* 1967; **113:** 311–20
8 Baker DW. Pulsed ultrasonic Doppler blood flow sensing. *IEEE Trans Biomed Engin* 1970; **17:** 170–85.
9 Beach KW. Physics and instrumentation for ultrasonic duplex scanning. In Strandness DE Jr (ed.) *Duplex Scanning in Vascular Disorders*, pp. 273–317. New York: Raven Press, 1993.
10 Strandness DE Jr (ed.) *Duplex Scanning in Vascular Disorders*, 2nd edn. New York: Raven Press, 1993.
11 Barber FE, Baker DW, Strandness DE Jr. Duplex scanner II for simultaneous imaging of artery tissues and flow. *Ultrasonics Symposium Proc IEEE* 1974; 74 (CH0896-ISU).
12 Strandness DE Jr. Extracranial arterial disease. In Strandness DE Jr (ed.) *Duplex Scanning in Vascular Disorders*, 2nd edn. pp. 113–57. New York: Raven Press, 1993.
13 Hamovici H, Zinicola N. Experimental renal artery stenosis: diagnostic significance of arterial hemodynamics. *J Cardiovasc Surg* 1962; **3:** 259–62.
14 Jacobsen HR. Ischemic renal disease: an overlooked clinical entity? *Kidney Int* 1988; **34:** 729–43
15 Strandness DE Jr. Hemodynamics of the normal arterial and venous system. In Strandness DE Jr (ed.) *Duplex Scanning in Vascular Disorders*, 2nd edn. pp. 45–79. New York: Raven Press, 1993.
16 Rittenhouse EA, Maitner W, Burr JW, Barnes RW. Directional arterial flow velocity: a sensitive index of changes in peripheral resistance. *Surgery* 1976; **79:** 350–5.
17 Norris DS, Pfeiffer JS, Rittgers SE, Barnes RW. Noninvasive evaluation of renal artery stenosis and renovascular resistance: experimental and clinical studies. *J Vasc Surg* 1984; **1:** 192–201
18 Strandness DE Jr. The renal arteries. In Strandness DE Jr (ed.) *Duplex Scanning in Vascular Disorders*, 2nd edn. pp. 197–215. New York: Raven Press, 1993.
19 Vaughan ED. Renovascular hypertension. *Kidney Int* 1985; **27:** 811–27.
20 Hoffman U, Edwards JM, Carter S *et al.* Role of duplex scanning for the detection of athrosclerotic renal artery disease. *Kidney Int* 1991; **39:** 1232–9.
21 Taylor DC, Moneta GL, Strandness DE Jr. Follow-up of renal artery stenosis by duplex ultrasound. *J Vasc Surg* 1989; **9:** 410–15.
22 Isaacson JA, Zierler RE, Bergelin RO, Strandness DE Jr. A method for minimizing variability in kidney length measurements during renal artery duplex scanning Abstract *J Vasc Tec.* 1994; **18:** 23–7.
23 Handa N, Fukunaga R, Uehara A *et al.* Echo-Doppler velocimeter in the diagnosis of hypertensive patients: the renal artery Doppler technique. *Ultrasound Med Biol* 1986; **12:** 945–952.
24 Martin B, Nanra RS, Wlodarczyk J. Renal hilar

Doppler analysis in the detection of renal artery stenosis. *J Vasc Tech* 1991; **15:** 173–80.
25 Stavros TA, Parker SH, Yakes WF *et al.* Segmental stenosis of the renal artery: pattern recognition of Tardus and Parvus abnormalities with duplex sonography. *Radiology* 1992; **184:** 487–92.
26 Isaacson JA, Zierler RE, Spitell PC *et al.* Noninvasive screening for renal artery stenosis: comparison of renal artery and renal hilar scanning. *J Vasc Tech* 1995 (submitted).
27 Meaney TF, Dustan HO, McCormack LJ. Natural history of renal arterial disease. *Radiology* 1968; **91:** 881–87.
28 Wollenweber J, Sheps SG, Davis GO. Clinical course of atherosclerotic renal vascular disease. *Am J Cardiol* 1968; **21:** 60–71.
29 Schreiber MJ, Pohl MA, Novick AJ. The natural history of atherosclerotic and fibrous renal artery disease. *Urol Clin North Am* 1984; **11:** 327–31.
30 Tollefson DF, Ernst CB. Natural history of atherosclerotic renal artery stenosis associated with aortic disease. *J Vasc Surg* 1991; **14:** 327–31.
31 Guzman RP, Zierler RE, Isaacson JA *et al.* Renal atrophy and arterial stenosis: a prospective study with duplex ultrasound. *Hypertension* 1994; **23:** 346–50.
32 Zierler RE, Isaacson JA. Natural history of atherosclerotic renal artery stenosis: a prospective study with duplex ultrasunography. *J Vasc Surg* 1994; **19:** 250–8.
33 Madias NE. Renovascular hypertension. *AKF Nephrol Lett* 1986; **3:** 27–42.
34 Kaplan NM. Renal vascular hypertension. In Kaplan NM (ed.) *Clinical Hypertension*, pp. 303–24. Baltimore: Williams and Wilkins, 1990.
35 Greene ER, Venters MD, Avasthi PS *et al.* Noninvasive characterization of renal blood flow. *Kidney Int* 1981; **20:** 523–9.
36 Avasthi PS, Voyles WF, Greene ER Noninvasive diagnosis of renal artery stenosis by echo-Doppler velocimetry. *Kidney Int* 1984; **25:** 824–829.
37 Edwards JM, Zaccardi MJ, Strandness DE Jr. A preliminary study of the role of duplex scanning in defining the adequacy of treatment of patients with renal artery fibromuscular dysplasia. *J Vasc Surg* 1992; **15:** 604–9.
38 Louie J, Isaacson JA, Zierler RE *et al.* Prevalence of carotid and lower extremity arterial disease in patients with renal artery stenosis. *Am J Hypertension* 1994; **7:** 436–9.

10

Intravascular ultrasound imaging of the renal artery

MICHAEL S BERKOBEN, STEVE J SCHWAB

Introduction

Renal angiography is the standard method used to delineate renal arterial anatomy. Most frequently performed because of a suspicion of renal artery stenosis, renal angiography is able to differentiate the two most common causes of renal artery stenosis – atherosclerosis and fibromuscular dysplasia – in the great majority of cases. In addition to providing a longitudinal outline of the diseased arterial lumen, angiography, with the help of commercially available software, can provide a measurement of the cross-sectional area of the stenotic segment. Contrast angiography, however, has two inherent limitations. Although able to silhouette the arterial lumen, angiography does not provide a full-thickness cross-sectional depiction of arterial wall composition and structure. Knowledge of the composition of a renal arterial lesion may have important diagnostic, prognostic and therapeutic implications. In addition, as we shall discuss below, the longitudinal perspective provided by angiography may obscure the extent of luminal narrowing. In recent years, there has been increasing interest in the use of intravascular ultrasound imaging in the evaluation of patients with coronary and peripheral arterial atherosclerosis. Because of differences in the acoustic impedances of the various constituents of atherosclerotic plaque, intravascular ultrasound imaging is able to provide a detailed depiction of plaque composition and structure. Experience with intravascular ultrasound imaging in the evaluation of renal arterial disease, however, is limited.

Principles of intravascular ultrasound imaging

Ultrasound is a high frequency mechanical wave motion that propagates through an elastic medium. It is produced by a mechanical disturbance or strain in the medium. In ultrasound imaging systems, ultrasound is produced by a transducer made of a certain type of crystal which can convert electrical energy into mechanical energy and vice versa. When an electric potential is applied across the face of the crystal, the face of the crystal becomes mechanically strained and resonates at a frequency determined by the crystal's thickness. This phenomenon is called the converse piezoelectric effect. The sound waves produced by the crystal propagate as pressure disturbances through the underlying material. Because the crystal can also convert mechanical energy into electrical energy, the transducer can also act as a receiver of ultrasound; when the face of the crystal is mechanically strained by ultrasound, an electrical potential develops across the face of the crystal. This phenomenon is called the piezoelectric effect.

The ultrasound waves produced by the transducer propagate as pressure disturbances through the underlying material. The resistance of the material to these pressure disturbances is called the acoustic impedance and is defined as the product of the mass density of the material and the speed of sound in the material. Reflection of ultrasound occurs when an ultrasound wave encounters an interface between materials with different acoustic impedances; a portion of the incident mechanical energy fails to cross the interface and returns as a reflected sound wave, or echo, which can be detected by the transducer. Because human tissue is composed of materials with different acoustic impedances, echoes may be used to characterize the structure and composition of human tissue.

In clinical ultrasound imaging, two types of echoes are of value.[1–3] When ultrasound waves encounter a large, smooth interface between materials with different acoustic impedances, specular or mirror-like echoes are produced. These reflected waves obey Snell's law of reflection: the angle of reflection equals the angle of incidence. Because the transducer both produces and receives ultrasound, it will detect echoes only from interfaces perpendicular to the ultrasound beam. In intravascular ultrasound imaging, specular echoes are produced at the interface of the lumen with the intima; at the interfaces between the layers of the normal arterial wall; and at the interfaces between lipid, fibrous tissue and calcium – the major constituents of atherosclerotic plaque. Because calcified tissue both reflects (because of its very high acoustic impedance) and absorbs ultrasound, acoustic shadowing is present behind calcified tissue. Because tissues contain internal structures (arterioles, venules, cylindrical structures such as smooth muscle and collagen and elastin), acoustic impedance mismatches also are present within tissues. Because these structures are of the same order of size as the ultrasound wavelength, the mechanical energy of the incident waves are transferred to the structures, which then act as point sources of ultrasound and scatter echoes in all directions. Scattered echoes, then, enable us to characterize the tissues themselves (Fig. 10.1). Lipid is echolucent and is represented as black on the B-mode echoreflective scale. Fibrous tissue is moderately echoreflective and is represented as gray.

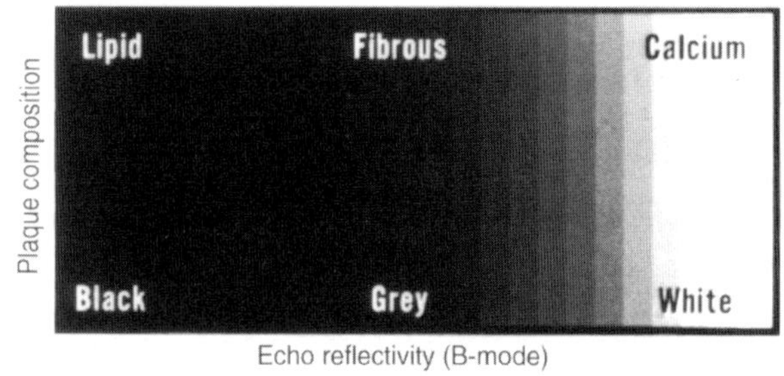

Figure 10.1. Echo reflectivity of the constituents of atherosclerotic plaque. Reprinted with permission from ref. 20.

Calcium is the most echoreflective and is represented as white.

To illustrate these ultrasonographic principles, intravascular ultrasound images of normal and diseased arteries will be described. A normal artery has a trilayered appearance (Fig. 10.2). Blood is transparent to ultrasound so that the lumen appears echolucent. The thin intima is easily imaged because of intense echoreflection from the collagen and elastin of the internal elastic membrane. Beyond the intima lies the media, more echolucent because of its smooth muscle content. Beyond the media lies the adventitia, more echoreflective because of its fibrous tissue (collagen and elastin) content. An artery with atherosclerotic plaque also has a trilayered appearance (Fig. 10.3). The plaque appears as an area of intimal thickening; the media underlying the plaque is frequently thinned. Fibrous plaque is echoreflective but may be distinguished from calcified plaque; fibrous tissue is not as intensely echoreflective as calcified tissue and causes no acoustic dropout. Fatty plaque appears echolucent. Intravascular ultrasound characterizations of atherosclerotic plaque correlate with histopathological findings.[4–7] Experience with intravascular ultrasound imaging of fibromuscular dysplasia is limited.

Intravascular ultrasound technology

In a typical intravascular ultrasound imaging system, a very small piezoelectric crystal is bonded to the tip of a mechanically rotated metal

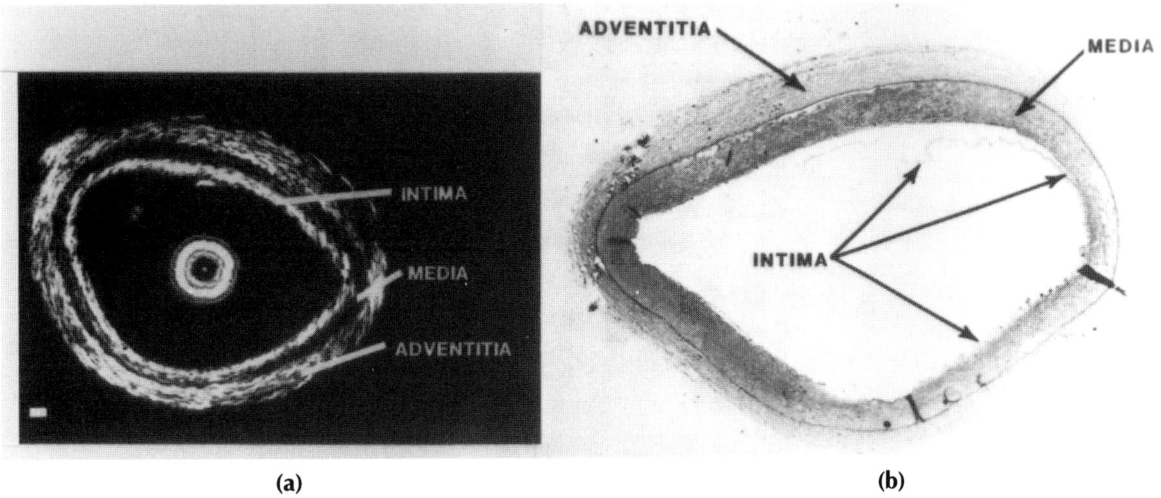

Figure 10.2. (a) Intravascular ultrasound image of normal human carotid artery. The echogenic circle seen within the lumen represents the ultrasound catheter. (b) Histologic section of a normal human carotid artery. Reprinted with permission from ref. 21.

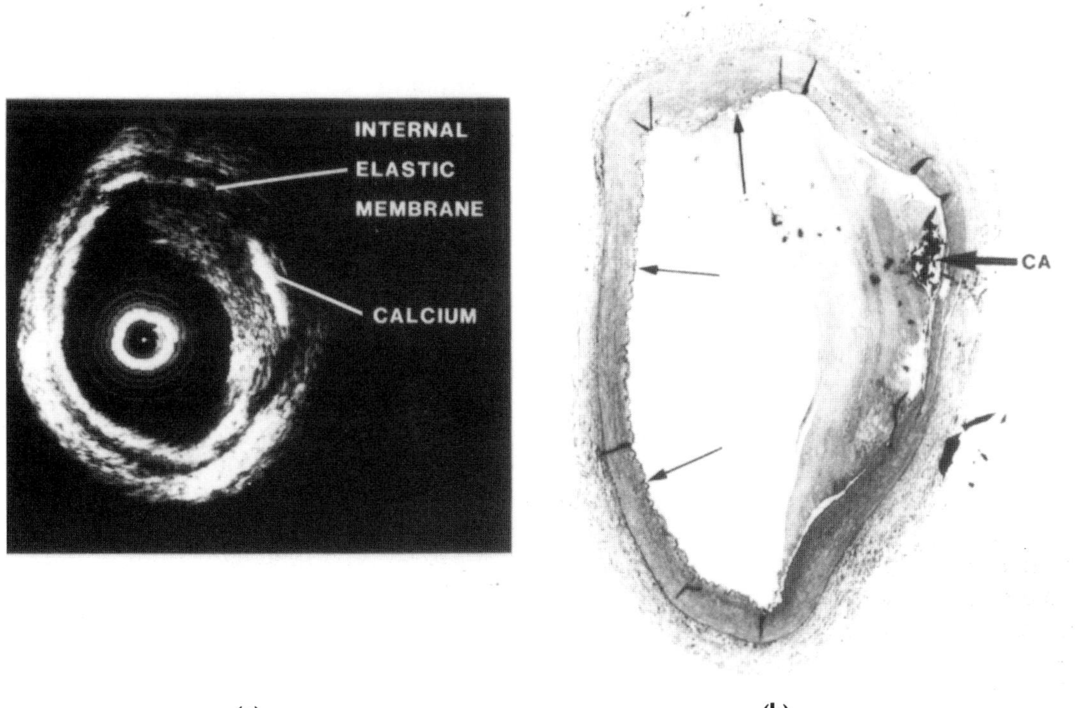

Figure 10.3. (a) Intravascular ultrasound image of diseased human carotid artery. Note the acoustic shadowing behind the calcium. Note also that the plaque is within the intima; the internal elastic membrane is seen behind the plaque. (b) Histologic section of diseased carotid artery. Reprinted with permission from ref. 21.

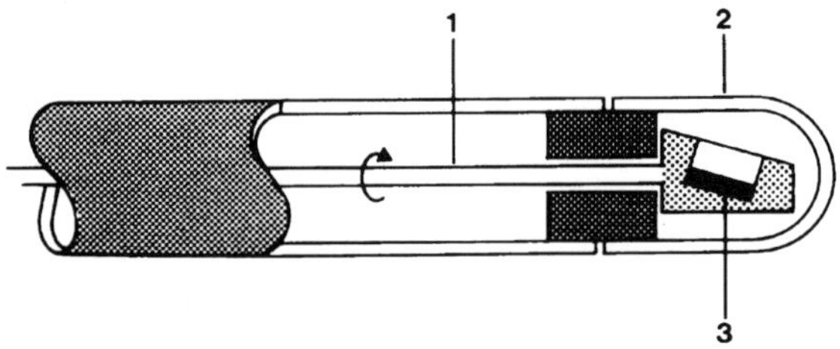

Figure 10.4. Rotating transducer. (1) Rotating shaft; (2) dome; (3) piezoelectric element. Reprinted with permission from ref. 22.

Table 10.1. Advantages of intravascular ultrasound over angiography

1	Allows differentiation of fibromuscular dysplasia from atherosclerotic plaque.
2	Allows detection of diffuse and circumferential atherosclerotic lesions.
3	Can provide accurate cross-sectional depictions of complex luminal shapes.
4	Allows evaluation of success of PTA.

core which is enclosed in 4–8 F catheter (Fig. 10.4). Selective cannulation of the renal artery is achieved by introduction of the ultrasound catheter through an angiography catheter.[8] As the crystal rotates through 360° on the metal core within a defined cross-sectional plane, a cross-sectional image of the arterial segment is obtained. Other imaging systems do not make use of a rotating transducer. The rotating mirror system consists of a stationary transducer and a rotating mirror which deflects the ultrasound beam through 360°.[9] The electronically switched phase array system consists of many small piezoelectric elements positioned along the circumference of the catheter tip.[10] Adjacent subgroups of elements may be sequentially activated by electronic switching, allowing a cross-sectional examination of the artery in the plane perpendicular to the catheter tip.

Advantages of intravascular ultrasound over angiography

Unlike contrast angiography, intravascular ultrasound can characterize vessel wall composition and structure and can provide a cross-sectional depiction of a stenotic segment. Based on the current state of knowledge of the diagnosis and treatment of renal artery stenosis, intravascular ultrasound offers four advantages over angiography – advantages in both the diagnosis and treatment of renal artery stenosis (Table 10.1). These advantages may make intravascular ultrasound an important adjunctive method for the evaluation of renal artery disease. Although these advantages are easily demonstrable in particular circumstances, it has yet to be demonstrated that they are clinically significant. To date, no large randomized trial has been conducted to determine if the routine use of intravascular ultrasound as an adjunct to angiography significantly affects patient management and significantly improves long-term percutaneous treatment results.

1 Intravascular ultrasound may allow the angiographer to distinguish fibromuscular dysplasia from atherosclerotic plaque. A 'string of beads' is the classic arteriographic appearance of medial fibroplasia; medial fibroplasia, however, accounts for only 60–70% of all cases of fibromuscular dysplasia.[11] Medial hyperplasia, due to increased smooth muscle in the media, and intimal hyperplasia, due to proliferation of mesenchymal cells and fibrous tissue in the intima, each account for approximately 5% of cases. Each can produce a single smooth proximal narrowing which can resemble atheromatous plaque.[12] In such cases, the angiographer must rely on non-specific criteria such as the younger age of the patient and the lack of atheromatous involvement of the aorta in order to distinguish these conditions from atherosclerosis. Although experience with intravascular ultrasound imaging of fibromuscular dysplasia is lacking, it seems likely that intravascular ultrasound's ability to provide cross-sectional depictions of arterial walls will prove helpful in cases in which the angiographic findings are equivocal.
2 Intravascular ultrasound may allow the angiographer to detect diffuse and circumferential atherosclerotic lesions that may be

missed by contrast angiography[13] (Fig. 10.5). The longitudinal silhouette provided by angiography allows estimation of the severity of stenosis based on the 'peak and valley' appearance of the affected artery; the percentage stenosis is determined by comparing the stenotic segment with an adjacent segment which is presumed to be normal. Because atherosclerosis is a diffuse process, however, the presumed normal segment may be diseased. The percent stenosis will therefore be underestimated. Should diffuse and circumferential atherosclerosis involve the length of the renal artery, the angiogram may be interpreted as being normal. Intravascular ultrasound overcomes these problems. The area enclosed by the intimal surface can be imaged because the more echoreflective intima appears distinct from the echolucent lumen. The normal intimal layer is thin; therefore, the area enclosed by the media approximates the original luminal area. The area enclosed by the media can be imaged because the more echoreflective intima appears distinct from the echolucent media. The diseased intimal layer is thick and is imaged as such by intravascular ultrasound. Comparison of the area enclosed by the intimal surface with the area enclosed by the media enables the angiographer to estimate the percentage of the original luminal area that is occupied by plaque.[9]

3 Intravascular ultrasound provides a more accurate cross-sectional depiction of luminal shape. Although orthogonal angiograms adequately depict most atherosclerotic lesions, irregular or asymmetric luminal narrowings will not be adequately depicted by orthogonal views, and angiography may markedly underestimate the extent of luminal narrowing.[14] By sweeping the ultrasound beam through 360° within a cross-sectional plane, intravascular ultrasound can image complex luminal shapes accurately.
4 Intravascular ultrasound may allow the angiographer to judge the success of percutaneous transluminal angioplasty (PTA). Successful balloon dilation increases luminal cross-sectional area by tearing the plaque from the lumen toward the media, allowing the outer arterial wall (media and adventitia) to dilate.[15–17] It is not known whether dissection (separation of the plaque from the media) is necessary for successful PTA. If intimal tearing does not occur, PTA may still be judged to be an angiographic success as transient stretching of the vessel wall will increase luminal cross-sectional area. Recoil of the vessel wall may occur within minutes to hours, however, resulting in early restenosis.[18] Intravascular ultrasound appears to be more sensitive than contrast angiography for the detection of tearing and dissection. In the case of arterial dissection, intravascular ultrasound will detect an oscillating intimal flap which separates the echolucent true and false lumens.[19]

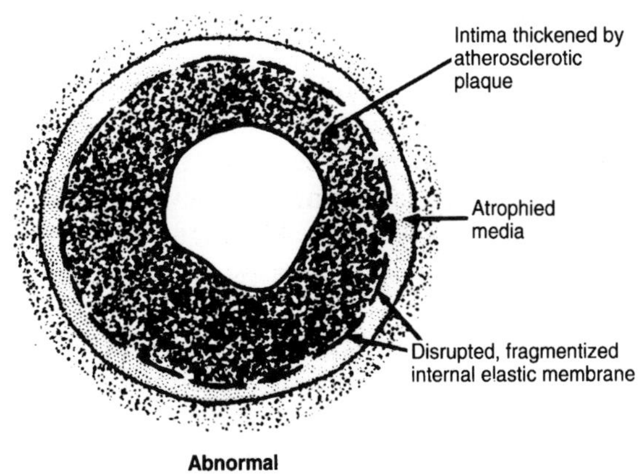

Figure 10.5. Diagram of concentric atherosclerotic plaque. Adapted with permission from ref. 23.

Clinical experience with intravascular ultrasound assessment of the renal artery

To date, there is one published report of clinical experience with intravascular ultrasound assessment of the renal artery.[8] Sheikh and co-workers performed digital angiography and intravascular ultrasound imaging of four renal artery segments in four normal subjects and of five renal artery segments in four consecutive subjects with renal artery stenosis who were referred for PTA. The five segments in the subjects with renal artery stenosis were imaged before and after PTA.

The ultrasound catheter was introduced through an 8 F angiography catheter. Intravascular ultrasound images were obtained during a single pass across the segment of interest; each imaging session added only 45–90 s to the length of the angiographic procedure. There was a good correlation between intravascular ultrasound and contrast angiography for measurement of lumen diameter (r=0.81) and for measurement of luminal cross-sectional area (r=0.83). Intravascular ultrasound demonstrated distinct intimal, medial and adventitial layers in the normal renal arteries (Fig. 10.6). Angiography identified atherosclerotic plaque in four of the five diseased segments and fibromuscular dysplasia in one. Intravascular ultrasound identified atherosclerotic plaque in three (Fig. 10.6) and fibromuscular dysplasia in two. In one of the lesions identified as atherosclerotic plaque by arteriography, intravascular ultrasound demonstrated thickening and increased echogenicity of the intima and media compatible with collagen and elastin deposition (Fig. 10.6); these were compatible with a diagnosis of fibromuscular

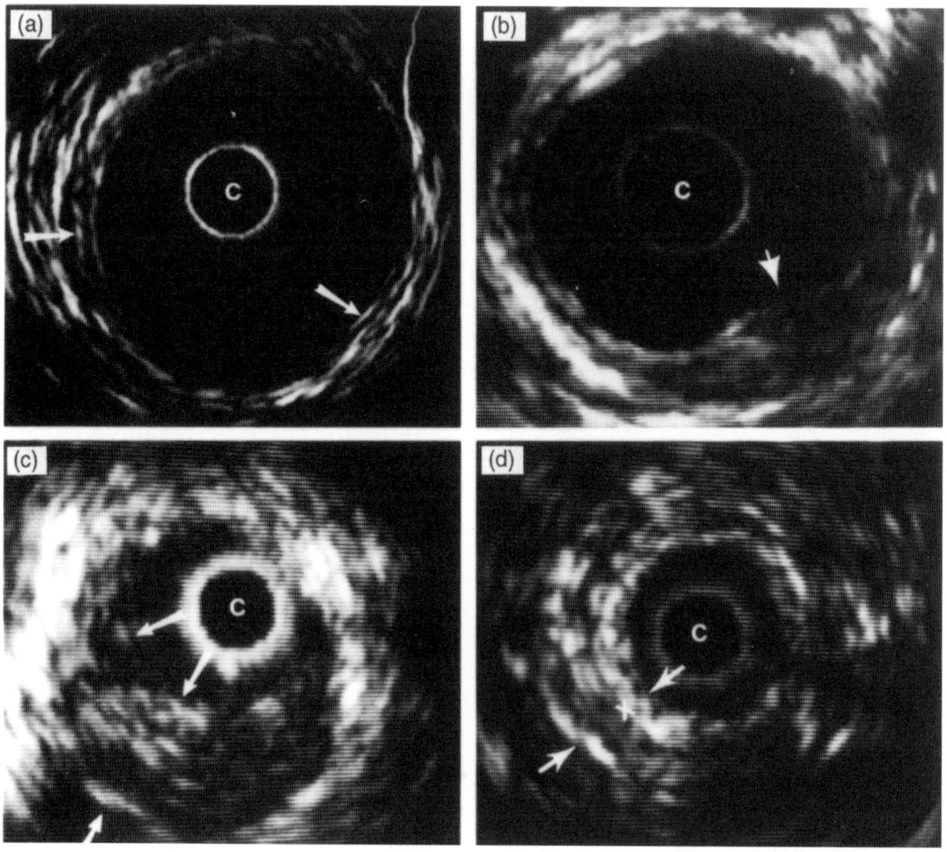

Figure 10.6. Intravascular ultrasound images of renal arteries. (a) A normal renal artery with a trilayered appearance. The echogenic circle within the arterial lumen represents the ultrasound catheter. (b) A renal artery with a small plaque indicated by the arrow. (c) Renal artery stenosis caused by atherosclerotic plaque. The plaque is hypoechoic and is indicated by the inner arrows. (d) Renal artery stenosis caused by fibromuscular dysplasia. The boundaries between the lumen and the intima and between the media and the adventitia are indicated by arrows. Elastin and collagen deposition in the intima and media result in the increased echogenicity of these layers. Reprinted with permission from ref. 8.

dysplasia. In addition, intravascular ultrasound's ability to identify diffuse, circumferential atherosclerotic plaque proved helpful. Arteriography identified a discrete stenosis in one segment; intravascular ultrasound identified diffuse, circumferential plaque at the site of stenosis as well as at an adjacent, angiographically normal segment. As a result, a larger angioplasty balloon was selected.

Intravascular ultrasound also enabled the investigators to gauge the success of PTA (Fig. 10.7). Three arterial wall dissections were detected by intravascular ultrasound; one dissection was detected by angiography. In addition, one PTA treatment judged to be an immediate angiographic success was judged by intravascular ultrasound to be inadequate because of elastic recoil. PTA was repeated using a larger balloon. Intravascular ultrasound thus prompted use of a larger balloon in two of the four patients with renal artery stenosis.

In summary, intravascular ultrasound was performed easily and safely in a small number of patients. Three of the four advantages of intravascular ultrasound discussed in the preceding section were found to be clinically useful.

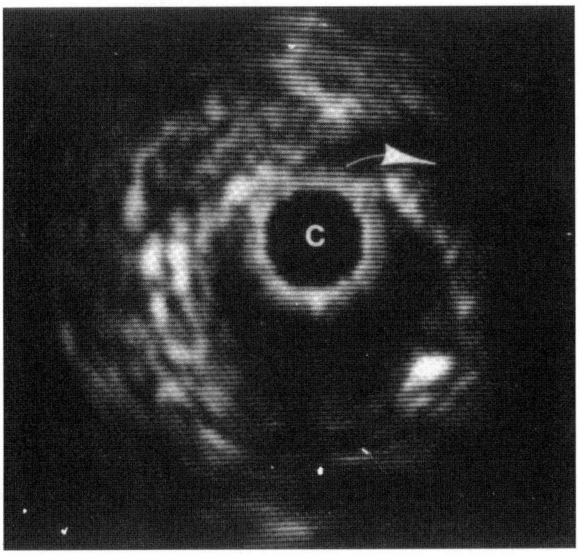

Figure 10.7. Intravascular ultrasound image obtained after PTA demonstrating dissection of the arterial wall. c = ultrasound catheter lumen. Reprinted with permission from ref. 8.

Intravascular ultrasound enabled the angiographer to distinguish fibromuscular dysplasia from atherosclerosis, to detect diffuse and circumferential atherosclerosis and to judge the success of PTA by detecting plaque disruption.

Potential uses of intravascular ultrasound

As intravascular ultrasound technology and knowledge of renal artery disease evolve, applications of intravascular ultrasound may evolve in lockstep. If we learn to correlate the clinical behavior of renal artery lesions with their morphologic characteristics, the morphologic characterization of renal artery lesions by intravascular ultrasound may prove invaluable. Intravascular ultrasound may allow the angiographer to predict the likelihood of progression of a lesion, to select the best intervention (PTA, atherectomy, stent placement or surgery) and to evaluate the response to intervention. Before the routine use of intravascular ultrasound in the assessment of renal artery disease is recommended now or in the future, a large randomized trial comparing angiography with angiography plus intravascular ultrasound must demonstrate that the addition of intravascular ultrasound to angiography significantly affects the management of patients and results in significant improvement in the long-term success rates of percutaneous treatments.

References

1 Goodsitt MM. The basic physics of ultrasound imaging. In Taveras JM (ed.) *Radiology: Diagnosis–Imaging–Intervention*, Vol. 1, Ch. 28. Philadelphia: JB Lipincott, 1993.
2 Cosgrove D. Ultrasound: general principles. In Grainger RG, Allison DJ (eds) *Diagnostic Radiology: An Anglo-American Textbook of Radiology*, 2nd edn, pp. 65–77. New York: Churchill Livingstone, 1992.
3 Linker DT, Yock PG. Tissue characterization in intra-arterial ultrasound: potential methods and clinical implications. In Tobis JM, Yock PG (eds) *Intravascular Ultrasound Imaging*, pp. 85–92. New York: Churchill Livingstone, 1992.
4 Gussenhoven EJ, Essed CE, Lancee CT *et al.*

Arterial wall characteristics determined by intravascular ultrasound imaging: an *in vitro* study. *J Am Coll Cardiol* 1989; **14:** 947–52.

5 Potkin BN, Bartorelli AL, Gessert JM *et al.* Coronary artery imaging with intravascular high-frequency ultrasound. *Circulation* 1990; **81:** 1575–85.

6 Nishimura RA, Edwards WD, Warnes CA *et al.* Intravascular ultrasound imaging: *in vitro* validation and pathologic correlation. *J Am Coll Cardiol* 1990; **16:** 145–54.

7 Moriuchi M, Gordon I, Honye J *et al.* Validation of intravascular ultrasound images. In Tobis JM, Yock PG (eds) *Intravascular Ultrasound Imaging*, pp. 57–70. New York: Churchill Livingstone, 1992.

8 Sheikh KH, Davidson CJ, Newman GE *et al.* Intravascular ultrasound assessment of the renal artery. *Ann Int Med*, 1991; **115:** 22–5.

9 Bom N, Lancee CT, Gussenhoven EJ *et al.* Basic principles of intravascular ultrasound imaging. In Tobis JM, Yock PG (eds) *Intravascular Ultrasound Imaging*, pp. 7–15. New York: Churchill Livingstone, 1992.

10 Bom N, Lancee CT, Van Egmond FC. An ultrasonic intracardiac scanner. *Ultrasonics* 1972; **10:** 72–6.

11 Harrison EG, McCormack LJ. Pathologic classification of renal arterial disease in renovascular hypertension. *Mayo Clin Proc*, 1971; **46:** 161–7.

12 Pickering TG. Renovascular hypertension: medical evaluation and non-surgical treatment. In Laragh JH, Brenner BM (eds) *Hypertension: Pathophysiology, Diagnosis, and Management*, pp. 1539–59. New York: Raven Press, 1990.

13 Waller BF. Coronary anatomy and pathology: what the angiogram does not reveal. In Tobis JM, Yock PG (eds) *Intravascular Ultrasound Imaging*, pp. 17–34. New York: Churchill Livingstone, 1992.

14 Nissen SE, Gurley JC. Quantitative assessment of coronary dimensions, lumen shape, and wall morphology by intravascular ultrasound. In Tobis JM, Yock PG (eds) *Intravascular Ultrasound Imaging*, pp. 71–83. New York: Churchill Livingstone, 1992.

15 Tobis JM, Honye J, Mahon DJ. Intravascular ultrasound imaging following coronary angioplasty. In Tobis JM, Yock PG (eds) *Intravascular Ultrasound Imaging*, pp. 199–218. New York: Churchill Livingstone, 1992.

16 Nishimura RA, Reeder GS. Intravascular ultrasound: research technique or clinical tool? *Circulation* 1992; **86:** 322–4.

17 Losordo DW, Rosenfield K, Pieczek A *et al.* How does angioplasty work? Serial analysis of human iliac arteries using intravascular ultrasound. *Circulation* 1992; **86:** 1845–58.

18 Waller BF. 'Crackers, breakers, stretchers, drillers, scrapers, shavers, burners, welders, and melters': the future of atherosclerotic coronary artery disease? A clinical-morphologic assessment. *J Am Coll Cardiol* 1989; **13:** 969–87.

19 Pandian NG, Kreis A, Brockway B *et al.* Intravascular high-frequency two-dimensional ultrasound detection of arterial dissection and intimal flaps. *Am J Cardiol* 1990; **65:** 1278–80.

20 Potkin BN, Keren G, Bartorelli AL *et al.* Morphologic characterization of human coronary atherosclerosis by high-frequency intravascular ultrasound. In Tobis JM, Yock PG (eds) *Intravascular Ultrasound Imaging*, pp. 47–55. New York: Churchill Livingstone, 1992.

21 Tobis JM, Mallery J, Mahon D *et al.* Intravascular ultrasound imaging of human coronary arteria *in vivo*: analysis of tissue characterizations with comparison to in vitro histological specimens. *Circulation* 1991; **83:** 913–26.

22 Bom H, ten Hoff H, Lancee CT *et al.* Early and recent intraluminal ultrasound devices. *Int J Cardiac Imaging* 1989; **4:** 79–88.

23 Waller BF. Anatomy, histology and pathology of the major epicardial coronary arteries relevant echocardiographic imaging techniques. *J Am Soc Echocardiogr* 1989; **2:** 232–52.

11

CT angiography and spiral angiography

ANDREW D PLATTS

Spiral CT in renal artery stenosis

The invention and production of computerized tonography (CT) scanners in England during the early 1970s had an immediate and appealing impact in the field of neuroradiology. It was soon predicted that the National Health Service within the United Kingdom would have to acquire at least five or six machines distributed around the country to cope with the inevitable demand that the availability of the technique would generate. There was no such limitation of imagination in other countries and the current reality of CT scanning equipment within all hospitals in the developed world is exactly that predicted by equipment manufacturers, particularly those in the United States of America. There was rapid technical development in CT scanning equipment with first generation machines being quickly superseded by second, third and fourth generation machines and latterly with electron beam devices.

Progress was also made in image reconstruction and processing software. Sophisticated three-dimensional (3D) reconstruction packages produce visually stunning images of bony anatomy, though with rather less pleasing demonstration of the soft tissues. During this stage of development, 3D or volume acquisition was not possible, the 3D data set was constructed from a stack of axially acquired data. While individual scan times were short, the rapid acquisition of a substantial number of axial images was limited by the heat load capacity of the X-ray tube. The most destructive influence on 3D imaging is respiratory movement. This is inescapable when the chest and abdomen are scanned and is unreliably countered by breath-holding techniques, it is very difficult to repeatedly suspend respiration in exactly the same phase.

The invention of spiral volume acquisition overcomes these problems. The patient is moved continually through the rotating X-ray beam to acquire a genuine 3D volume of data within the time constraint of a single breath-hold. Images can therefore be generated without any degradation caused by respiratory movement. Movement artifact does, of course, persist from both cardiovascular pulsation and intestinal peristalsis but this is generally of small amplitude and does not intrude on the final images. The essential requirements for the production of spiral scans are a continually rotating X-ray source, usually based upon slip-ring technology, and smooth patient translation through the emergent fan beam of X-rays. Initial systems were limited by the heat capacity of the X-ray tube but these have been overcome in the current generation of machines where high heat capacity tubes are combined with powerful generators.

The weakness of CT angiography (CTA) is imposed by the physics of radiation absorption; CT can only detect differences in electron density. Unlike magnetic resonance imaging (MRI) there is no inherent ability to detect flow, vessels

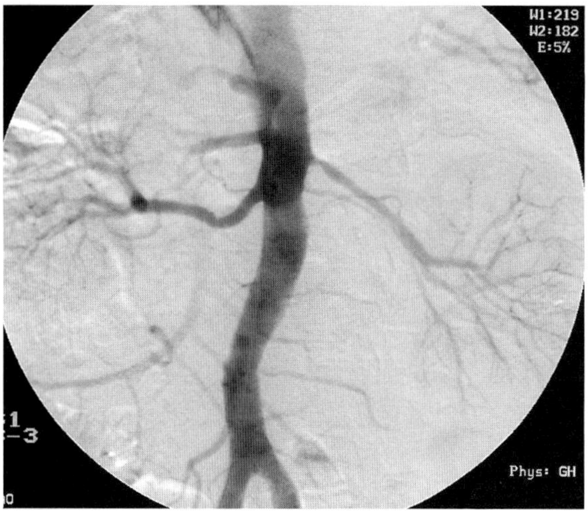

Figure 11.1. Intra-arterial DSA renal artery stenosis. Proximal RAS on the left, ? small lower pole artery on the left, normal right renal artery.

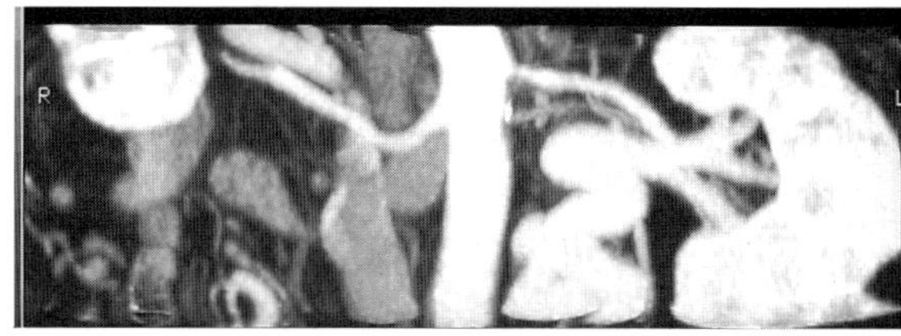

Figure 11.2. 3-D CTA renal artery stenosis. Frontal thick slab MIP confirms left RAS and also suggests small lower pole branch on the left.

can only be demonstrated when they are opacified by some form of contrast agent. This is currently exclusively performed by using a large bolus of positive contrast medium given by intravascular injection.

The production of CTA requires careful planning and cooperation between technician and patient. The area to be demonstrated must be planned on a digital projection image or axial data set to calculate the length that the patient must travel through the scanner. The collimation or thickness of the X-ray beam must then be selected, the thinner the beam the higher the spatial resolution but with some loss of contrast resolution leading to an inevitable increase in 'noise'. The pitch must be set so that the length of scan acquisition at the desired slice width can be accomplished within the time constraint of a patient's breath-hold. These decisions having been made and set within the machine, a calculation, estimate or guess of the time taken for the injected bolus of contrast to reach the plane of imaging must be made. Some authors describe using an arbitrary delay of 17–25 s after the start of the peripheral intravenous contrast injection before the scan run is started and have found this to be quite reliable.[1] Some form of bolus tracking is likely to help reduce the number of scans that have to be repeated because of inappropriate timing.[2] Some equipment now comes with the ability to generate a time – density curve from a sequence of static axial images acquired after a small test dose of contrast injection. The optimum time delay after the start of the main injection bolus can therefore be calculated.[2,3] Some equipment now employs a 'fluoro' mode where the spiral acquisition is preceded by a sequence of static axial images at the starting point of the run. When contrast is recognized on the instantly reconstructed axial section, the spiral acquisition is triggered.

The speed of movement of the patient through the X-ray beam is normally slower than the velocity of opacified blood through the vessel under investigation. The contrast injection must

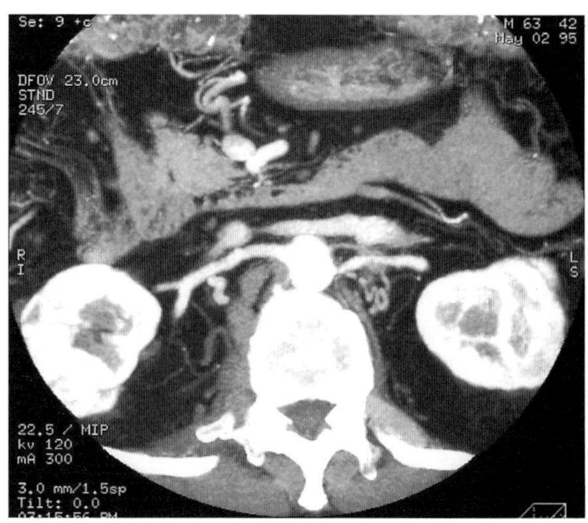

Figure 11.3. 3-D CTA renal artery stenosis. Craniocaudal thick slab MIP confirms left RAS and the presence of the accessory vessel by showing its more anterior origin thus excluding the possibility that it is a lumbar vessel.

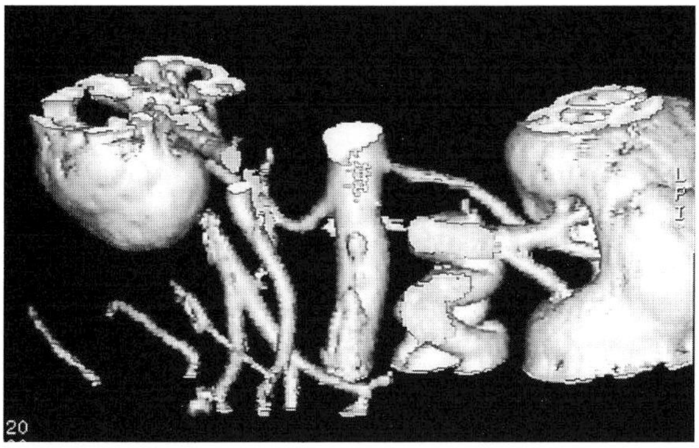

Figure 11.4. 3-D CTA renal artery stenosis. Frontal surface shaded display. The accessory artery on the left has been lost by the threshold being set too high to include it. Incidentally there is a left gonadal vein varix.

therefore be over a long duration, often 20–30 s, and a high dose of intravenous contrast given to ensure that there is marked opacification of the flowing blood (> 50 Hounsfield units). This typically requires a bolus of 130–150 ml of contrast given at 3–5 ml/s. If all these criteria are successfully fulfilled, the scanner will acquire a data set from a volume of tissue from which images of sufficiently high resolution can be generated.

The first stage of image reconstruction has traditionally been to produce a series of axial images which form the basis of postprocessing decisions. With conventional CT, axially acquired images that are reconstructed in orthogonal or arbitrary directions are always degraded to some extent by a step-like artifact imposed by the finite thickness of the axial sections (slice thickness). This is normally suppressed by a smoothing algorithm, though this inevitably degrades the integrity of the data to some extent. When a 3D volume of data is acquired with spiral CT the images are not degraded in this way. Image degradation caused by patient respiration is eliminated by acquiring the data in a single breath-hold but artifacts from vessel pulsation, peristalsis and the movement of the patient through the gantry require sophisticated software programs (algorithms) to produce high resolution, thin slice images. Individual images generated from a volume acquisition are now almost indistinguishable from those from a conventionally acquired axial scan.

Examination of these planar reconstructions may provide sufficient information on which to base a diagnosis,[2] but it is increasingly becoming clear that more sophisticated forms of image reformatting and display may allow a clearer understanding of the anatomy and morphology of vascular pathology. The two most commonly employed techniques are surface-shaded display (SSD) or maximum intensity projection (MIP), the latter technique imported from MR angiography. A brief description of these techniques may help in understanding the origin of artifacts and a clear understanding that with CTA it is not a matter of 'what you see is what you get' but rather 'what you see is not necessarily what they have got'.

Surface-shaded display

This is the method by which data are extracted from the volume set and projected. A 3D effect is created by using proximity shading and second point illumination shading to add a false perception of depth.

The first step in producing the image is to restrict the volume to be reconstructed by using a threshold technique. Pixels (picture elements) below or above a range that includes the diagnostic data are discarded from the reconstruction. The remaining data are reformatted as a 3D projected image and artificial perception of depth is added. The image or 3D model can normally be rotated in any plane on the monitor of the workstation so that the origin of the renal arteries can be projected free from overlying vessels. Artifacts are, however, generated by the reconstruction technique firstly by the thresholding method. The threshold cannot normally be set to completely exclude calcification from the contrast within vessels, and therefore a heavily calcified plaque which encroaches upon the lumen of the vessel will be included in the surface rendition to obscure any stenosis. The reconstruction algorithm normally uses some form of connectivity process so that areas of image inhomogeneity caused by 'noise' and other factors are bridged. This, however, allows

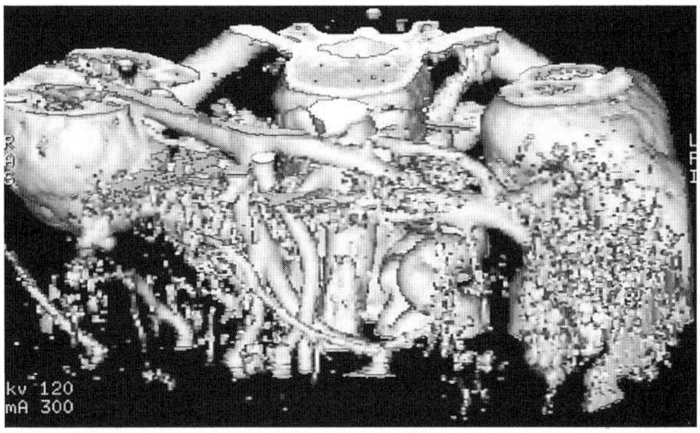

(a)

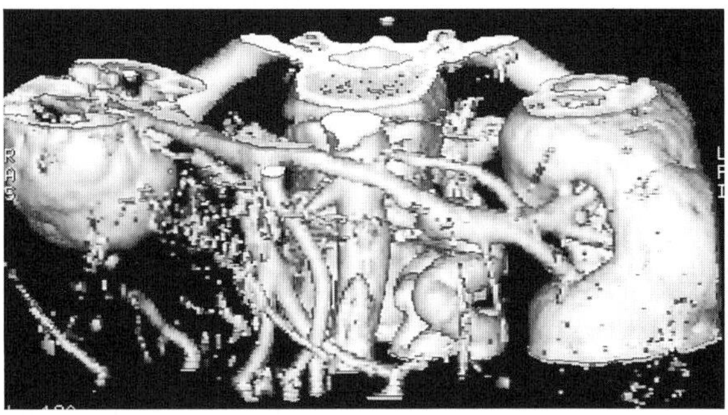

(b)

Figure 11.5. Surface-shaded display. (a, b) Two initial images produced by increasing the lower threshold to reveal the underlying vascular anatomy.

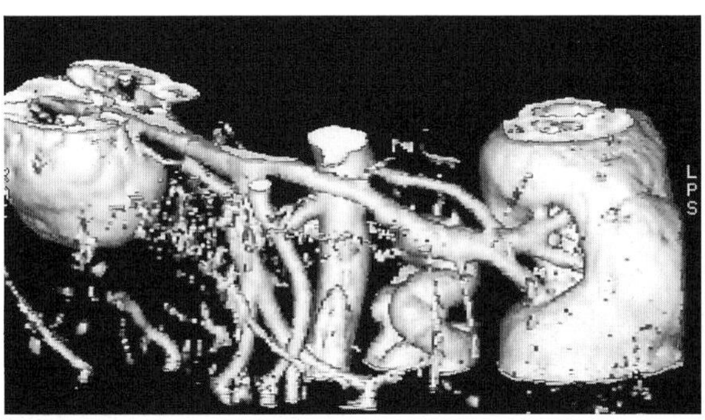

Figure 11.6. The bony anatomy has been removed by selective deletion of that part of the image by including it within an ROI. Removal of unconnected 'free floaters' resulted in image 11.4.

for cross-bridging between vessels and between vessels and bone. The contrast within arteries and veins that lie close together may be fused to obscure a stenosis or generate artifactual areas of apparent dilatation. Setting the threshold too high will cause the edges of vessels to be lost and produce artifactual narrowing of the vessel, too low a setting will cause the reconstructed vessel to appear artifactually large. Manual post-processing techniques can be added to the surface-shaded display, the operator can manually tag calcified plaques to remove them from the reconstruction or to display them in a different color. This is time consuming and the resultant image is obviously operator dependent.

Maximum intensity projection

This image processing technique was imported from MR angiography and is used to improve contrast resolution.[4] This is achieved by creating an image from the maximum intensity of any pixel within the data block along the ray of observation. Normal CT reconstruction results in an averaging of pixel density and therefore decreased contrast resolution. An MIP reconstruction is, however, unable to demonstrate, for instance, the difference between a volume that is entirely occupied by bone density pixels and a volume of similar size that contains a single pixel of calcium density. The reconstructed MIP can be observed from differing angles but this does not convey any benefit, a posterior projection merely being a reversal of a frontal projection. The MIP technique can itself cause artifacts. A vessel passing obliquely through the image volume might increase the pixel density above the threshold level in some areas though not in others and thus produce areas of discontinuity. If two vessels cross the pixel density is not doubled and they cannot be separated by rotating the reconstructed image. This may be overcome by producing an MIP image at a different angle so that, for example, branches of the superior mesenteric artery are not confused with accessory renal arteries. On a superior/inferior MIP projection jejunal branches will be thrown forwards from the aorta though overlap it on an anteroposterior projection.

An upper threshold of a maximum intensity projection cannot be used so that if bone or

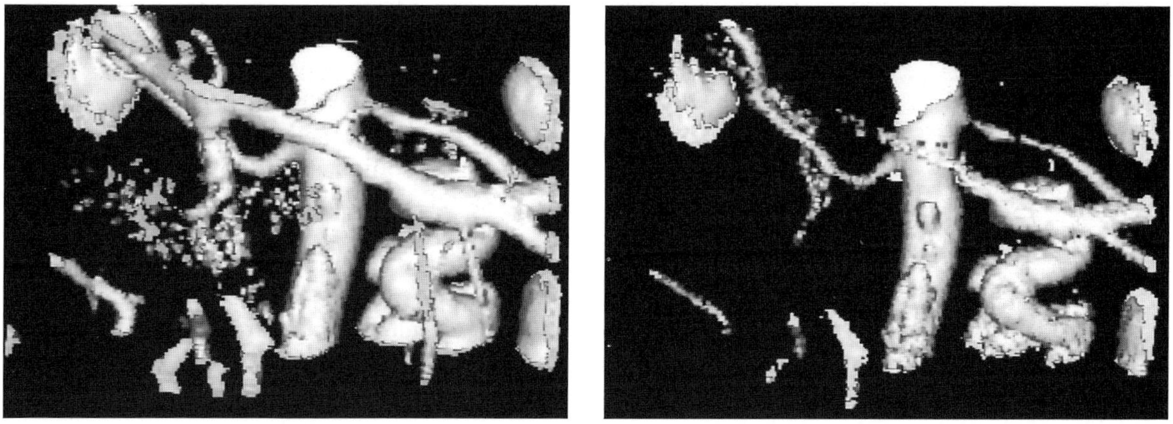

(a) (b)

Figure 11.7. Surface shaded display. (a, b) Altering the threshold of the reconstruction model can make the stenosis inconspicuous (a) or the vessels artefactually small with occluded segments.

calcium overlap a vessel, the vessel will be obscured. A wide variety of pre-MIP manipulations can be performed to increase the utility of the technique. The simplest initial move is to reduce the volume of the data block by performing an inner or outer deletion of data; a good example of this is to take a volume of data such as an opacified aorta viewed from above and to include it within a region of interest (ROI) without including the spine. The data outside the region of interest are discarded and an MIP performed on the remaining data will only show the structures that were within the ROI. Because the volume of data is reduced the computing time will be reduced and the image will be produced more rapidly. An inner deletion is achieved by placing an ROI around areas of data to be discarded. The spine, for example, can be removed

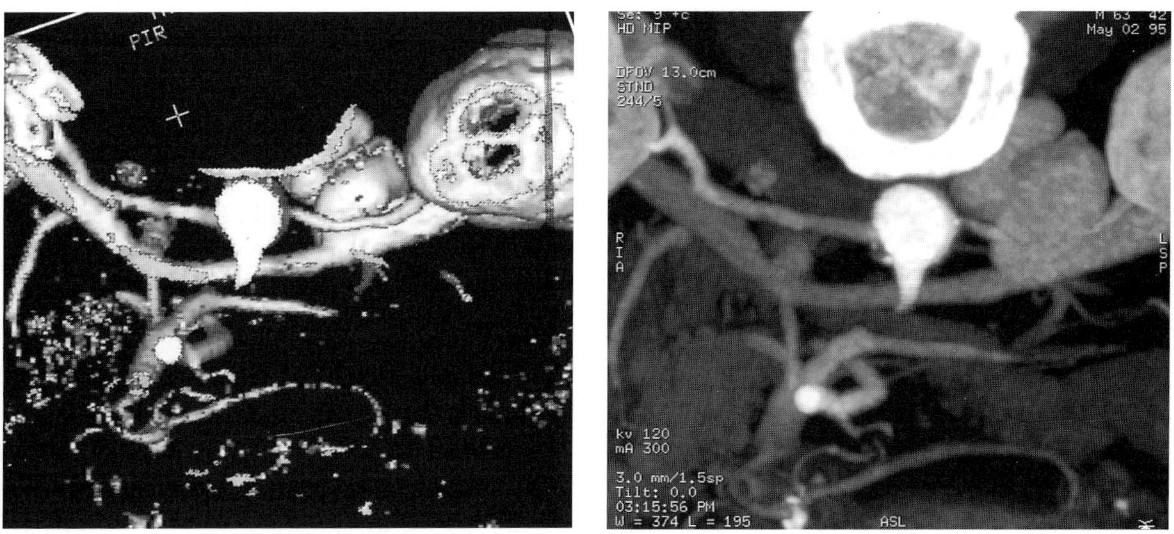

(a) (b)

Figure 11.8. (a,b) Craniocaudal SSD and 3D volume MIP show the angle at which the vessels originate from the aorta – information valuable to the angiographer to enable the planning of oblique projections.

by viewing the data block from above and drawing an ROI around the spine and then deleting all the data enclosed within it. Any subsequent MIP projections will not be obscured by the image of the spine. If a satisfactory image cannot be generated by altering the threshold level and performing inner and outer extractions then more sophisticated methods of deleting unwanted data can be applied. Seeding techniques employ the manual deposition of a 'seed' point on an image and any pixels that lie adjacent to that point and of a similar density will be deleted.[5] The computer can grow the deletion until any pixels of a set range of density that lie in contact to those already deleted are removed throughout the volume. This is used with varying degrees of success but if, for instance, the pixel density of bone is close to that of contrast within a vessel and a branch vessel touches bone, e.g. a lumbar vessel lying close to vertebral body, the seeding process will extend from the bone and into the arterial system removing both the vessels and the bone. With modern multitasking workstations many techniques can be tried independently until a satisfactory image is produced. If all else fails manual editing can be performed, a region of interest is drawn by hand around the area of interest on each image throughout the axial image set to produce a 3D volume. This can be extraordinarily time consuming but may result it very accurate reformatted images.

The rate at which automatic reprocessing algorithms are being developed suggests that acceptable and repeatable images will soon be automatically produced without utilizing current labor-intensive and rather arbitrary techniques.

Image display

The 3D image of data can currently only be projected in two dimensions, either on a television monitor or hard copy film, the false perception of depth can be added to SSD images by generating gray scale, traditionally utilizing proximity weighting and a secondary point of illumination, either of these are capable of producing artifacts. With MIP there can be no depth display in the images themselves, but by producing multiple thin slab MIPs or MIPs at multiple oblique angles and constructing a cine loop, depth impression can be simulated.

Interpretation of spiral CTA

At the end of all this processing what are we looking at? A standard CT scan reconstructed image is an unreal representation of anatomy in the same way that a map differs from an aerial photograph. Artifacts add or subtract data and reconstruction algorithms massage that data to add further artifact but improve the esthetic quality to the image. Despite these constraints, it is possible to produce relatively accurate images of the vascular tree, including the renal arteries, from spiral acquired volume CT scans. When these are compared with the current gold standard for arterial imaging, intra-arterial angiography, early studies suggest that CTA is in the order of 90% sensitive and 80% specific for major renal artery stenosis by combining a variety of projection and reconstruction techniques.[3]

The place of CTA in the investigation of patients suspected to have significant renal artery stenosis is yet to be defined. The risk of temporary or permanent deterioration in renal function caused by the substantial contrast burden indicates that CTA should only be performed when there is a strong suspicion of renal arterial disease. Protagonists of the technique protest that it is non-invasive though this is an argument that is difficult to sustain. Any patient with significantly impaired renal function who receives a bolus of 150 ml of intravenous contrast should probably have their renal function protected by infusion of dopamine. Despite these concerns, CT angiography already provides information of unquestionable value. Axial images demonstrate the angle at which the renal arteries arise from the aortic lumen. If this is performed prior to diagnostic arteriography they can be used to plan the angle of oblique images and so remove any possibility of obscuring the ostium of the renal artery by failing to have the origin in profile. CTA, particularly MIP or planar images, gives some indication of the quality of vessel from which it is planned to take a graft prior to surgery. If revascularization of the left kidney is planned, for example, a heavily calcified 'pipe-stem' splenic artery virtually rules out this vessel as a suitable conduit. The presence of multiple renal arteries can clearly be shown on SSD images and thus remove any doubt generated by conventional angiographic studies caused by overlap of jejunal or other branches.

Conclusion

CT angiography holds enormous potential for the investigation of renal arterial disease. Current restraints upon its routine utilization center around the requirement of a substantial contrast bolus. Developments in blood pool opacifying contrast agents using iodized lipid emulsion or perflourocytylbromides are awaited with great expectation. Sophisticated automatic image reconstruction algorithms will aid the rapid production of reliable images, but it remains conceivable that other innovations in CT, including investigation of the CT nephrogram or bolus tracking through the renal artery may have a major impact.

References

1 Rubin GD, Dake MD, Napel SA *et al.* Three-dimensional spiral CT angiography of the abdomen: initial clinical experience. *Radiology* 1993; **186:** 147–52.
2 Galinski M, Prokop M, Chavan A *et al.* Renal artery stenoses: spiral CT angiography. *Radiology* 1993; **189:** 85–92.
3 Rubin GD, Dake MD, Napel S *et al.* Spiral CT of renal artery stenosis: comparison of three-dimensional rendering techniques. *Radiology* 1994; **190:** 181–9.
4 Napel S, Marks MP, Rubin GD *et al.* CT angiography with spiral CT and maximum intensity projection. *Radiology* 1992; **185:** 607–10.
5 Cline HE, Dumoulin CL, Hart HR *et al.* 3D Reconstruction of the brain from magnetic resonance images using a connectivity algorithm. *Magn Reson Imaging* 1987; **5:** 345–52.

PART III

Renal Vascular Hypertension

12

The renin–angiotensin system

JD SWALES

Introduction

The concept that chemical compounds could circulate in the blood and elevate blood pressure is an old one, originating with the original observations of Richard Bright on chronic renal failure.[1] Bright's hypothesis which was subsequently developed by George Johnson[2] was based upon the premise that toxic substances were retained by the failing kidney, and that these caused structural changes in the blood vessels. It was Brown-Sequard who was responsible for the revolutionary suggestion that the kidneys could regulate activities of the tissues of the body through an internal secretion as well as through secretion of waste products.[3] Brown-Sequard was exclusively interested in how the kidney could modify the manifestations of uremia. He did not appreciate that the kidneys might have an important effect upon the circulation. The link between blood pressure and an internal secretion from the kidneys was made by Tigerstedt and his co-worker Bergman.[4] Extracts of rabbit renal cortex produced a prolonged pressor action when injected into normal rabbits. The active material was termed 'renin' and was found to be a water-soluble, non-dialyzable substance which was insoluble in alcohol and destroyed by boiling. These experiments proved difficult to reproduce in other hands, largely because the purification procedures used by Tigerstedt were not adhered to. As a result 'renin' lost credibility until Goldblatt produced hypertension in dogs by constriction of both renal arteries.[5] Like those who preceded him and indeed like many who followed him, Goldblatt was working on an erroneous hypothesis, i.e. that the narrowed arterial lumina observed in the renal arteries of patients with essential hypertension was a primary cause of elevated blood pressure. Although he did not recognize at first that renin was an excellent candidate as a cause of high blood pressure, the clinical importance of Goldblatt's observations was quickly appreciated and within 3 years the first report was published of hypertension cured by unilateral nephrectomy.[6]

The biochemistry of the renin–angiotensin system was elucidated over the next 20 years.[7] This laid the basis for many physiological and clinical studies which continue to the present day. The complexity of the system in terms of its regulation, expression in different tissues and sites of action has been only fully revealed over the last decade with the application of the tools of modern molecular biology. Remarkably, although so much is known about the system and its role in elevation of blood pressure, there are still fundamental unanswered questions about its mode of action in the pathogenesis of elevated blood pressure and other circulatory diseases.

The renin–angiotensin system

Classically, renin is an enzyme synthesized in the juxtaglomerular cells of the kidney as prorenin. After activation renin is secreted into the circulation where it acts upon a substrate, angiotensinogen, to generate the decapeptide angiotensin I which is converted by the dipeptidylhydrolase enzyme angiotensin converting enzyme into the active component of the system, angiotensin II. This is rapidly degraded by aminopeptidases to smaller molecular weight peptides. Although these have been shown to have some activity in *in vitro* systems their biological significance is still debatable although their contribution to measured angiotensin II levels in some radioimmunoassay systems for angiotensin II poses technical problems where separation is not carried out.[8]

Renin

In the juxtaglomerular cells of the kidney the first protein product in the formation of renin is pre-prorenin. This is a 45 kDa protein consisting of a signal peptide and prorenin sequence.[9] The signal peptide is cleaved in the rough endoplasmic reticulum and the glycosylated product (prorenin) passes through the Golgi complex where the prosegment is cleaved to yield the active protein renin (38 kDa). The renin molecules coalesce to form granules which are then extruded into the extracellular space by exocytosis. Not all prorenin is activated; some is released from smaller vesicles also by exocytosis. This mechanism is probably constitutive, i.e. not subject to physiological regulation whilst renin secretion is controlled by a number of physiological stimuli[9] (see below).

Renin belongs to the family of aspartyl proteases. These are enzymes which contain 2-aspartyl residues at the active site of the enzyme which lies in a cleft situated between two lobes.[10] The unique feature of renin which distinguishes it from the other aspartyl proteases is its high specificity, as the only known natural substrate is angiotensinogen. Renin is also species specific with molecular weights in different species varying between 36 and 40 kDa. This is reflected in function in that primate renin does not react with mouse or rat angiotensinogen and vice versa. Likewise the pH optimum for the renin–angiotensinogen reaction is also species dependent. Thus, the pH optimum for the human renin–human angiotensinogen reaction lies between 6.0 and 6.5 whilst with rat angiotensinogen the optimum is pH 5–5.5 and with pig and substrate angiotensinogen the optimum is in the alkaline range (pH 8).

The renin gene has been cloned and sequenced in a number of species.[11] The basic structure consists of nine coding regions (exons) separated by eight non-coding regions (introns). In addition the human gene contains a minute exon (Va) which codes for three amino acids of unknown significance. In man the renin gene is situated on chromosome 1. Regulatory sequences are found upstream in the five prime flanking region.

These sequences contain cAMP, glucocorticoid and estrogen-responsive elements. In addition there are negative regulatory sequences which reduce gene expression.

The identification of the renin gene sequence has enabled specific probes to be devised which can be used to evaluate renin gene expression as renin mRNA. Studies using these techniques have shown that renin mRNA synthesis occurs several hours after renin secretion has been stimulated so replenishing stores of renin.[12] It has to be borne in mind, however, that renin mRNA codes for pre-prorenin and changes in subsequent processing of this molecule could have a major impact on the relationship between the amount of renin mRNA and active renin.

Renin secretion

Stimulation of sympathetic efferent activity to the kidney increases renin secretion independently of changes in renal blood flow and glomerular filtration. This effect is mediated through β-adrenergic receptors.[13] In addition there are probably inhibitory α-adrenoreceptors. The response to stimulation of both receptors is of course sensitive to associated changes in perfusion pressure, blood flow and glomerular filtration which may all be influenced by changes in sympathetic activity.[9] Sodium loading inhibits and sodium depletion stimulates renin gene expression and renin secretion.[14] The major sensor for changes in sodium balance is probably a specialized segment of the early distal tubule, the macula densa.[15] Perfusion of this segment with high or low salt solutions in isolated glomeruli elicits the appropriate changes in renin secretion.[16] Sodium potassium chloride cotransport is important in mediating the responsiveness of the macula densa and this effect may be mediated by chloride rather than sodium ions.[17] The importance of this ion transport pathway is emphasized by the fact that inhibitors such as frusemide or ethacrynic acid elicit a renin secretory response independently of changes in sodium balance.[18] The macula densa mechanism is not the exclusive receptor for changes in sodium balance. Thus, renin secretion from hydronephrotic kidneys still respond to chronic changes in salt balance although the macula densa mechanism is destroyed in this preparation.[19]

Reduction in renal perfusion pressure stimulates renin secretion and increased renal perfusion pressure inhibits secretion. This response is seen in isolated glomeruli in the absence of the macula densa mechanism.[20] The change in renin secretion in response to altered perfusion pressure probably reflects a similar smooth muscle mechanism to that which mediates the contractile response to increased pressure i.e. autoregulation. Both are probably mediated by stretch-activated calcium channels. Over the normal autoregulatory range of renal artery pressure, i.e. that range over which flow is maintained constant, the juxtaglomerular cells are protected from any change in pressure. Outside this autoregulatory range, a threshold for stimulation or inhibition of renin secretion exists.[21] Both thresholds are well within the normal fluctuations in systemic arterial pressure suggesting that changes in renin secretion play an important part in the physiological regulation of blood pressure. This clearly has important implications in determining the blood pressure response to renal artery stenosis.

Renin secretion is under feedback inhibition by angiotensin II.[22] Inhibition of angiotensin II formation by agents which do not have any other actions upon the juxtaglomerular apparatus, e.g. angiotensin converting enzyme inhibitors, produces increased renin secretion therefore.[14] There is evidence that both systemically generated angiotensin II and locally generated angiotensin II within the kidney ('short feedback loop') are important in this respect.[23] It would be anticipated that other vasoactive substances influence renin secretion bearing in mind the vascular nature of the juxtaglomerular apparatus. This appears so.[9, 23] In some cases there is evidence for direct effects at least *in vitro*. Thus, atrial natriuretic peptide inhibits renin secretion as does the potent vasoconstrictor family of peptides, the endothelins. On the other hand, vasodilator prostanoids such as PGE2 and PGI2 stimulate renin secretion *in vitro*. The latter may be important local mediators of renin secretion. By contrast endothelial derived relaxant factor (EDRF) has been reported to have both stimulatory and inhibitory actions *in vitro*. Identifying the role of these potentially important mediators *in vivo* presents formidable difficulties because direct effects are likely to be modified by multiple indirect effects influencing electrolyte excretion and hemodynamics. Elucidation of the cellular mechanism of renin secretion may help to solve some of these problems.[9, 23, 24] Thus, increased intracellular cyclic AMP causes increase in renin synthesis and secretion associated with enhanced transcription of the renin gene mediated by cAMP responsive regulatory elements flanking the renin gene (see above). Paradoxically increased intracellular calcium inhibits renin secretion. This may account for the fact that calcium channel blockers cause little increase in renin secretion despite giving rise to activation of the sympathetic nervous system in some cases.

Angiotensinogen

The specific substrate for renin is angiotensinogen which is 60 kDa protein. The human gene has been cloned and sequenced and is situated on chromosome 1.[11] It consists of five coding regions (exons) separated by four non-coding regions (introns). The primary site of angiotensinogen gene expression is the liver but it is also expressed in a number of other tissues[25, 26] (see below). Transcription of the angiotensinogen gene and angiotensinogen secretion by the liver is stimulated by angiotensin II, glucocorticoids, estrogen, thyroid hormones and androgen. Upstream regulatory elements responsive to these factors have been identified flanking the angiotensinogen gene.[11]

Renin releases the decapeptide angiotensin I by splitting the angiotensinogen molecule at the amino terminal end between a leucine and valine residue in man and between a leucyl-leucine residue in other species such as the rat or mouse. The reaction is a first order one, i.e. angiotensin I generation is linearly related to the renin concentration. The reaction rate is also determined by the angiotensinogen concentrations, although the reaction rate flattens out at high concentrations. The normal plasma angiotensinogen concentration is well below the V_{max} so that changes in both angiotensinogen and renin concentrations *in vivo* influence the generation of angiotensin I in plasma.[27]

An interesting suggestion has been made to explain the evolution of the renin angiotensinogen reaction.[28] It has been postulated that angiotensinogen was originally a protease inhibitor analogous for instance to α_1-antitrypsin. On these grounds it has been suggested that renin might react with another unknown substrate, a reaction which is at least at some point in evolution inhibited by angiotensinogen.

Angiotensin converting enzyme

Angiotensin converting enzyme (ACE) is a zinc metalloproteinase.[29, 30] Most is membrane bound. It exists in two forms, one the endothelial form has a molecular weight of 50–180 kDa, whilst a testicular form of about 90 kDa exists. There is only one ACE gene and the origin of the two gene products lies in two different transcription start sites.

Angiotensin converting enzyme is widely distributed in most body tissues lying both within cells and on the outer surface of the cell with the catalytic domain facing the extracellular milieu.[30] In addition, it is present in plasma, probably as a result of release of the membrane-bound form. Angiotensin converting enzyme cleaves the histidyl-leucine fragment from the carboxypeptidase terminus of angiotensin I. *In vivo* concentrations of angiotensin I are well below the Km for angiotensin converting enzyme so that angiotensin II formation is directly and linearly related *in vivo* to the concentration of angiotensin I.[27] Since most ACE is membrane bound it is difficult to address the important issue of how far ACE concentrations are rate limiting *in vivo*, particularly for the local conversion of angiotensin I to angiotensin II which occurs in most tissue beds.

Unlike renin, ACE is promiscuous for substrates. Activity for synthetic tripeptides at one end of the range extending to the β-subchain of insulin at the other has been demonstrated. One of the most important natural substrates is bradykinin which is also cleaved at the C-terminal end of the molecule. As a result inhibition of ACE causes both reduction in angiotensin II and enhanced sensitivity to bradykinin.[31]

Angiotensin II degradation

Angiotensin II is destroyed by a variety of non-specific peptidases. Amongst these aminopeptidase A is present in high concentrations in plasma and removes the aspartate residue at the N-terminal end of the angiotensin II molecule to give rise to Des-Asp-angiotensin II.[32]

Prolylendopeptidase forms angiotensin 1–7 heptapeptide from angiotensin I. Action of peptidases on the angiotensin I molecule may therefore give rise to potentially biologically active peptide fragments through an 'alternative pathway' bypassing angiotensin II.[33]

The actions of angiotensin II

The renin–angiotensin system has been conserved throughout vertebrate evolution. Although its role has changed (and probably multiplied) during biological evolution, it is clearly of major importance in circulatory homeostasis. The system has been implicated in other processes such as fetal development, reproduction and inflammatory responsiveness. This review will however be confined to the circulatory role of the system.

Angiotensin II receptors

The actions of angiotensin II are mediated through cell surface membrane-bound receptors, although possible receptors at other sites have been described (see below). Binding studies using non-peptide angiotensin II receptor antagonists have defined several subtypes of angiotensin II receptor.[34] Of these the AT1 and AT2 receptors have been defined and the regulatory gene sequenced. The AT1 receptor binds specifically to losartan (Dup753) whilst the AT2 receptor is blocked by the amidazopyridine PD123177. The functions of the AT2 receptors are uncertain. However, increased expression of AT2 receptors has been demonstrated in association with tissue repair and they have been implicated in prenatal kidney development where they constitute the sole renal receptor.[35] In general AT2 receptors are much more abundant in the fetus and neonate than the adult although they have been demonstrated in tissues such as the heart, aorta and kidney.[35] AT1 receptors are coded by two distinct genes and the gene products are accordingly distinguished as AT1A and AT1B. For the AT1A receptor, mRNA is present in the kidney, aorta, liver, adrenal glands, uterus, ovary, spleen and lung and to a lesser extent in the central nervous system;[34] AT1B receptor RNA is detectable in the kidney, adrenal gland and pituitary gland.[34]

The AT1 subclasses of receptor mediate the classical actions of angiotensin II. Local responsiveness is regulated not merely by changes in concentration of angiotensin II but also by changes in activity of the receptors. This is downregulated by, for instance, angiotensin II and by sodium depletion in vascular smooth muscle cells.[34] On the other hand sodium depletion increases receptors in the adrenal zona glomerulosa cells.[36] Three mechanisms are involved in the regulation of angiotensin receptor activity. These are internalization and recycling within the membrane, regulation of angiotensin receptor gene expression and changes in binding affinity.[34] It should be emphasized, however, that changes in responsiveness to angiotensin II can also be mediated by any alteration downstream from receptor binding. Alterations in responsiveness of signal transduction pathways and structural changes[37] giving rise to increased force generation may all cause an increase in response to angiotensin II although the further downstream the changes are, the more likely the alteration is to be associated with general hyperreactivity to other pressor agonists. The distinction between specific enhanced responsiveness to angiotensin II and enhanced responsiveness due to a generalized increase in reactivity is one which is often ignored in the literature on hypertension.

Angiotensin II receptor binding activates a number of signal transduction pathways.[34] Activation of phospholipase A2 stimulates eicosanoid metabolism through release of arachidonic acid, phospholipase C activates the phosphoinositide system, phospholipase D produces sustained increased in phosphatidic acid (the second messenger role of which is unknown) and activation of adenylate cyclase generates cyclic AMP.

The immediate effect of angiotensin II on vascular smooth muscle is contraction mediated by the phosphoinositide pathway, release of intracellular calcium and activation of myosin light chain kinase.[34, 38] Long-term stimulation of vascular smooth muscle in tissue culture leads to increased protein synthesis and hypertrophy.[39] *In vivo* angiotensin II also has a mitogenic action, i.e. it produces hyperplasia.[40, 41] This is associated with early expression of proto-oncogenes and later expression of cytokine growth factors.[34] It has not been possible to show a mitogenic response of vascular smooth muscle cells to angiotensin II in tissue culture studies. This appears to be due to the complexity of the responses elicited by angiotensin II. It has been suggested for instance that it stimulates antiproliferative as well as proliferative pathways, the former including enhanced expression of TGF-β.[34] Angiotensin II has also been shown in some tissue culture systems to increase the production of extracellular matrix.[42] *In vivo* studies have shown that aldosterone increases collagen tissue in the heart in experimental hypertension.[43] How far this is true in peripheral blood vessels is unknown. However, the prevention of myointimal proliferation by ACE inhibitors after experimental balloon arterial injury in rats emphasizes the potential importance of either angiotensin II or bradykinin in regulation of arterial stricture;[44] although so far it has not been possible to demonstrate this phenomenon in man.

The renin–angiotensin system and aldosterone

The AT1 receptors situated in the adrenal zona glomerulosa stimulate the conversion of corticosterone to aldosterone through the phosphoinositide pathway.[45] Other important regulators are serum potassium and adrenocorticotrophic hormone (ACTH). Evidence for the importance of angiotensin II in the human subject *in vivo* is provided by the action of ACE inhibitors in lowering plasma aldosterone. Sodium depletion has contrasting effects upon vascular and adrenal sensitivity to angiotensin II. Whilst the contractile response of arteries is reduced, the secretory response of the adrenal zona glomerulosa is increased. The response of the renal vasculature as well as the adrenal cortex is lost in some human subjects with essential hypertension (non-modulators).[46] Non-modulators appear to be a genetically distinct group of patients with essential hypertension. The cellular mechanism which accounts for this abnormality is uncertain. It may relate to abnormal receptor regulation or to generation of abnormally large quantities of angiotensin II at these tissue sites.

The renin–angiotensin system and the autonomic nervous system

Angiotensin II facilitates neurotransmission in the autonomic efferents supplying the cardiovascular system.[47, 48] This appears to be an indirect effect enhancing the neurotransmitter release produced by sympathetic nerve stimulation rather than being a direct effect. The site of action appears to be prejunctional angiotensin II receptors. Circulating angiotensin II may also reach areas of the brain which lie outside the blood–brain barrier and which are concerned with blood pressure maintenance.[48, 49] The most important of these is probably the area postrema which lies close to both the vagal nucleus and the nucleus of the solitary tract. Angiotensin II infused through the vertebral artery produces pressor effects probably through these pathways. More rostral areas (the circumventricular organs) may also play an important role in blood pressure regulation in response to circulating angiotensin II. It is also possible that locally generated angiotensin II within the central nervous system plays a role in blood pressure regulation in less accessible sites. Strongest evidence for this is based upon demonstration of renin gene expression,[50, 51] within the central nervous system, and upon the blood pressure lowering effect of intraventricular infusions of inhibitors in experimental renovascular hypertension in some studies.[52]

Renin, angiotensin and the kidney

Angiotensin II has multiple direct and indirect effects on sodium balance.[53] Changes in renal perfusion pressure and glomerular filtration rate will modify sodium balance through alterations in the tubular load of sodium. Stimulation of aldosterone secretion will have an antinatriuretic effect through direct increase in distal renal tubular reabsorption. Other intrarenal mechanisms may also be involved in mediating the response to angiotensin II, however. Thus, efferent arteriolar vasoconstriction may help to sustain glomerular filtration rate whilst at the same time changing the physical forces in the peritubular circulation inducing mesangial cell contraction and modifying sodium reabsorption.[54] In addition angiotensin II has a direct effect causing increased sodium and water reabsorption by isolated proximal tubules. There are also less well-documented putative effects on sodium reabsorption by the distal tubule. Under most circumstances activation of the renin–angiotensin system is associated with sodium and water retention. Under some circumstances however, as for instance when hypertension is associated with marked elevation of angiotensin II in malignant hypertension, natriuresis and diuresis occur probably as a result of hemodynamic changes producing a pressure natriuresis.[55] In experimental (Goldblatt two-kidney, one-clip) hypertension in the rat associated with malignant change, severe sodium depletion produced as a result of pressure natriuresis can have an adverse effect upon survival. This can be reversed by saline infusions.[56] Contrasting effects may be seen in renal artery stenosis where antidiuresis and antinatriuresis beyond the renal artery stenosis are counterbalanced by diuresis and natriuresis from the opposite side, again presumably reflecting differences in renal perfusion pressure. As a result there is a negative relationship between exchangeable sodium and blood pressure.[57] Angiotensin II may also have actions in other parts of the kidney. It has thus been suggested that efferent arteriolar vasoconstriction leads to decreased medullary blood flow, increased reabsorption of water and urinary concentration.[53]

The renin-angiotensin system and elevated blood pressure

The well-defined actions of the circulating renin–angiotensin system interact with blood pressure control systems at several points. It is not surprising therefore that the blood pressure response to angiotensin II is a complex one. The immediate response to infusions of angiotensin II is a rapid rise in blood pressure associated with generalized vasoconstriction as a result of direct action. If high dose infusions are continued blood pressure declines back to baseline values as a result of tachyphylaxis associated probably with down-regulation of receptors.[58] More modest pressor doses of angiotensin II result in sustained blood pressure elevation. The response to initially subdepressor infusions of angiotensin II is of equal possible importance. Blood pressure progressively rises over a period of days despite the fact that plasma concentrations of angiotensin II remain within the 'normotensive range'.[59, 60]

The slow pressor response to acutely subpressor doses of angiotensin II could clearly be of great importance in the genesis of renovascular hypertension. The mechanism is unfortunately still debatable. Sodium retention is obviously a prime candidate and sodium depletion diminishes and sodium loading enhances the effect,[61] although sodium balance studies have not demonstrated significant sodium retention.[60] However, the sensitivity of such balance methods in rats is not great and minor degrees of sodium retention enhancing the pressor response to angiotensin II seem to be a likely component. The trophic actions of angiotensin II on resistance vessels are clearly another possible candidate.[62] However, discontinuing infusions causes a rapid decline in blood pressure which is not consistent with reversal of such trophic change[58]. Nevertheless, vascular hypertrophy could act as an amplifying mechanism, modifying the response to, for instance, sodium retention. Influence upon central nervous system cardiovascular centers (see above) has also been postulated although this is not consistent with the absence of signs of sympathetic nerve activity[63] and the failure of sympathectomy to prevent the slow pressor effect.[64]

The extra-renal renin–angiotensin system

The endocrine functions of the renin–angiotensin system have been well defined although there is still debate about the physiological relevance of specific actions, e.g. the interaction with the sympathetic nervous system and the trophic effects of angiotensin II. Angiotensin II is generated locally within tissue beds since most converting enzyme is bound to the vascular endothelium. There is now strong evidence that the complete renin–angiotensin system performs a paracrine and perhaps autocrine role, i.e. locally active renin and angiotensinogen generate angiotensin I which is then converted to angiotensin II by tissue-bound ACE.[65] Support for this suggestion comes from several sources. The earliest work suggested that renin-like activity was present in aortic homogenates as well as in other tissues.[66] These studies were controversial as the specificity of the biochemical techniques used was low. A variety of acid proteases such as cathepsin D make a contribution to angiotensinogenase activity of tissue homogenates.[67] The low pH optimum for activity suggested that such acid proteases were probably responsible. It was subsequently possible to demonstrate that renin-like activity at the optimal pH for renin in aortic homogenates is almost totally abolished by bilateral nephrectomy.[68] On the other hand, when renin was injected into bilaterally nephrectomized rats aortic homogenate activity increases and the pH optimum was consistent with that of the injected renin.[69] The renin which was taken up appeared to be tightly bound and cleared at a much slower rate than plasma renin. The blood pressure rise produced by renin injections was much more closely correlated with renin taken up by arterial tissue than by renin in the circulation.[69] Nevertheless, the blood pressure rise could be corrected by infusion of an angiotensin II antagonist. Further experiments indicated that renal renin was tightly bound in the interstitial space of the aortic wall outside the albumen accessible space.[69] Renin synthesis has also been identified by binding of fluorescent labelled antibodies both *in vivo*[70] in cultured arterial smooth muscle cells, vascular endothelial cells and adrenal cells.[71–73] These latter studies have to be viewed with care, however, as phenotypic changes may occur in tissue culture and biochemical properties may therefore be changed.

Our information in this area has been enormously increased by the newer techniques of molecular biology. Probes for the renin gene can be constructed from radiolabeled RNA or DNA sequences complementary to part of the sequence of the renin gene. A sensitive and specific development of this technique (RNAase protection assay) demonstrated specific renin messenger RNA in aorta, adrenal gland, heart, spleen, liver and brain extracts.[74] Angiotensinogen-specific RNA has been detected by Northern blotting in a variety of tissues including liver, brain, blood vessels and heart.[75] In some tissues such as the heart the message is low and there appear to be marked differences between different strains and whether the messenger RNA can be detected or not. In addition it should be borne in mind that the presence of renin messenger RNA does not necessarily imply that active renin is present. Prorenin is not necessarily processed or extruded as it is in the juxtaglomerular cell. Despite this, the presence of significant quantities of renin-specific mRNA in cardiovascular and other tissues suggests that the system is performing a physiological function, although this is not necessarily identical with that performed by the 'classical' renin–angiotensin system.

Other groups have approached the problem by examining the capacity of isolated tissue beds to release angiotensin II. Although there are substantial discrepancies in the quantity of angiotensin II reported as being released there is consistent evidence for the release of angiotensin II into tissue venous effluent from the isolated rat hindlimb.[76] One group has reported that ACE inhibitors have little influence on production of this but that the protease inhibitor N-acetylpepstatin has a dose-dependent inhibitory effect suggesting that angiotensin II is produced by an alternative pathway.[77] Although release of angiotensin II persists at a stable level in this preparation, there is a close correlation between plasma renin and angiotensin II release suggesting that uptake of renin and subsequent tight binding is responsible for this phenomenon. In addition, local release is increased in rats infused with renin.[78] In rats bilateral nephectomy produced a 59–78% decrease in tissue angiotensin II levels indicating again that the large proportion of tissue-derived angiotensin II is produced as a result of kidney-derived renin.[79] The persistence of significant levels of angiotensin II in plasma and tissues of nephrectomized rats, however, indicated that a small proportion is produced by local mechanisms.[79]

Admiraal and co-workers have conducted analogous studies in man.[80] After adjustment for angiotensin I extraction rates, tissue formation of angiotensin I measured across the renal, antecubital, femoral and hepatic beds for instance accounted for 40% of angiotensin I appearing in the hepatic venous effluent.

Functional responses can also be used to demonstrate local angiotensin generation. For instance infusion of angiotensin II antiserum is effective in lowering angiotensin II infusion-induced hypertension, but is not effective in lowering blood pressure in nephrectomized rats infused with renin or in a renin-dependent model such as the Goldblatt two-kidney, one-clip hypertensive rat.[81, 82] On the other hand, the competitive antagonist saralasin is much more effective at lowering blood pressure in these models even when it is infused into rats pretreated with large doses of angiotensin II antisera.[82] These experiments suggest enhanced access of the angiotensin II antagonist compared with antiserum. Isolated resistance vessels can be studied in an analogous fashion. Juul *et al.* used resistance vessels from the rat femoral bed[83] and Bund *et al.* used resistance vessels obtained from human skin biopsies.[84] Both groups showed vessels constricted in a dose-dependent manner to synthetic tetradecapeptide renin substrate, angiotensin I and angiotensin II. These responses could be inhibited by saralasin. However, response to angiotensin I but not substrate was inhibited by captopril. The specific renin inhibitor, H261, and a polyclonal renin antibody had only a small effect on the human blood vessels whereas in both preparations the non-specific protease inhibitor aprotonin had an inhibitory effect on the contractile response to tetradecapeptide substrate. This implies that angiotensin II can be generated in the blood vessel wall by alternative pathways to those of the classic renin–angiotensin–aldosterone system. However, tetradecapeptide substrate is susceptible to non-specific hydrolysis in vascular preparations and the relevance of these studies to a vascular renin–angiotensin system in which the full size angiotensinogen molecule participates is open to question.[85]

These studies indicate that there are systems within the arterial wall which transcribe the renin gene and may produce locally active renin. These systems have to be distinguished from uptake and tight binding of kidney-derived renin which also can generate angiotensin II either from locally synthesized angiotensinogen or from angiotensinogen derived from the circulation. In addition it is important to discriminate between renin and other proteases which may generate angiotensin II perhaps at local intracellular sites of low pH. Such activity may be an *in vitro* artifact or alternatively may have an important physiological role.

Functional role of tissue renin–angiotensin systems

It is important to distinguish between the renin uptake system within the arterial wall and putative local synthesis of renin. In studies of a number of hypertensive models (DOC salt, early Goldblatt two-kidney, one-clip and late Goldblatt two-kidney, one-clip), together with other preparations in which renin was stimulated or suppressed, there was a close relationship between plasma and aortic wall renin. In no steady-state model have we been able to detect inappropriately high or low aortic renin.[65] Only temporarily following injection of renin is the relationship between aortic and plasma renin disturbed. This is consistent with the close relationship between the blood pressure fall produced by angiotensin II antagonism and concurrent plasma renin and angiotensin II levels.

With the qualifications mentioned above, molecular biological studies of renin gene expression can be used to assess the activity of local renin synthetic systems. Apart from the possibility that translational or post-translational events may modify renin it is also possible that changes observed in such studies are due to changes in mRNA stability rather than due to alterations of gene transcription. Although findings are by no means consistent it is clear that the conventional regulators of renal renin synthesis and release, i.e. feedback inhibition by angiotensin II, changes in sodium balance and perfusion pressure, do not operate on renin gene expression in extrarenal tissues in the same manner as in the juxtaglomerular apparatus of the kidney.[74]

The role of the extrarenal renin angiotensin system in blood pressure homeostasis is wholly unknown. Nevertheless there is now convincing evidence that it is of importance. Thus, DNA markers at the rat renin locus have been found to cosegregate with blood pressure in several genetically hypertensive rat strains which do not consistently have any evidence of activation of the renin–angiotensin system.[86] Further, a transgenic model in which the mouse REN-2 gene was introduced into the rat developed severe hypertension despite reduction of plasma renin–angiotensin I and angiotensin II levels.[87] On the other hand plasma prorenin and adrenal renin were elevated. Angiotensin II release from the isolated hindquarters of this transgenic model was increased and not reduced by bilateral nephrectomy (although levels were reduced in bilaterally nephrectomized control rats).[88]

Fewer studies have been carried out on the extrarenal renin–angiotensin system in experimental renovascular hypertension. Although some earlier investigations suggested that arterial renin-like activity was elevated this was not well characterized and may well have been a reflection of other proteases perhaps influenced by trophic changes. We were unable to demonstrate any dissociation between plasma renin activity and aortic renin activity in either the early or chronic phases of Goldblatt two-kidney hypertension.[65] Likewise extra renal renin gene expression was not elevated in either early or chronic phase Goldblatt two-kidney hypertension with one possibly illuminating exception.[89] In chronic Goldblatt two-kidney hypertension despite normality of renin levels, adrenal renin gene expression was increased.[89] In addition, renal renin gene expression in the clipped kidney was sustained at an increased level despite restoration of plasma renin to normal, suggesting a dissociation between storage of renin in the juxtaglomerular apparatus and release. The possible role of adrenal renin in regulation of aldosterone release suggests that elevated mineralocorticoid activity might be sustained in the chronic phrase of Goldblatt hypertension and could play an important role in sustaining blood pressure despite normal renin levels. Unfortunately, steroid activity was not measured in these studies.

The processes by which the extra renal renin–angiotensin system maintains hypertension are unknown. It seems unlikely that the system simply contributes to the circulating pool of angiotensin II although the studies of Campbell *et al.* suggest that it may make a minor contribution.[79] The most likely explanation is that the system subserves a paracrine function either in the blood vessel wall, the adrenal gland or the central nervous system. Hypertension could then result from either local constrictor or trophic effects in the resistance vessel wall, mineralocorticoid effects in the adrenal or modification of central regulation of blood pressure. Re and his colleagues demonstrated apparently specific chromosomal intracellular nuclear receptors for angiotensin II which appeared to regulate gene transcription although the specific genes were not identified.[90] This suggests that angiotensin II generated either by classical or alternative pathways intracellularly may have quite distinct effects from those mediated by the AT receptor family.

Identification of the regulation and the functional role of the extrarenal renin–angiotensin system is of major importance with the development of specific inhibitors exhibiting major differences in tissue accessibility and sites of action within the system.

Role of the renin–angiotensin system in renovascular hypertension

Goldblatt's original preparation employed bilateral renal arterial constriction.[5] In later studies renal arterial constriction on one side was combined with contralateral nephrectomy (Goldblatt one-kidney, one-clip hypertension).[91] Some species such as the rat develop severe hypertension when one renal artery is clipped and the other left untouched (Goldblatt two-kidney, one-clip hypertension). Early studies frequently combined more than one preparation. It subsequently became clear that there are important differences betweeen Goldblatt one-kidney, one-clip hypertension and Goldblatt two-kidney, one-clip hypertension. In the one-kidney model in the rat for instance renal renin,[92] juxtaglomerular granulation[93] and plasma renin[94] were found to be reduced whilst in the two-kidney model these indices of renin–angiotensin activation were increased.[92–94] These differences are related to the different impact of the two procedures on sodium balance.[95] The ischemic kidney in Goldblatt one-kidney one-clip hypertension retains sodium until the natriuretic effect of raised renal perfusion pressure balances the sodium-retaining action of renal ischemia. When the opposite kidney remains *in situ* it undergoes perfusion pressure natriuresis and diuresis so that a slight negative balance occurs as blood pressure becomes elevated. Elevated angiotensin II levels modify the pressure natriuresis curve however, limiting pressure natriuresis.[96, 97] Although the renal effects of angiotensin II could therefore maintain and amplify peripheral pressor effects, it is noteworthy that sodium depletion either acutely or dietetically does not produce blood pressure reduction and may indeed raise blood pressure in Goldblatt two-kidney, one-clip hypertension.[98, 99] In man, severe renovascular hypertension has been described in association with reduced exchangeable sodium levels presumably as a result of pressure natriuresis.[57] By contrast the Goldblatt one-kidney, one-clip model is associated with sodium retention.[95] Reversal of renovascular hypertension in these two models by removal of the constricting clip restores sodium balance to normal, i.e. the Goldblatt one-kidney, one-clip model undergoes natriuresis and the Goldblatt two-kidney, one-clip model undergoes sodium retention.[100]

Although it was originally argued that blood pressure was the response to reciprocal mechanisms in the two models, i.e. sodium retention and renin hypersecretion,[101] the changes in the renin–angiotensin system during the development of renovascular hypertension indicate a much more complicated sequence of processes. The initial response to renal artery constriction is a temporary rise in blood pressure and renin secretion.[102] This is sometimes termed actue or Phase I response. Blood pressure then rises gradually over a period of days or weeks depending upon the degree of renal artery constriction and the species investigated. In this early or Phase II response in the Goldblatt two-kidney model renin is elevated although there are marked species differences with high renins often seen in the rat[103] but only modest elevations of renin in the dog[104, 105] or the rabbit.[106] This may relate to the difficulty in producing substantial blood pressure rises within the Goldblatt two-kidney, one-clip preparation in these species perhaps as a result of the rapid development of collaterals. The sheep on the other hand readily develops Goldblatt hypertension.[107] After blood pressure has been elevated for a period of time renin hypersecretion becomes less apparent. The duration of hypereninemia in early or Phase II hypertension is variable depending upon the species and indeed probably the strain, being of only a few days' duration in the dog or rabbit but several weeks in the rat. In the chronic or Phase III stage of hypertension in the two-kidney, one-clip model plasma renin levels are normal or near normal.[108, 109] Correction of renovascular hypertension by removal of the clip in this model causes a fall to normal levels in the early phase: in the chronic phase a small fall may still be seen despite the fact the plasma renin levels are normal preoperatively.[98] This presumably reflects the response of the ischemic kidney to increased perfusion pressure.

Despite the apparent normality of the renin–angiotensin system in the chronic phase of two-kidney, one-clip hypertension, there is evidence that the system is still potentially hyperresponsive. Increased renin gene expression in the ischemic kidney has already been discussed (see above). Renin measurements obtained under situations of stress may still be high.[100, 111] Hyperresponsiveness of the juxtaglomerular apparatus can also be shown in man by the increased renin responsiveness in patients with renovascular hypertension to ACE inhibition.[112] The fall in renin levels which occur as early phase Goldblatt two-kidney, one-clip hypertension evolves into chronic phase Goldblatt two kidney hypertension appears therefore to reflect posttranscriptional processing of renin and renin secretion rather than gene transcription. Despite earlier suggestions, the fall in renin levels are not due to sodium retention. Thus, even when chronic phase Goldblatt two-kidney hypertension is reversed by removal of the renal artery clip sodium retention occurs in association with the fall in blood pressure,[100] indicating a sustained negative balance from the earliest phases of blood pressure elevation. There is strong evidence that renin hypersecretion is an essential feature of the earliest phases of blood pressure elevation in the Goldblatt two-kidney, one-clip model. Thus, inhibition of the renin–angiotensin system before renal artery constriction prevents the development of hypertension.[113, 114] However, inhibition by a competitive antagonist of angiotensin II in established two-kidney one-clip hypertension has a diminishing impact on blood pressure with the passage of time.[110] There is a close correlation between the depressor effect of angiotensin II antagonism and circulating renin levels,[110] indicating that the antagonist is lowering blood pressure through the 'classical' circulating renin–angiotensin system and that measures of circulating renin (and angiotensin II) provide a measure of activity of the renal system. This is consistent with the evidence discussed above that vascular uptake of renin in steady-state conditions reflects plasma concentrations. By contrast ACE inhibitors retain a blood pressure lowering effect in chronic Goldblatt two-kidney, one-clip hypertension, despite normality of circulating renin levels, perhaps indicating a role for other vasodepressor mechanisms.[115] Angiotensin converting enzyme inhibitors do not lower blood pressure in Goldblatt one-kidney, one-clip hypertension.[116]

The reasons for the decline in renin levels as two-kidney, one-clip hypertension enters the chronic phase is unknown. The antagonist infusion studies indicate that this decline in plasma levels parallels a decline in the role which renin is playing in blood pressure maintenance. This view is strongly supported by experiments in which renovascular hypertension in the two-kidney, one-clip rat model is reversed by removal of the renal artery clip during infusions of ACE inhibitors or angiotensin antagonists.[117] In the earlier phases of hypertension these inhibitors of the renin–angiotensin system may lower the preoperative baseline blood pressures depending upon the duration of hypertension but in the early and chronic phase normalization of blood pressure occurs within 6–12 h of unclipping despite continued inhibition of the renin–angiotensin system.

This evidence would argue strongly against developing hyperresponsiveness to angiotensin II as a mechanism for the maintenance of hypertension even when plasma angiotensin II levels were normal. When attempts are made to maintain blood pressure at preoperative levels following removal of the renal artery clip pharmacological doses of angiotensin II are required.[118] Interestingly, when the infusions of angiotensin II are discontinued under these circumstances the pattern of blood pressure fall over several hours mirrors that observed when the clip is removed in this model, suggesting that a precipitate fall in angiotensin II levels activates the same mechanisms that are involved in the reversal of hypertension with renal artery deconstriction, although such a fall in angiotensin II is not a *sine qua non* for this response.[118]

This is not to say that hyperresponsiveness to angiotensin II does not occur. Angiotensin II infusion studies in dogs with Goldblatt hypertension indicates a progressive increase in sensitivity when dose–response relationships between blood pressure and angiotensin II are plotted.[119] A similar phenomenon can be demonstrated in man in a situation where renin hypersecretion is undeniably the cause of hypertension i.e. in patients with renin-secreting tumors.[120] When angiotensin II levels are plotted against blood pressure and dose–response curves compared with normal subjects, the angiotensin II levels in patients with renin-secreting tumors were too low to explain the blood pressure elevation. Although some studies in Goldblatt hypertension in the rat have suggested specific enhancement of angiotensin II pressor responsiveness,[121] in most investigations angiotensin II hypersensitivity is part of a general increase in reactivity caused by increased wall to lumen ratio in the resistance vasculature.[122] Thus, vascular responsiveness in the isolated blood-perfused hind limb in response to angiotensin II and noradrenaline are increased. In the chronic model reversal of hypertension by removal of the constricting clip only partially reverses hyperreactivity even after an interval of several weeks, while in the early phase reactivity is almost completely normalized suggesting structural changes as a result of long-standing hypertension are responsible.[122]

There has been considerable discussion in the literature as to whether the renin–angiotensin system has a specific trophic action.[120, 123] If so, this might contribute to vascular hyperreactivity and the maintenance of hypertension. The obvious experimental approach is to block the renin–angiotensin system and study arterial structure. Unfortunately, most studies in the literature do not distinguish between the blood pressure lowering action of renin–angiotensin blockade and blockade of specific effects of angiotensin II on structure. The experiment reported by Griffin demonstrated that blood pressure lowering by hydralazine did not cause regression of resistance vessel hypertrophy induced by angiotensin II in rats (see above). Owens examined smooth muscle hypertrophy in arterial tissue from spontaneously hypertensive rats treated with a variety of blood pressure lowering agents.[124] The ACE inhibitor captopril proved more effective in reducing vascular hypertrophy than other vasodilators despite equal lowering of blood pressure. In other studies ACE inhibitors in doses insufficient to lower blood pressure inhibited smooth muscle growth in the one-kidney one-clip rat model.[125] It is still possible, however, that differential hemodynamic effects (for instance on pulse pressure or on specific tissue beds) could account for these changes despite the absence of an overall change in mean blood pressure which is a fairly crude measure of hemodynamic action of antihypertensive drugs. Harrap and co-workers administered an ACE inhibitor to spontaneously hypertensive rats and in another group of animals maintained blood pressure by increasing sodium intake while the ACE inhibitor was administered.[126] Reduction in blood pressure was associated with correction of the increased resistance vessel wall to lumen ratio but this effect was blocked when blood pressure was maintained despite suppression of the renin– angiotensin system, indicating that the correction of trophic changes observed was the effect of lowered blood pressure and not the reduction in angiotensin II.

It appears therefore that although the renin–angiotensin system is a major participant in the earliest phases of Goldblatt two-kidney, one-clip hypertension not hyperactivity of the renin–angiotensin system or hyperresponsiveness to angiotensin II or trophic changes in the vasculature can explain the maintenance of hypertension in the chronic model. Similarly sodium retention cannot be envoked as a complementary process. The processes observed during reversal of chronic renovascular hypertension by removal of the constricting clip support these conclusions. Blood pressure falls in animals with normal preoperative renin levels within a period of time far too short to be explained by regression of trophic changes and further more the fall cannot be inhibited by blockade of the renin–angiotensin system.[117] Despite this, reversal in either the Goldblatt two-kidney or the one-kidney model even during the chronic phase is associated with a dramatic fall in total peripheral vascular resistance.[127] In the rat there may be strain differences, however, in the response to surgical correction. Some studies have reported that in the chronic Phase III stage of hypertension blood pressure is sustained when surgical correction is attempted either by nephrectomy or unclipping.[128] However, most reports of this phenomenon are early and based upon indirect blood pressure measurement in which a significant stress component may be observed. Renin secretory hyperresponsiveness which is retained in the chronic phase (see above) may therefore cause spurious elevation of blood pressure even after surgical correction. Hemodynamic studies provide unequivocal evidence for major reduction in vascular resistance well before any changes in structure would be expected.[127] Assessment of resistance vessel wall to lumen ratio confirms that reversal is a slow and partial process over many weeks in the rat.[129, 130] This is consistent with observations in man where surgical correction of renovascular hypertension is frequently observed as an immediate and sustained response to surgery: such a response is often independent of either preoperative or postoperative renin levels.

In an attempt to identify the mechanism which could have such a powerful effect on peripheral vascular resistance, studies have been carried out in which reversal of hypertension by renal artery deconstriction has been attempted during continuous infusion of inhibitors. Inhibition of cyclo-oxygenase, the kinin system or endogenous opioid systems failed to have any impact upon the pattern of blood pressure fall.[131, 132] The only maneuver which was successful was chemical removal of the renal medulla.[133] This procedure produces modest hypertension in rats, probably as a result of removal of the renomedullary interstitial cells. These secrete a potent vasodepressor lipid, medullipin 1 which is converted in the liver into the active compound medullipin 2.[134] Secretion of medullipin appears to be a renal homeostatic system which results in blood pressure lowering when renal perfusion pressure is increased.[135] Decrease of renal perfusion pressure inhibits the release of medullipin.[135] Release of medullipin, therefore, as a result of increased renal perfusion pressure resulting from renal artery deconstriction may cause the acute reduction in peripheral vascular resistance observed. Angiotensin II also inhibits medullipin secretion by renomedullary interstitial cells[134] and the fall in angiotensin II by corrective surgery may therefore play an indirect role particularly when blood pressure is lowered by removal of the ischemic kidney rather than by removal of the constricting clip. However, this is clearly not an essential feature of a process which occurs despite continued blockade of the renin–angiotensin system.

The role of the extrarenal renin–angiotensin system in renovascular hypertension remains unclear. The only clearcut evidence for a sustained abnormality is the increased renin gene expression in the ischemic kidney and in the adrenal glands.[89] Whether this latter is part of a generalized trophic response in the adrenals as a result of hyperreninemia in the early phase of Goldblatt hypertension is uncertain. If so, it may represent a secondary change rather than directly participating in blood pressure elevation although it may be associated with secondary aldosteronism. The absence of changes in other tissues in Goldblatt hypertension contrasts sharply with, for instance, the spontaneously hypertensive rat where the majority of extrarenal tissues exhibit increased renin gene expression during the phase of development of hypertension.[136] On current evidence there would seem to be no occasion to invoke increased activity of the extrarenal system in renovascular hypertension. Greater knowledge of its regulation and function, however, may necessitate revision of this opinion.

References

1 Bright R. Tabular view of the morbid appearances in 100 cases connected with albuminous urine with observations. *Guy's Hosp Rep* 1836; **1:** 380–400.

2 Johnson G. *On Diseases of the Kidney, Their Pathology, Diagnosis and Treatment.* London: Parker and Sons, 1852.

3 Brown-Sequard CE. Importance de la secretion interne des reins demonstrée par les phenomenes de l'anurie et de l'uremie. *Arch Physiol Norm Path* 1893; **5:** 778–86.

4 Tigerstedt R, Bergman PG. Niere and Kreislauf. *Scand Arch Physiol* 1989; **7–8:** 223–71.

5 Goldblatt H, Lynch J, Hanzal RF, Summerville WW. Studies on experimental hypertension. 1. The production of persistent elevation of systolic blood pressure by means of renal ischaemia. *J Exp Med* 1934; **59:** 347–57.

6 Butler AM. Chronic pyelonephritis and arterial hypertension. *J Clin Invest* 1937; **16:** 889–97.

7 Swales JD. *Classic Papers in Hypertension: Blood Pressure and Renin.* London: Science Press, 1987.

8 Nussberger J, Buhler K, Waeber B, Brunner HR. Identification and quanitation of angiotensins. *J Cardiovasc Pharmacol* 1986; **8:** (Suppl. 10) s23–s28.

9 Hackenthal E, Nobiling R. Renin secretion and its regulation. In JD Swales (ed.) *Textbook of Hypertension*, pp. 232–44. Oxford: Blackwell, 1994.

10 Inagami T. Renin: purification, structure and function. In Robertson JIS, Nicholls MG (eds) *The Renin–Angiotensin System. Biochemistry, Physiology and Pathophysiology and Therapeutics*, pp. 4.1–4.17. London: Gower, 1993.

11 Bader M, Paul M, Fernandez-Alfonso M *et al.* Molecular biology and biochemistry of the renin—angiotensin system. In Swales JD (ed.) *Textbook of Hypertension*; pp. 214–32. Oxford: Blackwell, 1994.

12 Chen M, Schnermann J, Malvin RL *et al.* Time course of stimulation of renal renin messenger RNA by furosamide. *Hypertension* 1993; **21:** 36–41.

13 Keeton TK, Campbell WB. The pharmacologic alteration of renin release. *Pharmacol Rev* 1980; **32:** 81–227.

14 Ludwig G, Suzuki F, Murakami K *et al.* Kidney renin mRNA renin secretion and plasma renin following adrenalectomy, salt depletion or enalapril treatment in the rat. *J Hypertension* 1986; **4:** S431-S433.

15 Vander AJ. Control of renin release. *Physiol Rev* 1967; **47:** 359–82.

16 Skott O, Briggs JP. Direct demonstration of macula densa mediated renin secretion. *Science* 1987; **237:** 1618–20.

17 Kotchen TA, Welch WJ, Lorenz JN, Ott CE. Renal tubular chloride and renin release. *J Lab Clin Med* 1987; **110:** 533–40.

18 Cooke CR, Brown TC, Zacherle BJ, Walker WG. Effect of altered sodium concentration in the distal nephron segments on renin release. *J Clin Invest* 1970; **49:** 1630–8.

19 Munter K, Hackenthal E. NaCl intake and

macula densa mechanism of renin secretion. *Arch Pharmacol* 1989; **339:** R71.

20 Bock HA, Hermle M, Brunner FP, Thiel G. Pressure dependent modulation of renin release in isolated perfused glomeruli. *Kidney Int* 1992; **41:** 275–80.

21 Finke R, Gross R, Hackenthal E *et al.* Threshold pressure for the pressure dependent renin release in the autoregulated kidney of conscious dogs. *Pfluger's Arch* 1983; **399:** 102–10.

22 Gibnbons GH, Dzau VJ, Farhie R, Barger AC. Interaction of signals influencing renin release. *Ann Rev Physiol* 1984; **46:** 291–308.

23 Hackenthal E, Paul M, Ganten D, Taugner R. Morphology, physiology and molecular biology of renin secretion. *Physiol Rev* 1990; **70:** 1067–116.

24 Kurtz A, Scholz H, Bruna della R. Molecular mechanisms of renin release. *J Cardiovasc Pharmacol* 1990; **16:** (Suppl. 4) S1–7.

25 Campbell DJ, Habener JF. Angiotensinogen gene is expressed in differentially regulated in multiple tissues of the rat. *J Clin Invest* 1986; **78:** 31–9.

26 Cassis LA, Saye J, Peach MJ. Location and regulation of rat angiotensinogen messenger RNA. *Hypertension* 1988; **11:** 591–6.

27 Poulsen K, Jacobsen J. Enzymic reactions of the renin–angiotensin system. In Robertson JIS, Nicholls MG (eds) *The Renin–Angiotensin System. Biochemistry Physiology, Pathophysiology and Therapeutics,* pp. 5.1–5.12. London: Gower, 1993.

28 Poulsen K, Jacobsen J. Is angiotensinogen a renin inhibitor and not the substrate for renin? *J Hypertension* 1986; **4:** 65–9.

29 Erdos EG. Angiotensin I converting enzyme and the changes in our concepts through the years. *Hypertension* 1990; **16:** 363–70.

30 Skidgel RA, Erdos EG. Biochemistry of angiotensin I converting enzyme. In Robertson JIS, Nicholls MG (eds) *The Renin–Angiotensin System, Biochemistry, Physiology, Pathophysiology and Therapeutics*, pp. 10.1–10.10. London: Gower, 1993.

31 Regoli D, Drapeau G, Rovero P *et al.* Conversion of kinins and their antagonists into beta 1 receptor activators and blockers in isolated vessels. *Eur J Pharmacol* 1986; **127:** 219–24.

32 Goodfriend TI, Peach MJ. Angiotensin III (desaspartic acid) angiotensin II. *Circ Res* 1975; **36–7:** (Suppl. 1) 38–48.

33 Goodfriend TI. Angiotensinase. In Robertson JIS, Nicholls MG (eds) *The Renin–Angiotensin System. Biochemistry, Physiology, Pathophysiology and Therapeutics*, pp. 11.1–11.5. London: Gower, 1993.

34 Griendling KK, Alexander RW. Cellular mechanisms of angiotensin II action. In Swales JD (ed.) *Textbook of Hypertension*, pp. 244–53. Oxford: Blackwell, 1994.

35 Grady EF, Sechila LA, Griffin CA, Schambelan M, Kalinyaka JE. Expression of ATII receptors in the developing rat foetus. *J Clin Invest* 1991; **88:** 921–33.

36 Aguilera G, Schirar A, Baukal A, Catt KJ. Angiotensin II receptors: properties and regulation in adrenal glomerulosa cells. *Circ Res* 1980; **46:** (Suppl. 11) 118–27.

37 Folkow B, Hallback M, Lundgren Y *et al.* Importance of adaptive changes in vascular design for establishment of primary hypertension studied in man and in spontaneously hypertensive rats. *Circ Res* 1973; **32:** (Suppl. 1) 2–16.

38 Smith JB. Angiotensin receptor signalling in cultured vascular smooth muscle cells. *Am J Physiol* 1986; **250:** F759–F769.

39 Geisterfer A, Peach MJ, Owens GK. Angiotensin II induces hypertrophy not hyperplasia of cultured rat aortic smooth muscle cells. *Circ Res* 1988; **62:** 749–56.

40 Paquet JL, Bandonim-Legros M, Brunelle G, Meyer P. Angiotensin II induced proliferation of aortic myocytes in spontaneously hypertensive rats. *J Hypertension* 1990; **8:** 565–72.

41 Daemen MJAP, Lombardi DM, Bosman FT, Schwartz SM. Angiotensin II induces smooth muscle cell proliferation in the normal and injured rat arterial wall. *Circ Res* 1991; **68:** 450–56.

42 Scott-Burden T, Hahn AWA, Resink TJ, Buhler FR. Modulation of extracellular matrix by angiotensin II: stimulated glucoconjugate synthesis and growth in vascular smooth muscle cells. *J Cardiovasc Pharmacol* 1990; **16:** (Suppl. 4) s26–s41.

43 Brilla CG, Pick R, Tan LB *et al.* Remodelling of the rat right and left ventricles in experimental hypertension. *Circ Res* 1990; **67:** 1355–64.

44 Powell JS, Clozel JP, Mueller RKM *et al.* Inhibitors of angiotensin converting enzyme prevent myointimal proliferation after vascular injury. *Science* 1989; **245:** 186–8.

45 Quinn SJ, Williams GH. Regulation of aldosterone secretion. *Ann Rev Physiol* 1988; **50:** 409–26.

46 Williams GH, Tuck ML, Sullivan JM *et al.* Parallel adrenal and renal abnormalities in the young patient with essential hypertension. *Am J Med* 1982; **72:** 907–14.

47 Zimmerman BG. Adrenergic facilitation by angiotensin: does it serve a physiologic function? *Clin Sci* 1981; **60:** 343–8.

48 Squire IB, Reid JL. Interactions between the renin–angiotensin system and the autonomic nervous system. In Robertson JIS, Nicholls MG (eds) *The Renin–Angiotensin System. Biochemistry, Physiology, Pathophysiology and Therapeutics*, pp. 37.1–37.16. London: Gower, 1993.

49 Buckley JP. Action of angiotensin on the central nervous system. *Fed Proc* 1972; **31:** 1332–7.
50 Samani NJ, Swales JD, Brammar WJ. Expression of the renin gene in extra-renal tissues of the rat. *Biochem J* 1988; **253:** 907–10.
51 Bunnemnan B, Fuxe K, Ganten D. Extra-renal renin systems: the brain. In Robertson JIS, Nicholls MG (eds) *The Renin–Angiotensin System. Biochemistry, Physiology, Pathophysiology and Therapeutics*, pp. 41.1–41.17. London: Gower, 1993.
52 Sweet CS, Columbo JM, Gaul SL. Central antihypertensive effects of inhibitors of the renin-angiotensin system in rats. *Am J Physiol* 1976; **231:** 1794–9.
53 Hall JE. Control of sodium excretion by angiotensin II: Intra-renal mechanism and blood pressure regulation. *Am J Physiol* 1986; **250:** R960–72.
54 Hall JE. Regulation of glomerular filtration rate and sodium excretion by angiotensin II. *Fed Proc* 1986; **45:** 1431–7.
55 Barraclough MA. Sodium and weater depletion with acute malignant hypertension. *Am J Med* 1966; **40:** 265–72.
56 Mohring J, Petri M, Szokol M *et al.* Effects of saline drinking on malignant course of renal hypertension in rats. *Am J Physiol* 1976; **230:** 849–57.
57 McAreavey D, Brown JJ, Cumming AMM *et al.* Inverse relation of exchangeable sodium and blood pressure in hypertensive patients with renal artery stenosis. *J Hypertension* 1983; **1:** 297–302.
58 Brown JJ, Chapuis G, Robertson JIS. The effect of prolonged intravenous infusion of angiotensin in the rabbit. *Clin Sci* 1964; **26:** 165–75.
59 Dickinson CJ, Lawrence JR. A slowly developing pressor response to small concentrations of angiotensin. *Lancet* 1963; **1:** 1354–6.
60 Brown AJ, Casals-Stenzel J, Gofford S *et al.* Comparison of fast and slow pressor effects of angiotensin II in the conscious rat. *Am J Physiol* 1981; **241:** H381–H388.
61 De Clue JW, Guyton AC, Cowley AW *et al.* Subpressor angiotensin infusions, renal sodium handling and salt induced hypertension in the dog. *Circ Res* 1978; **43:** 503–12.
62 Griffin SA, Brown WCB, Macpherson F *et al.* Angiotensin II causes vascular hypertrophy in part by a non-pressor mechanism. *Hypertension* 1991; **17:** 626–35.
63 Goldsmith SR, Hasking FJ. Sub-pressor angiotensin II infusions do not stimulate sympathetic activity in humans. *Am J Physiol* 1990; **258:** H179–H182.
64 Li P, Jackson ED. Enhanced slow pressor response to angiotensin II in spontaneously hypertensive rats. *J Pharmacol Exp Ther* 1989; **251:** 909–21.
65 Swales JD, Samani NJ. Vascular renin and hypertension: uptake versus synthesis. *Am J Hypertension* 1990; **3:** 890–92.
66 Gould LB, Skeggs LT, Kha JR. The presence of renin activity in blood vessel walls. *J Exp Med* 1964; **119:** 389–90.
67 Dzau VJ. Multiple pathways of angiotensin production in the blood vessel wall: evidence, possibilities and hypotheses. *J Hypertension* 1989; **7:** 933–6.
68 Thurston H, Swales JD, Bing RF *et al.* Vascular renin-like activity and blood pressure maintenance in the rat: studies of the effect of changes in sodium balance, hypertension and nephrectomy. *Hypertension* 1979; **1:** 643–9.
69 Loudon M, Bing RF, Thurston H, Swales JD. Arterial wall uptake of renal renin and blood pressure control. *Hypertension* 1983; **5:** 629–34.
70 Swales JD, Abramovici A, Beck F *et al.* Arterial wall renin. *J Hypertension* 1983; **1:** (Suppl. 1) 17–22.
71 Re R, Falloon JT, Dzau V *et al.* Renin synthesis by canine aortic smooth muscle cells in culture. *Life Sci* 1992; **30:** 99–106.
72 Lilly LS, Pratt RE, Alexander RW. Renin expression by vascular endothelial cells in culture. *Circ Res* 1985; **57:** 312–18.
73 Naruse M, Takii Y, Inagami T. Renin exists in high concentrations in the adrenal gland of the rat. *Biomed Rev* 1981; **2:** 583–6.
74 Samani NJ, Swales JD, Brammar WJ. Expression of the renin gene in extra-renal tissues of the rat. *Biochem J* 1988; **253:** 907–10.
75 Campbell DJ, Habener JF. Angiotensinogen gene is expressed differently and regulated in multiple tissues of the rat. *J Clin Invest* 1986; **78:** 31–9.
76 Hilgers KF, Kuczer AM, Wilhelm MJ. Angiotensin formation in the isolated rat hindlimb. *J Hypertension* 1989; **7:** 789–98.
77 Seito H, Nakamaru M, Ogihara T *et al.* Renin inhibitor and converting enzyme inhibitors suppress vascular angiotensin II. *Hypertension* 1989; **13:** 749–53.
78 Kato H, Iwai N, Inui H *et al.* Regulation of vascular angiotensin release. *Hypertension* 1993; **21:** 446–54.
79 Campbell DJ, Kladis A, Duncan AM. Nephrectomy, converting enzyme inhibition, and angiotensin peptides. *Hypertension* 1993; **22:** 513–22.
80 Admiraal PJJ, Derkx FHHM *et al.* Metabolism and production of angiotensin in different vascular beds in subjects with hypertension. *Hypertension* 1990; **15:** 44–55.
81 Thurston H, Swales JD. Action of angiotensin antagonists and antiserum upon the pressor response to renin: further evidence for the local generation of angiotensin II. *Clin Sci Mol Med* 1974; **46:** 273–6.

82 Thurston H, Swales JD. Comparison of angiotensin II antagonists and antiserum infusion with nephrectomy in the rat with two kidney Goldblatt hypertension. *Circ Res* 1974; **35:** 325–9.
83 Juul B, Aalkjaer C, Mulvany MJ. Contractile effects of tetra-decapeptide renin substrate in rat femoral vessels. *J Hypertension* 1987; **5:** (Suppl. 2) s7–s10.
84 Bund SJ, Aalkjaer C, Heagerty AM *et al.* The contractile effects of porcine tetra-deca-peptide renin substrate in human resistance vessels: evidence of activation by vascular wall renin and serine proteases. *J Hypertension* 1989; **7:** 741–6.
85 Campbell DJ, Ziogas J, Kladis A. Metabolism of tetra deca peptide angiotensinogen and angiotensin I and II by isolated perfused rat hind limbs. *Clin Exp Pharmacol Physiol* 1990; **17:** 335–50.
86 Samani NJ. Molecular genetics of susceptibility to the development of hypertension. *Br Med Bull* 1994; **50:** 260–71.
87 Mullins JJ, Peters J, Ganten D. Fulminant hypertension in transgenic rats harbouring the mouse Ren-2 gene. *Nature* 1990; **344:** 541–4.
88 Hilgers KF, Peters J, Veelken R *et al.* Increased vascular angiotensin formation in female rats harboring the mouse Ren 2 gene. *Hypertension* 1992; **19:** 687–91.
89 Samani NJ, Brammar WJ, Swales JD. Renal and extra-renal renin messenger RNA levels in experimental hypertension. *Clin Sci* 1991; **80:** 339–44.
90 Re RN, Vizard DL, Bryan SE. Angiotensin II receptors in chromatin fragments generated by micrococcal nuclease. *Biochem Biophys Res Commun* 1984; **119:** 220–5.
91 Wilson C, Byrom FB. Renal changes in malignant hypertension. *Lancet* 1939; **1:** 136–9.
92 Regoli D, Brunner H, Peters G, Gross F. Changes in renin content in kidneys of renal hypertensive rats. *Proc Soc Exp Biol Med* 1962; **109:** 142–5.
93 Heptinstall RH. The role of the juxtaglomerular apparatus in experimental hypertension in the rat. *Lab Invest* 1965; **14:** 2150–9.
94 Mikshe LW, Mikshe U, Gross F. Effect of sodium restriction on renal hypertension and renin activity in the rat. *Circ Res* 1970; **27:** 973–84.
95 Swales JD, Thurston H, Queiroz FP, Medina A. Sodium balance during the development of experimental hypertension. *J Lab Clin Med* 1972; **80:** 539–47.
96 Hall JE, Guyton AC, Smith MJ Jr, Coleman TG. Blood pressure and renal function during chronic changes in sodium intake: role of angiotensin. *Am J Physiol* 1980; **239:** F271–F280.
97 Hall JE, Mizelle HL, Woods LL. The renin–angiotensin system and long-term regulation of arterial pressure. *J Hypertension* 1986; **4:** 387–97.
98 Thurston H, Swales JD. Influence of dietary sodium restriction upon two models of renal hypertension. *Clin Sci Mol Med* 1976; **51:** 275–9.
99 Taquini CH, Basso GN, Taquini AC. Influence of sodium on experimental renovascular hypertension in rats. *Clin Sci* 1980; **59:** (Suppl. 6) 149S–151S.
100 Thurston H, Bing RF, Swales JD. Reversal of two kidney one clip renovascular hypertension in the rat. *Hypertension* 1980; **2:** 256–65.
101 Gavras H, Brunner HR, Vaughan ED, Laragh JH. Angiotensin, sodium interaction in blood pressure maintenance of renal hypertensive and normotensive rats. *Science* 1973; **180:** 1369–72.
102 Miller ED, Samuels AI, Haber E, Barger AC. Inhibition of angiotensin conversion and prevention of renal hypertension. *Am J Physiol* 1975; **228:** 448–53.
103 Mohring J, Mohring B, Naumann HJ *et al.* Salt and water balance and renin activity in renal hypertension of rats. *Am J Physiol* 1975; **228:** 1847–55.
104 Watkins BE, Davis JO, Hanson RC *et al.* Incidence and pathophysiological changes in chronic two kidney hypertension in the dog. *Am J Physiol* 1976; **231:** 954–60.
105 Masaki Z, Ferrario CM, Bumpus FM *et al.* The cause and the effect of Sar^1-THR^3-angiotensin II in a new model of two kidney hypertension in conscious dogs. *Clin Sci Mol Med* 1977; **52:** 163–70.
106 Lohmier TE, Davis JO. Renin–angiotensin–aldosterone system in experimental renal hypertension in the rabbit. *Am J Physiol* 1976; **230:** 311–18.
107 Blair-West JR, Coghlan JP, Denton DA *et al.* Renin, angiotensin, aldosterone system and sodium balance in experimental renal hypertension. *Endocrinology* 1968; **83:** 1199–209.
108 MacDonald GJ, Boyd GW, Peart WS. Effect of angiotensin II blocker. 1. SAR-8-Ala angiotensin II on renal artery clip hypertension in the rat. *Circ Res* 1975; **37:** 640–6.
109 Russell GI, Bing RF, Thurston H, Swales JD. Surgical reversal of two-kidney, one clip hypertension during inhibition of the renin– angiotensin system. *Hypertension* 1982; **4:** 69–76.
110 Bing RF, Russell GI, Swales JD, Thurston H. Effect of 12 hour infusions of saralasin or captopril on blood pressure in conscious rats. Relationship to plasma renin, duration of hypertension and effect of unclipping. *J Lab Clin Med* 1981; **98:** 302–10.
111 Oates HF, Stokes GS. Renin stimulation caused by blood collection techniques in the rat. *Clin Exp Pharmacol Physiol* 1974; **1:** 495–500.
112 Case DB, Laragh JH. Reactive hyperreninaemia

in renovascular hypertension after angiotensin blockade with saralasin or converting enzyme inhibitor. *Ann Int Med* 1979; **91:** 153–60.

113 DeForrest JM, Knappenberger RC, Antonaccio MJ *et al.* Angiotensin II is a necessary component for the development of hypertension in the two kidney one clip rat. *Am J Cardiol* 1982; **49:** 1515–17.

114 Freeman RH, Davis JO, Watkins BE *et al.* Effects of continuous converting enzyme blockade on renovascular hypertension in the rat. *Am J Physiol* 1979; **236:** F21–F24.

115 Wallis ECH, Balmforth AJ, Morton JJ. Effect of chronic and acute captopril infusion on blood pressure in the two kidney one clip hypertensive rat. *J Hypertension* 1985; **3:** 607–12.

116 Freeman RH, Davis JO, Watkins BE *et al.* Effects of continuous converting enzyme blockade on renovascular hypertension in the rat. *Am J Physiol* 1979; **236:** F21–F24.

117 Russell GI, Bing RF, Thurston H, Swales JD. Surgical reversal of two kidney one clip hypertension during inhibition of the renin-angiotensin system. *Hypertension* 1982; **4:** 69–76.

118 Kumar A, Bing RF, Swales JD, Thurston H. Delayed reversal of Goldblatt hypertension by angiotensin II infusion in the rat. *Am J Physiol* 1984; **246:** H811–H817.

119 Brown JJ, Casals-Stenzel J, Cumming AMM *et al.* Angiotensin II, aldosterone and arterial pressure: a quantitative approach. Arthur C. Corcoran Memorial Lecture. *Hypertension* 1979; **1:** 159–79.

120 Lever AF. Slow pressor mechanisms in hypertension: a role for hypertrophy of resistance vessels. *J Hypertension* 1986; **4:** 515–24.

121 Collis MG, Van Houtte PM. Increased renal vascular reactivity to angiotensin II but not to nerve stimulation or exogenous norepinephrine in renal hypertensive rats. *Circ Res* 1978; **42:** 744–52.

122 Mistry M, Bing RF, Swales JD, Thurston H. The role of vascular hypertrophy in early and chronic renovascular hypertension. *J Hypertension* 1983; **1:** (Suppl. 2): 79–81.

123 Schelling P, Fischer H, Ganten D. Angiotensin and cell growth: a link to cardiovascular hypertrophy. *J Hypertension* 1991; **9:** 3–15.

124 Owens GK. Influence of blood pressure on the development of aortic medial smooth muscle hyperttrophy in spontaneously hypertensive rats. *Hypertension* 1987; **9:** 178–87.

125 Wang DH, Prewitt RL. Captopril reduces aortic and microvascular growth in hypertensive and normotensive rats. *Hypertension* 1990; **15:** 68–77.

126 Harrap SB, Mitchell GA, Casley DJ *et al.* Angiotensin II, sodium and cardiovascular hypertrophy in spontaneously hypertensive rats. *Hypertension* 1993; **21:** 50–5.

127 Russell GI, Bing RF, Swales JD, Thurston H. Haemodynamic changes induced by reversal of early and late renovascular hypertension. *Am J Physiol* 1983; **245:** H734-H740.

128 Brown JJ, Cuesta V, Davies DL *et al.* Mechanism of renal hypertension. *Lancet* 1976; **1:** 1219–21.

129 Lundgren Y, Weiss L. Cardiovascular design after 'reversal' of longstanding renal hypertension in rats. *Clin Sci* 1979; **57:** (Suppl. 5), 19–21.

130 Watt PAC, Thurston H. The regression of resistance vessel hypertrophy with reversal of renovascular hypertension in the rat. *J Hypertension* 1990; **81:** (Suppl. 3) S123.

131 Russell GI, Bing RF, Swales JD, Thurston H. Indomethacin or aprotinin infusion. Effect on infusion of chronic two kidney one clip hypertension in the conscious rat. *Clin Sci* 1982; **62:** 361–6.

132 Edmunds ME, Russell GI, Bing RF *et al.* Failure of naxolone to influence surgical reversal of two kidney one clip hypertension in the rat. *Proc Soc Exp Biol Med* 1987; **184:** 107–12.

133 Swales JD, Bing RF, Edmunds ME *et al.* Reversal of renovascular hypertension: role of the renal medulla. *Can J Physiol Pharmacol* 1987; **65:** 1566–71.

134 Muirhead EE. Renomedullary vasodepressor lipid: medullipin. In Swales JD (ed.) *Textbook of Hypertension*, pp. 341–59. Oxford: Blackwell, 1994.

135 Muirhead EE, Brooks B, Byers LW *et al.* Secretion of medullipin I by isolated kidneys perfused under elevated pressure. *Clin Exp Pharmacol Physiol* 1991; **18:** 409–17.

136 Samani NJ, Swales JD, Brammar WJ. A widespread abnormality of renin gene expression in the spontaneously hypertensive rat: modulation in some tissues with the development of hypertension. *Clin Sci* 1989; **77:** 629–36.

13

Epidemiology and clinical manifestations

ROBERT WILKINSON

Introduction

A great deal of confusion arises in the consideration of renovascular hypertension (RVH) because many studies do not clearly separate patients with renal artery stenosis (RAS) due to atheroma from those due to fibromuscular dysplasia (FMD). The epidemiology of the two conditions is quite different and is therefore dealt with separately. The two conditions have many clinical features in common and I have therefore considered them together for this section.

Epidemiology

Fibromuscular dysplasia

Age and sex

Fibromuscular disease of the renal arteries is predominantly a disease of young women although it does occur in men, who represent about 25% of patients. It is unusual before the age of 16[1] but may be seen in younger children with neurofibromatosis. The average age of patients with FMD in the United States Cooperative Study of Patients with Renovascular Hypertension was 32.6 ± 11.8 years,[2] whereas patients with essential hypertension were older at onset (35.1 ± 11.1 years).

The diagnosis is not uncommonly made in middle-aged patients but in this situation it is not known whether it is a recent development or whether it is long-standing but undiagnosed. Interestingly, in these older patients the sex distribution seems to be more even.[3]

Geographic and racial differences

In Western populations FMD accounts for only one-third of all patients with RAS[4] although in young people almost all are due to this. In Asian populations the pattern is quite different because Takayasu's arteritis is much more common, and in one study in India 61% of patients with renal artery stenosis had this condition,[5] whereas in Western Europe it is extremely rare.

A lower prevalence of RVH in black compared with white hypertensives has been reported[6] in a study in which 123 patients with grade III or IV retinopathy were subjected to angiography: 7% of black and 43% of white patients had stenoses. However, in a study of black and white patients selected for study on clinical grounds the incidence of RVH did not differ.[7] Nevertheless, the observation that FMD may be familial[8] suggests that there may also be true racial differences. In the US Cooperative Study only 10% of patients with RAS due to FMD were black compared with 29% of essential hypertensives.

Family history

In patients with RAS due to FMD a family history of hypertension and its complications is less common than in essential hypertension or atheromatous RAS[2] and this is often used as a clue to the diagnosis. However, there have been several reports of familial cases of fibromuscular dysplasia,[8, 9] and this together with the association of FMD with neurofibromatosis[10] and the report of its occurrence in a patient with Turner's syndrome[11] strongly suggests the importance of genetic factors in FMD. In the families studied by Rushton[8] 60% of families had between one and eleven affected relatives in addition to the propositus. Vertical transmission was observed suggesting an autosomal dominant trait with variable penetrance.

Prevalence of RAS due to FMD

The prevalence of FMD affecting the renal vessels in patients with hypertension is not known because systematic full investigation of unselected populations with all grades of hypertension has not been undertaken. In one study of 819 consecutive autopsies nine cases of FMD affecting the renal artery were found but these patients were not all hypertensive, neither can they be considered to represent the normal population since they had reached autopsy.

In clinical studies the prevalence of RVH has been reported to be between 1 and 5%.[12, 13] In the US Cooperative Study one-third of 884 patients with RVH had FMD and two-thirds atheroma.[4, 14] If this proportion applies in the other clinical studies of hypertensives then approximately 12 would have FMD, a figure in broad agreement with the autopsy series.

In patients with malignant hypertension up to 30% may have RVH[6] and in young people this will almost always be due to FMD.

The prevalence of RVH is also increased in patients with hypertension which is resistant to drug therapy.[15, 16]

Natural history of RAS due to FMD

Progression of FMD

Fibromuscular dysplasia may be considered as a low grade arteritis analogous to Takayasu's arteritis. Although the renal arteries are most commonly affected many other vessels including the carotids, coronaries, abdominal aorta, femoral, iliac, popliteal, axillary, brachial and even retinal arteries may be involved.[17] However, unlike Takayasu's arteritis FMD is not accompanied by systemic illness and erythrocyte sedimentation rate is usually normal. The condition usually develops in young women and progresses often over several years; we have observed new lesions developing in previously unaffected vessels[18] (Fig. 13.1). It has been suggested that the progress of the disease is arrested around the menopause[1] implying that when the diagnosis is made at this age the changes may be long-standing and the risk of further progression small. However Goncharenko has reported progression in all types of FMD and in all age groups.[3]

Occlusion of the renal artery

The natural history of FMD depends on the histological type. Medial fibroplasia results in bands of fibrosis separated by dilated segments giving rise to the classical string of beads appearance, it also affects cerebral and hepatic arteries, it rarely progresses to occlusion but well-documented cases of renal artery occlusion have been reported.[19] Perimedial fibroplasia gives rise to multiple tight stenoses without aneurysmal dilatation between them and is more likely to progress to occlusion.[20] Intimal fibroplasia and medial hyperplasia are much less common, both usually cause a single stenosis which may progress to occlusion. However the risk of progression to occlusion is much lower in FMD than it is in atheromatous RAS in whom up to 17% occlude over a 3–4 year period.[21, 22]

Collateral circulation

In addition to renal artery occlusion being less common in FMD than in atheromatous RAS (ARAS) uremia is rare. It has been suggested that this is because collaterals develop much more readily in younger patients than in the generally older patients with ARAS.[1]

Renal artery aneurysm

Multiple small aneurysms are an intrinsic part of FMD but not uncommonly a larger aneurysm,

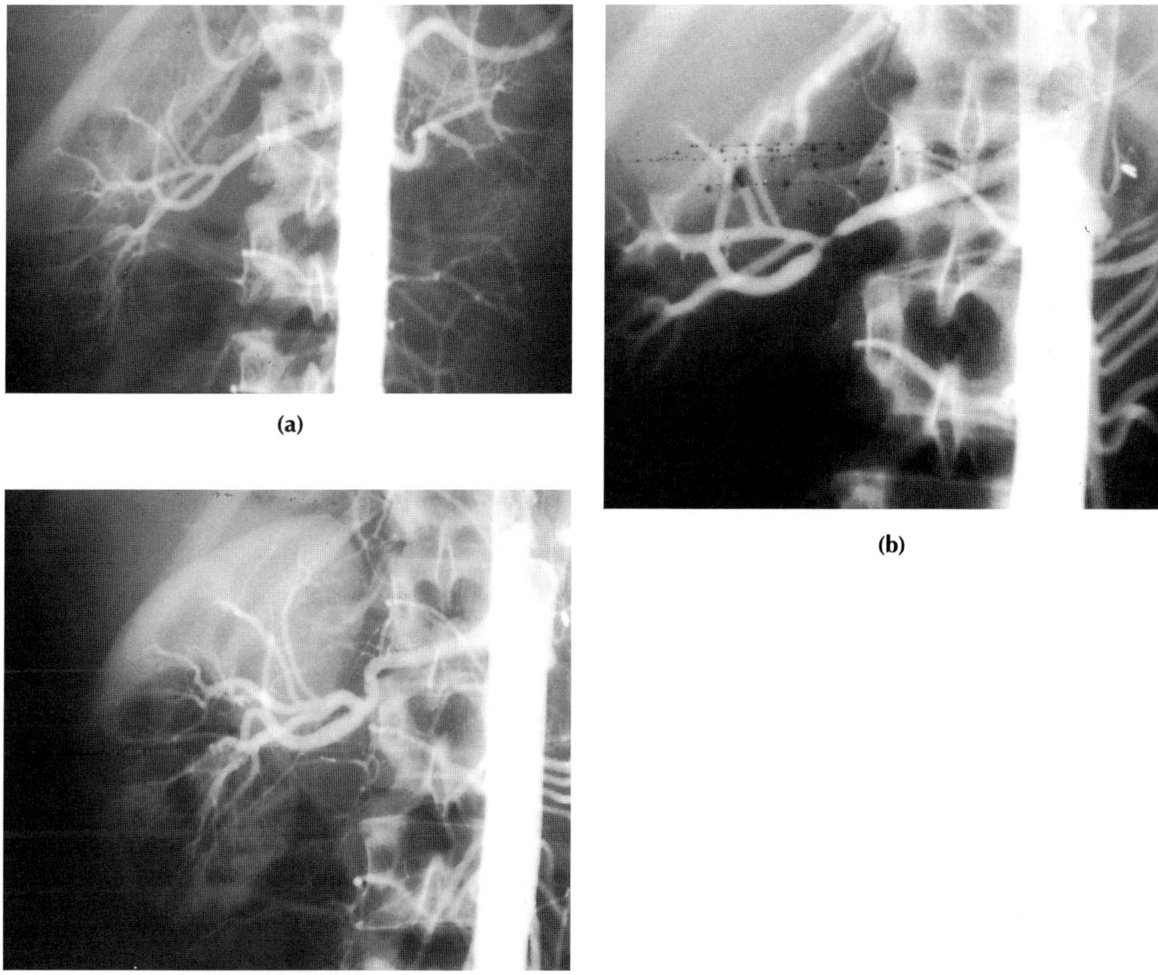

(a) (b) (c)

Figure 13.1. (a) A single stenosis at the bifurcation of the left renal artery in a girl aged 18 years, probably due to intimal fibroplasia or medial hyperplasia, causing severe hypertension. Nephrectomy followed unsuccessful reconstruction. (b) Hypertension recurred 5 years later and stenosis had developed in the previously normal right renal artery. (c) The right renal artery stenosis was subsequently treated by percutaneous transluminal angioplasty. From refs 18, 87, with permission.

usually fusiform develops (Fig. 13.2). Dissection of the aneurysm may very occasionally occur but rupture is rare although the risk of rupture is increased in pregnancy. Usually intervention is reserved for those aneurysms exceeding 2 cm in diameter and in which the wall is not calcified, although women of child-bearing potential should also be considered for surgery. Even in the absence of concomitant RAS renal artery aneurysms are thought to cause hypertension; the mechanisms suggested for this include renal ischemia due to turbulent flow, compression of the renal artery, emboli from thrombus within the aneurysm and, rarely, the formation of an arteriovenous fistula.

Body habitus

Obesity is a major contributory factor to the elevation of blood pressure in essential hypertension and reduction in body weight results in a useful reduction in blood pressure. In the US

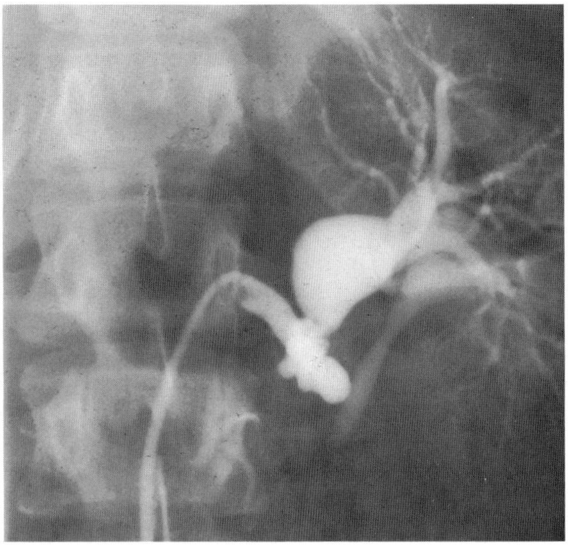

Figure 13.2. Fusiform aneurysm of the renal artery in a girl of 16 years presenting with severe hypertension and an epigastric bruit. From ref. 87, with permission.

Cooperative Study[2] 38% of essential hypertensives but only 11% of patients with FMD were classified as obese. This probably reflects the younger age of the patients with FMD as well as the major contribution of obesity to the elevation of blood pressure in the essential hypertensives.

Cigarette smoking

The association of ARAS with smoking is to be expected in view of the increased prevalence of atheroma in other vessels in smokers and has in fact been documented.[23, 24] However the observation by the same groups of an increased incidence of smoking in patients with FMD was more surprising. The mechanism by which cigarette smoking might lead to FMD is not known.

Neurofibromatosis

Renal artery stenosis is an uncommon feature of neurofibromatosis arising as the result of intimal proliferation. It usually occurs in children under the age of 16 years but 30% of cases occur in adults[10] and it may be accompanied by coarctation of the abdominal aorta and by renal artery aneurysm.[25]

Takayasu's arteritis

Renal artery stenosis may develop as a consequence of Takayasu's arteritis which is a chronic inflammatory disease affecting the wall of the aorta and its large branches and leading to their stenosis or occlusion. It affects mainly young woman, the female to male ratio is 2.8:1, and although rare in Western populations is a common cause of RAS in Asian and African patients with RVH.[5]

Middle aortic syndrome

This is a very rare syndrome which consists of stenosis of the abdominal aorta and its major branches but usually sparing the iliac arteries (Fig. 13.3). We have seen only three patients with this condition from a population of 3 million in the north of England over the past 25

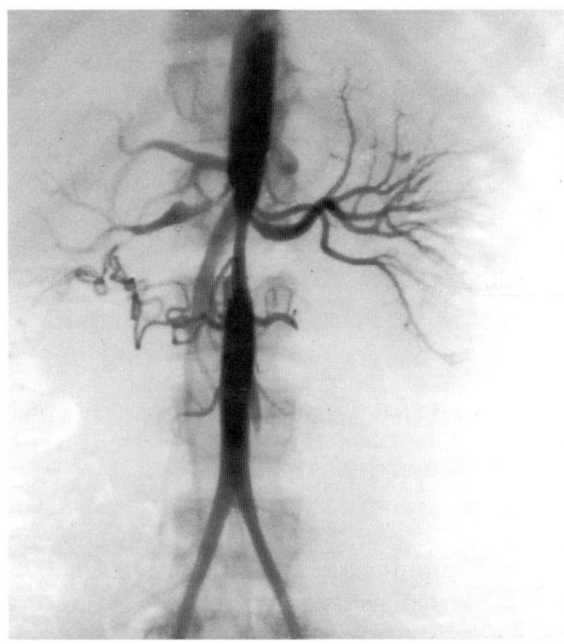

Figure 13.3. The middle aortic syndrome. This young woman was found to be hypertensive at the age of 18 years at routine examination while taking an estrogen-containing contraceptive pill. There was a loud systolic epigastric bruit and femoral pulses were delayed. The angiogram shows bilateral renal artery stenosis and stenosis of the abdominal aorta. CT scan showed that the aortic wall was very thin, making angioplasty hazardous.

years. It may be a variant of Takayasu's arteritis, it usually affects children but may occur in young adults.[26] The aortic wall may be thin making angioplasty hazardous.

Dissecting aneurysm of the aorta

Renal artery stenosis or occlusion may arise as a complication of aortic dissection but pre-existing RAS due to FMD or atheroma may in fact have preceded the dissection and predisposed the patient to dissection through hypertension. Rackson *et al.* found RAS in about one-fifth of hypertensives who develop dissection.[27]

External compression of the renal artery

It is uncommon for renal artery stenosis to be due to external compression but it has been reported in association with tumors, including pheochromocytoma.[28] It should be remembered, however, that both pheochromocytoma and intimal proliferation leading to RAS are recognized complications of neurofibromatosis and both may coexist.[29] Other tumors may cause renal artery compression as may a retroperitoneal hematoma. Fibrous bands are said to be responsible for external compression of the renal artery but I have not observed this over a period of 25 years.

Renal arteriovenous fistula

Arteriovenous fistulas within the kidney usually develop as a complication of needle biopsy and most of these close spontaneously. Fistulas may follow injury or surgery and approximately one-quarter are congenital.

Clinical presentation is with persisting hematuria following biopsy or injury or with hypertension often with a systolic and diastolic bruit raising the suspicion of RAS. Hypertension is thought to be due to ischemia of renal tissue beyond the fistula. Diagnosis is made by renal angiography which shows early filling of the renal vein, the fistula itself and ischemia of renal parenchyma beyond the fistula (Fig. 13.4).

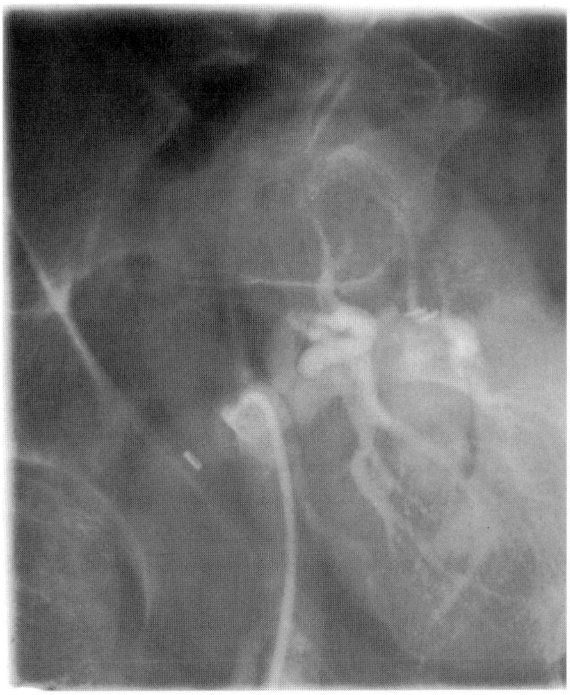

Figure 13.4. Renal arteriovenous fistula complicating renal biopsy in a renal transplant recipient. Contrast can be seen in the arteries and there is early venous filling. From ref. 87, with permission.

Radiation arteritis

In patients treated with radiotherapy for conditions such as seminoma of the testis in which upper abdominal para-aortic glands are irradiated RAS may develop as a late complication. This should be considered as an alternative to post radiation nephritis when hypertension occurs following radiotherapy since it is treatable by angioplasty.[30]

Atheromatous renal artery stenosis

Age and sex

The mean age at diagnosis of patients with renovascular hypertension due to ARAS is around 50 years[2] and two-thirds are male. Patients presenting with renal failure due to ARAS are usually older.

Race

In the US Cooperative Study of RVH[2] only about 7% of patients with ARAS were black but it may be that this was an artifact due to the method of recruitment, and others have reported no difference in the incidence of RAS in black and white patients.[7]

Prevalence of ARAS

A precise figure for the prevalence of ARAS in patients with hypertension cannot be given. The prevalence increases with age so that the overall prevalence usually quoted of between 1 and 5% in the hypertensive population[12, 13] is difficult to apply to individuals. In contrast to FMD in which the renal artery lesion is almost always the cause of the associated hypertension, in ARAS the stenosis is in many cases incidental to the hypertension or may be part of the vascular complications of hypertension rather than its cause. As will be discussed, ARAS is often an incidental finding in normotensive patients with peripheral vascular disease and coronary artery disease so that the prevalence of true RVH may be much less than that of ARAS. Not until a reliable test for the assessment of the functional significance of RAS becomes available will it be possible to determine the true prevalence of renovascular hypertension due to ARAS.

The generally accepted estimates for the prevalence of renovascular hypertension in adult hypertensives is 1% in the general population of hypertensives,[31] 5% in hospital-based populations and up to 40% in patients referred to hypertension clinics.[32] This last high figure reflects the higher prevalence of RVH in patients with more severe and drug-resistant hypertension and with other clinical features suggesting a secondary cause who are therefore more likely to be referred to a specialist clinic. In two-thirds of these patients the RAS is due to atheroma.

Natural history of ARAS

Atheromatous RAS is a progressive condition. Between 8 and 17% of stenoses progress to occlusion in 3–4 years and progression does not seem to be influenced by the quality of blood pressure control.[21, 22] In keeping with this arteriographic progression 12% of patients initially non-azotemic develop a degree of renal failure over 42 months[33] and 40% of patients with unilateral disease progress to bilateral involvement over 4 years.[21] One-third of all lesions have been shown to progress over a period of 4 years,[21, 34] unfortunately there is no means of predicting which lesions will progress. The patients with greatest risk of progressing to renal failure are those with impaired function at presentation, those with high grade stenosis to both kidneys or to a single functioning kidney, or with a 75–99% narrowing to either kidney. All of these conclusions are based on retrospective studies which of course are limited by the problem of selection of survivors and of compliant patients for follow-up. Two recent prospective studies have however broadly confirmed the retrospective findings. Zierler *et al.*,[35] in a Doppler ultrasound study of renal arteries with initial stenosis of less that 60%, showed progression to a stenosis of greater that 60% or to occlusion in 23% of arteries at 1 year and 42% of arteries at 2 years. In patients with initial narrowing of more than 60%, 5% progressed to occlusion at 1 year and 11% by 2 years.[35] In keeping with these Doppler findings Guzman *et al.*[36] reported a reduction in renal length of more than 1 cm over 1 year in 19% of patients with greater than 60% RAS.

There are no studies published to date to indicate whether lipid-lowering therapy influences the progression of ARAS.

Survival of patients with ARAS

The majority of patients with ARAS have evidence of vascular disease elsewhere and it is this, rather than the direct consequences of progression of RAS, which limits survival. In a joint study of patients attending the Glasgow and the Newcastle Hypertension Clinics we found that the survival of hypertensives with ARAS was 83% at 5 years and 67% at 10 years, compared with 90 and 79% respectively in essential hypertensives with death occurring mainly from coronary or cerebrovascular disease rather than renal failure.[37] A similar reduction in survival to 67% at 5 years compared with 92% in the general population has been reported by Wollenweber *et al.*[33] Pattison *et al.*[38] also reported a death rate from myocardial infarction of nearly 30% over the 5 years following renal artery angioplasty.

Thus, although renovascular disease undoubtedly progresses, death may occur from coronary or cerebrovascular disease before the renal disease reaches a critical stage with regard to either hypertension or renal function.

Aneurysm of the aorta

As discussed in relation to FMD, as well as aortic dissection causing renal artery narrowing pre-existing RAS, whether due to atheroma or FMD, by causing hypertension may be the cause of the dissection. In addition, ARAS often accompanies abdominal aortic aneurysm and the combination greatly increases the risks of surgical treatment.

Body habitus

In the US Cooperative Study of RVH[2] patients with ARAS were less likely to be obese than comparable patients with essential hypertension, 17 vs 38% being classified as being obese. This may be explained by the greater prevalence of cigarette smoking in ARAS[23, 24] since smokers tend to be lighter than non-smokers.[39]

Clinical manifestations of renovascular hypertension

Functionally significant RAS from whatever cause has the same clinical consequences, and stenosis due to FMD and to atheroma will therefore be considered together.

Severity of hypertension

Hypertension in patients with RVH is usually more severe and resistant to treatment than in essential hypertension[6, 16] but this is not invariable. In women investigated because of hypertension complicating pregnancy we have found RAS even though the blood pressure following pregnancy was often only very mildly elevated.[40] Furthermore in the US Cooperative Study[2] although the level of blood pressure and the severity of retinopathy was greater in patients with ARAS than in essential hypertensives, the latter did not differ from patients with FMD in these characteristics.

Duration of hypertension prior to diagnosis

In the US Cooperative Study[2] the mean duration of hypertension prior to diagnosis was longer in essential hypertension (3.1 years) than in patients with ARAS (1.9 years) or FMD (2.0 years), indicating more rapid progression of hypertension in RAS. This more rapid progression provides a useful clinical clue to the presence of RAS (Fig. 13.5).

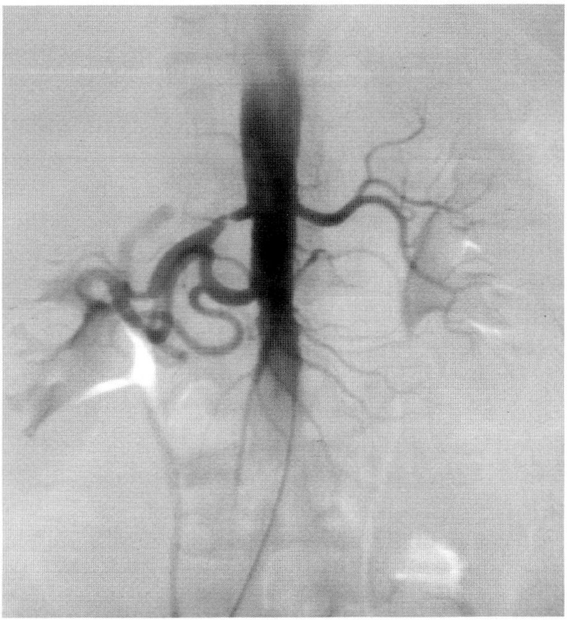

Figure 13.5. Rapid development of malignant hypertension due to renal artery stenosis in a woman of 60 years. She presented with moderate hypertension, blood pressure 180/110 mmHg, without retinopathy at routine medical examination; 6 weeks later she complained of persistent severe headache worst in the morning, blood pressure was 220/126 mmHg and fundoscopy revealed hemorrhages and exudates. IVU was normal but because of the rapid worsening of hypertension renal angiography was performed and revealed a tight right renal artery stenosis.

Hypertensive retinopathy

Hypertension due to RAS is often more severe than essential hypertension and as discussed above develops more rapidly. These two characteristics combine to make fundal hemorrhages and exudates more likely[2] since there is less time for hypertrophy of the smooth muscle of the resistance vessels to develop. The relatively thin walled resistance vessels cannot resist the high intraluminal pressure which is therefore transmitted, through to the capillary beds of the retina causing exudates and hemorrhages and to the glomerular capillaries causing proteinuria and hematuria. Approximately one-third of patients with retinal hemorrhages and exudates prove to have RVH[6] whereas only 1–5% of the total hypertensive population have RVH. Investigation of patients with severe retinopathy is therefore worthwhile.

Left ventricular hypertrophy

The pathogenesis of left ventricular hypertrophy (LVH) is not fully understood. Growth factors including angiotensin II and catecholamines are thought to be important as well as the direct effect of systolic pressure load in increasing left ventricular mass.[41–43] If angiotensin II is important then it would seem probable that LVH would be greater in patients with renovascular hypertension than in essential hypertension, especially since hypertension is also usually more severe. In fact in the US Cooperative Study there was no difference in the prevalence of electrocardiographic evidence of LVH between patients with essential hypertension and those with renovascular hypertension due to either atheroma or FMD.[2] In addition, even with echocardiographic assessment there was no difference in LV mass between matched patients with essential and renovascular hypertension.[44] Furthermore, a comparison of the echocardiographic changes in patients with unilateral RVH with those in patients with primary aldosteronism showed almost identical degrees of LVH[45] suggesting that it is the level of blood pressure rather than of angiotensin II which determines LVH.

Epigastric bruit

An epigastric systolic bruit is audible in only 50–60% of patients with RVH and in up to 10% of essential hypertensives. The presence of a systolic bruit therefore only increases the chances of finding RVH in an otherwise unselected hypertensive patient from around 1% to approximately 5%. If exclusively systolic bruits were disregarded and only systolic-diastolic bruits were considered to be significant then the specificity of the bruit for RVH increased to 99.5% being audible in only 2 of 379 patients with essential hypertension. However the sensitivity of the presence or absence of a bruit for the diagnosis of RVH fell to only 39%.[46] If applied to an unselected group of hypertensives in whom the prevalence of RVH is around 1%,[31] then the presence of a systolic-diastolic bruit has a positive predictive value of approximately 50% for RVH. If the prevalence of RVH in the population screened is around 5%, as it is in the older population, then the positive predictive value of a systolic-diastolic bruit rises to around 80%.

Vascular disease elsewhere

Atheromatous RAS is found in up to 50% of patients undergoing angiography for peripheral vascular disease many of whom are normotensive.[47, 48] It has also been reported in a high proportion of hypertensive patients who undergo coronary angiography,[49] and in one study 15% of these patients had significant and 15% non-significant RAS. Atheroma of the carotids and mesenteric vessels is also associated with an increased prevalence of renal artery stenosis.[50] In the US Cooperative Study 20% of patients with ARAS had a history of clinically manifest arterial occlusive disease in the brain, heart or limbs[2] compared with 10% of patients with essential hypertension or FMD. Fibromuscular dysplasia, although much less common and usually confined to the renal arteries, can affect all other arteries. The carotids are most commonly involved but lesions of the brachial, iliac, mesenteric, coronary and retinal arteries have been described.[51–53] Evidence of disease in any vascular bed should therefore raise the suspicion of RVH in a patient with hypertension, conversely it should be remembered that up to one-third of patients with FMD will have involvement of other vascular beds.[53]

Proteinuria

Proteinuria is more common in RVH than in essential hypertension[2] but is usually of mild degree. Nephrotic range proteinuria in the absence of specific glomerular pathology may occur.[54] Heavy proteinuria may be corrected by revascularization of the kidney[55] or by angiotensin converting enzyme (ACE) inhibitors which were shown to reduce membrane pore size.[56] This suggests that angiotensin II was responsible for the increased permeability of the glomerular membrane and resultant proteinuria. The effect of ACE inhibitors on proteinuria appears to be specific and not simply a consequence of lowering blood pressure since the same reduction in blood pressure on treatment with nifedipine and frusemide did not reduce proteinuria.[57]

Fluid retention

In RAS glomerular filtration falls less than renal plasma flow so the filtration fraction is increased. This protection of glomerular filtration rate (GFR) is achieved by baroreceptor-mediated release of renin from the wall of the afferent arteriole which acts locally on angiotensinogen to produce angiotensin I which is converted by angiotensin converting enzyme present within the kidney to produce angiotensin II which preferentially constricts the efferent arteriole.[58, 59] The increase in filtration fraction is achieved despite a reduction in the glomerular capillary ultrafiltration coefficient (K_f) by angiotensin II because of the increase in filtration pressure.[59] This increase in filtration fraction results in an increase in the oncotic pressure of plasma leaving the glomerulus and going on to the peritubular capillaries and this facilitates absorption of fluid from the proximal tubule. This movement of fluid is also encouraged by the reduced hydrostatic pressure in the peritubular capillaries resulting from efferent arteriolar constriction.[60] In addition angiotensin has a direct antinatriuretic effect on the proximal tubular epithelium.[61] The result of these humoral and hemodynamic changes within the kidney is therefore preservation of GFR despite reduction in renal plasma flow but at the cost of sodium retention (Fig. 13.6).

In patients with unilateral RAS and a normal contralateral kidney, sodium balance is maintained by contralateral pressure natriuresis[62, 63] despite the ipsilateral increased proximal sodium reabsorption and the bilateral increase in distal tubular sodium reabsorption resulting from angiotensin-stimulated aldosterone secretion.

However, in patients with bilateral disease or with a single functioning kidney RAS can lead to clinically significant fluid retention which is often resistant to diuretics. The patient presents clinically with recurrent pulmonary edema or other manifestations of cardiac failure despite echocardiographic evidence of normal cardiac function, although heart disease is undoubtedly a contributing factor in some patients, as well as a degree of renal impairment which in other circumstances would be insufficient to cause fluid retention.[64, 65] Correction of the RAS can be very effective in correcting fluid overload and in improving renal function.

Hypokalemia

Hyperreninemia leads to hypokalemia through secondary hyperaldosteronism in approximately 15% of patients.[66] In a patient with hypertension and hypokalemia, secondary aldosteronism due to renal artery stenosis is more likely than primary aldosteronism. A clinical clue in making the distinction is that in secondary aldosteronism plasma sodium tends to be below 140 mmol/l whereas it is usually above this level in primary aldosteronism. However, to make the distinction between the two with confidence it is necessary to measure plasma renin and aldosterone levels. In practice this is seldom undertaken in the acute phase of presentation of severe hypertension as it may cause confusion since severe hypertension, even if the result of primary aldosteronism,

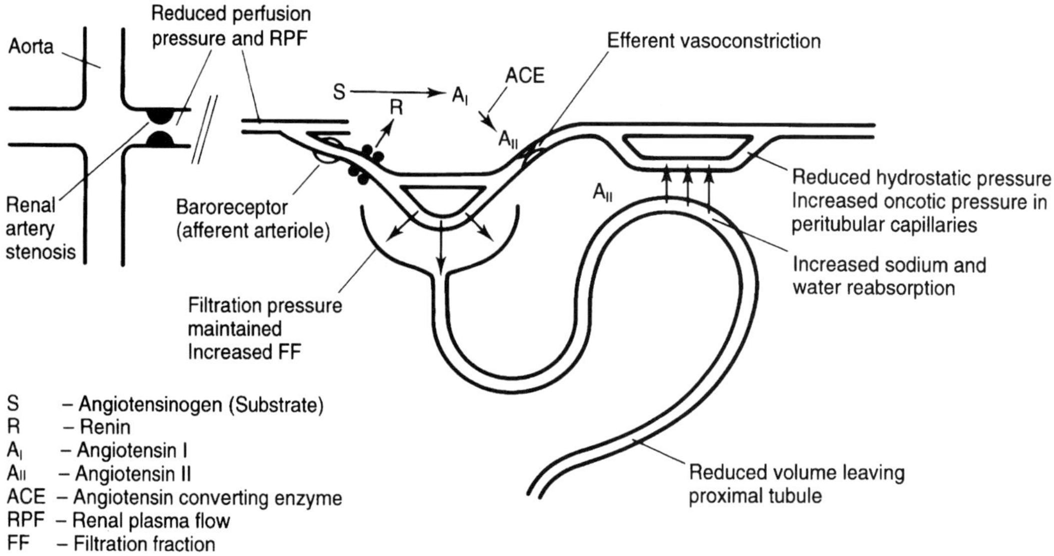

Figure 13.6. Intrarenal hemodynamic and humoral changes in RAS leading to fluid retention. In addition to hydrostatic and osmotic gradients facilitating proximal tubular sodium reabsorption, angiotensin II acts directly on the proximal tubular cells to stimulate sodium reabsorption. Redrawn from ref. 88 with permission.

may itself lead to secondary aldosteronism by causing damage to small vessels in the kidney. In this situation, since there is no urgency in establishing the cause of hypertension, the usual approach is to control blood pressure with drugs and then after a period of several months with controlled pressure, if hypokalemia persists, to undertake measurements of renin and aldosterone to exclude primary aldosteronism. Other causes of severe hypertension would of course usually be sought before this.

Impaired renal function

Impairment of renal function in a patient with hypertension, especially in the absence of proteinuria or hematuria, should raise the suspicion of renal vascular disease. In one study 66% of patients with ARAS presented with definite impairment of renal function.[67] However, the true prevalence of impairment of renal function in renovascular hypertension is not known since patients subjected to angiography have always been subjected to some sort of selection and a raised plasma creatinine is often one of the criteria for selection. The more common experience is that renal impairment is much less common and Maxwell[66] reported that 15% of patients with ARAS had impaired renal function and elevation in serum creatinine was even less common in FMD affecting only 2% of patients. The comparative rarity of elevation in plasma creatinine despite a marked reduction in renal plasma flow is explained by the angiotensin-mediated increase in filtration fraction already discussed in relation to fluid retention in RAS.

The importance of the role of angiotensin II is demonstrated by the effect of ACE inhibitors in inducing renal failure in patients with RAS affecting a single functioning kidney or with bilateral disease.[68, 69] The rise in plasma creatinine following treatment with ACE inhibitors is a valuable clue to the presence of RAS although not all patients who develop renal impairment will be found to have RAS.[70] Although renal failure occurs in less than 1% of patients treated with ACE inhibitors[71] around 5% of all patients presenting with acute renal failure to 1 unit had failure from this cause.[72] The renal failure which occurs with ACE inhibitors is usually reversible and only rarely and in very frail patients leads to death.[73] However, there have been reports of renal artery occlusion in patients treated with a combination of ACE inhibitors and diuretics,[74] although it is difficult to be certain that this was not simply a non-specific effect of lowering the blood pressure.

Reduced perfusion is not the only factor responsible for the deterioration in renal function in RAS since many patients show no immediate improvement in renal function following correction of stenosis and no change in the rate of deterioration of function.[75] Microembolization from atheromatous plaques may be important,[75] but there is rarely direct histological proof of this. It may be that progressive renal damage is due to tubular ischemia due to angiotensin-induced efferent arteriolar constriction rather than to microembolism since ischemic changes have been reported to affect proximal tubules to a greater extent than the glomeruli.[76]

RAS in association with primary antiphospholipid antibodies

Circulating antibodies directed against anionic phospholipids are common (25–50%) in systemic lupus erythematosis and other autoimmune diseases[77] and are very uncommon (1–2%) in the general population.[78] A characteristic 'primary antiphospholipid syndrome' (APS) has been described in patients with antiphospholipid antibodies (APA) but no other evidence of underlying autoimmune disease, and is characterized by recurring venous and arterial thrombosis, thrombocytopenia, hemolytic anemia, recurrent fetal loss and skin lesions.[79] In the kidney APS has usually been associated with renal vein thrombosis and with thrombosis in glomerular capillaries which is observed in about one-quarter of cases.[80] There have, however, been more recent reports of renal artery stenosis in this syndrome.[81–84] The changes in the renal vessels may be those of fibromuscular dysplasia or of non-specific damage to the vessel wall. The prevalence of APA inpatients presenting with hypertension and found to have RAS is not known, nor conversely is the proportion of patients with the APS who have RAS. It would seem sensible to check all patients with RAS for APA and to consider treatment with aspirin in those found to be positive since renal infarction appears to be common in those patients with RAS who have APA.[84]

A variant of this condition referred to as the 'catastrophic antiphospholipid syndrome' in which there is diffuse thrombosis in the kidney and other organs has been described but in this condition the thrombi are usually in small vessels.[85]

Raised anticardiolipin antibodies have been described in the majority of patients with Takayasu's arteritis.[86]

The value of clinical features in identifiying RVH

In the US Cooperative Study of RVH[2] there were no differences in clinical characteristics which reliably separated patients with renal hypertension from essential hypertensives. Although differences between the two groups were observed, the overlap was large. The features which make renovascular disease more likely are listed in Table 13.1.

A smaller study of 100 patients showed that, apart from renal artery bruit, only resistant hypertension was useful as a clue to the presence of RVH.[16] Perhaps the most common clinical clue now is the development of impaired renal function with ACE inhibitors. Since up to 30% of patients with malignant hypertension may have RVH,[6] investigation is worthwhile in these

Table 13.1. Clinical features suggesting renovascular hypertension[a]

Onset before age 30 or after age 50 years
Absence of family history of hypertension
Shorter duration of hypertension or recent worsening
More severe hypertension and retinopathy
Resistance to therapy
Symptoms or signs of vascular disease elsewhere
Elevation of plasma creatinine especially if following ACE inhibitors
Epigastric bruit
Hypokalemia
Neurofibromatosis

[a]These features individually have a low predictive value, but taken together are useful in selecting patients for further investigation.

patients provided that they would be suitable for intervention if the diagnosis were to be confirmed. Although RAS is an uncommon complication of neurofibromatosis it should be borne in mind if a patient with this condition develops hypertension as well as the more classically associated pheochromocytoma.

Acknowledgments

I am grateful to Mrs Sheila Davidson and Mrs Rita Grieveson for their invaluable help in collecting material and in preparing this manuscript.

References

1 Bergentz SE. Natural history of renal artery stenosis. *Ann Chir Gynaecol* 1992; **81**(2): 98–101.
2 Simon N, Franklin SS, Bleifer KH, Maxwell MH. Clinical characteristics of renovascular hypertension. *JAMA* 1972; **220(9):** 1209–18.
3 Goncharenko V, Gerlock AJ, Shaff MI, Hollifield JW. Progression of renal artery fibromuscular dysplasia in 42 patients as seen on angiography. *Radiology* 1981; **139:** 45–51.
4 Bookstein JJ, Abrams HL, Buenger RE *et al.* Radiologic aspects of renovascular hypertension: II. The role of urography in unilateral renovascular disease. *JAMA* 1972; **220:** 1225–30.
5 Chugh KS, Jain S, Sakhuja V *et al.* Renovascular hypertension due to Takayasu's arteritis among Indian patients. *Quart J Med* 1992; **85:** 833–43.
6 Davis BA, Crook JE, Vestal RE, Oates JA. Prevalence of renovascular hypertension in patients with grade III or IV hypertensive retinopathy. *N Engl J Med* 1979; **301:** 1273–6.
7 Svetkey LP, Kadir S, Dunnick NR *et al.* Similar prevalence of renovascular hypertension in selected black and whites. *Hypertension* 1991; **17:** 678–83.
8 Rushton AR. The genetics of fibromuscular dysplasia. *Arch Int Med* 1980; **140:** 233–16.
9 Galdstein K, Rushton AR, Kidd KK. Penetrance estimates and recurrence risks for fibromuscular dysplasia. *Clin Genet* 1980; **17:** 115–6.
10 Muller-Wiefel DE. Renovaskulare Hypertension bei Neurofibromatose von Recklinhausen. *Monats Kinderheilk* 1978; **126:** 113–18.
11 Lancman M, Mesropian H, Serra P, Granillo R. Turner's syndrome, fibromuscular dysplasia, and stroke. *Stroke* 1991; **22:** 269–71.
12 Danielson M, Damstrom BG. Prevalence of primary and secondary hypertension. *Acta Med Scand* 1981; **290:** 451–5.
13 Lewin A, Blaufox MD, Castle H *et al.* Apparent prevalence of curable hypertension in the Hypertension Detection and Follow-up Program. *Arch Int Med* 1985; **145:** 424–7.
14 Bookstein JJ *et al.* Radiologic aspects of renovascular hypertension: I. Aims and methods of the radiology study group. *JAMA* 1972; **220:** 1218–24.
15 Ying CY, Tifft CP, Gavras H, Chobanian AV. Renal vascularization in the azotemic hypertensive patient resistant to therapy. *New Eng J Med* 1984; **231:** 1070–5.
16 Svetkey LP, Helms MJ, Dunnick NR, Klotman PE. Clinical characteristics useful in screening for renovascular disease. *South Med J* 1990; **83:** 743–7.
17 Meire FM, De Laey JJ, Van Thienen MN, Schuddinck L. Retinal manifestations in fibromuscular dysplasia. *Eur J Ophthalmol* 1991; **1(2):** 63–8.
18 Jones EOP, Wilkinson R, Taylor RMR. Contralateral renal artery fibromuscular dysplasia after nephrectomy for renal artery stenosis. *Br Med J* 1978; **1:** 825.
19 Stinchcombe SJ, Manhire AR, Bishop MC, Gregson RHS. Renal arterial fibromuscular dysplasia: acute renal infarction in three patients with angiographic evidence of medial fibroplasia. *Br J Radiol* 1992; **65:** 81–4.
20 Forster JH, Dean RH, Pinkerton JA, Rhamy RK. Ten years experience with the surgical management of renovascular hypertension. *Ann Surg* 1973; **177:** 755.
21 Schreiber MJ, Pohl MA, Novick AC. The natural history of atherosclerotic and fibrous renal artery disease. *Urol Clin North Am* 1984; **11:** 383–92.
22 Bergentz SE, Bergqvist D, Weibull H. Changing concepts of renovascular surgery. *Br J Surg* 1989; **76:** 429–30.
23 Nicholson JP, Teichman SL, Alderman MH *et al.* Smoking and renovasuclar hypertension. *Lancet* 1983; **2:** 765–6.
24 Mackay A, Brown JJ, Cumming AMM *et al.* Cigarette smoking and renal artery stenosis. *Br Med J* 1979; **2:** 770.
25 Kuo JY, Okada Y, Takeuchi H *et al.* Neurofibromatosis associated with renovascular hypertension due to stenosis and aneurysm of the left renal segmental artery: report of a case. *Urol Int* 1989; **44:** 177–80.
26 Kaufman JJ. The middle aortic syndrome: report of a case treated by renal autotransplantation. *J Urol* 1973; **109:** 711.
27 Rackson ME, Lossef SV, Sos TA. Renal artery stnosis in patients with aortic dissection: increased prevalence. *Radiology* 1990; **177:** 555–8.
28 Alvestrand A, Bergstrom J, & Wehle B. Pheochromocytoma and renovascular hypertension. A case report and review of the literature. *Acta Med Scand* 1977; **202:** 231–6.

29 Muller-Wiefel DE. Renovaskulare Hypertension bei Neurofibromatose von Recklinghausen. *Monatas Kinderheilk* 1978; **126:** 113–18.
30 Milutinovic J, Darcy M, Thompson KA. Radiation-induced renovascular hypertension successfully treated with transluminal angioplasty; case report. *Cardiovasc Intervent Radiol* 1990; **13:** 29–31.
31 Berglund G, Anderson O, Wilhelmson L. Prevalence of primary and secondary hypertension. *Br Med J* 1976; **2:** 554–6.
32 Derkx FHM, Schalekamp MADH. Renal artery stenosis and hypertension. *Lancet* 1994; **344:** 237–9.
33 Wollenweber J, Sheps S, Davis G. Clinical course of atherosclerotic renovascular disease. *Am J Cardiol* 1968; **21:** 60–71.
34 Dean R, Kieffer R, Smith B *et al.* Renovascular hypertension. *Arch Surg* 1981; **116:** 1408–15.
35 Zierler RE, Bergelin RO, Isaacson JA, Strandness DE. Natural history of atherosclerotic renal artery stenosis: a prospective study with duplex ultrasonography. *J Vasc Surg* 1994; **19:** 250–8.
36 Guzman RP, Zierler RE, Isaacson JA *et al.* Renal atrophy and arterial stenosis: a prospective study with duplex ultrasound. *Hypertension* 1994; **23:** 346–50.
37 Isles C, Main J, O'Connell J *et al.* Survival associated with renovascular disease in Glasgow and Newcastle: a collaborative study. *Scot Med J* 1990; **35:** 170–3.
38 Pattison JM, Reidy JF, Rafferty MJ *et al.* Percutaneous transluminal renal angioplasty in patients with renal failure. *Quart J Med* 1992; **85:** 883–8.
39 Wannamethee G, Shaper AG. Body weight and mortality in middle aged British men: impact of smoking. *Br Med J* 1989; **299:** 1497–502.
40 Sellars L, Siamopoulos KC, Wilkinson R. Prognosis for pregnancy after correction of renovascular hypertension. *Nephron* 1985; **39:** 280–1.
41 Kromer EP, Riegger GA. Effects of long-term angiotensin converting enzyme inhibition on myocardial hypertrophy in experimental aortic stenosis in a rat. *Am J Cardiol* 1988; **62:** 161–3.
42 Laks MN. Norepinephrine – the myocardial hypertrophy hormone? *Am Heart J* 1976; **91:** 674–5.
43 Schunkert H, Dzau VJ, Tang SS *et al.* Increased rat cardiac angiotensin converting enzyme, activity and mRNA expression in pressure overload left ventricular hypertrophy. *J Clin Invest* 1990; **86:** 1913–20.
44 Vensel LA, Devereux RB, Pickering TG *et al.* Cardiac anatomy and function in renovascular hypertension produced by unilateral and bilateral renal artery stenosis. *Am J Cardiol* 1986; **58:** 575–82.
45 Suzuki T, Abe H, Nagata S *et al.* Left ventricular structural characteristics in unilateral renovascular hypertension and primary aldosteronism. *Am J Cardiol* 1988; **62** (17): 1224–7.
46 Grim Ce, Luft FC, Weinburger MH, Grim CM. Sensitivity and specificity of screening tests for renal vascular hypertension. *Ann Int Med* 1979; **91:** 617–22.
47 Holley KE, Hunt JC, Brown AL *et al.* Renal artery stenosis. *Am J Med* 1964; **37:** 14–18.
48 Dunstan HP, Humphries AW, De Wolfe VG, Page IH. Normal arterial pressure in patients with renal artery stenosis. *JAMA* 1984; **187:** 138–42.
49 Vetrovec GW, Cowley MJ, Landwehr DM, Parker VE. High prevalence of renal artery stenosis in hypertensive patients with coronary artery disease. *J Am Coll Cardiol* 1984; **3:** 518.
50 Harding MB, Smith LR, Himmelstein SI *et al.* Renal artery stenosis – prevalence and associated risk factors in patients undergoing routine cardiac catherterisation. *J Am Soc Nephrol* 1992; **2:** 1608–16.
51 James TN. Morphologic characteristics and functional significance of focal fibromuscular dysplasia of small coronary arteries. *Am J Cardiol* 1990; **65:** 12G–22G.
52 Reilly JM, McGraw DJ, Sicard GA. Bilateral brachial artery fibromusclar dysplasia. *Ann Vasc Surg* 1993; **7:** 483–7.
53 Luscher TF, Keller HM, Imhof HG *et al.* Fibromuscular hyperplasia: extension of the disease and therapeutic outcome. *Nephron* **44**(suppl. 1): 109–14.
54 Berlyne GW, Tarill AS, Baker SBC. Renal artery stenosis and the nephrotic syndrome. *Quart J Med* 1964; **33:** 325–35.
55 Zimbler MS, Pickering TG, Sos TA, Laragh JH. Proteinuria in renovascular hypertension and the effects of renal angioplasty. *Am J Cardiol* 1987; **590:** 406–8.
56 Remuzzi A, Schieppati A, Battaglia C, Remuzzi G. Angiotensin-converting enzyme inhibition ameliorates the defect in glomerular size selectivity in hyponatremic hypertensive syndrome. *Am J Kidney Dis* 1989; **14:** 170–7.
57 Holman ND, Donker AJ, van der Meer J. Disappearance of renin-induced proteinuria by an ACE-inhibitor: a case report. *Clin Nephrol* 1990; **34:** 70–71.
58 Ichikawa I, Miehle JF, Brenner BM. Reversal of renal cortical actions of angiotensin II by verapamil and manganese. *Kidney Int* 1979; **16:** 137.
59 Blantz R, Konnen KS, Tucker BJ. Angiotensin II effects upon the glomerular microcirculation and ultrafiltration coeffient of the rat. *J Clin Invest* 1976; **57:** 419.
60 Ichikawa I, Brenner BM. Importance of efferent arteriolar vascular tone in regulation of proximal tubule fluid reabsorption and glomerulotubular balance in the rat. *J Clin Invest* 1980; **65:** 1192.
61 Schuster VL, Kokko GP, Jacobson HR. Angiotensin II directly stimulates transport in

rabbit proximal convoluted tubules. *J Clin Invest* 1984; **73:** 507.

62 Selkurt EE, Womack I, Dailey WN. Mechanism of natriuresis and diuresis during elevated renal artery pressure. *Am J Physiol* 1965; **209:** 95–9.

63 Kimura G, London GM, Safar ME, *et al.* Split intrarenal hemodynamics in renovascular hypertension. *Clin Invest Med* 1991; **14:** 559–65.

64 Messina LM, Zelenock GB, Yao KA, Stanley JC. Renal revascularization for recurrent pulmonary oedema in patients with poorly controlled hypertension and renal insufficiency: a distinct subgroup of patients with arteriosclerotic renal artery occlusive disease. *J Vasc Surg* 1992; **15:** 73–80.

65 Pickering TG, Devereux RB, James GD, *et al.* Recurrent pulmonary oedmea in hypertension due to bilateral renal artery stenosis: treatment by angioplasty or surgical revascularistation. *Lancet* 1988; **ii:** 551–2.

66 Maxwell MH, Bleifer KH, Franklin SS, Varady P. Cooperative study of renovascular hypertension: Demographic analysis of the study. *JAMA* 1972; **220:** 1195.

67 Canzanello VJ *et al.* Percutaneous transluminal renal angioplasty in the management of atherosclerotic renal vascular hypertension: results in 100 patients. *Hypertension* 1989; **13:** 163–72.

68 Hricik DE, Browning PJ, Kopelman R *et al.* Captopril-induced functional renal insufficiency in patients with bilateral renal artery stenosis or renal artery stenosis in a solitary kidney. *N Engl J Med* 1983; **308:** 373–6.

69 Farrow PR, Wilkinson R. Reversible renal failure during treatment with captopril. *Br Med J* 1979; **1:** 1680.

70 Mimran A, Ribstein J, DuCailar G. Converting enzyme inhibitors and renal function in essential and renovascular hypertension. *Am J Hypertension* 1991; **4**(Suppl. 1)**:** 7S–14S.

71 Inman WHW, Rawson NSB, Wilton LV *et al.* Post marketing surveillance of enalapril I: results of prescription event monitoring. *Br Med J* 1988; **297:** 826–9.

72 Kalra PS, Mamtora H, Holmes AM, Waldeck S. Renovascular disease and renal complications of angiotensin-converting enzyme inhibitor therapy. *Quart J Med* 1990; **282:** 1013.

73 Speirs CJ, Dollery CT, Inman WHW. Post marketing surveillance of enalapril II: investigation of the potential role of enalapirl in deaths with renal failure. *Br Med J* 1988; **297:** 830–2.

74 Postma CT, Hoefnagels WH, Barentsz JO, *et al.* Occlusion of unilateral stenosed renal arteries – relation to medical treatment. *J Human Hypertens* 1989; **3:** 185–90.

75 Dean RH, Tribble RW, Hansen KJ *et al.* Evolution of renal insufficiency in ischemic nephropathy. *Ann Surg* 1991; **213:** 446–55.

76 Marcussen N. Atubular glomeruli in renal artery stnosis. *Lab Invest* 1991; **65:** 558–65.

77 Love PE, Santoro SA. Antiphospholipid antibodies: anticardiolipin and the lupus anticoagulant in systemic lupus erythematosis (SLE) and in non-SLE disorders. Prevalence and clinical significance. *Ann Int Med* 1990; **112:** 682–98.

78 Rosove MH, Brewer PMC. Antiphospholipid thrombosis: clinical course after the first thrombotic event in 70 patients. *Ann Int Med* 1992; **117:** 303–8.

79 Alarcon-Segovia D, Sanchez-Guerrero J. Primary antiphospholipid syndrome. *J Rheumatol* 1989; **16:** 482–8.

80 Amigo MC, Garcia-Torres R, Robles M *et al.* Renal involvement in primary antiphospholipid syndrome. *J Rheumatol* 1992; **19:** 1181–5.

81 Asherson RA, Noble GE, Hughes GRV. Hypertension, renal artery stenosis and primary antiphospholipid syndrome. *J Rheumatol* 1991; **18:** 1413–15.

82 Kleinknecht D, Bobrie G, Meryer O *et al.* Recurrent thrombosis and renal vascular disease in patients with lupus anticoagulant. *Nephrol Dial Transplant* 1989; **4:** 854–8.

83 Mandreoli M, Zuccala A, Zucchelli P. Fibromuscular dysplasia of the renal arteries associated with antiphospholipid antibodies: two case reports. *Am J Kidney Dis* 1992; **20:** 500–3.

84 Mandreoli M, Zucchelli P. Renal vascular disease in patients with primary antiphospholipid antibodies. *Nephrol Dial Transplant* 1993; **8:** 1277–80.

85 Asherson RA. The catastrophic antiphospholipid syndrome. *J Rheumatol* 1992; **19:** 508–12.

86 Misra R, Aggarwal A, Chag M *et al.* Raised anticardiolipin antibodies in Takayasu's arteritis. *Lancet* 1994; **343:** 164–5.

87 Wilkinson R. Renal and renovascular hypertension. In Swales JD (ed.) *Textbook of Hypertension*. Oxford: Blackwell, 1994.

88 Wilkinson R. Renovascular hypertension. In *Current Practice in Surgery*, Vol. 2. London: Longman, 1990.

14

Peripheral and renal vein renin testing

THOMAS G PICKERING

The renin–angiotensin system plays a major role in the development of renovascular hypertension, and this can be exploited for diagnostic purposes. Although the demonstration of an anatomical renal artery stenosis is the *sine qua non* of the diagnostic evaluation, it is often not sufficient on its own, because there are many patients who have such a stenosis who do not have renovascular hypertension. Renin measurements may be of great value in establishing that the stenosis is causing renal ischemia.

The role of the renin–angiotensin system in experimental renovascular hypertension

The classic experiments on the production of renovascular hypertension were published in 1934 by Goldblatt *et al.*[1] who demonstrated that persistent hypertension could be produced in dogs by constricting both renal arteries, or one if the other kidney was removed. Goldblatt postulated that a humoral mechanism could be responsible for the hypertension, which was later confirmed by numerous other workers. Despite the early work suggesting that hypersecretion of renin by the ischemic kidney was directly responsible for the raised blood pressure, later studies indicated that other factors were responsible for the maintenance of the hypertension, because the hyperreninemia often did not persist. Nethertheless, the overwhelming bulk of evidence favors a predominant role for the two limbs of the renin–angiotensin system: vasoconstriction and sodium retention.[2]

Two experimental models of renovascular hypertension

The physiological mechanisms underlying renovascular hypertension in experimental animal models differ according to whether the contralateral kidney is intact (two-kidney, one-clip model), or removed (one-kidney, one-clip model) as summarized in Table 14.1. In the two-kidney, one-clip model, plasma renin activity (PRA) is high, and blockade of the renin–angiotensin system, whether by angiotensin antibody, saralasin, or angiotensin converting enzyme (ACE) inhibitors produce a bigger fall of pressure in two-kidney, one-clip rats than in one kidney rats, suggesting a greater degree of renin dependency in two-kidney hypertension.[2–5] The simplest explanation for the difference between one- and two-kidney hypertension is that in the latter case the contralateral kidney can excrete sodium normally, thereby preventing sodium retention.

In the one-kidney, one-clip model there is an expansion of the plasma volume occurring as a result of sodium retention, with normal plasma renin levels. If a converting enzyme inhibitor is given, blood pressure falls little if at all.[3] If the

Table 14.1. Comparison of animal and human models of renovascular hypertension

	Animal	Human
	Two-kidney, one-clip	Unilateral stenosis
Renin	High	High
Plasma volume	Normal	Normal
Blood pressure response to ACE inhibition	Decrease	Decrease
	One-kidney, one-clip	Bilateral stenosis
Renin	Normal	Normal/high
Plasma volume	High	?High
Blood pressure response to ACE inhibition	No change	Decrease

animals are maintained on a low sodium diet throughout, the rise of pressure still takes place, but the mechanism is different: renin levels remain elevated, but there is no sodium retention or increase of plasma volume.[6] These findings are consistent with experiments done by Gavras *et al.* in rats, who found that acute saralasin infusion lowered the blood pressure of one-kidney, one-clip hypertensive rats only if they were sodium depleted.[7] Thus it appears that this type of hypertension may be either renin dependent or volume dependent according to the sodium intake.

As the blood pressure rises following clipping, there is also a rise of peripheral PRA, but there is a closer correlation between renal vein renin activity from the ischemic kidney and blood pressure than between peripheral PRA and pressure.[8] The renin content of the contralateral kidney is correspondingly diminished.[9] These changes occurring in rats appear to parallel what has been observed in man.

Pathophysiology of renovascular hypertension in man

An important question is whether the pathophysiology of the two common human patterns can be equated with the two animal models described above. The resemblance between unilateral human renal artery stenosis and the one-clip, two-kidney model is close, since both are clearly dependent on increased secretion of renin by the ischemic kidney. What is much less clear is what occurs when there are bilateral stenoses. Relatively little information is available concerning peripheral renin levels, although two studies have reported that renin may be high in patients with both unilateral and bilateral disease.[10,11] Consistent with this finding, patients with bilateral renal artery stenosis are just as likely to show a decrease of blood pressure when given converting enzyme inhibitors.[11] The pattern of renal vein renin is also the same as in unilateral disease, and in patients with bilateral renal artery stenosis the renins tend to lateralize to the most ischemic kidney.[12]

In addition to this evidence of hypersecretion of renin in patients with bilateral renovascular disease a number of circumstantial pieces of evidence suggest that there may also be an increased effective blood volume. Firstly, in patients with bilateral disease the cardiac output is usually higher than in patients with unilateral disease.[13] Second, as described in more detail below, we have found that recurrent pulmonary edema is more common in patients with bilateral than unilateral disease.[14] Third, successful revascularization by angioplasty in a patient with bilateral renal artery stenosis or a solitary kidney is frequently followed by a diuresis, which is not seen in patients with unilateral disease.[15]

The overall picture in patients with bilateral renal artery stenosis is thus a mixed one, with both renin and volume factors typically being involved (Table 14.1). In this respect it differs from the one-kidney animal model, which is more highly dependent on volume factors. The most likely reason for this is that bilateral disease almost never develops symmetrically in the two kidneys, as witnessed by the common finding of unequal kidney sizes, and asymmetrical renal vein renin patterns. All bilateral cases presumably start out with unilateral disease. During the early stages of unilateral involvement there may well be parenchymal disease developing in the contralateral kidney, which would impair the pressure natriuresis by which the contralateral kidney normally maintains the classic high renin–normal volume pattern of unilateral renal artery stenosis. This volume retention would be further exacerbated when the second stenosis develops in the contralateral renal artery.

The renin–angiotensin system and the control of intrarenal hemodynamics in renovascular hypertension

The clinical observation that converting enzyme inhibitors may cause a deterioration of renal function in some patients with renovascular hypertension can be accounted for by animal studies which have demonstrated the important effects of angiotensin on intrarenal hemodynamics.[16] One of the most important intrarenal effects of angiotensin II is to decrease renal blood flow, with a smaller decrease of glomerular filtration rate (GFR). Thus, filtration fraction increases.[17] It has been proposed that these changes are brought about by a vasoconstriction of both afferent and efferent arterioles, with the predominant effect being on the latter. Thus in the normal kidney, particularly when renin levels are high, angiotensin blockade increases renal blood flow, with less consistent changes of GFR.[18] In the ischemic kidney GFR is maintained by angiotensin II-mediated efferent vasoconstriction, so that angiotensin blockade lowers it. This effect provides the rationale for captopril renography.

Diagnosis of renovascular hypertension

Renovascular hypertension is almost certainly underdiagnosed in clinical practice. Extensive screening of all hypertensive patients is impractical, but a number of clinical clues should increase the clinician's suspicion of its presence.

There is no perfect screening test for its detection. A large number of tests have been proposed, which can be classified in two categories. First, those that can be done in a physician's office, which are relatively simple to perform and inexpensive, but which do not indicate which kidney is involved. Measurement of peripheral PRA and the captopril test come into this category. Second, are those tests such as renal vein renin measurement which provide anatomical or functional information about each kidney. Ideally, one or more of these tests should be done following the first stage test.

Peripheral plasma renin activity

Since the renin–angiotensin system plays a central role in the genesis of renovascular hypertension it might be expected that the measurement of PRA might be a useful screening test for its diagnosis. In practice, it is of limited value, however. One problem is that renin secretion is influenced by many antihypertensive drugs: β-blockers inhibit it, while diuretics and ACE inhibitors increase it. Since it is also affected by the level of salt intake, this too should ideally be evaluated.

In the absence of antihypertensive medication, a high PRA, measured in the morning in the seated position and indexed against sodium excretion, is present in about 75% of patients with proven renovascular hypertension.[19,20] However, its predictive value in the absence of clinical clues of renovascular hypertension is low. Plasma renin activity is normal in some patients with renovascular hypertension, but rarely, if ever, low. Furthermore a high renin measurement is characteristic of about 20% of patients with essential hypertension. Further workup of patients in whom a high renin is the only clue to renovascular hypertension is often disappointing. While such patients may have a positive captopril test, it is likely to be a false positive (see below).

Despite these limitations, a PRA measurement may still have value as a screening test in patients presenting with refractory hypertension and on multiple drugs. If these include ACE inhibitors, a low or normal renin virtually excludes the possibility of renovascular hypertension, as does the finding of a low renin on any other medications.

Captopril test

Case and Laragh[21] were the first to show that the reactive rise of renin following administration of captopril is greater in patients with renovascular than with essential hypertension. This study was followed by a much larger survey by Müller *et al.*[22] of 246 patients with a variety of conditions, including essential and renovascular hypertension, with and without azotemia. Many of the patients were studied while taking antihypertensive medication (see Fig. 14.1). Arteriography was performed in all 56 cases with renovascular hypertension, and in 54 of the remaining cases, none of whom were considered to have renovascular disease by other criteria. The criteria which were found *post hoc* to be the most reliable for distinguishing patients with renovascular hypertension were a post-captopril renin of more than 12 ng/ml/h, an absolute increase of 10 ng/ml/h or more, and a percentage increase of 150% or more, or 400% if the baseline renin was below 3. In this series the sensitivity and specificity of this test was better than 95%.[22]

Another large study was conducted by Derkx *et al.*[23] They took 179 patients, all of whom had severe or refractory hypertension and were less than 40 years old. Sodium intake was controlled, and antihypertensive medication discontinued for 2 weeks prior to the test. With their criterion for a positive test being a post-captopril renin of 200 μU/l or more, they found a sensitivity of 93% and a specificity of 84%. It should be noted that since the absolute values of renin measurements may vary from one laboratory to another, it may be preferable to use a percentage change (as proposed by Müller *et al.*) for defining the normal range.

Subsequent studies have for the most part confirmed the value of the captopril test, but they have also found lower sensitivity and specificity,[22–30] as shown in Table 14.2.

The overall sensitivity is approximately 74%, and specificity 89%. Differences in the reported accuracy of the test may be attributed to a number of factors, including the assay used, varying criteria for defining renovascular hypertension, and the position of the patient during the test.

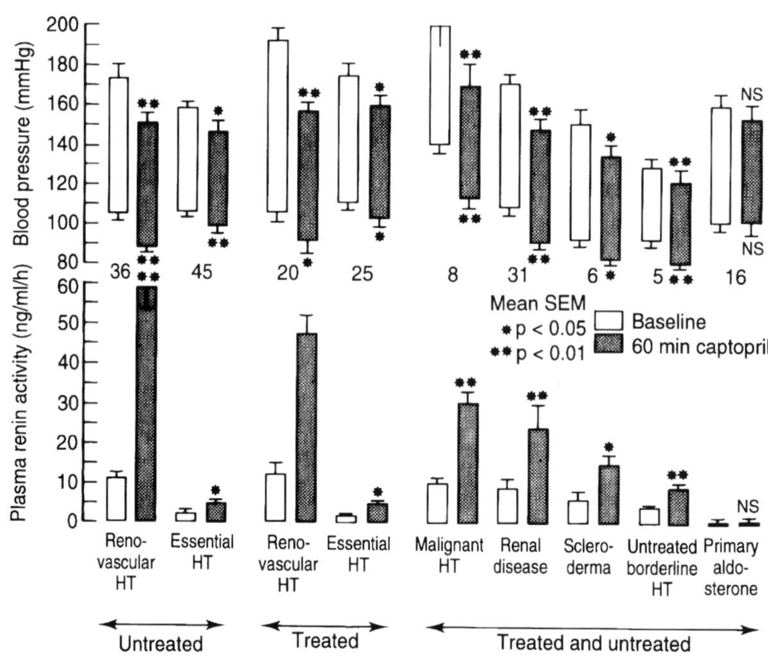

Figure 14.1. Seated blood pressure and PRA before and after a single dose of captopril in groups of various types of treated and untreated hypertensive patients. Note that the discrimination between essential and renovascular hypertension is better for the renin respose than for the blood pressure response. From ref. 22, with permission.

Table 14.2. Sensitivity and specificity of the captopril test

Investigator	No of patients	Sensitivity	Specificity
Müller *et al.*[22]	246	100	95
Derkx *et al.*[23]	179	93	84
Frederickson *et al.*[24]	100	100	80
Gosse *et al.*[25]	114	73	84
Hansen *et al.*[26]	47	91	89
Postma *et al.*[27]	149	38	93
Svetkey *et al.*[28]	66	73	72
Thibonnier *et al.*[29]	65	40	100
Elliott *et al.*[30]	100	76	58

Thus the low sensitivity reported by Postma *et al.*[27] may have occurred because their patients were studied supine (which would result in a lower increase of renin following captopril administration). Furthermore, their citerion for renovascular hypertension was a renal artery stenosis of 50% or greater. Most experts would not consider a stenosis to be hemodynamically significant until it reaches 75%.

An important consideration in the evaluation of the captopril test (as in any screening test) is the prevalence of disease in the population being studied. When the prevalence is low, as for example with renovascular disease in the general population, a relatively high proportion of the positive test results will be false positives. This was exactly the finding of a study conducted by Gerber *et al.*[31] in 108 uncomplicated and consecutive patients who underwent captopril testing. Nine patients had a positive test, but all turned out to be false positives when further evaluated with renal vein renin measurement and digital intravenous angiography. Eight of these nine patients had a high baseline peripheral PRA.

Most investigators have found the test to be less reliable in patients who are azotemic. It does not discriminate between patients with unilateral bilateral disease, both of which groups usually show a positive response,[11,22] although others have found that it is still reliable.[30]

The test is generally regarded as safe, the main hazard being an excessive fall of blood pressure in patients with very high renins who are also volume depleted. Although it is well recognized that ACE inhibitors can impair renal function in patients with bilateral renal artery stenoses,[32] this is rarely if ever a problem with acute testing.

Captopril testing in children

Although any kind of hypertension is relatively uncommon in children, a large proportion of cases are the result of renal artery stenosis, usually from some variety of fibromuscular dysplasia. Since there is a reluctance to perform arteriography in these patients, non-invasive screening tests are particularly useful. Two studies have explored its use. Hamed *et al.*[33] performed it in 49 children who were either hypertensive or who had scarred kidneys secondary to vesicoureteric reflux, and concluded that it might differentiate the renovascular patients from others. Gauthier *et al.* used it in 20 consecutive hypertensive children and adolescents, nine of whom subsequently had a renal arteriogram.[34] The predictive value of a positive test was only 43%, leading to the conclusion that it was not of sufficient accuracy to be used as a screening test.

Renal vein renin determinations

In patients with unilateral renal artery stenosis, the ischemic kidney typically secretes an increased amount of renin, causing an elevation in the systemic levels, and suppression of renin secretion by the contralateral kidney. This results in a marked asymmetry in PRA in the two renal veins, which can be expressed either as the ratio of PRA in the two renal veins (with an upper limit of normal usually taken as 1.5:1 or 2:1), or by comparing the increment of PRA between the renal vein (V) and renal artery (A) separately on each side, expressed as (V-A/A[19] In practice, the PRA measured in the inferior vena cava distal to the renal veins can be substituted for the arterial level. The normal increment is 25%; in patients with renovascular hypertension it is typically 50% or more in the ischemic kidney, and zero in the contralateral kidney.

In patients with stenoses of both renal arteries, the pattern of renal vein renins often shows the same degree of asymmetry as in patients with unilateral stenosis, and usually lateralizes to the kidney which shows the greatest degree of stenosis on the arteriogram[12] (Fig. 14.2). The most marked asymmetry is seen in patients who have complete occlusion of one renal artery. Extreme elevations of renal vein renin may represent low flow through the kidney rather than hypersecretion of renin.

Numerous studies have examined the sensitivity and specificity of renal vein renin measurements, in many cases using the outcome from surgery rather than the presence or absence of renal artery stenoses as the dependent variable. The earlier results were reviewed by Marks and Maxwell, whose figures gave a sensitivity of 64% and a specificity of 87% in patients with unilateral disease.[35] The most common error is a false negative, i.e. the finding of a normal renal vein renin ratio in a patient whose hypertension is improved by surgery or angioplasty. More recent studies have attempted to improve the accuracy by using maneuvers to stimulate renin secretion, most usually captopril.

In patients with refractory hypertension and a non-functioning kidney who are candidates for nephrectomy the demonstration of an exaggerated renin secretion from the affected kidney is advisable before surgery can be recommended.

Renal vein renin with captopril stimulation

Just as captopril stimulation may be used to enhance the difference in peripheral PRA between patients with essential and renovascular hypertension, so may it be used to increase the asymmetry of renin secretion between the normal and ischemic kidneys when there is a renal

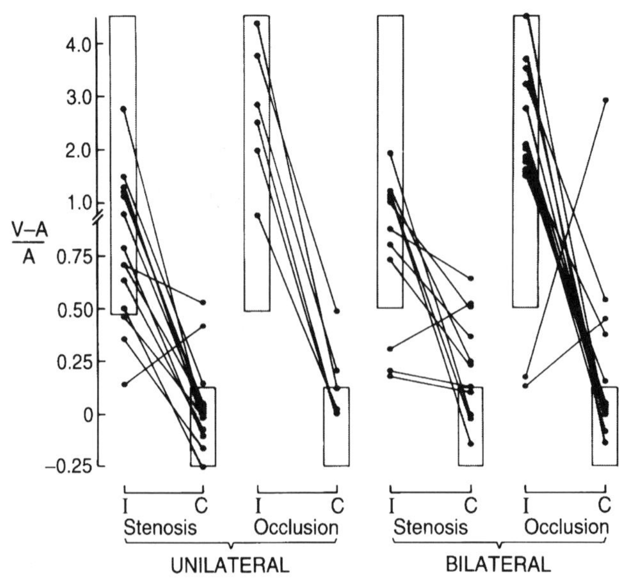

Figure 14.2. Renal vein renin patterns in patients with stenosis of one or both renal arteries. I: most ischemic kidney (as judged by arteriography); C: contralateral kidney; O: occluded renal artery. From ref. 12, with permission.

Table 14.3. Sensitivity and specificity of renal vein renins before and after captopril

Investigator	No. of patients	Sensitivity Pre	Sensitivity Post		Specificity Pre	Specificity Post
Lyons *et al.*[37]	26	43	86		80	100
Thibonnier *et al.*[38]	37	69	91		100	100
Simon *et al.*[39]	43	44	61	(unilateral)	62	96
		17	92	(bilateral)	93	90
Svetkey *et al.*[28]	66	–	64		–	73
Roubidoux *et al.*[40]	133	–	65		–	52

artery stenosis. In essential hypertension the renal vein renin ratio is unaffected by captopril, while in renovascular hypertension it tends to be enhanced.[36] This occurs partly because the renin secretion from the ischemic kidney is stimulated, but also to a lesser extent by further suppressing secretion from the contralateral kidney.[36]

As shown in Table 14.3, most studies have found that captopril stimulation improves the accuracy of the test. Four studies reported measurements made before and after captopril, in all of which the post-captopril ratios were better at predicting the presence of a stenosis. The lowest accuracy was reported in the study of Svetkey *et al.* who compared the utility of several diagnostic tests, including the captopril test and renal vein renins measured after captopril. For the latter they reported a sensitivity of 64% and a specificity of 73%.[28] Another study from the same group related the captopril-stimulated renal vein renins to outcome following angioplasty.[37] In 133 patients the sensitivity was 65% and specificity 52%, leading the authors to conclude that the test was insufficiently reliable to be used routinely. The main problem was the high false positive rate, which was 48%. This may be in part attributable to the relatively low prevalence of renal artery stenosis (16%) in this population.

Conclusions

Renin measurements continue to have an important place in the evaluation of patients with suspected and confirmed renovascular hypertension. Measurement of peripheral PRA is of limited value as a screening test on its own, but may be helpful in patients with either extremely high or extremely low values. Measurement of renin after captopril stimulation with the oral captopril test has received mixed reviews, but remains the only procedure that has the capability of being used as a general screening test. Nevertheless, its use cannot be recommended in all patients with hypertension, since there is likely to be a high proportion of false positives, particularly in patients with high renin hypertension. It may be of greatest value in patients in whom there are clinical clues to the presence of renovascular disease, and in whom peripheral PRA is normal. It is of unproven value in children.

Renal vein renin measurements as traditionally performed have been found to have an unacceptably high false negative rate. Their reliability can be increased by making the measurements after captopril, but the test still cannot distinguish between unilateral and bilateral disease, and may now have a high false positive rate. In selected patients, however, it may still be of value.

Renal vein renin testing has been largely surpassed by captopril renography as a measure of functional ischemia, but even this is less than ideal.[41,42] There is unfortunately no ideal screening test for diagnosing renovascular hypertension, and the available tests are best utilized in patients in whom there is a moderate level of clinical suspicion of its presence.[43] When the index of suspicion is low, none of the tests can be recommended, whereas when it is high it may be appropriate to proceed straight to angiography.

References

1 Goldblatt H, Lynch J, Hanzal RF, Summerville WW. Studies on experimental hypertension. I. The production of persistent elevation of systolic blood pressure by means of renal ischemia. *J Exp Med* 1934; **59:** 347–78.

2 Laragh JH, Sealey JE, Buhler FR *et al.* The renin axis and vasoconstriction volume analysis for understanding and treating renovascular and renal hypertension. *Am J Med* 1975; **58:** 4–13.

3 Bengis RG, Coleman TG. Antihypertensive effect of prolonged blockade of angiotensin formation in benign and malignant one- and two-kidney Goldblatt hypertensive rats. *Clin Sci* 1979; **57:** 53–62.

4 Brunner HR, Kirshman JD, Sealey JE, Laragh JH. Hypertension of renal origin: evidence for two different mechanisms. *Science* 1971; **174:** 1344–6.

5 Gavras H, Brunner HR, Vaughan ED, Jr, Laragh JH. Angiotensin-sodium interaction in blood pressure maintenance of renal hypertensive and normotensive rats. *Science* 1973; **180:** 1369–72.

6 Rocchini AP, Barger AC. Renovascular hypertension in sodium-depleted dogs: role of renin and carotid sinus reflex. *Am J Physiol* 1979; **236:** H101–107.

7 Gavras H, Brunner HR, Thurston H, Laragh JH. Reciprocation of renin dependency in renal hypertension. *Science* 1979; **188:** 1316–17.

8 Leenen FHH, DeJong W, DeWied D. Renal venous and peripheral plasma renin activity in renal hypertension in the rat. *Am J Physiol* 1973; **225:** 1513–18.

9 DeJong W. Release of renin by rat kidney slices; relationship by plasma renin after desoxycorticosterone and renal hypertension. *Proc Soc Exp Biol Med* 1969; **130:** 85–8.

10 Bianchi C, Bonadio M, Andriole VT. Influence of postural changes on the glomerular filtration rate in nephroptosis. *Nephron* 1976; **16:** 161–72.

11 Derkx RHM, Tan-Tjiong HL, Wenting GJ *et al.* Captopril test for diagnosis of renal artery stenosis. In Glorioso N *et al.* (eds) *Renovascular Hypertension*, pp. 295–315. New York: Raven Press, 1917.

12 Pickering TG, Sos TA, James GD *et al.*. Comparison of renal vein renin activity in hypertensive patients with stenosis of one or both renal arteries. *J Hypertension* 1985; **3:** (Suppl. 3) S291-3.

13 Vensel LA, Devereux RB, Pickering TG *et al.* Cardiac structure and function in renovascular hypertension produced by unilateral and bilateral renal artery stenosis. *Am J Cardiol* 1986; **58:** 575–82.

14 Pickering TG, Herman L, Sotelo JE *et al.* Recurrent pulmonary edema as a manifestation of renovascular hypertension and its treatment by renal revascularization. *Circulation* 1987; **76:** (Suppl. IV): 274.

15 Sutters M, Al-Kutoubi MA, Mathias CJ, Peart S. Diuresis and syncope after renal angioplasty in a patient with one functioning kidney. *Br Med J* 1987; **295:** 527–8.

16 Navar LG, Rosivall L. Contribution of the renin–angiotensin system to the control of intrarenal hemodynamics. *Kidney Int* 1984; **25:** 857–68.

17 Lohmeier TE, Cowley AW. Hypertensive and renal effects of chronic low level intrarenal angiotensin infusion in the dog. *Circ Res* 1979; **44:** 154–60.

18 Hollenberg NK, Swartz SL, Passan DR, Williams Ga. Increased glomerular filtration rate after converting-enzyme inhibition in essential hypertension. *N Engl J Med* 1979; **301:** 9.

19 Vaughan ED Jr, Bühler FR, Laragh JH *et al.* Renovascular hypertension: renin measurements to indicate hypersecretion and contralateral suppression, estimate renal plasma flow, and score for surgical curability. *Am J Med* 1973; **55:** 402–14.

20 Vaughan ED Jr, Carey RM, Ayers CR *et al.* A physiologic definition of blood pressure response to renal revascularization in patients with renovascular hypertension. *Kidney Int* 1979; **15:** S83-S92.

21 Case DB, Laragh JH. Reactive hyperreninemia in renovascular hypertension after angiotensin blockade with saralasin or converting enzyme inhibitor. *Ann Int Med* 1979; **91:** 153–60.

22 Müller FB, Sealey JE, Case CB *et al.* The captopril test for identifying renovascular disease in hypertensive patients. *Am J Med* 1986; **80:** 633–44.

23 Derkx FHM, Tan-Tjiong HL, Wenting GJ *et al.* Schalekamp MADH. Captopril test for diagnosis of renal artery stenosis. In Glorioso N, Laragh JH, Rappelli A (eds) *Renovascular Hypertension*, pp. 295–304. New York: Raven, 1987.

24 Frederickson ED, Wilcos CS, Bucci CM *et al.* A prospective evaluation of a simplified captopril test for the detection of renovascular hypertension. *Arch Int Med* 1990; **150:** 569–72.

25 Gosse P, Dupas JY, Reynaud P *et al.* Captopril test in the detection of renovascular hypertension in a population with low prevalence of the disease. A prospective study. *Am J Hypertension* 1989; **2:** 191–3.

26 Hansen PD, Gardeal P, Fruergaard P. The captopril test for identification of renovascular hypertension: value and immediate adverse effects. *J Intern Med* 1990; **228:** 159–63.

27 Postma CT, Van der Steen PH, Hoefragels WH *et al.* The captopril test in the detection of renovascular disease in hypertensive patients. *Arch Int Med* 1990; **150:** 625–8.

28 Svetkey LP, Himmelstein SI, Dunnick NR *et al.* Prospective analysis of strategies for diagnosing renovascular hypertension. *Hypertension* 1989; **145:** 247–57.
29 Thibonnier M, Sassano P, Joseph A *et al.* Diagnostic value of a single dose of captopril in renin- and aldosterone-dependent, surgically curable hypertension. *Cardiovasc Rev Rep* 1982; **3:** 1659–67.
30 Elliott WJ, Martin WB, Murphy MB. Comparison of two noninvasive screening tests for renovascular hypertension. *Arch Int Med* 1993;**153:** 755–64.
31 Gerber LM, Mann SJ, Muller FB *et al.* Response to the captopril test is dependent on baseline renin profile. *J Hypertension* 1994; **12:** 173–8.
32 Hricik DE, Browning PJ, Kapelman R *et al.* Captopril-induced functional renal insufficiency in patients with bilateral renal-artery stenoses or renal-artery stenosis in a solitary kidney. *N Engl J. Med* 1983; **308:** 373.
33 Hamed RM, Balfe JW, Ellis G. Use of the captopril test to assess renin responsiveness in children with hypertension and renal disease. *Child Nephrol Urol* 1991; **11:** (1) 10–4.
34 Gauthier B, Trachtman H, Frank R, Pillari G. Inadequacy of captopril challenge test for diagnosing renovascular hypertension in children and adolescents. *Pediatr Nephrol* 1991; **5:** (1) 42–4.
35 Marks LS, Maxwell MH. Renal vein renin. Value and limitations in the prediction of operative results. *Urol Clin North Am* 1975; 2: 311–25.
36 Tomoda F, Takata M, Ohashi S *et al.* Captopril-stimulated renal vein renin in hypertensive patients with or without renal artery stenosis. *Am J Hypertension* 1990; **3:** 918–26.
37 Lyons DF, Streck WF, Kem DC *et al.* Captopril stimulation of differential renins in renovascular hypertension. *Hypertension* 1983; **5:** 615–22.
38 Thibonnier M, Joseph A, Sasano P *et al.* Improved diagnosis of unilateral renal artery lesions after captopril administration. *JAMA* 1984; **251:** 56–60.
39 Simon G, Coleman CC. Captopril-stimulated renal vein renin measurements in the diagnosis of atherosclerotic renovascular hypertension. *Am J Hypertension* 1994; **7:** (1) 1–6.
40 Roubidoux MA, Dunnick NR, Klotman PE *et al.* Renal vein renins: inability to predict response to revascularization in patients with hypertension. *Radiology* 1991; **178:** 819–22.
41 Postma CT, van Oijen AH, Barentsz JO *et al.* The value of tests predicting renovascular hypertension in patients with renal artery stenosis treated by angioplasty. *Arch Int Med* 1991, **151:** (8) 1531–5.
42 Mann SJ, Pickering TG, Sos TA *et al.* Captopril renography in the diagnosis of renal artery stenosis: accuracy and limitations. *Am J Med* 1991; **90:** 30–40.
43 Mann SJ, Pickering TG. Detection of renovascular hypertension. State of the Art: 1992. *Ann Int Med* 1992; **117:** 845–53.

15

Captopril renography

JOSEPH V NALLY Jr

Introduction

Hypertension affects nearly 50 million Americans and poses a tremendous risk for cardiovascular morbidity and mortality. Renovascular hypertension (RVH) remains a leading cause of potentially correctable hypertension. Although RVH may affect only 1–3% of an unselected hypertensive population, up to 15–30% of appropriately screened patients referred to a subspecialty center for problematic hypertension may prove to have renovascular disease. Advances in percutaneous renal angioplasty, renal artery stenting and renovascular surgical techniques have renewed interest in developing better screening tests to identify patients with potentially correctable hypertension and/or renal dysfunction secondary to renovascular disease. The combination of radionuclide studies of the kidney with angiotensin converting enzyme (ACE) inhibition using captopril has shown promise for improving the non-invasive detection of significant stenosis of the renal artery. This review will focus upon both the alterations in renal physiology of renal artery stenosis (RAS) which are clinically relevant to the interpretation of captopril renography in the evaluation of the hypertensive patient and the results of the pertinent clinical studies.

Pathophysiology of RAS

Constricting the main renal artery leads to a cascade of important hemodynamic and humoral events within the kidney distal to the stenosis.[1,2] Initially, there is a vasodilatation distal to the stenosis in an attempt to maintain renal blood flow. If stenosis is significant, reduction in ipsilateral renal artery perfusion pressure stimulates renin release from the juxtaglomerular apparatus and augments intrarenal angiotensin A II production. In the systemic circulation, A II promotes both systemic vasoconstriction and aldosterone secretion with its attendant sodium retention. The increase in total peripheral resistance and salt retention may both contribute to an elevation of mean arterial pressure (Fig. 15.1). Within the affected kidney, the A II-dependent renal vasoconstriction attenuates the fall in renal perfusion pressure and also affects the glomerular filtration rate (GFR) by

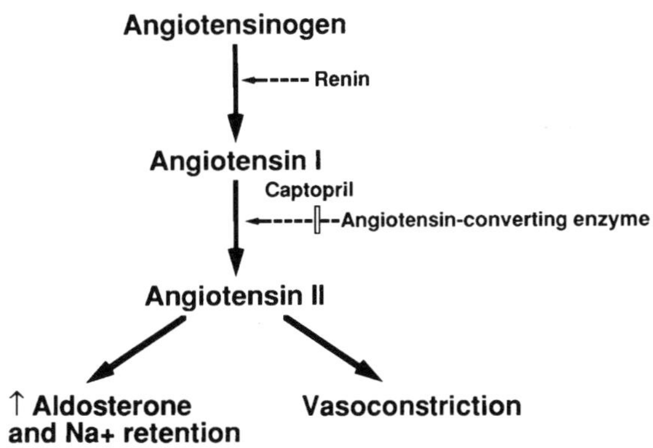

Figure 15.1. Renin–angiotensin system.

modulating vascular resistance of the afferent and efferent renal arterioles. Angiotensin A II exerts a powerful influence on maintaining GFR by inducing preferential efferent arteriolar vasoconstriction to maintain transcapillary pressures within the glomerulus that maintains the GFR of the affected kidney. Challenge with ACE inhibitors has been used as a pharmacologic probe to attenuate A II production and assess the humoral and hemodynamic responses to the pharmacological challenge.

Rationale for ACE inhibition

Understanding the effects of ACE inhibition upon the kidney ipsilateral to the stenosis as well as on the contralateral kidney is crucial in anticipating the changes in the radionuclide studies of the kidney following ACE inhibition.

Renovascular hypertension appears to be dependent on renin secretion from the juxtaglomerular apparatus of the underperfused, stenotic kidney and is partially maintained by participation of the contralateral kidney which demonstrates an abnormal pressure–natriuresis relationship in which a new set point of sodium homeostasis is attained at a higher level of mean arterial pressure. As seen in Fig. 15.1, inhibition acts to interrupt the renin–angiotensin–aldosterone pathway by preventing the conversion of the decapeptide angiotensin I (A I) to the octapeptide A II so that both the vasoconstrictor-hemodynamic and aldosterone-stimulating effects of A II are blocked. Hence, ACE inhibition acts as a pharmacologic probe to investigate the role of A II in the pathophysiology of RAS.

The provocative challenge of the ACE inhibitor captopril has been studied in two fashions. As seen in Fig. 15.1, the administration of the ACE inhibitor blocks the conversion of A I to A II so that the concentration of plasma renin activity, which is proximal to the blockade, may increase. In fact, patients with RVH have a marked hyperreninemic response to captopril stimulation compared with patients with essential hypertension. This pathophysiology forms the basis of the captopril plasma renin activity test as described in Chapter 16. Secondly, effective blockade of the renin–angiotensin cascade with the ACE inhibitor markedly attenuates the generation of A II which has measurable effects on both systemic blood pressure and intrarenal hemodynamics and function. The latter effect forms the pathophysiologic basis of the provocative captopril renography studies. An understanding of the effect of ACE inhibition upon renal hemodynamics and function is critical to understanding and interpreting captopril renography. The effects of ACE inhibition upon renal function are schematically represented in Fig. 15.2. A reduction in renal perfusion pressure

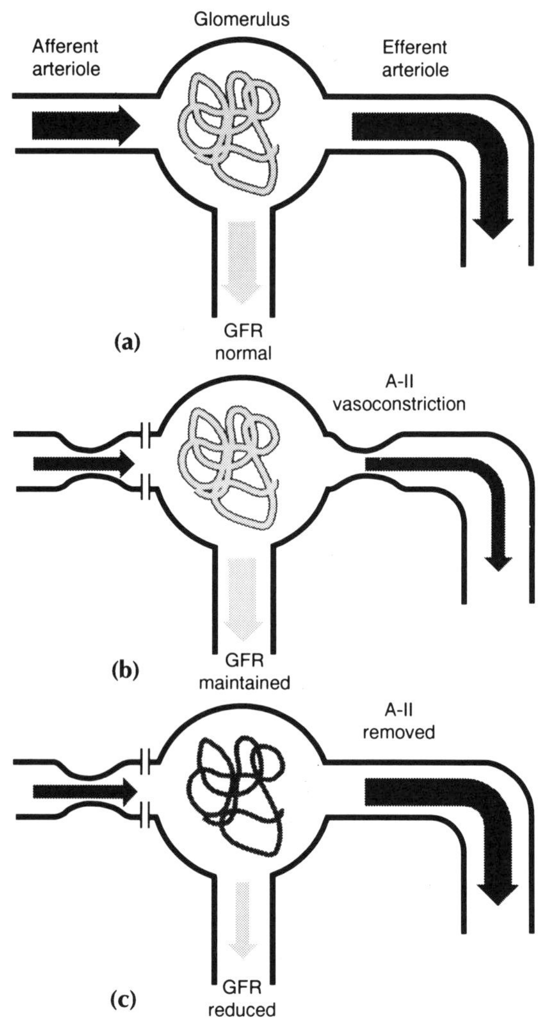

Figure 15.2. Schematic effect of captopril on renal function. (a) Normal. (b) Renal artery stenosis. (c) Renal artery stenosis plus. See text for details.

results in preferential A II-mediated vasoconstriction of the efferent arteriole in an attempt to maintain GFR of the stenotic kidney (Fig. 15.2b). Angiotensin converting enzyme inhibition blocks the formation of A II and consequently reduces the postglomerular efferent resistance and thereby decreases the GFR of the kidney distal to the stenosis (Fig. 15.2). This decrease in individual kidney function may be assessed non-invasively using radionuclide studies.

In most experimental and human forms of unilateral RAS, the GFR of the stenotic kidney falls approximately 30% after ACE inhibition.[3, 4] In contrast, the contralateral normal kidney exhibits an increase in GFR, urine flow and sodium excretion despite a reduction in mean arterial blood pressure. For example, in a canine model of unilateral renal artery stenosis (Fig. 15.3a), captopril lowered mean arterial pressure and produced striking alterations in the time–activity curves of technetium–99 m (^{99}Tc) diethylenetriaminepentaacetic acid (DTPA) (Fig. 15.3b) renograms.[3] The change is correlated with a 30% reduction of GFR in the kidney distal to the stenosis. Angiotensin converting enzyme inhibition did not reduce effective renal plasma flow (ERPF) in the affected kidney and the ERPF of the contralateral kidney rose by 22% despite a 20% reduction in arterial pressure. The changes in the renogram were reversible (Fig. 15.3c) and did not occur when mean arterial pressure was lowered with the non-specific vasodilator sodium nitroprusside (Fig. 15.3d). These expected

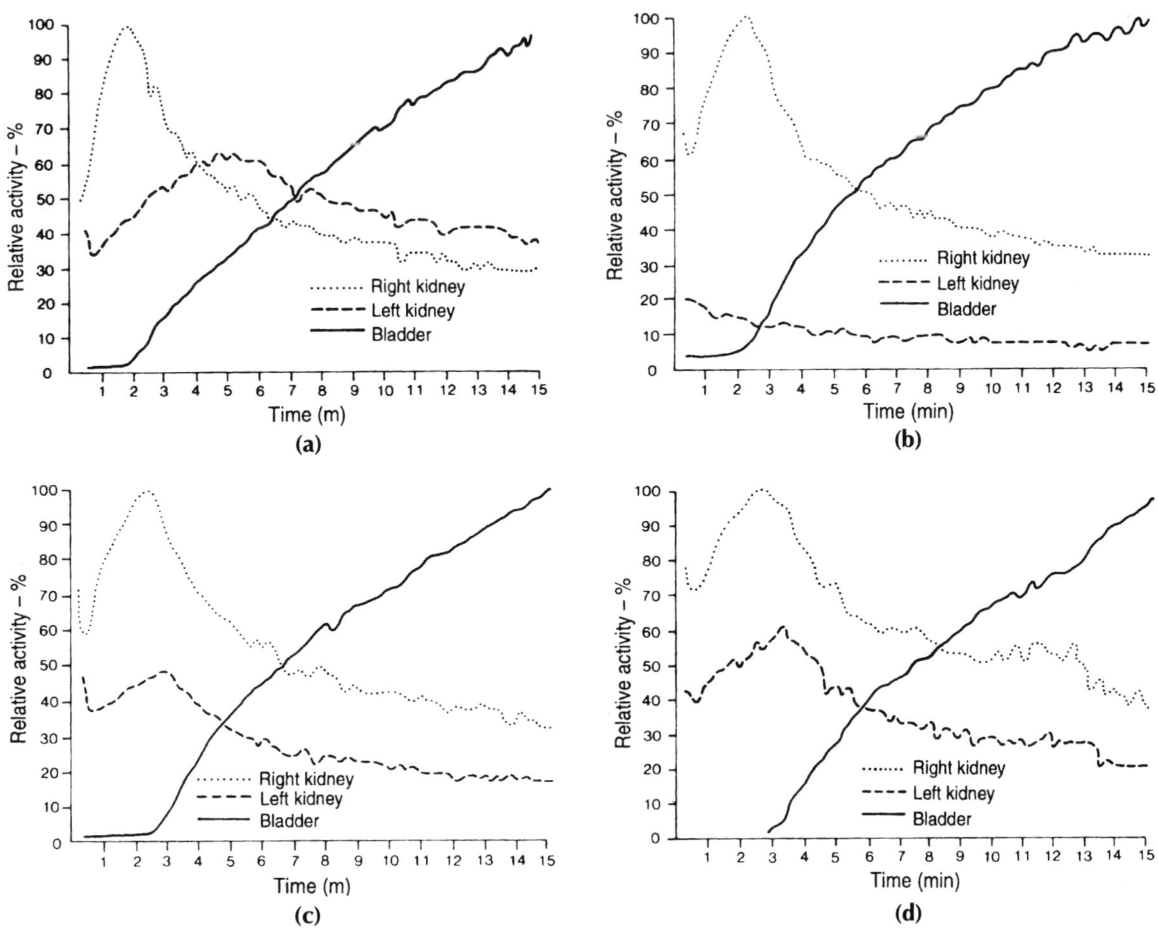

Figure 15.3. ^{99}Tc DTPA studies in a canine model of unilateral RAS. (a) RAS alone. (b) RAS plus captopril. (c) recovery. (d) RAS plus nitroprusside. See text for details.

physiologic changes within the stenotic and contralateral kidneys are the basis of the asymmetry of renal function following ACE inhibition (detected by renal radionuclide studies) which should enhance the non-invasive diagnosis of unilateral RAS.

With bilateral RAS, detection of stenosis may be more complex for two reasons. First, the exaggerated asymmetry of renal function after ACE inhibition may be attenuated as both kidneys behave in the 'clipped' fashion. In a canine model of bilateral RAS, captopril lowered mean arterial pressure and produced striking changes in the time–activity curve of each kidney. The changes in the renogram were more pronounced in the more severely stenotic kidney and correlated with a greater reduction in GFR and enhanced renal vein renin determinations of that kidney following captopril stimulation.[5] Clinical studies of patients with bilateral RAS by Mann *et al.*[6] suggest that captopril renography may be less sensitive in identifying stenosis of the contralateral, less stenotic kidney. Secondly, coexisting renal insufficiency secondary to advanced renovascular disease might compromise the ability of some radionuclides (e.g. ^{99}Tc DTPA) to assess accurately the changes in renal function. Furthermore, in a solitary kidney with stenosis, the issue of degree of renin dependency of blood pressure and renal function remain controversial. Overall, attention should be given to the type, degree and location of RAS when interpreting the clinical studies of captopril renography.

Clinical observations

Understanding the pathophysiologic basis for captopril renography permits one to review critically the clinical utility of this combined technology as a screening test to detect or exclude potentially reversible hypertension attributed to RAS. The following questions must be addressed. Which patients should be selected for study? How should the patients be prepared? What are the most appropriate radionuclides and ACE inhibitors to be employed? What are the most helpful diagnostic criteria and how accurately are they applied? The remainder of this chapter will focus upon patient preparation, test methodology and accuracy and limitations of the captopril-stimulated radionuclide studies.

Table 15.1. Clinical clues to the presence of renovascular disease

Abrupt onset of hypertension before age 30 or after age 55
Severe hypertension (diastolic blood pressure >120 mmHg)
Accelerated or malignant hypertension (with Grade II or IV retinopathy)
Hypertension refractory to triple-drug therapy
Moderate hypertension and diffuse vascular disease (carotid, coronary, peripheral vascular disease)
Epigastric bruit (especially systolic-diastolic)
Moderate hypertension and unexplained azotemia
Azotemia induced by ACE inhibitor therapy

Before delving into the specifics, two important reminders are appropriate. First, it is critical to distinguish between renovascular hypertension and RAS. Renal artery stenosis is the mere presence of anatomic stenosis of the renal artery (usually > 70%). It is common in the elderly population with or without hypertension and may not be the etiology of the hypertension in patients with RAS. In contrast, true RVH is defined as an elevated blood pressure caused by renal hypoperfusion, usually due to anatomic RAS and activation of the renin–angiotensin system. Ideally, the hypertension should be ameliorated by the correction of RAS. Secondly, the predictive value of any screening test is a function of the accuracy (sensitivity and specificity) of the test, as well as the prevalence of the disease within the population to be screened.[7, 8] Captopril renography should be applied only to those hypertensive patients thought to have a moderate suspicion of RVH based upon the usual clinical clues as outlined in Table 15.1.

Captopril renography

When renography was introduced over three decades ago, considerable optimism accompanied the development of the renogram for the non-invasive detection of RAS. Unfortunately, results with conventional renography with iodine-131 (^{131}I) orthoiodohippurate (OIH) did not exceed those of the hypertensive intravenous pyelogram with a sensitivity and specificity of approximately 75 and 85% respectively.[7] In a seminal observation, Majd and colleagues in the United States observed over a decade ago that pretreatment with the ACE inhibitor captopril markedly altered the renogram in several patients with RAS.[9] The pioneering work of Geyskes, Oei and colleagues in Europe suggested that captopril-stimulated renography offered great promise as a non-invasive screening tool and predictor of blood pressure response in their series of hypertensive patients.[10] The initial optimism for this combined technique led to larger controlled series of captopril renography which are now available for critical review. The clinical protocols and diagnostic criteria often vary from center to center. Special focus must be given to patient preparation and test methodology, as well as the accuracy and limitations of the test.

Patient preparation

The radionuclide study should be performed in well-hydrated patients who have ingested an ad lib salt diet.[11] Recommendations regarding the use of antihypertensive medications prior to testing have been evolving since many referring physicians find it unacceptable to discontinue medications. The studies of Setaro *et al.* have provided some important data on this matter.[12] The chronic use of ACE inhibitors appears to significantly reduce the sensitivity (97–70%) without reducing specificity. It is recommended that ACE inhibitors be withheld for 3–5 days before study. Diuretics appear to have a marginal effect on diminishing sensitivities. The effect of other classes of antihypertensive agents was minimal. These authors conclude that other antihypertensive agents may be administered up to the morning of the study without adversely affecting the efficacy of the captopril renogram clinical protocol.

Clinical protocol

On the day of study, vigorous oral hydration (water 10 mg/kg po) is encouraged. After insertion of a peripheral venous catheter for sampling and/or injection, baseline blood pressure is measured and measurements are repeated at 15–20 min intervals, although clinically significant hypotension is unusual. Captopril (25–50 mg crushed po) is administered, and a conventional radionuclide study of the kidney is begun 60 min post-captopril. A baseline non-stimulated radionuclide study may be obtained on a separate day for comparison.

A second approach is to administer intravenous enalapril at 0.04 mg/kg up to a maximum of 2.5 mg i.v. over 3–5 min and then perform the radionuclide study 10–15 min after the i.v. enalapril.[13] This procedure is advocated by some in order to improve patient through-put and avoid potential problems with delayed gastric emptying or poor absorption. Similarly, a few centers advocate the use of furosemide with the ACE inhibitor-stimulated renogram.[14] When tubular agents such as ^{99}Tc mercaptoacetyltriglycine (^{99}Tc MAG_3) or ^{131}I OIH are used, the diagnosis of RVH is primarily based on cortical retention in the proximal tubules. Furosemide is a loop diuretic that acts distally to the proximal tubules where ^{99}Tc MAG_3 and OIH are secreted. The disadvantage of furosemide is volume depletion and a greater risk of severe hypotension. If furosemide is used, an intravenous line should be considered for supplemental hydration. The protocol for furosemide intravenous hydration is described by Erbslöh-Möller.[14]

Choice of radionuclide

The majority of captopril renography studies to date have been performed with either ^{99}Tc (DTPA) or ^{131}I OIH using a medium energy collimator and conventional software.[15] More recently, ^{99}Tc MAG_3 has become clinically available for renography. In contrast to OIH and MAG_3, DTPA is excreted by the kidney solely via glomerular filtration. Because of the superior imaging capabilities of the ^{99}Tc compared ^{131}I labeling, the early phase of the ^{99}Tc DTPA and MAG_3 studies offer index of renal perfusion and kidney size. On the other hand, OIH and MAG_3 are handled by the kidney like paraaminohippurate (PAH) and are excreted by both glomerular filtration and tubular secretion–a physiology that could be advantageous for renal imaging, especially for patients with renal dysfunction. Unfortunately, the ^{131}I label suffers from suboptimal imaging characteristics. However, initial successful results with either ^{99}Tc DTPA or ^{131}I OIH have been reported for captopril renography. More recently, ^{99}Tc MAG_3 may become the radionuclide of choice because it offers both the advantageous technetium labeling characteristics and optimal renal handling and excretion. To date, the results of ^{99}Tc MAG_3 for captopril renography have been quite promising from the studies of Dondi and a subset of patients in the European Multicenter Captopril Trial.[16, 17] Unfortunately, ^{99}Tc MAG_3 is more costly than the other two agents, but the use of ^{99}Tc MAG_3 may be more cost effective with appropriate scheduling to 'cluster' these renal studies.

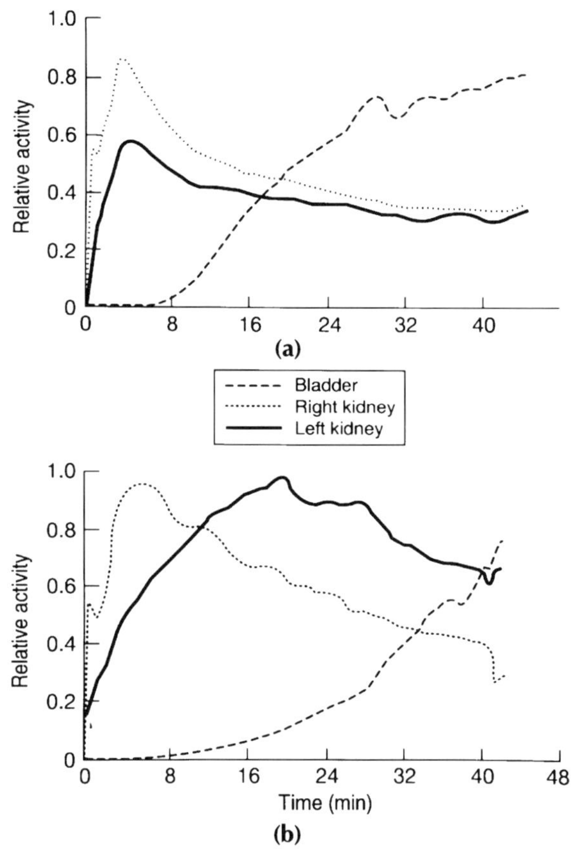

Figure 15.4. Renogram of patient with unilateral left renal artery stenosis. (a) ^{99}Tc DTPA time–activity curves during baseline. (b) ^{99}Tc DTPA time–activity following captopril stimulation.

Diagnostic interpretation

The existing clinical and renographic results must be interpreted with some caution since the protocols are complex and the diagnostic criteria are not well standardized. The Consensus Panel on Captopril Renography suggested in 1990 that both the scintigraphic images and computer-generated time–activity curves provide helpful information about renal size, perfusion and excretory capacity.[18] Two categories of diagnostic criteria for RAS include: (1) asymmetry of renal size and function and (2) specific captopril-induced changes in the renogram. Such abnormalities following ACE inhibition include: (1) delayed time to maximal activity ($T_{max} \geq 11$ min); (2) significant asymmetry of peak activity of each kidney; (3) marked cortical retention of radionuclide; and (4) marked reduction in calculated GFR of the ipsilateral kidney. Figure 15.4 depicts a classic example of changes in the time–activity curves with captopril in a patient with renal artery stenosis on the left. In addition, Fig. 15.5 highlights the importance of close scrutiny of the scintigraphic images before and after captopril in a patient with segmental changes of the right nephrogram. This patient had two renal arteries on the right with severe RAS of the superior artery. Note the absence of radionuclide in the superior aspect of the right kidney with captopril. Surgical correction of the lesion resulted in normalization of his hypertension.

Critical review on the interpretative data of captopril renography should focus on two important questions. (1) Does captopril renography accurately identify patients with RVH? (2) Is captopril renography predictive of a response of blood pressure (or renal function) following successful intervention?

Table 15.2 represents a synopsis of the captopril renography studies in hypertension patients suspected of RVH. The table summarizes the number of patients studied with and without renovascular disease (RAS or RVH), radionuclide

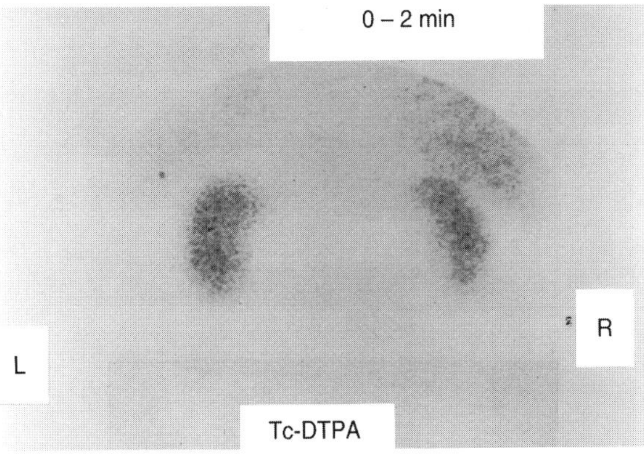

(a)

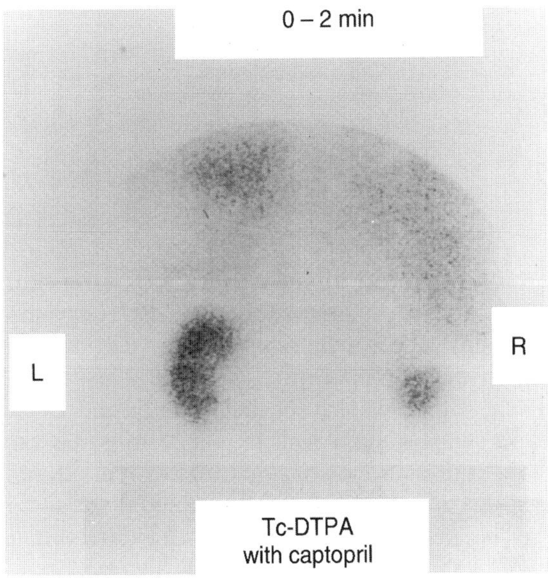

(b)

Figure 15.5. Scintigram of patient with segmental right RAS. (a) ^{99}Tc DTPA baseline. (b) ^{99}Tc DTPA following captopril. See text for details.

employed, sensitivity, specificity and positive predictive response of blood pressure to intervention. Different diagnostic criteria as well as different patient populations may account for some variations in results. Overall, the accuracy of captopril renography in identifying patients with renovascular disease appears to be quite acceptable with the sensitivity of approximately 90–93% (range 83–94%) and a specificity of approximately 93–98% (range 85–100%). The most useful criteria appear to be a diminished uptake of the radionuclide and prolonged T_{max} of the kidney (i.e. delayed excretion or cortical retention) after captopril. Furthermore, most investigators in the collaborative Consensus Panel recommended that a single post-captopril study is adequate for screening, as sensitivity and specificity of the single stimulated study are similar to those summarized above.

Initially, changes after captopril were postulated to be the hallmark of hemodynamically significant RAS.[2] In fact, the Consensus Panel suggested in 1991 that tests be interpreted as high, low or indeterminate probability based upon captopril-induced changes.[18] However, in a well-executed study by Mann *et al.*,[6] captopril-induced changes with ^{99}Tc DTPA were only observed in 51% of their cases. These changes alone were not very sensitive, but they were quite specific. Importantly, captopril did increase overall sensitivity with ^{99}Tc DTPA (from 71 to 91% respectively) without adversely affecting specificity (94–95% respectively). Furthermore, other reports of Geyskes,[10] Fommei *et al.*,[17] Setaro [12] and Elliott [21] also suggest that captopril response is predictive of a cure or improvement in blood pressure in 80–90% of cases in response to a technically successful intervention such as percutaneous transluminal angioplasty or revascularization (see Table 15.2). In contrast, a positive captopril renogram did not correlate with successive blood pressure control in the patients of Mann *et al.*[6] Unfortunately, data concerning the preservation or improvement of GFR of the stenotic kidney following intervention are not available.

The presence of bilateral RAS, solitary kidney RAS or renal dysfunction may adversely affect the accuracy of captopril renography. Many investigators have excluded patients with moderately compromised renal function with serum creatinines exceeding 2.5–3 mg%. In patients with mild renal impairment, Fommei *et al.*[17] report a reduction in the positive predictive value from 88 to 57% in patients enrolled in the European Multicenter Captopril Trial; whereas, Setaro *et al.*[12] noted a minimal reduction in sensitivity and specificity in patients with serum creatinines >1.5 mg%. In the report of Mann *et al.*[6] patients with bilateral RAS tended to have more azotemia than unilateral RAS patients, yet

Table 15.2. Sensitivity, specificity and predictive value of captopril renography

Investigator	No. of patients studied	No. of patients with renovascular disease	Radionuclide	Sensitivity	Specificity	Positive predictor of blood pressure response[a]
Geyskes *et al.*[22]			OIH (47)	–	–	
	94	94	MAG_3 (47)	–	–	91% (53/58)
Sfakianakis *et al.*[13]			OIH	100	100	–
	36	18	DTPA	100	73	–
Erbslöh-Möller *et al.*[14]	50	28	OIH	96	95	91% (10/11)
Svetkey *et al.*[20]			DTPA	74	44	
	140	31	OIH	71	41	
Setaro *et al.*[12]	94	44	DTPA	91	94	83% (15/18)
			DTPA	94	95	69% (11/16)
Mann *et al.*[6]	55	35	OIH	83	85	82% (9/11)
Fommei *et al.*[17]			DTPA (380)	83	91	
	472	259	MAG_3 (74)	83	100	93% (40/43)
Dondi *et al.*[16]	102	54	MAG_3	90	92	–
Elliott *et al.*[21]	100	59	DTPA	92	80	96% (51/53)
Dondi *et al.*[19]			DTPA (38)			
	51	32	MAG_3 (13)	87	93	97% (32/33)

[a] The positive values are based on the blood pressure response (improved or cured) in patients who underwent revascularization.

the diagnostic accuracy of captopril renography was comparable. Importantly, these authors noted that captopril renography was capable of identifying the more stenotic kidney as abnormal, but the status of the contralateral kidney (normal vs RAS) could not be ascertained with certainty. Overall, approximately a third of the RAS patients had bilateral RAS and the overall accuracy of the combined procedure appears to be adequate for clinical screening.

Captopril renography may offer advantages and some disadvantages compared with other non-invasive screening techniques. In the studies of Elliot *et al.*,[21] the sensitivity and specificity of both captopril renography and the captopril plasma renin activity (PRA) test were examined in 150 patients screened for RVH. Overall, captopril renography was more sensitive (92 vs 76%) and more specific (80 vs 58%) in patients with angiographically proven RAS. Moreover, the captopril renogram may offer information regarding the anatomic involvement of the individual kidney which is not available from the captopril PRA test. Captopril renography may share some advantages and limitations with duplex ultrasonography of the renal arteries.[23] Both appear to offer advantages as they appear to be safe, non-invasive and less costly compared with invasive angiography. Both appear to be reasonably sensitive and specific for detecting RAS although the two modalities have not been compared in a controlled, blinded fashion. Theoretically, captopril may offer more functional information about the hemodynamic impact of RAS which might be predictive of response to intervention. Accuracy of duplex ultrasonography may be technology and operator dependent such that its results must be validated within a given center. However, duplex ultrasonography may offer a potential advantage over captopril renography for the detection of RAS in those patients with significant azotemia or proteinuric renal disease.

Summary

Precise recommendations regarding the clinical procedures, radionuclide of choice and diagnostic criteria for RVH are somewhat difficult given the lack of rigorous standardization of these complex protocols. Nevertheless, review of the available data indicates that provocative captopril renography appears to be a safe and effective means of non-invasively screening hypertensive patients for renovascular disease. A normal study after captopril suggests with a reasonable degree of certainty that potentially reversible RVH is unlikely. A positive captopril renogram in an appropriately screened hypertensive patient with preserved renal function suggests that renovascular disease is likely, with sensitivity and specificity in excess of 90%. Although there may be confounding variables such as renal dysfunction, type and location of RAS, etc., a positive captopril renogram might also imply cure or improvement in blood pressure control with successful intervention. Whether captopril renography might predict stabilization of individual kidney function following intervention is speculative and deserves further study.

References

1 Anderson WP, Dentol KM, Woods RL *et al.* Angiotensin II and the maintenance of GFR and renal blood flow during renal artery narrowing. *Kidney Int* 1990; **38:** (Suppl. 30) S109-S113.

2 Nally JV. Renal physiology of renal artery stenosis. *Am J Hypertension* **4:** 1991, 669S-674S.

3 Nally JV, Clarke HS Jr, Grecos GP *et al.* Effect of captopril on ^{99m}Tc-diethylenetriaminepentaacetic acid renograms in two-kidney, one-clip hypertension. *Hypertension* 1986; **8:** 685–93.

4 Ploth DW. Angiotensin-dependent renal mechanisms in two-kidney, one-clip renal vascular hypertension. *Am J Physiol* 1983; **245:** F131-F141.

5 Nally JV, Bedoya LA, Park CH *et al.* Captopril-stimulated renography versus renal vein renins in two-kidney, two-clip hypertension. *Contrib Nephrol* 1990; **79:** 176–80.

6 Mann SJ, Pickering TG, Sos TA *et al.* Captopril renography in the diagnosis of renal artery stenosis: accuracy and limitations. *Am J Med* 1991; **90:** 30–40.

7 Davidson RA, Wilcox CS. Newer tests for the diagnosis of renovascular disease. *JAMA* 1992; **268:** 3353–8.

8 Mann SJ, Pickering TG. Detection of renovascular hypertension. *Ann Int Med* 1992; **117:** 845–53.

9 Majd N, Potter BN, Guzzetta PC *et al.* Effect of captopril on efficacy of renal artery stenosis [abstract]. *J Nucl Med* 1983; **24:** P23.

10 Geyskes GG, Oei HY, Puylaert CABJ *et al.* Renography with captopril: changes in a patient with hypertension and unilateral renal artery stenosis. *Arch Int Med* 1986; **146:** 1705–8.

11 Black HR, Bourgoignie JJ, Pickering T *et al.* Report of the working party group for patient selection and preparation. *Am J Hypertension* 1991; **4:** 745S–746S.

12 Setaro JF, Saddler MC, Chen CC *et al.* Simplified captopril renography in diagnosis and treatment of renal artery stenosis. *Hypertension* 1991; **18:** 289–98.

13 Sfakianakis GN, Bourgoignie JJ, Daffe D *et al.* Single dose captopril scintigraphy in the diagnosis of renovascular hypertension. *J Nucl Med* 1987; **28:** 1383–92.

14 Erbslöh-Möller B, Dumas A, Roth D *et al.* Furosemide ^{131}I-hippuran renography after angiotensin-converting enzyme inhibition for the diagnosis of renovascular hypertension *Am J Med* 1991; **90:** 23–40.

15 Blaufox MD, Dubovsky EV, Hilson AJW *et al.* Report of working party on radionuclide of choice: captopril renogram consensus conference. *Am J Hypertension* 1991; **4:** 747S-748S.

16 Dondi M. Captopril renal scintigraphy with ^{99m}Tc-mercaptoacetyltriglycine (^{99m}Tc-MAG_3) for detecting renal artery stenosis. *Am J Hypertension* 1991; **4:** 737S–740S.

17 Fommei E, Ghione S, Hilson AJW *et al.* Captopril radionuclide test in renovascular hypertension: European multicenter study. In O'Reilly PH, Taylor A and Nally JV (eds) *Radionuclides in Nephrourology*, Vol. 1 Blue Bell, PA: Field and Wood Medical Periodicals, in press.

18 Nally JV, Chen C, Fine E *et al.* Diagnostic criteria of renovascular hypertension with captopril renography – a consensus statement. *Am J Hypertension* 1991; **4:** 7495–525.

19 Dondi M, Fanti S, De Fabritiis A *et al.* Prognostic value of captopril renal scintigraphy in renovascular hypertension. *J Nucl Med* 1992; **33:** 2040–4.

20 Svetkey LP, Wilkinson R Jr, Dunnick NR *et al.* Captopril renography in the diagnosis of renovascular disease. *Am J Hypertension* 1991; **4:** 711S–715S.

21 Elliott WJ, Martin WB, Murphy MB. Comparison of two noninvasive screening tests for renovascular hypertension. *Arch Int Med* 1993, **153:** 755–64.

22 Geyskes GG, deBruyn AJG. Captopril renography and the effect of percutaneous transluminal angioplasty on blood pressure in 94 patients with renal artery stenosis. *Am J Hypertension* 1991; **4:** 685S–689S.

23 Nally JV, Olin JW, Lammert GK. Advances in noninvasive screening for renovascular disease. *Cleve Clin J Med* 1994; **61:** 328–36.

24 Nally JV, Black HR. State-of-the-art review: captopril renography – pathophysiological considerations and clinical observations. *Sem Nucl Med* 1992; **92:** 85–91.

16

Screening and diagnosis in renovascular hypertension

FRANK J ALBERS AND LAURA P SVETKEY

Introduction

Renovascular hypertension (RVH) carries substantial morbidity, yet it is ultimately a curable disease. While uncommon compared with essential hypertension, renovascular disease still afflicts a substantial number of patients: using conservative estimates of prevalence, this disease affects 300 000 people in the United States and over 750 000 in Europe. Early identification of renovascular hypertension with appropriate intervention may save years of antihypertensive therapy, reduce the morbidity associated with long-standing hypertension, and help reduce the incidence of renal failure. For these reasons there continues to be great effort exerted in improving diagnosis. Unfortunately there is no single accurate or effective screening test to identify this disease.

Numerous factors combine to obfuscate the early recognition of renovascular hypertension. The natural history of the disease is largely unknown. While stenosis of one or both renal arteries is a necessary component of the disease, the anatomic lesion alone is insufficient to define renovascular hypertension.[1,2,3] There is a continuum in the progression of renal artery stenosis (RAS) and its pathophysiologic effects on the kidney. Correlation between the degree of stenosis and its ischemic effect is poor,[4,5] although it is suggested the lesion must have at least a 60% luminal narrowing to affect blood flow.[6] Conversely, an insignificant renal artery stenosis may eventually progress, often to total occlusion.[7–10] It is also evident that renovascular disease causes involution of renal mass and deterioration in renal function over time.[7,10–12] These data emphasize the progressive nature of renovascular disease and the heterogeneous correlation between anatomic appearance and physiologic effect.

Concomitant renal insufficiency also complicates the detection of RVH. Intrinsic renal disease can affect the typical hyperreninemic state present in the earlier stages of significant renal artery stenosis, and it can alter the response to angiotensin converting enzyme inhibition. Thus these two factors affect the reliability of functional tests used in screening. In addition, renal insufficiency is a relative contraindication to intravenous contrast dye exposure due to the increased risk of acute renal failure in this circumstance. Obviously renal insufficiency poses a dilemma for the clinician: the most reliable test to detect an anatomic lesion (arteriography) is relatively contraindicated yet functional studies are less reliable. The conundrum is worsened by the fact that renovascular disease may be contributing to the renal insufficiency itself, and left untreated, it can result in end-stage renal disease.

Renovascular hypertension cries out for an effective and reliable screening test to aid in its detection. Unfortunately the ideal test does not yet exist. Even the gold standard of renal arteriography falls well short of the goal due to its invasive nature, intravenous contrast exposure, cost, and its inability to discern a functionally significant renal artery lesion from an incidental one. We shall attempt to review the current diagnostic tests for renovascular hypertension and propose a schema for the diagnosis of this disease.

Predictive value of tests

Tests in clinical medicine help refine the physician's suspicion for the disease of interest. A pretest suspicion (probability) is first established through historical and physical observation, then diagnostic tests help support or refute this pretest likelihood. To interpret test results appropiately, one must have some knowledge of the operating characteristics of the test. Some features, namely sensitivity and specificity (defined in Fig 16.1), are inherent to the test itself, and these remain fixed independent of the population tested.[14] Alterations in test protocol or in interpretation criteria can change sensitivity and specificity. The clinical usefulness of a test is determined by its predictive value (Fig. 16.1). In contrast to sensitivity and specificity, the predictive values vary with the prevalence of the disease in the population tested.[15] The positive predictive value of a test can be enhanced by increasing the prevalence, or pretest probability, of the disease (Fig. 16.2). When pretest suspicion of disease is high, a positive diagnostic test helps confirm this probability while a negative test is of little benefit. On the other hand, when pretest probability is low, a negative diagnostic test helps exclude the disease.

Among unselected hypertensives, the pretest probability of RVH is low, and what is needed is a screening test with which to 'rule out' RVH. An adequate screening test must have very high sensitivity, be easy to perform, and have benefits that far outweigh the risks and cost to the patient. At this time there are no screening tests available for RVH that fulfill these requirements. Although the overall prevalence of RVH is low, clinical selection can be used to increase pretest probability. Application of findings from the history and physical exam can serve to select a population in whom the prevalence of RVH is comparatively higher. This will serve to increase the pretest probability of the disease and thereby make diagnostic tests more effective.

		Disease of Interest	
		Present	Absent
Test Result	Positive	a	b
	Negative	c	d

a = true positives
b = false positives
c = false negatives
d = true negatives

Sensitivity
- likelihood test will be positive when disease is present
- true positive rate
- sensitivity = a/(a+c)

Specificity
- likelihood test will be negative when disease is absent
- true negative rate
- specificity = d/(b+d)

Positive Predictive Value (PV+)
- probability disease is present given a positive test
- PV+ = a/(a+b)

Negative Predictive Value (PV−)
- probability disease is absent given a negative test result
- PV− = d/(c+d)

Figure 16.1. Definitions for operating characteristics of clinical tests and their derivation through the use of a 2 × 2 table.

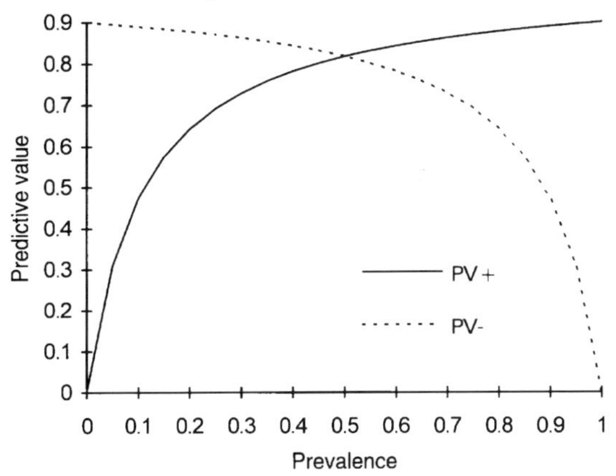

Figure 16.2. Relation between predictive values and prevalence of disease for a test having a sensitivity of 90% and a specificity of 90% (PV+, positive predictive value; PV–, negative predictive value).

Clinical Features

Epidemiology

The prevalence of RVH is not known with precision, but available data suggest it occurs in 1–5% of the general hypertensive population.[16–18] At first glance this small proportion implies the disease is rare until one realizes that hypertension affects approximately 15% of the general population in Western societies.[19] Renovascular hypertension could therefore affect over a quarter of a million people in the United States alone. The lack of accurate screening tests makes it very difficult to determine the precise number of patients afflicted with this process. Prevalence could actually be underestimated, especially considering that clinically unsuspected RAS has been found frequently in some studies.[1] Nevertheless consistent results over the years makes the general estimate of 5% of the hypertensive population a reasonable assumption. Another important issue is the question of varying racial prevalence of renovascular disease. It has previously been suggested that RVH is all but non-existent in the black population.[20] Evaluation of these data indeed shows a lower incidence of the disease in blacks; however, because hypertension affects a greater proportion of the black population, the absolute number of blacks with renovascular disease may be substantial. When clinical selection criteria are applied to blacks, the prevalence of RVH is comparable with that in the clinically selected white population.[21] Therefore race alone is not useful in discriminating the subset of patients with secondary vascular hypertension.

History and symptoms

Without a sensitive and inexpensive screening test, it remains critical to select the patient subgroup in whom there is a higher prevalence of renovascular disease (i.e. to increase the pretest probability). The most reasonable and cost-effective means through which to accomplish this selection is a knowledgeable clinician with a high suspicion for the disease. Unfortunately, it has been quite difficult to discern clinical findings that accurately predict renovascular disease.[22–24] To clarify the clinical differences between essential and renovascular hypertension, the Cooperative Study of Renovascular Hypertension was established.[25, 26] In this multicenter study, a large cohort of hypertensive patients was evaluated for RVH as defined by surgical cure of high blood pressure. Systematic evaluation and uniform data acquisition then allowed retrospective comparison of the clinical characteristics of patients with renovascular disease to those with documented essential hypertension. Several differences in the groups became apparent. Those patients with RVH had a biphasic age distribution that was significantly different from the group with primary disease. The known duration of hypertension was also shorter in the former. Another item of importance was the higher prevalence of known pre-existent vascular disease in the patients with atherosclerotic RVH.

These criteria remain the dominate historical selection characteristics to assess patients for renovascular disease, and they are usually applied in a collective fashion, i.e. patients are usually selected for study because they have one or more of the pertinent findings. Unfortunately there are few studies that attempt to determine which of these criteria are of true benefit in the detection of RVH. Age at onset of hypertension is used as a selection criterion because patients with fibromuscular dysplasia tend to be younger while those with atheromatous RAS are older than patients having essential hypertension (Table 16.1). Recent diagnosis (within 2 years) is also a significant discriminating factor in the Cooperative Study. This relatively early detection possibly relates to the characteristics of the blood pressure since patients with renovascular disease may have a higher incidence of uncontrollable or accelerated hypertension, leading to earlier evaluation for secondary causes. The predictive value of these selection characteristics for renovascular disease is low[27] (Table 16.1), supporting other authors' contention that the age at onset of hypertension has no useful role in screening.[28]

The pattern of blood pressure elevation is advocated as a useful indicator of secondary causes of hypertension (Table 16.1). The Cooperative Study supports this notion.[26] There is a higher incidence of rapid increase in blood pressure, loss of previous control, or uncontrolled pressure on several antihypertensive agents in patients with renovascular disease compared with essential hypertension. Prospective studies, however, show that refractory hypertension (uncontrolled on three or more drugs) along with the pattern of blood pressure elevation are poor predictors for RVH.[27, 29] Patients' concern about labile blood pressure as well as the clinician's frustration in obtaining hypertension control may prompt evaluation of this group for RAS, making these features more common (and less selective) in the population referred for study.

Numerous investigations suggest that there is also an increased prevalence of renovascular disease in those patients with vascular disease elsewhere. Analysis of almost 300 autopsies in both hypertensive and normotensive patients has found a 22.3% overall prevalence of significant (>50%) renal artery stenosis.[3] In those cases with aortic atherosclerosis, the association with renovascular disease increases to 40%. Patients undergoing aortography for aortic aneurysm, aorto-occlusive disease, or lower extremity occlusive disease also have up to a 39% prevalence of severe stenosis in one or both renal arteries.[2] Besides the correlation with peripheral

Table 16.1. Association between selected clinical features and RVH

Characteristic	Prevalence of characteristic among all hypertensives (%)	Prevalence of characteristic in population with RVH (%)	Prevalence of RVH in population with characteristic (%)	Study
Onset hypertension <25 or >45 years	23	31	45	Simon *et al.* [26]
	41	12	6	Svetkey *et al.* [27]
Diagnosis of hypertension within	14	22	52	Simon *et al.* [26]
2 years	18	25	13	Svetkey *et al.* [27]
Accelerated hypertension[a]				
Refractory hypertension	15	19	42	Simon *et al.* [26]
Refractory hypertension	59	38	6	Svetkey *et al.* [27]
Loss of blood pressure control	39	75	19	Svetkey *et al.* [27]
Rapid elevation in blood pressure	39	62	16	Svetkey *et al.* [27]
Atherosclerotic vascular disease	11	13	40	Simon *et al.* [26]
	64[b]	85[c]	17[c]	Harding *et al.* [1]
			39[c]	Olin *et al.* [2]
Unexplained pulmonary edema		9		Messina *et al.* [30]
		24		Pickering *et al.* [31]
Abdominal bruit	21	49	78	Simon *et al.* [26]
	10	39	92	Grim *et al.* [32]
	18	56	56	Svetkey *et al.* [27]
Hypertensive retinopathy	14	18	44	Simon *et al.* [26]
			31	Davis *et al.* [33]

[a] Subcategories of accelerated hypertension defined in text and in Table 16.5.
[b] Represents prevalence within the entire study population, with and without hypertension.
[c] Data reported for anatomically significant RAS, not necessarily RVH.

vascular disease, renovascular lesions may also be associated with coronary artery disease. In a study of over 1000 patients undergoing coronary angiography, concurrent renal arteriography demonstrates a 15% prevalence of significant RAS despite a low clinical suspicion of renovascular disease.[1] Other authors suggest an association between renovascular disease and pulmonary edema independent of coronary artery disease. Patients with RAS and recurrent acute pulmonary edema have resolution of congestive heart failure after correction of the renovascular lesion independent of improvement in blood pressure control or renal function.[30, 31] It is important to note in all these investigations that the correlations are simply between anatomic renal arterial lesions and the associated conditions of interest. There is no established relationship between these findings and renovascular hypertension. Nevertheless in evaluating an individual patient for RVH, one must keep in mind the possible association between renovascular disease and peripheral vascular disease, coronary artery disease or poorly explained pulmonary edema (Table 16.1).

Signs

Physical signs appear to have greater positive predictive value for renovascular disease than do historical features. Unfortunately, the absence of these findings does not preclude renal arterial disease. In other words the physical examination can help support RVH, but alone it cannot exclude the disease. There has been great attention to abdominal or flank bruits as predictive features for RAS. Again the Cooperative Study is the first to demonstrate this correlation (Table 16.1).[26] Grim *et al.*[32] have used retrospective data to establish a sensitivity of 39% and a specificity of 100% for abdominal or flank bruits in detecting RVH. This study suggests a continuous systolic-diastolic bruit is of particular use and lends a higher predictive value than bruits with only systolic components. A prospective study specifically evaluating the use of clinical features in predicting RVH[27] also shows that the highest correlation between selection criteria and presence of RAS occurs with abdominal or flank bruits, in this case without a distinction between systolic and diastolic bruits. Table 16.1 shows that abdominal bruits are fairly infrequent in the general hypertensive population, but of those patients with bruits, a high proportion have renovascular disease. Therefore, we feel that any abdominal or flank bruit is important in the overall patient evaluation for RVH, but its absence does not exclude this condition.

The only other physical finding that is clearly useful in predicting RVH is retinopathy. Retrospective analysis shows that Grade III or IV hypertensive retinopathy has a high association with underlying renovascular disease.[26, 33] Thirty-one percent of patients demonstrating this sign have RVH.[33] Like bruits, this sign, a reflection of the severity of hypertension, raises the clinical suspicion of RVH, but its absence does not rule it out. Other physical findings suggesting diffuse atherosclerotic vascular disease help support the historical data, but these signs lack specificity for renal arterial lesions. Bruit, severe retinopathy and other evidence of vascular disease are suggestive of RVH but are not sufficient to establish the diagnosis.

Hypertension and azotemia

Clinical findings suggesting renovascular disease in patients with renal insufficiency have been difficult to establish. Many studies find no correlation between RAS and renal insufficiency[1, 26] while others purposely exclude patients with renal insufficiency due to the risk of radiographic contrast exposure during evaluation. Jacobson[34] has helped focus attention on ischemic nephropathy as a cause of progressive azotemia with or without RVH. The association of bilateral RAS (or stenosis in a solitary kidney) with acute renal failure induced by angiotensin converting enzyme inhibitors is now well established.[35–37] In a large study of patients with refractory hypertension (uncontrolled on three agents) and renal insufficiency (creatinine >133 μmol/l), approximately one-third of the subjects have critical stenoses of both renal arteries or of the artery in a solitary kidney.[38] Otherwise unexplained progressive renal insufficiency may also herald renovascular disease. Patients with RVH treated medically have a progressive deterioration in renal function in comparison with patients undergoing renal artery revascularization.[10] Several scenarios should then raise the suspicion of RVH in patients with renal insufficiency.[34] (1) acute renal failure precipitated by treatment with angiotensin converting enzyme inhibitors; (2) acute renal failure induced by rapid control of hypertension; (3) progressive azotemia in patients with refractory hypertension, and (4) unexplained progressive azotemia in the elderly hypertensive patient. Further study is required to determine the reliability and predictive power of these clinical features in the detection of renovascular disease.

Functional diagnostic studies

General considerations

The classic studies by Goldblatt in the 1930s[39, 40] established the kidney's central role in the pathophysiology of hypertension. The discovery of renin and its involvement in the production of angiotensin II confirmed the suspicion of a humoral mechanism involving the kidney in the pathogenesis of hypertension. Further evaluation in the two-kidney, one-clip animal model demonstrated a central role of this mechanism in the generation of RVH. Tests were developed to evaluate perfusion of and renin production in the ischemic kidney. These assays of renal function were then applied in the diagnosis of renovascular disease.

Peripheral renin levels

Renin/sodium profiling

There is extensive investigation of renin–angiotensin activity in attempts to distinguish patients with RVH from those with essential hypertension. These studies are fraught with difficulties, some of which are predictable from the animal model. In the two-kidney, one-clip rat, renin secretion and angiotensin levels vary with time.[41] Although renin levels are high within days after clipping the renal artery, eventually the animals develop sodium retention, increase in total body volume and suppression of both renin production and systemic angiotensin II levels. Correction of the renal artery stenosis or resection of the ischemic kidney generally corrects or at least improves the hypertension, but, after several weeks, hypertension is not dependent on renin production and kidney revascularization has no effect on blood pressure. However, even when hypertension has become irreversible in this model, the renin–angiotensin system can be restimulated through volume depletion with resultant malignant hypertension.[41]

In humans, the duration of RAS and volume status are generally unknown, and as in the Goldblatt animal, these can markedly affect the renin level at any given time. Therefore, it is not surprising that a single measure of plasma renin activity (PRA) does not distinguish patients with RVH from those with essential hypertension.[42] To compensate for these factors, Laragh[43, 44] has done extensive work profiling renin levels under standard conditions (e.g. supine vs upright position) indexed to sodium excretion. His work categorizes patients with essential hypertension into those with low, normal and high renin states. Despite these refinements, renin profiling has not helped select a population having a high prevalence of renovascular disease.[42, 45–47]

Captopril renin test

The ability of the renin assay to identify patients with RVH may be improved through modulation of hemodynamics in the poststenotic kidney with use of angiotensin-converting enzyme inhibitors. In this situation, blockade of angiotensin II production potentiates renin generation within the ischemic kidney.[45, 48, 49] Thus the diagnostic accuracy of renin determination as a predictor for renovascular hypertension should be improved through the use of converting enzyme inhibitors (CEI).

In 1988 Müller's group[50] performed a retrospective analysis of patients in whom peripheral PRA was assayed after captopril administration. Patients with renovascular hypertension were defined according to the criteria of the Cooperative Study of Renovascular

Hypertension.[25] These authors combined three parameters of the PRA response to captopril that successfully distinguished patients with renovascular hypertension from those with essential hypertension. An important aspect of this study was the unreliable response of this test in patients with renal disease: PRA had no predictive value in this group.

Other authors have since applied the captopril test in a prospective manner with variable results. The sensitivity of this test in the diagnosis of renovascular hypertension ranges between 38 and 100% with a specificity 76–95% (Table 16.2).[51–55] The question remains why there are such wide variations in the results of this assay. There are numerous potential explanations for these discrepancies. As noted earlier, absolute PRA and its alteration in response to CEI are heavily dependent on volume status, sodium intake and perhaps duration of stenosis. In the setting of volume contraction there will be a false elevation of baseline renin activity. For this reason it is quite important that the patient be off all diuretics and on a normal sodium diet for several days before the test. Certain antihypertensive agents (e.g. β-blockers) can also affect renin production. Ideally a patient should, therefore, be off all diuretics and other antihypertensive agents for 2 weeks prior to testing. Clearly many of the patients suspected of renovascular hypertension will not tolerate such a long respite off antihypertensive medications. In this circumstance the patient should be converted to short-acting agents with minimal effects on PRA, such as nifedipine, during the drug holiday, and no agents should be taken the day of the test. Variations among assays for PRA have also complicated interpretation of the test, hindering its widespread application. Therefore, if the captopril test is used, results from the local laboratory should be converted to values that correspond to the originally described diagnostic criteria.[50] Given the numerous factors that can influence results of the captopril renin test, it is imperative that it be performed following a uniform protocol.[52]

Despite the variable sensitivity and specificity of the captopril renin test, one very consistent finding is its high negative predictive value (Table 16.2).[29, 51–55] This characteristic represents the strength of this particular diagnostic procedure. In those patients for whom there is a relatively low clinical suspicion of renovascular disease, a negative captopril renin test has a negative predictive value >95% (Table 16.2) and should circumvent further testing. In contrast, a positive captopril test in this population implies only a 11–27% likelihood of RVH. Despite this low positive predictive value, a positive captopril test may provide justification for further diagnostic evaluation. It must be re-emphasized that this test is not interpretable in patients having renal insufficiency (creatinine >124 μmol/l)[50] or in those patients who are volume depleted.[56]

In summary, the captopril renin test does not fit the requirements for an adequate screening test due to its low sensitivity. On the other hand, the test is low risk and relatively inexpensive. It is most effective in *excluding* RVH in the low suspicion group. A negative captopril test under these circumstances avoids further evaluation for renovascular disease. Large prospective studies using uniform protocols and renin

Table 16.2. Characteristics of the captopril renin test as evaluated in prospective studies determining functionally significant RAS

Study	Sensitivity %	Specificity %	Prevalence %	Assume 5% PV+ %	Prevalence PV– %	Assume 20% + %	Prevalence PV– %
Svetkey *et al.*[53]	58	76	22	11	97	38	88
Postma *et al.*[54]	38	95	24	27	97	64	86
Frederickson *et al.*[52]	100	80	29	21	100	56	100
Gosse *et al.*[55]	73	84	11	19	98	53	92

In Tables 16.2–16.4 PV+: position predictive value.
PV–: negative predictive value.

activity assays, along with well-defined test outcome criteria are needed to determine the value of this test in the diagnosis of RVH.

Renal vein renins

Theoretically, steady-state peripheral renin activity should be determined solely by renin production and renal plasma flow.[46] Therefore, measurement of renin activity closer to its source (i.e. in the renal vein) could improve our ability to uncover renin-dependent (renovascular) hypertension. However, unstimulated renal vein renin (RVR) determination does not distinguish renovascular from essential hypertension.[45] Maneuvers to stimulate renin production have variable success in improving performance.[57–60] The logical choices to stimulate renin production are angiotensin II receptor inhibitors such as saralasin or angiotensin converting enzyme inhibitors such as captopril. The studies of Re and others[61–64] suggest that renal vein renins RVR can successfully predict response to revascularization in patients having known unilateral renal artery stenosis. The benefit of RVR determination is questionable in bilateral renal artery stenosis.[65, 66] There is little information about renal vein renin determination in *screening* for renovascular disease, i.e. when renal vascular anatomy is unknown. Recent data suggest that RVR ratios do not have adequate sensitivity (64%) nor specificity (73%) in detection of RVH.[29] In addition, the technique suffers from its invasive nature as well as an unacceptably high number of false negative results. In summary, despite its theoretical advantage as a functional indicator for significant renal hypoperfusion, RVR ratio determination in the screening and diagnosis of RVH is not useful.

Renography

Technetium-labeled diethylenetriamenepentaacetic acid (^{99}Tc DTPA) is currently the dominant tracer used in renography. This agent is eliminated strictly through glomerular filtration without any significant tubular secretion or reabsorption (similar to inulin). Thus ^{99}Tc DTPA can allow scintigraphy to indirectly assess overall renal function and compare the relative contribution of each kidney. Static renography using ^{99}Tc DTPA is of little use in screening for RAS; however, the application of CEI to this technique has markedly improved its predictive value in the diagnosis of renovascular disease.[67–69] The Goldblatt two-kidney, one-clip hypertension model predicts that CEI use should decrease the glomerular filtration rate (GFR) and filtration fraction (FF) in the clipped kidney while GFR is unaffected in the non-clipped kidney,[41, 45] and this action can be detected with renography.[69]

Evaluation for renovascular disease using ^{99}Tc DTPA involves the acquisition of baseline renal scintigraphic images with assessment of computer-generated time–activity curves. Later the test is repeated after an oral or intravenous dose of CEI. Tracer uptake with calculated GFR estimates are compared between kidneys under both conditions, and a ratio >1.5 of the unaffected:affected kidney is consistent with unilateral RAS.[70] Delay in tracer appearance or prolongation in time to maximal tracer activity (T_{max}) under the influence of CEI also indicates a functionally significant RAS.[70] The specificity of these criteria is dependent on a reasonably normal baseline renogram. To compensate for a suboptimal baseline study, the Working Party in Diagnostic Criteria of Renovascular Hypertension with Captopril Renography recommends comparison of captopril-induced shifts in the pattern of time–activity curves.[71, 72] The advantage of this technique is simplicity of application and more uniform interpretation. However, these test criteria are not yet validated through prospective testing.

All forms of renography are potentially affected by renal insufficiency. This is especially true for renography using radiolabels that are excreted primarily through glomerular filtration, e.g. DTPA, making them less reliable for detection of renal artery stenosis. The use of radiolabeled substances excreted primarily through tubular secretion, such as ^{121}I-orthoiodohippurate (OIH) and ^{99}Tc mercaptoacetyltriglycine (MAG_3), may help overcome this limitation. These agents are scintigraphically detected as they accumulate in renal cortical tubules, and they dissipate as tubular flow moves them into the collecting system. In the setting of significant renovascular disease, pretreatment with CEI will reduce tubular flow rate of the affected kidney, resulting in delayed elimination of these agents.[73] Since renal plasma flow is maintained in renal insufficiency, this technique may have advantages over DTPA renography in this subset of patients. Recommendations concerning blood flow scintigraphy await prospective validation of this technique.

Overall the application of CEI renography in diagnosing RVH is encouraging but not yet definitive. Available investigations show relatively good sensitivity and specificity in detection of RAS, but for RVH the test has poor specificity (Table 16.3).[74] Different definitions for a positive test, variations in the definition of the disease and inclusion of patients with renal insufficiency undoubtedly contribute to these variable results. Prospective studies in detecting the anatomic lesion, i.e. RAS, show good operating characteristics of CEI renography, with sensitivity of 89–94% and specificity of 89–96% (Table 16.3).[28, 70, 75, 76] Setaro[28] achieves these results even in patients with renal insufficiency, but other studies do not support reproducible findings in this subset of patients.[70, 75] The sensitivity of CEI renography in diagnosing the hemodynamic lesion, i.e. renovascular hypertension, remains good, but specificity falls dramatically (17–81%) (Table 16.3).[28, 29, 70, 72, 73, 77] Despite the drop-off in specificity, negative predictive value remains high in a clinically selected population. Therefore, a normal CEI renogram result should preclude further testing. In contrast, abnormal CEI renography with a normal baseline study increases the suspicion of RAS sufficiently to warrant further evaluation via angiography (Table 16.3). An abnormal baseline study makes interpretation of CEI renography much more difficult. Many authors designate an abnormal baseline renogram as a positive test and proceed to angiography, but this approach serves to increase false positive results. Further investigation is needed to clarify the interpretation of CEI renography in this circumstance.

While there are some limitations to its efficacy in detecting renovascular disease, CEI renography is an attractive diagnostic test for several reasons: it is non-invasive, it does not require radiographic contrast material, and it allows continuation of antihypertensives during testing. Another benefit of renography is its potential in predicting outcome of therapeutic intervention. There are several retrospective studies in which there is limited predictive value of renography in detecting RAS; however, the operating characteristics of the test improve

Table 16.3. Results of captopril renography in detecting renovascular disease

	Sensitivity (%)	Specificity (%)	Prevalence (%)	Assume 5% PV+ (%)	Prevalence PV− (%)	Assume 20% PV+ (%)	Prevalence PV− (%)
Renal artery stenosis							
Prospective Studies							
Setaro *et al.* [28]	90	96	48	52	99	84	98
Mann *et al.* [70]	94	95	64	50	100	83	99
Dondi *et al.* [75]	89	89	33	30	99	67	97
Retrospective Studies							
Fommei *et al.* [76]	83	85	31	23	99	58	95
Renovascular hypertension							
Prospective Studies							
Setaro *et al.* [28]	83	81	53	19	99	53	95
Svetkey *et al.* [29]	91	50	18	9	99	31	96
Mann *et al.* [70]	58	17	76	4	88	15	61
Retrospective studies							
Geyskes *et al.* [77]	87	89	44	30	99	67	96
Fommei *et al.* [72]	93	67	73	13	99	41	97
Erbslöh-Möller *et al.* [73]	96	92	70	38	100	74	99

dramatically when predicting blood pressure response to revascularization, i.e. RVH.[67, 76, 78, 79] At this point broad prospective studies are still needed to determine the overall usefulness of CEI renography. Obviously it is not indicated as a screening test in the unselected hypertensive population due to its variable sensitivity and its cost. However, it may be quite beneficial in selected patients. Better consensus about testing procedure and diagnostic criteria is needed to allow more widespread application of this technique. Its use in patients with renal insufficiency is probably inappropriate. Converting enzyme inhibitor renography using markers removed by tubular secretion, namely OIH or MAG_3, may be more efficacious in this subgroup of patients.

Anatomic diagnostic studies

General considerations

The majority of work in diagnosing renovascular hypertension has been devoted to the detection of the requisite anatomic lesion. All of these tests, however, suffer from their inability to correlate a significant stenosis with a physiologic effect. Therefore none of the anatomic tests at this time have value in predicting response to therapy. These tests as a group also suffer from cost and technical considerations: they are difficult to perform, are difficult to interpret, are invasive, are expensive, have the inherent risk of intravenous contrast exposure, or all the above. Efforts to minimize one of these deficiencies tends to exacerbate another. Tests having great simplicity often are insensitive for detection of RAS, while improvements in sensitivity and specificity are accompanied by increased complexity or increased invasiveness.

Intravenous urography

Maxwell[80] first demonstrated the potential efficacy of rapid sequence intravenous urography in the detection of renovascular disease. A significant RAS should reduce renal arterial blood flow and cause hyperconcentration of urine, resulting in a delayed early nephrogram and concentration of contrast material in the affected kidney compared with the contralateral organ. An obvious drawback of this test is the necessity of unilateral disease to induce a positive result. Bilateral RAS will not be detected. Retrospective evaluation of this test suggests that it has high predictive value for both RAS and RVH;[32, 81, 82] however, prospective evaluation shows a sensitivity of 59% and specificity of 89% in the diagnosis of RAS as well as a sensitivity of 60% and specificity of 63% in detecting RVH (Table 16.4).[83] Newer imaging techniques using intravenous contrast can detect more specifically lesions within the renal vasculature. Technical advances, its questionable sensitivity and its inability to detect bilateral stenosis have relegated urography to the annals of medical history in the diagnosis of renovascular disease.

Ultrasonography/duplex

Since its inception, renal ultrasonography has been employed in screening for nephrologic disease. Disproportionate renal size on ultrasonography is often touted as a sign of significant unilateral renal ischemia. Studies are available that demonstrate progressive loss of renal mass in the setting of ischemic renal disease.[7, 10] In fact with known significant RAS, prospective evaluation of renal size via ultrasonography shows gradual loss of renal mass over time.[12] However, ultrasonographic size comparison is insufficiently sensitive for use in screening for renovascular disease since substantial RAS can be present in normal-sized kidneys. In addition, size determination via ultrasound is highly dependent on the imaging technique.[12] Therefore, comparative renal size does not have utility in prospective screening for RAS or RVH.

Duplex and Doppler sonography is a useful technique in evaluating the renal arteries. Vascular stenosis alters the flow characteristics within vessels, increasing flow velocity through the stenotic lesion and causing poststenotic turbulence. Studies have established Doppler criteria that correlate well with RAS of more than 60%.[84, 85] Investigators with substantial experience in this technique have obtained impressive

Table 16.4. Prospective evaluation of anatomic tests in the diagnosis of RAS.

Study	Sensitivity (%)	Specificity (%)	Prevalence (%)	Assume 5% Prevalence PV+ (%)	Assume 5% Prevalence PV− (%)	Assume 20% Prevalence PV+ (%)	Assume 20% Prevalence PV− (%)
Rapid sequence urography							
Thornbury *et al.*[83]	59	89	60	22	98	58	90
Thornbury *et al.*[83b]	60	63	92	8	97	29	86
Doppler/duplex sonography							
Flow characteristics[a]							
Hansen *et al.*[87]	93	100	59	100	100	100	98
Taylor *et al.*[88]	84	97	33	63	99	89	96
Berland *et al*[c89]	0	37	27	0	88	0	60
Waveform pattern[a]							
Stavros *et al.*[91]	95	97	30	59	100	87	99
Kleiwer *et al.*[92]	57	67	30	8	97	30	86
Intravenous DSA							
Dunnick *et al.*[101]	100	93	27	42	100	78	100
Smith *et al.*[102]	87	83	41	21	99	56	96
Clark and Alexander[103]	88	100	40	100	99	100	97
Campbell *et al.*[104]	83	96	29	52	99	84	96

[a] Flow characteristics refers to peak systolic velocity and renal:aortic ratios in determining significant renal artery stenosis. Waveform pattern refers to tradus parvus morphology in detecting RAS.
[b] Data reported in detection of RVH.
[c] Study restricted duration of procedure. Technically inadequate results reported as negative tests.

data using duplex ultrasound in the detection of RAS both in retrospective[86] and prospective studies (Table 16.4).[87–89] Sensitivity in detection of > 60% RAS is between 84 and 95% with specificities of 81–98%. Obvious benefits with this imaging procedure are its non-invasive nature and relatively low cost. Since duplex sonography provides information about flow, it has the added potential benefit of detecting physiologically significant lesions rather than simple anatomic stenoses.

However, as with all diagnostic tests in this arena there are substantial problems with the application of duplex sonography in diagnosing RAS. The technique is very operator dependent since the entire length of the renal artery must be evaluated, and adequate Doppler information can only be assessed when the transducer is at the appropriate angle to the vessel of interest. This serves to make duplex renal sonography very time consuming and susceptible to technical errors. In fact, even those centers having great success with the technique have a 10–12% technical failure rate.[84, 86] Concerns about the use of this test in clinical practice are underscored by a study that limited the duration of the procedure to that expected for abdominal ultrasonography. In this prospective study, duplex ultrasound had a sensitivity of 0% and a specificity of 37% (Table 16.4).[89] This technique cannot yet be advocated for widespread use.

Despite these limitations, simplification of duplex renal sonography may help overcome its shortfalls in diagnosing renovascular disease. It is known that significant arterial stenosis alters the waveform transmitted downstream.[90] This altered waveform can be detected in the segmental renal arteries which are technically easier to visualize. Stavros[91] suggests that waveform pattern recognition (early systolic peak) can be used in detection of > 60% renal artery stenoses with a sensitivity of 95% and specificity of 97% (Table 16.4). Unfortunately, these excellent results have not been supported by any subsequent studies.[92] Detection of the early systolic peak effectively excludes significant renal artery stenosis, but an altered waveform does not confirm renovascular disease. Therefore, the false positive rate for this technique can be quite high. Prospective studies are needed to further clarify the role of waveform pattern recognition in the diagnosis of renovascular disease. Overall, duplex sonography of the renal arteries and segmental renal artery waveform recognition hold great potential, but they cannot be recommended for the diagnosis of renovascular disease except in those centers well experienced in the technique.

Computerized tomography and magnetic resonance imaging

Spiral, or helical, computerized tomography (spiral CT) is a newer technique that produces anatomically contiguous tomographic images.[93] Computerized reconstruction of these data allows evaluation of intra-abdominal vessels, specifically of the aorta and its branches.[94] This technique offers the advantage of non-invasive detection of renovascular disease as well as characterization of the blood vessel wall using minimal intravenous contrast. Spiral CT has shown good correlation with standard angiography[95, 96] in detecting known renal artery stenosis, but spiral CT has far greater interobserver variability than does arteriography.[96] There are yet no prospective studies evaluating the efficacy of this procedure in predicting renovascular disease. At this point spiral computerized angiography offers no advantage over other available diagnostic tests.

Magnetic resonance imaging of blood vessels may be a viable alternative to angiography in some circumstances. The advantages of a non-invasive technique of imaging the renal arteries without the need for intravenous contrast is self-evident. Studies comparing magnetic resonance angiography (MRA) with standard arteriography have shown good correlation in detection of stenoses within the main renal arteries.[97–99] Unfortunately, these studies all consistently show that MRA is useful only in evaluating the proximal 3 cm of the renal artery, suggesting that significant distal or branch lesions can be missed entirely. Severity of stenosis tends to be overestimated using MRA,[97] which may reduce the specificity of this technique. MRA holds promise in the detection of the anatomic lesion, but no prospective evaluation of MRA in the detection of renovascular disease has yet been published. This technique offers great future potential but it cannot be currently advocated in the diagnosis of RVH.

Angiography

Direct imaging of the renal arteries using intravascular contrast remains the definitive method of detecting RAS. Developments in computer-enhanced radiographic imaging allow the application of digital subtraction angiography to evaluate the renal arteries. Intravenous digital subtraction angiography (DSA) possesses the advantages of lower cost, lower complication rate and decreased invasiveness compared with standard arteriography. Unfortunately it has its limitations. Intravenous DSA is affected by body morphology and bowel activity, with obesity and increased bowel gas preventing adequate imaging of vessels. There may also be suboptimal visualization of the renal vasculature when cardiac output is poor. Overlying vessels can obscure the arteries of interest. The combination of these factors results in technically uninterpretable studies in about 7% of cases.[100] Despite these technical problems, intravenous DSA has good efficacy in diagnosing renal artery stenosis. Prospective evaluation shows sensitivities and specificities of 83–100% of intravenous DSA in detecting RAS of greater than 50% (Table 16.4).[29, 100–104] It is important to recognize that in all these studies, technically inadequate or non-diagnostic studies are either excluded from analysis or counted as positive tests. Intravenous DSA may serve to exclude patients from further evaluation when the test is normal, but the clinician must be warned that this technique can miss some lesions due to technical problems.

Intra-arterial digital subtraction imaging of the renal arteries is performed through intra-aortic contrast injection proximal to the renal arteries. This variation of the technique uses less contrast than intravenous DSA and has better correlation with conventional angiography in detecting renal artery lesions.[105] The primary advantage of this technique over standard arteriography is through minimizing contrast exposure: adequate visualization of the renal arteries can be accomplished with as little as 50 ml of contrast; therefore, this technique is potentially advantageous in renal insufficiency.

Evaluation strategy

Currently available tests for the diagnosis of RAS and RVH are either too invasive or lack sufficient sensitivity and specificity for effective use in screening large unselected populations. It is imperative to categorize patients as to the clinical suspicion of renovascular disease. This categorization accomplishes two purposes: it helps direct the most appropriate diagnostic test by clarifying the pretest probability for the disease, and it improves the predictive value of a diagnostic test by increasing the prevalence of the disease in the subpopulation tested. It is clear that applying a combination of clinical criteria to hypertensive patients selects a subpopulation with about a 20% prevalence of RVH.[27, 29] However, not all clinical characteristics are equally important in predicting RAS and RVH. Abdominal bruits are consistently associated with renovascular disease and their presence suggests a high probability of this condition.[27, 32]

Over 30% of patients with Grade III or IV hypertensive retinopathy have RVH.[33] Acute renal failure after converting enzyme inhibition strongly suggests critical renal artery stenosis. These three conditions are major features in predicting RAS and possibly RVH (Table 16.5). Features such as blood pressure control, age at diagnosis of hypertension and unexplained pulmonary edema are associated with RVH when used in combination, but as individual criteria, they do not have sufficient power to suggest RVH (Table 16.5). We define these as minor features in predicting RVH. Atherosclerotic vascular disease (ASVD) in the form of peripheral vascular disease, coronary artery disease or cerebrovascular disease is strongly associated with renal artery stenosis, but it is not very specific. Atherosclerotic vascular disease alone does not help the clinician predict renovascular disease. When other minor clinical features suggesting RVH are present along with ASVD, the suspicion for RAS is greatly increased. We recommend separating patients according to suspicion for RVH into high (>20%), intermediate (6–20%), and low (≤5%) probability groups based on these clinical characteristics (Table 16.5). The presence of one major finding places a patient into the high suspicion group. Evident ASVD along with a minor finding establishes an intermediate level of probability. A single minor characteristic does not increase suspicion for RVH above that in the general population with hypertension; however, the presence of several

Table 16.5. Establishing pretest probability for RVH through the application of clinical features

High suspicion (> 20%)	Intermediate suspicion (6–20%)	Low suspicion (≤5%)
One or more *major features*	More than one *minor feature* *OR* One *minor feature* PLUS *Atherosclerotic vascular disease*	One or no *minor features*
Major features	**Atherosclerotic vascular disease**	**Minor features**
Abdominal bruit	Peripheral vascular disease	Refractory hypertension: Uncontrolled on maximal dose of three or more drugs
Grade III or IV hypertensive retinopathy	Coronary artery disease	
Acute renal failure with use of angiotensin converting enzyme inhibitors	Cerebrovascular disease	Unexplained loss of previous blood pressure control
		Rapid elevation in blood pressure Sudden >15% increase in systolic or diastolic blood pressure
		Unexplained episodes of pulmonary edema
		Diagnosis of hypertension at age <25 or >45 years

minor characteristics may increase the probability of renovascular disease to the intermediate suspicion level.

Once the clinician completes this broad categorization and generates a level of suspicion for RVH, the patient should then have his/her renal function evaluated. This subcharacterization is important since tests dependent upon renin activity or on the effect of CEI in the diagnosis of RVH are markedly altered by renal dysfunction. Renal insufficiency is also a relative contraindication to intravenous contrast dye exposure since diagnostic tests that require contrast have increased morbidity in this setting. Obviously the next most appropriate diagnostic test for RAS can be changed in the setting of renal dysfunction. For this purpose, we choose a serum creatinine level > 124 μmol/l (1.4 mg/dl) as indicative of renal insufficiency.

Our diagnostic strategy is summarized in Fig. 16.3. When clinical evaluation places a patient into the low suspicion category, the probability of RVH is no different from the general hypertensive population. The captopril renin test can be useful in this low prevalence population with normal renal function. While a positive captopril test does not diagnose renovascular disease, a normal test confirms the low suspicion for this condition and should prevent further diagnostic evaluation. It is reasonable to follow these patients with medical management of their blood pressure, but patients should be reassessed on a regular basis for clinical features of renovascular disease.

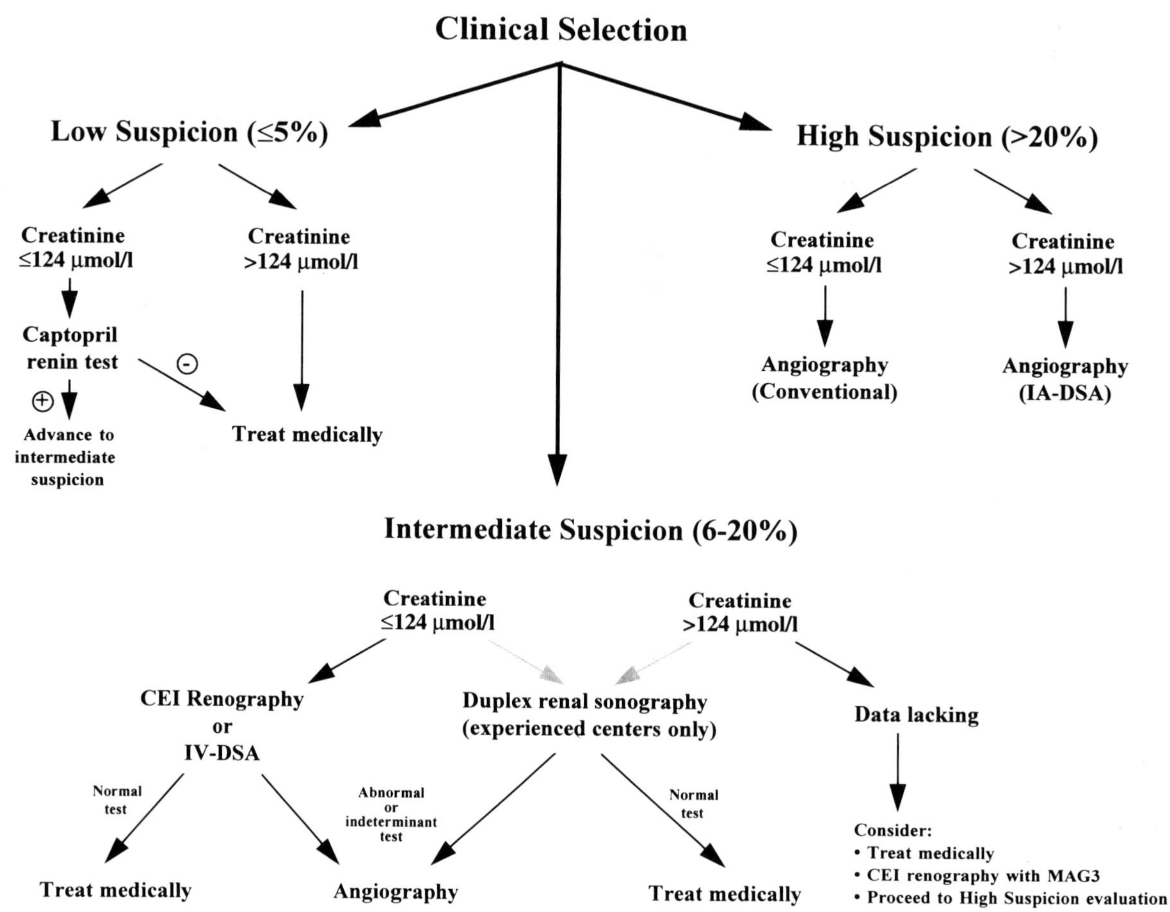

Figure 16.3. Proposed schema for the diagnosis of RVH.

For best results the captopril renin test must be performed when the patient is off antihypertensive medications for a short time. A positive captopril renin test only minimally increases the suspicion for RVH (positive predictive value ≈ 20%), and further evaluation should be performed according to the paradigm for the intermediate risk group. Patients with renal insufficiency in the low suspicion category should not have further testing for RVH since blood pressure elevation may be the result of the renal dysfunction and the low likelihood of detecting significant renovascular disease in this subgroup does not warrant the expense or the risk of testing. (Again we emphasize this procedure is for evaluation of RVH; evaluation for vascular disease causing renal dysfunction is discussed in other chapters.)

The combination of hypertension with an abdominal bruit, with Grade III or IV hypertensive retinopathy, or with acute renal failure after converting enzyme inhibition is highly suggestive of renovascular disease and places the patient into the high prevalence population (Fig. 16.3). Those patients with normal renal function (and no other contraindications for intravenous contrast) should proceed directly to renal arteriography. There is no advantage in performing other preliminary testing in this group: the lesser predictive value of other tests, even in attempts to define a *physiologically* active lesion, does not warrant their risk or expense in this situation. Patients with a high clinical suspicion of renovascular disease and renal insufficiency pose a dilemma. These patients have relative contraindications for angiography and intravenous contrast exposure, yet non-invasive testing is poorly characterized and has poor predictive value in this group. Ultrasonography with renal artery duplex/Doppler may be useful in avoiding arteriography, but duplex sonography can only be recommended for centers experienced in this technique. In the final analysis the clinician must determine the risk of vascular imaging and possible intervention vs the risk of continued medical management for an individual patient. Once the decision is made to proceed with diagnostic vascular imaging in patients with renal dysfunction, we recommend intra-arterial digital subtraction angiography which provides optimal vascular imaging while minimizing dye exposure to as little as 50 ml.

As noted above, atherosclerotic vascular disease with a single minor feature of RVH or the presence of several minor clinical features (Table 16.5) classifies the patient as intermediate probability for renovascular disease (Fig. 16.3). This group is the most difficult to evaluate. Arteriography cannot be justified as the initial diagnostic test since the great majority of patients will be subjected to potential morbidity only to find normal renal arteries. The subgroup of patients with normal renal function should undergo ^{99}Tc DTPA CEI renography (according to the protocol of Setaro[28] or intravenous digital subtraction renal arteriography. Renal artery duplex sonography is a viable option but only at those centers with extensive experience in this technique. One should select the appropriate test with great attention to the particular strengths of the institution performing the procedure. Independent of the type of test used, a normal result should preclude any further diagnostic evaluation. If the test result is positive or equivocal, the patient should proceed to arteriography in anticipation of further intervention. For those patients with renal insufficiency and an intermediate probability of RVH, accurate data are not available to offer further recommendations. In this group ^{99}Tc DTPA CEI renography can be unreliable. There is a theoretical advantage for MAG_3 captopril/furosemide renography in this population, but no prospective evaluation is available. Duplex renal sonography may be ideal for these patients, but operator variability determines the accuracy of the test and limits its widespread application. Intravenous DSA cannot be used in the setting of renal dysfunction because it requires a substantial amount of intravenous contrast. Pending more definitive data, we recommend MAG_3 renography in this subgroup of patients according to the protocol of Sfakianakis.[106] A normal test prevents further evaluation. An indeterminate test does not help the clinician confirm or exclude renovascular disease. A positive test result should increase the suspicion of, but does not confirm, renovascular disease: it should prompt consideration of further invasive testing with evaluation of the risks and potential benefits.

In summary, diagnostic testing for renovascular disease should only be performed in a clinically selected patient population. The level of suspicion for RVH helps determine which diagnostic test is performed, although the presence of renal insufficiency also influences this decision. The particular strengths of the testing institution should help direct selection of the most appropriate diagnostic procedure. Since RVH is a retrospective diagnosis made after treating an anatomic lesion, we recommend emphasis on the detection of RAS in the appropriate clinical setting and intervention when feasible. There is yet no definitive test for RVH, but advances in our understanding of renal pathophysiology and developments in renovascular imaging may eventually produce a non-invasive, reliable and relatively inexpensive procedure that can accurately predict this condition. In the meantime, careful consideration of the patient and of the currently available tests can frequently lead to appropriate diagnosis and treatment.

References

1 Harding MB, Smith LR, Himmelstein SI *et al.* (1992) Renal artery stenosis: prevalence and associated risk factors in patients undergoing routine cardiac catheterization. *J Am Soc Nephrol* 1992; **2:** 1608–16.

2 Olin JW, Melia M, Young JR *et al.* Prevalence of atherosclerotic renal artery stenosis in patients with atherosclerosis elsewhere. *Am J Med* 1990; **88:** 1-46–1-51.

3 Holley KE, Hunt JC, Brown AL *et al.* Renal artery stenosis: a clinical-pathologic study in normotensive and hypertensive patients. *Am J Med* 1964; **37:** 14–22.

4 Shipley RE, Gregg DE. The effect of external constriction of a blood vessel on blood flow. *Am J Physiol* 1944; **141:** 289–96.

5 Levin DC, Beckmann CF, Serur JR. Vascular resistance changes distal to progressive arterial stenosis: a critical reevaluation of the concept of vasodilator reserve. *Invest Radiol* 1980; **14:** 120–8.

6 Haimovici H, Zinicola N. Experimental renal-artery stenosis. Diagnostic significance of arterial hemodynamics. *J Cardiovasc Surg* 1962; **3:** 259–62.

7 Schreiber MJ, Pohl MA, Novick AC. The natural history of atherosclerotic and fibrous renal artery disease. *Urol Clin North Am* 1984; **11:** 383–92.

8 Meaney TF, Dustan HP, McCormack LJ. Natural history of renal arterial disease. *Radiology* 1968; **91:** 881–7.

9 Wollenweber J, Sheps SG, Davis GD. Clinical course of atherosclerotic renovascular disease. *Am J Cardiol* 1968; **21:** 60–71.

10 Dean RH, Kieffer RW, Smith BM *et al.* Renovascular hypertension: anatomic and functional changes during drug therapy. *Arch Surg* 1981; **116:** 1408–15.

11 Dean RH, Tribble RW, Hansen KJ *et al.* Evolution of renal insufficiency in ischemic nephropathy. *Ann Surg* 1991; **213:** 446–55.

12 Guzman RP, Zierler RE, Isaacson JA *et al.* Renal atrophy and arterial stenosis: a prospective study with duplex ultrasound. *Hypertension* 1994; **23:** 346–50.

13 Cronin RE. Radiocontrast media-induced acute renal failure. In Schrier RW, Gottschalk CW (eds) *Diseases of the Kidney*, pp. 1187–201. Boston, Toronto and London: Little, Brown, 1993.

14 Griner PF, Mayewski RJ, Mushlin AI, Greenland P. Selection and interpretation of diagnostic tests and procedures. I. Principles of test selection and use. *Ann Int Med* 1981; **94:** 559–63.

15 Griner PF, Mayewski RJ, Mushlin AI, Greenland P. Selection and interpretation of diagnostic tests and procedures. II. Principles of test interpretation. *Ann Int Med* 1981; **94:** 565–70.

16 Gifford RW Jr. Evaluation of the hypertensive patient with emphasis on detecting curable causes. *Milbank Mem Fund Q* 1969; **47:** 170–86.

17 Danielson M, Dammström BG. The prevalence of secondary and curable hypertension. *Acta Med Scand* 1981; **209:** 451–5.

18 Bech K, Hilden T. The frequency of secondary hypertension. *Acta Med Scand* 1975; **197:** 65–9.

19 Ward R. Familial aggregation and genetic epidemiology of blood pressure. In Laragh JH, Brenner BM (eds) *Hypertension: Pathophysiology, Diagnosis, and Management*, pp. 81–100. New York: Raven Press, 1990.

20 Keith TA III. Renovascular hypertension in black patients. *Hypertension* 1982; **4:** 438–43.

21 Svetkey LP, Kadir S, Dunnick NR *et al.* Similar prevalence of renovascular hypertension in selected blacks and whites. *Hypertension* 1991; **17:** 678–83.

22 Perera GA, Haelig AW. Clinical characteristics of hypertension associated with unilateral renal disease. *Circulation* 1952; **6:** 549–52.

23 Perloff D, Sokolow M, Wylie EJ *et al.* Hypertension secondary to renal artery occlusive disease. *Circulation* 1961; **24:** 1286–304.

24 Moser RJ Jr, Caldwell JR. Abdominal murmurs, an aid in the diagnosis of renal artery disease in hypertension. *Ann Int Med* 1962; **56:** 471–83.

25 Maxwell MH, Bleifer KH, Franklin SS, Varady PD. Cooperative study of renovascular hypertension: demographic analysis of the study. *JAMA* 1972; **220:** 1195–204.
26 Simon N, Franklin SS, Bleifer KH, Maxwell MH. Clinical characteristics of renovascular hypertension. *JAMA* 1972; **220:** 1209–18.
27 Svetkey LP, Helms MJ, Dunnick NR, Klotman PE. Clinical characteristics useful in screening for renovascular disease. *South Med J* 1990; **83:** 743–7.
28 Setaro JF, Saddler MC, Chen CC *et al.* Simplified captopril renography in diagnosis and treatment of renal artery stenosis. *Hypertension* 1991; **18:** 289–98.
29 Svetkey LP, Himmelstein SI, Dunnick NR *et al.* Prospective analysis of strategies for diagnosing renovascular hypertension. *Hypertension* 1989; **14:** 247–57.
30 Messina LM, Zelenock GB, Yao KA, Stanley JC. Renal revascularization for recurrent pulmonary edema in patients with poorly controlled hypertension and renal insufficiency: a distinct subgroup of patients with arteriosclerotic renal artery occlusive disease. *J Vasc Surg* 1992; **15:** 73–82.
31 Pickering TG, Herman L, Devereux RB *et al.* Recurrent pulmonary oedema in hypertension due to bilateral renal artery stenosis: treatment by angioplasty or surgical revascularization: *Lancet* 1988; **2:** 551–2.
32 Grim CE, Luft FC, Weinberger MH, Grim CM. Sensitivity and specificity of screening tests for renal vascular hypertension. *Ann Int Med* 1979; **91:** 617–22.
33 Davis BA, Crook JE, Vestal RE, Oates JA. Prevalence of renovascular hypertension in patients with grade III or IV hypertensive retinopathy. *N Engl J Med* 1979; **301:** 1273–6.
34 Jacobson HR. Ischemic renal disease: an overlooked clinical entity? *Kidney Int* 1988; **34:** 729–43.
35 Fotino S, Sporn P. Nonoliguric acute renal failure after captopril therapy. *Arch Int Med* 1983; **143:** 1252–3.
36 Hollenberg GG, Clarkson AR, Woodroffe AJ, Farris J. Medical therapy of renovascular hypertension: efficacy and safety of captopril in 269 patients. *Cardiovasc Res* 1983; **4:** 852–76.
37 Hricik DE, Browning PJ, Kopelman R *et al.* Captopril-induced functional renal insufficiency in patients with bilateral renal artery stenoses or renal artery stenosis in a solitary kidney. *N Engl J Med* 1983; **308:** 373–6.
38 Ying CY, Tifft CP, Gavras H, Chobanian AV. Renal revascularization in the azotemic hypertensive patient resistant to therapy. *N Engl J Med* 1984; **311:** 1070–5.
39 Goldblatt H, Lynch J, Hanzal RF, Summerville WW. Studies on experimental hypertension. I. The production of persistent elevation of systolic blood pressure by means of renal ischemia. *J Exp Med* 1934; **59:** 347–79.
40 Goldblatt H. Studies on experimental hypertension. V. The pathogenesis of experimental hypertension due to renal ischemia. *Ann Int Med* 1937; **11:** 69–103.
41 Ploth DW. Angiotensin-dependent renal mechanisms in two-kidney, one-clip renal vascular hypertension. *Am J Physiol* 1983; **245:** F131–F141.
42 Vaughan ED Jr. Renovascular hypertension. *Kidney Int* 1985; **27:** 811–27.
43 Laragh JH, Baer L, Brunner HR *et al.* Renin, angiotensin, and aldosterone system in pathogenesis and management of hypertensive vascular disease. *Am J Med* 1972; **52:** 633–52.
44 Brunner HR, Laragh JH, Baer L *et al.* Essential hypertension: renin and aldosterone, heart attack and stroke. *N Engl J Med* 1972; **284:** 441–9.
45 Wilcox CS. Use of angiotensin-converting-enzyme inhibitors for diagnosing renovascular hypertension. *Kidney Int* 1993; **44:** 1379–90.
46 Sealey JE, Bühler FR, Laragh JH, Vaughan ED Jr. The physiology of renin secretion in essential hypertension: estimation of renin secretion rate and renal plasma flow from peripheral and renal vein renin levels. *Am J Med* 1973; **55:** 391–401.
47 Vaughan ED Jr, Bühler FR, Laragh JH *et al.* Renovascular hypertension: renin measurements to indicate hypersecretion and contralateral suppression, estimate renal plasma flow, and score for surgical curability. *Am J Med* 1973; **55:** 402–14.
48 Wilcox CS, Dzau VJ. Effect of captopril on the release of the components of the renin-angiotensin system into plasma and lymph. *J Am Soc Nephrol* 1992; **2:** 1241–50.
49 Jonker GJ, de Zeeuw D, Huisman RM *et al.* Angiotensin converting enzyme inhibition improves diagnostic procedures for renovascular hypertension in dogs. *Hypertension* 1988; **12:** 411–19.
50 Müller FB, Sealey JE, Case DB *et al.* The captopril test for identifying renovascular disease in hypertensive patients. *Am J Med* 1986; **80:** 633–44.
51 Gaul MK, Linn WD, Mulrow CD. Captopril-stimulated renin secretion in the diagnosis of renovascular hypertension. *Am J Hypertension* 1989; **2:** 335–40.
52 Frederickson ED, Wilcox CS, Bucci CM *et al.* A prospective evaluation of a simplified captopril test for the detection of renovascular hypertension. *Arch Int Med* 1990; **150:** 569–72.
53 Svetkey LP, Wilkinson R Jr, Dunnick NR *et al.* Captopril renography in the diagnosis of renovascular disease. *Am J Hypertension* 1991; **4:** 711S–715S.
54 Postma CT, van der Steen PHM, Hoefnagels

WHL *et al.* The captoril test in the detection of renovascular disease in hypertensive patients. *Arch Int Med* 1990; **150:** 625–8.
55 Gosse P, Dupas JY, Reynaud P *et al.* Captopril test in the detection of renovascular hypertension in a population with low prevalence of the disease: a prospective study. *Am J Hypertension* 1989; **2:** 191–3.
56 Case DB, Laragh JH. Reactive hyperreninemia in renovascular hypertension after angiotensin blockade with saralasin or converting enzyme inhibitor. *Ann Int Med* 1979; **91:** 153–60.
57 Cohen EL, Rovner DR, Conn JW. Postural augmentation of plasma renin activity. Importance in diagnosis of renovascular hypertension. *JAMA* 1966; **197:** 973–8.
58 Strong CG, Hunt JC, Sheps SG *et al.* Renal venous renin activity: enhancement of sensitivity of lateralization by sodium depletion. *Am J Cardiol* 1971; **27:** 602–11.
59 Kaneko Y, Ikeda T, Takeda T, Ueda H. Renin release during acute reduction of arterial pressure in normotensive subjects and patients with renovascular hypertension. *J Clin Invest* 1967; **46:** 705–16.
60 Wilson HM, Wilson JP, Slaton PE *et al.* Saralasin infusion in the recognition of renovascular hypertension. *Ann Int Med* 1977; **87:** 36–42.
61 Re R, Novelline R, Escourrou MT, Athanasoulis C *et al.* Inhibition of angiotensin-converting enzyme for diagnosis of renal-artery stenosis. *N Eng J Med* 1978; **298:** 582–6.
62 Pickering TG, Sos TA, Vaughan ED Jr, *et al.* Predictive value and changes of renin secretion in hypertensive patients with unilateral renovascular disease undergoing successful renal angioplasty. *Am J Med* 1984; **76:** 398–404.
63 Thibonnier M, Joseph A, Sassano P *et al.* Improved diagnosis of unilateral renal artery lesions after captopril administration. *JAMA* 1984; **251:** 56–60.
64 Lyons DF, Streck WF, Kem DC *et al.* Captropril stimulation of differential renins in renovascular hypertension. *Hypertension* 1983; **5:** 615–22.
65 Tomoda F, Takata M, Ohashi S *et al.* Captopril-stimulated renal vein renin in hypertensive patients with or without renal artery stenosis. *Am J Hypertension* 1990; **3:** 918–26.
66 Roubidoux MA, Dunnick NR, Klotman PE *et al.* Renal vein renins: inability to predict response to revascularization in patients with hypertension. *Radiology* 1991; **178:** 819–22.
67 Oei HY, Geyskes GG, Roos GC *et al.* Diagnosis of unilateral renal artery stenosis by captopril renography. (Abstract.) *Eur J Nucl Med* 1984; **9:** A24.
68 Jackson B, McGrath BP, Matthews PG *et al.* Differential renal function during angiotensin converting enzyme inhibition in renovascular hypertension. *Hypertension* 1986; **8:** 650–4.
69 Nally JV, Clarke HS, Grecos GP, *et al.* Effect of captopril on 99mTc-diethylenetriaminepentaacetic acid renograms in two-kidney, one clip hypertension. *Hypertension* 1986; **8:** 685–93.
70 Mann SJ, Pickering TG, Sos TA *et al.* Captopril renography in the diagnosis of renal artery stenosis: accuracy and limitations. *Am J Med* 1991; **90:** 30–40.
71 Nally JV Jr, Chen C, Fine E *et al.* Diagnostic criteria of renovascular hypertension with captopril renography: a consensus statement. *Am J Hypertension* 1991; **4:** 749S–752S.
72 Fommei E, Mezzasalma L, Ghione S *et al.* European captopril radionuclide test multicenter study. Preliminary results. Inspective renographic analysis. *Am J Hypertension* 1991; **4:** 690S–679S.
73 Erbslöh-Möller B, Dumas A, Roth DS *et al.* Furosemide-[131] I-hippuran renography after angiotensin-converting enzyme inhibition for the diagnosis of renovascular hypertension. *Am J Med* 1991; **90:** 23–9.
74 Davidson R, Wilcox CS, Diagnostic usefulness of renal scanning after angiotensin converting enzyme inhibitors. *Hypertension* 1991; **18:** 299–303.
75 Dondi M, Monetti N, Fanti S *et al.* Use of technitium-99m-MAG$_3$ for renal scintigraphy after angiotensin-converting enzyme inhibition. *J Nucl Med* 1991; **32:** 424–8.
76 Fommei E, Ghione S, Palla L *et al.* Renal scintigraphic captopril test in the diagnosis of renovascular hypertension. *Hypertension* 1987; **10:** 212–20.
77 Geyskes GG, Oei HY, Puylaert CBAJ *et al.* Renovascular hypertension identified by captopril-induced changes in the renogram. *Hypertension* 1987; **9:** 451–8.
78 Dondi M, Fanti S, DeFabritiis A *et al.* Prognostic value of captopril renal scintigraphy in renovascular hypertension. *J Nucl Med* 1992; **33:** 2040–4.
79 Datseris JE, Bomanji JB, Brown EA *et al.* Captopril renal scintigraphy in patients with hypertension and chronic renal failure. *J Nucl Med* 1994; **35:** 251–4.
80 Maxwell MH, Gonick HC, Wiita R, Kaufman JJ. Use of the rapid-sequence intravenous pyelogram in the diagnosis of renovascular hypertension. *N Eng J Med* 1964; **270:** 213–20.
81 Bookstein JJ, Abrams HL, Buenger RE *et al.* Radiologic aspects of renovascular hypertension. Part I. Aims and methods of the radiology study group. *JAMA* 1972; **220:** 1218–24.
82 Bookstein JJ, Abrams HL, Buenger RE *et al.* Radiologic aspects of renovascular hypertension. Part II. The role of urography in unilateral renovascular disease. *JAMA* 1972; **220:** 1225–30.
83 Thornbury JR, Stanley JC, Fryback DG.

Hypertensive urogram: a nondiscriminatory test for renovascular hypertension. *Am J Roentgenol* 1982; **138:** 43–9.

84 Kohler TR, Zierler RE, Martin RL *et al.* Noninvasive diagnosis of renal artery stenosis by ultrasonic duplex scanning. *J Vasc Surg* 1986; **4:** 450–6.

85 Desberg AL, Paushter DM, Lammert GK *et al.* Renal artery stenosis: evaluation with color Doppler flow imaging. *Radiology* 1990; **177:** 749–53.

86 Hoffman U, Edwards JM, Carter S *et al.* Role of duplex scanning for the detection of atherosclerotic renal artery disease. *Kidney Int* 1991; **39:** 1232–9.

87 Hansen KJ, Tribble RW, Reavis SW *et al.* Renal duplex sonography: evaluation of clinical utility. *J Vasc Surg* 1990; **12:** 227–36.

88 Taylor DC, Kettler MD, Moneta GL *et al.* Duplex ultrasound scanning in the diagnosis of renal artery stenosis: a prospective evaluation. *J Vasc Surg* 1988; **7:** 363–9.

89 Berland LL, Koslin DB, Routh WD, Keller FS. Renal artery stenosis: prospective evaluation of diagnosis with color duplex US compared with angiography. Work in progress. *Radiology* 1990; **174:** 421–3.

90 Kotval PS. Doppler waveform parvus and tardus: a sign of proximal flow obstruction. *J Ultrasound Med* 1989; **8:** 435–40.

91 Stavros AT, Parker SH, Yakes WF *et al.* Segmental stenosis of the renal artery: pattern recognition of tardus and parvus abnormalities with duplex sonography. *Radiology* 1992; **184:** 487–92.

92 Kleiwer MA, Tupler RH, Carroll BA *et al.* Renal artery stenosis: analysis of Doppler waveform parameters and tardus parvus pattern. *Radiology* 1993; **189:** 779–87.

93 Rubin GD, Dake MD, Napel SA *et al.* Three-dimensional spiral CT angiography of the abdomen: initial clinical experience. *Radiology* 1993; **186:** 147–52.

94 Rubin GD, Walker PJ, Dake MD *et al.* Three-dimensional spiral computed tomographic angiography: an alternative imaging modality for the abdominal aorta and its branches. *J Vasc Surg* 1993; **18:** 656–66.

95 Galanski M, Prokop M, Chavan A *et al.* Renal artery stenoses: spiral CT angiography. *Radiology* 1993; **189:** 185–92.

96 Rubin GD, Dake MD, Napel S *et al.* Spiral CT of renal artery stenosis: comparison of three-dimensional rendering techniques. *Radiology* 1994; **190:** 181–9.

97 Kim D, Edelman RR, Kent KC *et al.* Abdominal aorta and renal artery stenosis: evaluation with MR angiography. *Radiology* 1990; **174:** 727–31.

98 Debatin JF, Spritzer CE, Grist TM *et al.* Imaging of the renal arteries: value of MR Angiography. *Am J Roentgenol* 1991; **157:** 981–90.

99 Loubeyre P, Revel D, Garcia P *et al.* Screening patients for renal artery stenosis: value of three-dimensional time-of-flight MR angiography. *Am J Roentgenol* 1994; **162:** 847–52.

100 Havey RJ, Krumlovsky F, delGreco F, Martin HG. Screening for renovascular hypertension: is digital-subtraction angiography the preferred noninvasive test? *JAMA* 1985; **254:** 388–93.

101 Dunnick NR, Svetkey LP, Cohan RH *et al.* Intravenous digital substraction renal angiography: use in screening for renovascular hypertension. *Radiology* 1989; **171:** 219–22.

102 Smith CW, Winfield AC, Price RR *et al.* Evaluation of digital venous angiography for the diagnosis of renovascular hypertension. *Radiology* 1982; **144:** 51–4.

103 Clark RA, Alexander ES. Digital subtraction angiography of the renal arteries: prospective comparison with conventional arteriography. *Invest Radiol* 1983; **18:** 6–10.

104 Campbell DR, Mason WF, Flemming BK, Fraser DB. Digital subtraction arteriography in the diagnosis of renovascular hypertension. *J Can Assoc Radiol* 1983; **34:** 261–3.

105 Kim D, Porter DH, Brown R *et al.* Renal artery imaging: a prospective comparison of intra-arterial digital subtraction angiography with conventional angiography. *Angiology* 1991; **42:** 345–57.

106 Sfakianakis GN, Bourgoignie JJ. Renographic diagnosis of renovascular hypertension with angiotensin converting enzyme inhibition and furosemide. *Am J Hypertension* 1991; **4:** 706S–710S.

17

Screening and diagnosis of renal vascular hypertension

RICHARD H DEAN

Introduction

Historically, evaluation of patients for renovascular occlusive disease has evolved through several screening methods. During respective eras, rapid sequence intravenous pyelography, peripheral plasma renin activity, infusion of angiotensin II antagonists, and radionuclide renography have been suggested as valuable screening tests to detect functionally significant renovascular disease. Nevertheless, none of these methods has survived close scrutiny or sustained use owing to a lack of sensitivity, specificity, or both. Although standard 'cut-film' renal arteriography has continued to be the most reliable method to identify renovascular lesions potentially causing renovascular hypertension (RVH), its cost and invasiveness have limited its widespread use for this purpose. This reluctance is augmented when renal insufficiency coexists due to the potential nephrotoxicity of contrast material in such patients. These limitations of arteriography as a screening tool have led to the continued search for an accurate non-invasive technique with which to base decisions regarding more invasive angiographic evaluation.

Currently the most popular screening tests to identify renal artery occlusive disease are renal duplex sonography and isotope renography before and after captopril ingestion or exercise. Prior to review of their use, however, a perspective on which hypertensive patient requires such screening diagnostic studies is appropriate. One could argue that the most important screening test is the medical history, physical examination and routine blood chemistries. Obviously, the accurate exclusion of some patients from further study by such simple measures allows a more reasoned approach to application of more complex screening tests in the remaining hypertensive population.

Clinical characteristics

Renovascular hypertension is a severe form of hypertension and probably represents only 1–5% of the entire hypertensive population. Because the renovascular form tends to be relatively severe, its prevalence in the large subpopulation of mildly hypertensive patients (untreated diastolic blood pressure less than 105 mmHg) is probably negligible. In contrast, however, it occurs frequently in the smaller group of severely hypertensive people. Hollifield investigated 137 patients with previously unrecognized hypertension who were discovered through a shopping center screening program (Table 17.1). Diagnostic study of these patients included arteriography and, when appropriate, renal vein renin assays and split renal function studies. In the more severely hypertensive group, none of the 13 black patients had RVH, whereas the disorder occurred in 9 of the 22 white patients (41%). Similarly, Davis and colleagues have shown a 31% incidence of RVH in 85 patients

Table 17.1. Results of screening 137 new hypertensive patients[a]

Diastolic blood pressure	No. of patients	No. with RVH	%
90–115 mmHg	102	0	
> 117 mmHg	35	9	26
Black	13	0	
White	22	9	41

From JW Hollifield (unpublished data).

initially evaluated at Vanderbilt University for malignant hypertension.[1]

In our experience, severe hypertension at the two extremes of life carries the highest probability of being of renovascular origin. Our review of the causes of hypertension in 74 children admitted for diagnostic evaluation over a 5-year period showed that in 78% of those less than 5 years old it had a correctable renovascular origin.[2] Interestingly, after childhood, the age group that is next most likely to have RVH is the elderly. In our center, 33% of patients over 60 years old admitted for evaluation have had the disorder. Certainly, these elderly patients represent the more severe spectrum of hypertension, for those with less severe levels most likely would not have been referred to our center.

On the basis of these data, it is inappropriate to view hypertensive patients as a homogeneous group with respect to the prevalence of RVH. Rather, the probability of finding a renovascular origin correlates with the severity of the hypertension. Accordingly, the search for the disease should be directed to the subset of patients with the more severe degree of hypertension. It must be remembered, however, that severity of hypertension is based on its level without medication and does not take into account the difficulty of its control by drug therapy.

Because of the relative infrequency of RVH in the entire hypertensive population, many reports have focused on the value of demographic factors, physical findings and screening tests to discriminate between it and essential hypertension as a basis for deciding to pursue further diagnostic study. Most frequently quoted among these are recent onset of hypertension, young age, lack of family history of hypertension and the presence of an abdominal bruit. The most complete study comparing the clinical characteristics of patients with RVH and those with essential hypertension was the Cooperative Study of Renovascular Hypertension.[3] In that study, the prevalence of certain clinical characteristics in 339 patients with essential hypertension was compared with their prevalence in 175 patients with RVH secondary to atherosclerotic lesions (91 patients) and fibromuscular dysplasia (84 patients). A summary of the differential points identified in that study is presented in Table 17.2. Although several characteristics show significant differences in prevalence between the two disorders, *none* of them has sufficient discriminative value to be used to exclude patients from further diagnostic investigation for RVH. Certainly, the finding of an epigastric bruit in a young white woman with malignant hypertension is strongly suggestive of a renovascular origin of the hypertension. However, the absence of such criteria does not exclude the presence of the disease, and such criteria should not be used to eliminate patients from further diagnostic study. Therefore, one should base the decision for diagnostic study on the severity of hypertension. Mild hypertension has a minimal chance of being renovascular in origin. In contrast, the more severe the hypertension the greater the probability that it is from a correctable cause. With this in mind, we submit all patients with diastolic blood pressure above 115 mmHg who would be acceptable candidates for operation to evaluation for a correctable origin of hypertension.

Diagnostic evaluation

The general evaluation of all hypertensive patients is outlined in Table 17.3. Electrocardiography is important to gauge the extent of secondary myocardial hypertrophy or associated ischemic heart disease. Serum electrolytes and serial serum

Table 17.2. Clinical considerations in hypertension and RVH[a]

	Essential hypertension (339 cases)		Renovascular hypertension: Arteriosclerotic (91 cases)		Renovascular hypertension: Fibromuscular (84 cases)	
	%	Years	%	Years	%	Years
History						
Average age <20 years	2	41	1	48	14	35
Average duration		3.1		1.9		2.0
<1 year	10		23		19	
>10 years	23		12		10	
Average age at onset		35		46		33[b]
>50 years	7		39		3[b]	
<20 years	12		2		16[b]	
Sex (female)	40		34		81	
Race (black)	29		7		10	
Acceleration of hypertension	13		23		14	
Family history						
Hypertension	67		68[b]		41	
Stroke 37			44[b]		22	
Neither of foregoing	19		30[b]		46	
Symptoms						
Nocturia	38		55		35	
Weakness, fatigue	32		49		42[b]	
Angina						
Headache						
All of foregoing	0		14		10	
Previous vascular occlusive disease	10		20		6	
Physical examination						
Body habitus						
Obese	38		17		11	
Thin	6		13[b]		30	
Fundi (Grades 3 and 4)	12		26		10[b]	
Bruit						
Abdomen	6		38		55	
Flank	1		8		20	
Abdomen or flank	7		41		57	

[a] From the Cooperative Study of Renovascular Hypertension.[3]
[b] Differences are statistically different at the 5% level except where so designated.

Table 17.3. General evaluation of patients with hypertension

History and physical examination
Hemogram, SMA-12, urinalysis, urine culture, serum potassium (3 times)
Electrocardiogram and chest X-ray
Analysis of 24-h urine collection for creatinine clearance, electrolytes, catecholamines, vanillylmandelic acid and 17-hydroxy steroids and ketosteroids
Creatinine clearance
Renal duplex sonography

SMA: Serum multiple analysis

potassium determinations can effectively exclude patients with primary aldosteronism if potassium levels are greater than 3.0 mg/dl. One must remember, however, that hypokalemia is most often due to salt-depleting diets and previous diuretic therapy. Estimation of renal function is mandatory. A rough gauge of excretory impairment can be obtained simply by measuring a serum creatinine. When this shows an impairment, a 24-h creatinine clearance measurement is appropriate. Finally, assessment of the urinary 17-hydroxy and ketosteroid and vanillylmandelic acid levels will effectively identify the rare patient with a pheochromocytoma or a functioning adrenal cortical tumor. These latter studies are performed only when some part of the medical history or initial assessment increase the suspicion of their presence.

Renal duplex sonography

Through continued improvements in probe design and duplex sonographic technology, imaging and Doppler-shift interrogation of deep abdominal vasculature has been introduced as a potentially accurate screening method to identify and quantify visceral and renal artery occlusive disease. Our clinical experience with its use has centered on evaluation of renovascular disease. We have evaluated the role of duplex sonography as an initial surface screening test, an intraoperative study to confirm technical success of reconstructive procedures and as a postoperative surveillance method to follow progression of disease and stability of reconstructions. This discussion will summarize the methods we use for these studies and our results to date.

Technically successful studies defined as a complete main renal artery interrogation from aortic origin to renal bilum should be obtained in almost 95% of cases. These results are ensured by proper patient preparation and method of examination. Details of the conduct of the procedure are covered elsewhere.[4]

Renal duplex sonography (RDS) criteria for critical renal artery stenosis are depicted in Table 17.4. Assuming that RA-PSV varied with the degree of renal artery stenosis and aortic PSV (i.e. inflow), most authors[5–8] have advocated the ratio of RA-PSV to aortic PSV (the renal–aortic ratio) to define critical renal artery stenosis. In contrast, we have found no relationship between RA-PSV and aortic PSV in the presence or absence of disease (Fig. 17.1). Focal RA-PSV 2 m/s or more in combination with distal poststenotic turbulence has proved to correlate highly with the angiographic presence of 60% or greater diameter-reducing stenosis of the renal artery.[4] In 122 kidneys with single renal arteries with renal angiography for comparison, RDS correctly identified 67 of 68 kidneys with normal and less than 60% renal artery stenosis, and 35 of 39 kidneys with 60–99% renal artery stenosis (Table 17.5). All 15 renal artery occlusions were correctly identified by failure to

Table 17.4. Doppler velocity criteria for B-scan defects

Defect	Criteria
< 60% diameter-reducing RA defect	RA-PSV from entire RA < 2.0 m/s
≥ 60% diameter-reducing RA defect	Focal RA-PSV ≥ 2.0 m/s and distal turbulent velocity waveform
Occlusion	Doppler-shifted signal from renal artery B-scan image
Inadequate study for interpretation	Failure to obtain Doppler samples from entire main renal artery

RA: Renal artery; RA-PSV: Renal artery peak systolic velocity

Table 17.5. Comparative analysis parameter estimates and their 95% confidence intervals

Group	*N*	Measure	Estimate	95% Confidence interval
All kidneys	142 (kidneys)	Sensitivity	0.88	(0.84–0.92)
		Specificity	0.99	(0.97–1.00)
		PV+	0.98[b]	(0.96–0.99)
		PV–	0.92[c]	(0.89–0.95)
	148 (kidneys)	Accuracy	0.91	(0.87–0.95)
Kidneys with single renal artery	122 (kidneys)	Sensitivity	0.93	(0.90–0.96)
		Specificity	0.98[b]	(0.96–1.00)
		PV+	0.98[c]	(0.96–1.00)
		PV–	0.94	(0.91–0 97)
	148 (kidneys)	Accuracy	0.91	(0.87–0.95)
Kidneys with multiple renal arteries	21 (arteries)	Sensitivity	0.67	(0.53–0.81)
		Specificity	1.00[a]	–
		PV+	1.00[a, b]	–
		PV–	0.79[c]	(0.68–0.90)
		Accuracy	0.86	(0.76–0.96)
	74 (subjects)	Sensitivity	0.93	(0.87–0.99)
All patients		Specificity	1.00*a*	–
		PV+	1.00[a, b]	–
		PV–	0.91[c]	(0.84–0.98)
		Accuracy	0.96	(0.91–1.00)

[a] Estimated standard error is zero, confidence level is inestimable.
[b] PV+, positive predictive value.
[c] PV–, negative predictive value.

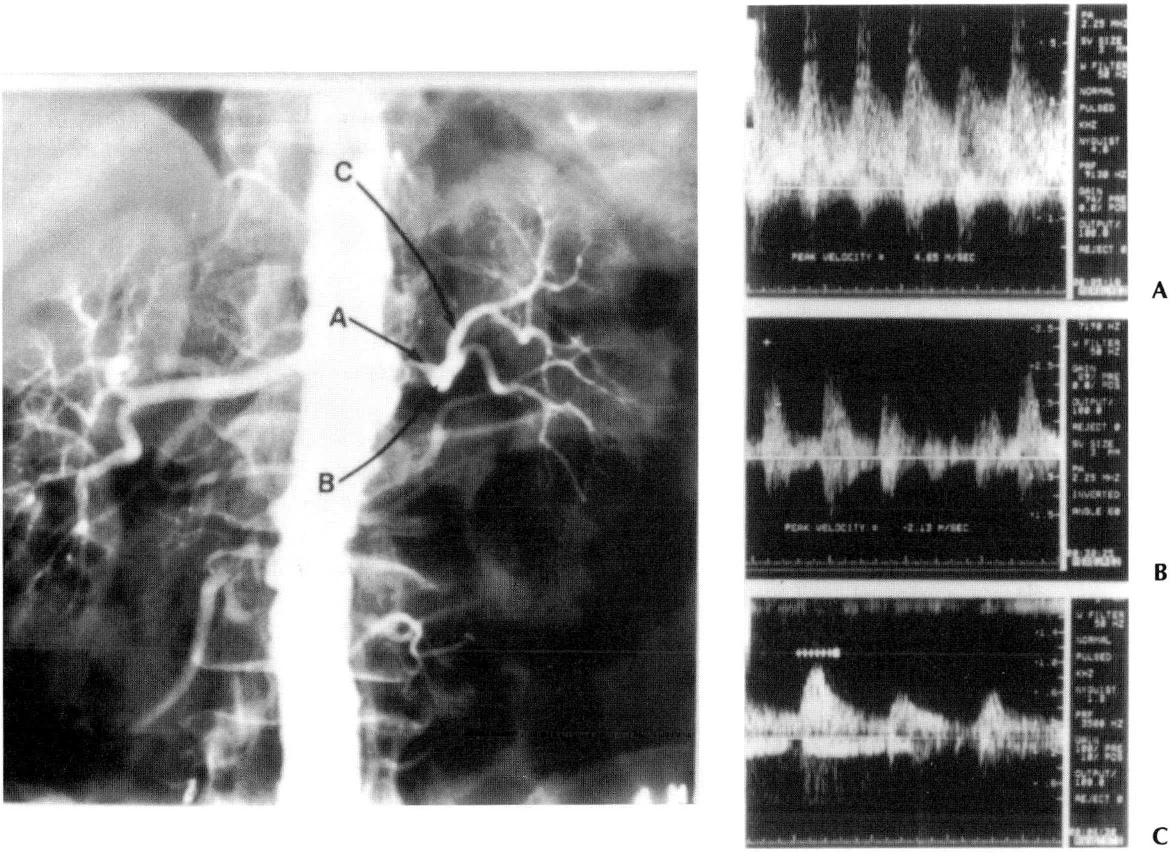

Figure 17.1. Radiographic cut-film angiogram demonstrating high grade left renal artery stenosis. (A) Doppler spectral analysis at the site of stenosis demonstrating focal increase in RA-PSV (4.6 m/s). (B) Distal spectral analysis demonstrating turbulent waveform-decreased RA-PSV with ragged spectral envelope and spontaneous bidirectional signals. (C) Spectral analysis several vessel diameters distal to stenosis demonstrating return of near normal waveform.

obtain a Doppler-shifted signal from an imaged renal artery. Using this methodology and criteria for interpretation, renal duplex was 93% sensitive and 98% specific, with a positive predictive value of 98% and a negative predictive value of 94 percent. Overall accuracy was 96% when compared prospectively with cut-film angiography.

Multiple or polar renal arteries pose a potentially serious limitation of surface RDS. Of the patients presenting to our institution for evaluation of RVH 19% have had polar renal arteries by angiography. Among these patients, 43% have had multiple vessels to both kidneys and 40% of all the multiple vessels have demonstrated 60% or greater diameter-reducing stenosis or occlusion. Because of variable polar vessel origin, small vessel size and compromised image quality associated with low frequency probes, identification of polar vessels and their associated disease is difficult. In our validity analysis of surface RDS, we identified only 1 of 43 polar arteries. Although Doppler color flow has enhanced recognition of multiple renal arteries, failure to identify these polar vessels and their associated disease constituted the largest single source of false negative studies.

The pertinence of RDS insensitivity to polar vessel disease relates to the prevalence of such disease within the patient population examined and the clinical indication for surface RDS. Fourteen percent of our patients who were submitted to repair for unilateral renovascular disease and presumed RVH have had only polar branch disease. We believe this group constitutes a significant minority of patients. Therefore, we proceed with conventional angiography in patients less than 60 years of age with poorly controlled hypertension despite multidrug therapy, even in the presence of a negative surface RDS. When RDS is used to screen for ischemic nephropathy and renal insufficiency, however, a negative RDS study effectively excludes significant RVD, since polar vessel disease alone does not account for renal insufficiency.[9]

Captopril renal scintigraphy

To grasp the basis of captopril renal scintigraphy (CRS) one must understand some of the components of renal excretory physiology and the importance of the renin—angiotensin system in maintenance of homeostasis. Glomerular filtration is governed partially by the relative tone of the afferent and efferent arterioles. During periods recognized by the juxtaglomerular apparatus of reduced blood pressure (e.g. proximal renal artery stenosis) increased renin is released which ultimately leads to an increase in the level of angiotensin II. Angiotensin II acts predominantly to vasoconstrict the efferent arteriole to maintain renal glomerular perfusion pressure and filtration. When an angiotensin II converting enzyme inhibitor such as captopril is given in this circumstance, an acute reduction in the amount of angiotensin II occurs. This, in turn, leads to a reduction in vasoconstriction of the efferent arteriole and a decrease in the glomerular filtration pressure. Therefore, CRS is a study which is composed of a baseline renogram and a repeat renogram performed after a dose of captopril. A test is considered positive when a normal baseline scan becomes abnormal after captopril administration by either an increase in the time to peak activity to more than 11 min or by a normal glomerular filtration ratio between the two sides increasing to greater than 1.5:1 (Fig. 17.2). In experienced hands this study is reported to be highly reliable.[10] Unfortunately, it is less reliable when significant parenchymal disease is present. For that reason, we have not relied on its results to stop workup in the azotemic group.

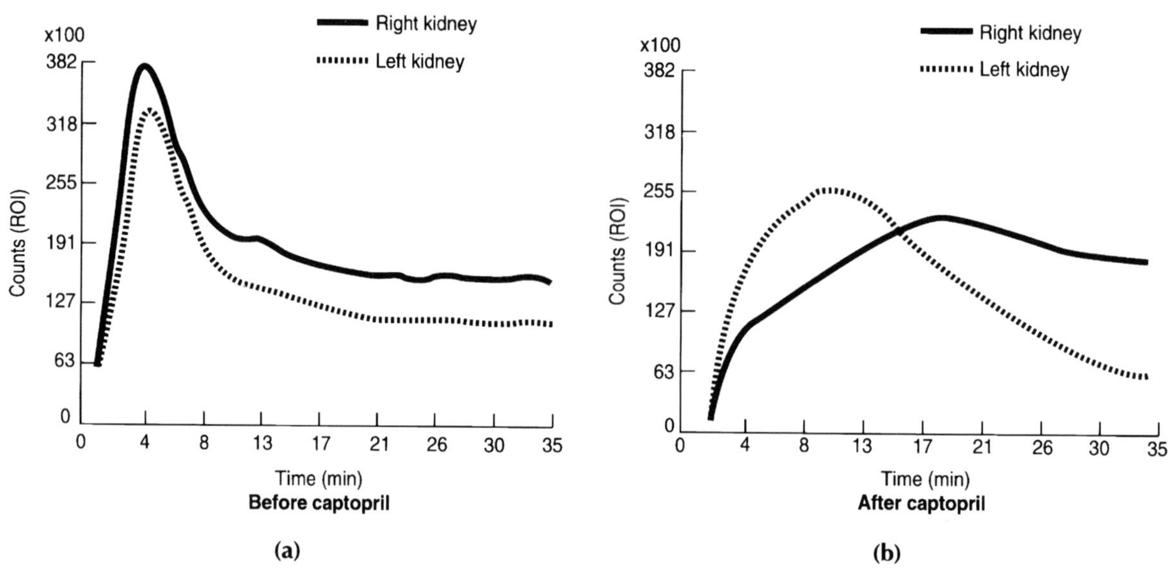

Figure 17.2. Captopril renal scintigraphy before (a) and after (b) captopril ingestion demonstrating the positive finding of a slowing of the rate of isotope clearance and time to peak radioactivity after captopril.

Renal arteriography

There continues to be controversy over the use of aortography and renal arteriography in the routine screening of hypertensive individuals. Some believe it should be reserved for select groups of patients. We do not share this conservative view and proceed with arteriography in circumstances summarized elsewhere in this chapter. Both aortography and selective renal arteriography using multiple projections may be necessary to examine adequately the entire renal artery. The proximal third of the left renal artery usually courses anteriorly, the middle third transversely and the distal third posteriorly, whereas the right renal artery pursues a more consistent posterior course. Lesions in the renal artery that are coursing anteriorly or posteriorly are frequently not seen or may appear insignificant in an anteroposterior (AP) aortogram. Oblique aortography or oblique selective renal arteriography will project these portions of the vessels in profile and identify the stenosis. Delicate septal lesions of fibromuscular dysplasia may be unrecognizable or appear insignificant in the AP projection, whereas in the oblique projection the true severity is demonstrated.

The introduction of digital subtraction angiography (DSA) has broadened enthusiasm for the use of angiography in screening for renovascular disease. Although the intravenous route of contrast injection for DSA was initially thought to be useful for this evaluation, this method provides such poor delineation that many fibromuscular dysplastic lesions are missed and one cannot evaluate branch vessels with any accuracy. In addition, the amount of contrast material used for intravenous DSA is contraindicated in patients with reduced renal function. In contrast, intra-arterial DSA can be performed as an outpatient procedure and is useful in some patients. Depending on resolution, however, even this technique can miss some lesions and inadequately define branch disease. For these reasons, we continue to primarily rely on standard cut-film arteriography for most evaluations.

Definitive functional studies

Two tests, renal vein renin assays and split renal function studies, have proven valuable in confirming the functional significance of renal artery stenosis. Neither have great value, however, when severe bilateral disease or disease in the renal artery supplying a single kidney is present. In these circumstances, the decision for operation is based on the severity of hypertension and the degree of renal insufficiency. Further, urologically performed split renal function studies are no longer done in any center studying patients with RVH. Therefore the reader is referred to earlier texts describing their use historically.[11]

Renal vein renin assays

When a unilateral obstructive lesion is found by renal arteriography, its functional significance should be evaluated. Most centers now rely on renal vein renin (RVR) assays to establish the diagnosis of RVH. Understanding the specifics of the performance of RVR assays is imperative in order for the test to provide valid results. There are many factors that affect the results of RVR assays that, if not properly managed, will lead to erroneous results.

The effect of antihypertensive medications and unrestricted sodium intake on renin release, and thereby RVR, is widely recognized. Many antihypertensive medications, especially those that function through β-adrenergic blockade, suppress renin output and can lead to false non-lateralization of RVR. Before one can consider that there is no drug interference in the release of renin, all such medications must have been withheld for at least 5 days prior to the measurement of RVR. Similar effects on renin levels are seen when sodium intake is not restricted. For this reason, the patient must be on no more than a 2 g sodium diet for at least 2 weeks prior to the study.

Probably the most common situation currently producing erroneous results of RVR assays is the chronic use of angiotensin converting enzyme (ACE) inhibitors. Since these drugs block angiotensin II production they also block the negative feedback mechanism controlling renin production. Consequently, renin activity will be too high to interpret in the effluent from both kidneys regardless of the presence or absence of renal artery lesions. For this reason, ACE inhibitors should be stopped at least 5 days prior to RVR assay. The preparation of patients for RVR assays in our center is summarized in Table 17.6.

The technical aspects of performing RVR assays cannot be overemphasized as a potential source of error. Since the left renal vein contains not only renal venous effluent but also adrenal, gonadal, and lumbar venous effluent, misplacement of the venous catheter into the origin of one of the non-renal branches or sampling in the proximal renal vein where a mixture from these other sources is present may dilute the renin activity coming from the kidney. This will lead to erroneously low measurements of renin activity and produce a false interpretation of RVR.

The time of sampling the two renal veins for renin activity is also a potential source of error in RVR assays. In studies performed with a single catheter, several minutes may elapse between sampling the two renal veins as the catheter is switched from one side to the other. Furthermore, catheter manipulation and patient discomfort may affect renin release. It is not surprising, therefore, that when the single catheter is employed, both false positive and false negative RVR ratios are frequent.

Several methods of stimulating renin release have been suggested over the past 15 years. These include tilting the patient to the upright posture during the study, stimulation with intravenous hydralazine, and, more recently, nitroprusside and captopril stimulation. Although all of these methods increase renin release, they also increase false positive determinations and reduce reliability of RVR assays to unacceptable levels.

Vaughn *et al.* stressed the importance of expressing RVR in relation to the systemic renin activity rather than simply evaluating the ratio of renin activity between the two renal veins.[11] In patients with RVH secondary to unilateral renal artery stenosis, one should find hypersecretion of renin from the ischemic kidney and suppression of renin secretion from the normal kidney. Through application of this hypothesis, Stanley and Fry have shown a statistically significant difference in the renal-systemic renin indices in patients who were cured of RVH by operation when compared with those who were only improved.[12] Although this method has appeal as a predictor of the extent of benefit, its value in patients with bilateral renal artery lesions is limited. Since both lesions may be producing RVH, both this method and RVR ratios have reduced validity as predictors of response to operation. Furthermore, the risk of hypertension is more directly related to its severity rather than its absolute presence or absence. If one bases the decision for operative management solely on whether or not absolute cure is to be expected, then many patients who would receive the benefit of reduction in severity of hypertension to a mild, easily controlled level would be dropped from consideration as operative candidates. Therefore, this method of RVR assay interpretation should be considered only as an additional predictive tool and not an alternative to the evaluation of RVR ratios.

Renal vein renin assays also may be spuriously unrevealing in patients with accessory or segmental renal artery stenosis if renal venous sampling is limited to the main renal vein. Since recognition of renin hypersecretion depends on sampling the ischemic areas of the kidneys, selective segmental venous sampling must be done in these patients. When segmental sampling is required, the renin activity from the segment sampled is compared with the simultaneously collected contralateral main renal vein sample to calculate the RVR ratio.

Table 17.6. Patient preparation for RVR assays

1	Chronic salt restriction (20 g sodium diet)
2	Discontinue all interfering antihypertensive drugs for at least 5 days prior to study
3	Oral furosemide (40 mg) diuresis night before the study
4	Nothing by mouth for 8 h prior to study
5	Strictly flat bed rest for 4 h before and during study
6	Prestudy sedation with intramuscular diazepam (5 mg)

Summary

In conclusion, one should approach the screening and diagnostic evaluation for RVH with some degree of patient individualization. In general, we limit our screening to patients with recent onset or accelerated hypertension, patients with poorly controlled hypertension and those with diastolic blood pressures greater than 115 mmHg under no treatment. Although we might obtain renal duplex sonography in any of these circumstances, in essentially all such instances we proceed to arteriography. When hypertension is less severe yet azotemia is present we are guided by the results of renal duplex sonography. In this situation, we reason that renal insufficiency requires global ischemia from a main renal artery stenosis to be present to explain the azotemia. Renal duplex sonography is highly accurate for identification or exclusion of such lesions of the main renal artery and can be used to dictate further evaluation.

When renovascular disease is identified by arteriography, RVR assays are used to investigate the importance of unilateral lesions. Except under unusual circumstances, unilateral lesions are only corrected when RVR assays lateralize to the involved side. In contrast, the decision for intervention for bilateral lesions is dictated by the severity of the hypertension or presence of azotemia and RVR assays are not obtained.

References

1 Davis BA, Crook JE, Vestal RE *et al.* Prevalence of renovascular hypertension in patients with grade III or IV hypertensive retinopathy. *N Engl J Med* 1979; **301:** 1273.

2 Lawson JD, Boerth RK, Foster JH *et al.* Diagnosis and management of renovascular hypertension in children. *Arch Surg* 1977; **112:** 1307.

3 Simon N, Franklin SS, Bleifer KH *et al.* Clinical characteristics of renovascular hypertension. *JAMA* 1972; **220:** 1209.

4 Hansen KJ, Tribble RW, Reavis S *et al.* Renal duplex sonography: evaluation of clinical utility. *J Vasc Surg* 1990; **12:** 227–36.

5 Norris CS, Pfeiffer JS, Rittgers SE, Barnes RW. Noninvasive evaluation of renal artery stenosis and renovascular disease. *J Vasc Surg* 1984; **1:** 192–201.

6 Kohler TR, Zierler RE, Martin RL *et al.* Noninvasive diagnosis of renal artery stenosis by ultrasonic duplex scanning. *J Vasc Surg* 1986; **4:** 450–6.

7 Taylor DC, Kettler MD, Moneta GL *et al.* Duplex ultrasound scanning in the diagnosis of renal artery stenosis: a prospective evaluation. *J Vasc Surg* 1988; **7:** 363–9.

8 Barnes RW. Utility of duplex scanning of the renal artery. In Bergan JJ, Yao JST (eds) *Arterial Surgery: New Diagnostic and Operative Techniques*, 1st edn, pp. 351–66 Orlando; Grune and Stratton, 1988.

9 Dean RH. Renovascular hypertension. *Curr Prob Surg* 1985; **22:** 6–67.

10 Meier GH, Sumpio B, Black HR, Gusberg RJ. Captopril renal scintigraphy: an advance in the detection and treatment of renovascular hypertension. *J Vasc Surg* 1990; **11:** 770–7.

11 Vaughn ED, Buhler FR, Larach JH *et al.* Renovascular hypertension: renin measurements to indicate hypersecretion and contralateral suppression, estimate renal plasma flow, and score for surgical curability. *Am J Med* 1973; **55:** 402.

12 Stanley JC, Fry WJ. Surgical treatment of renovascular hypertension. *Arch Surg* 1977; **112:** 1291.

18

Renovascular hypertension in children

MJ DILLON, JE DEAL

Introduction

Renovascular hypertension can be defined as hypertension resulting from a lesion (or lesions) that impairs blood flow to a part, or all, of one or both kidneys. It constitutes between 5 and 25% of cases of secondary hypertension in children,[1] in contrast to the prevalence of renovascular disease in selected hypertensive adults which is less than 1%.[2] It tends to present more commonly in younger children and at major pediatric centers seeing large numbers of patients, 8–10% of patients referred for evaluation and treatment of hypertension have renovascular disease.[3–6] It is potentially curable, second only to coarctation of the aorta as a cause of surgically remediable hypertension in children.[7, 8] The most common abnormality is some form of renal artery stenosis and it is interesting that the first published case of renovascular hypertension treated operatively was a 5½-year-old hypertensive boy in whom nephrectomy resulted in blood pressure normalization.[9] Recent reviews of childhood renovascular hypertension have been published.[10, 11]

Etiology

The most common abnormality causing renovascular disease in children is fibromuscular dysplasia which is reported in 70% of affected patients.[7, 8, 12–15] This is in marked contrast to the situation affecting adults where atherosclerosis accounts for 60% of cases of renovasular disease.[15] Fibromuscular dysplasia may affect only the intima (intimal hyperplasia), but usually the media, as the predominant layer of the arterial wall is involved. The lesions result in areas of arterial narrowing alternating with aneurysmal sections giving rise to a 'string of beads' appearance (Fig. 18.1). The causes are unknown, but it is interesting to speculate on whether uncontrolled release of 'growth factors' plays a role in the development of the lesions. However, there are many causes of renovascular disease, in addition to fibromuscular dysplasia, seen in childhood.

Intimal hyperplasia occurs in association with neurofibromatosis[16–20] and there are also familial cases of fibromuscular dysplasia without this association.[21] Renal artery stenosis is also seen in association with idiopathic hypercalcemia,[22] Marfan's syndrome,[23] the rubella syndrome,[24] Takayasu's disease,[25] Klippel–Trenaunay–Weber syndrome[26] and the Feuerstein–Mims syndrome.[6] Renovasular hypertension has also been reported following systemic vasculitis and in children with renal artery aneurysms[21] (Fig. 18.2), arteriovenous fistula,[27] renal artery disruption after trauma,[7] following neonatal renal artery thrombosis associated with umbilical artery catheterization,[28] renal artery embolization from thrombosis of the ductus arteriosus,[28] following abdominal radiation[29, 30] and due to external compression of the renal arteries due to renal masses, such as pheochromocytomar[31] or

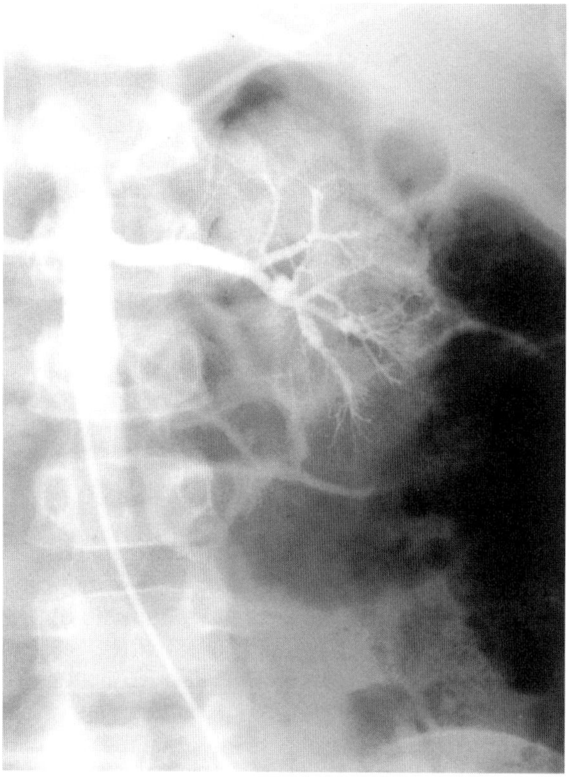

Figure 18.1. Left selective renal angiogram showing 'string of beads' appearance due to fibromuscular dysplasia in child with renovascular hypertension.

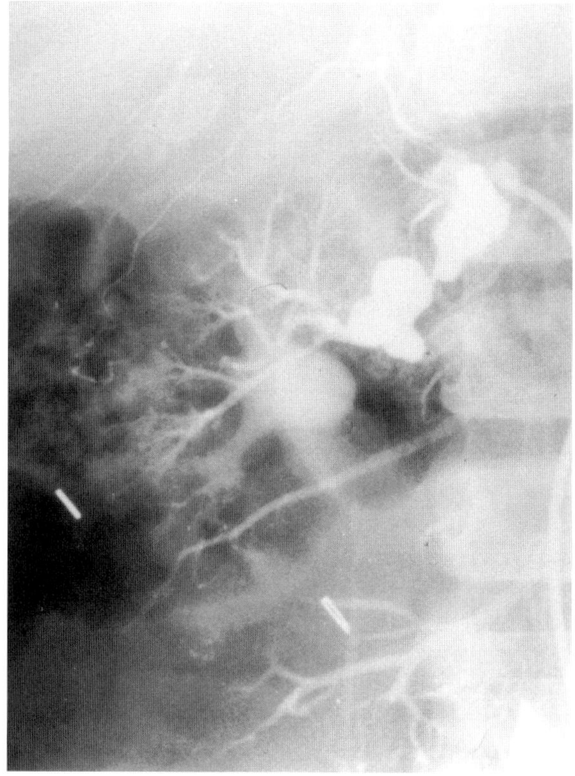

Figure 18.2. Aneurysmal dilatation of right renal artery in child with the Klippel–Trenaunay–Weber syndrome.

hilar lymph nodes.[6] Renal tumors, such as Wilm's, can produce hypertension secondary either to encroachment on the renal artery or to renin secretion by the tumor itself.[32]

Anatomical presentations

Although a main renal artery may be affected in isolation, it is common to have bilateral disease (Fig. 18.3). Intrarenal arterial involvement is also common and may occur in isolation or be associated with the main renal artery disease. It may affect a single branch vessel (Fig. 18.4) or involve the peripheral renal vasculature extensively (Fig. 18.5). Of 54 patients reviewed at the Hospital for Sick Children, London,[6] 38 had bilateral disease; of these the main arteries alone were involved in 7, the main and intrarenal vessels in 13 and intrarenal vessels alone in 18. Unilateral disease occurred in 16 patients; the distribution of the lesions was as follows: main in 6 patients, main and intrarenal in 4, intrarenal alone in 6.

Children with renovascular hypertension often have other abnormalities involving the mesenteric, splenic and hepatic vessels. A substantial number of these individuals have neurofibromatosis Type 1 (NF-1).[33] Of considerable importance is the association of renovascular disease with abdominal coarctation (middle aortic syndrome)[34] or with intracranial arterial disease.[6, 35] In the series reported from the Hospital for Sick Children[6] 11 of 54 patients (20%) with renovascular disease had coarctation of the abdominal aorta (Fig. 18.6); 9 of 16 with renovascular disease and neurological disease, who underwent cerebral arteriography, had intracranial arterial disease (Fig. 18.7).[6, 35]

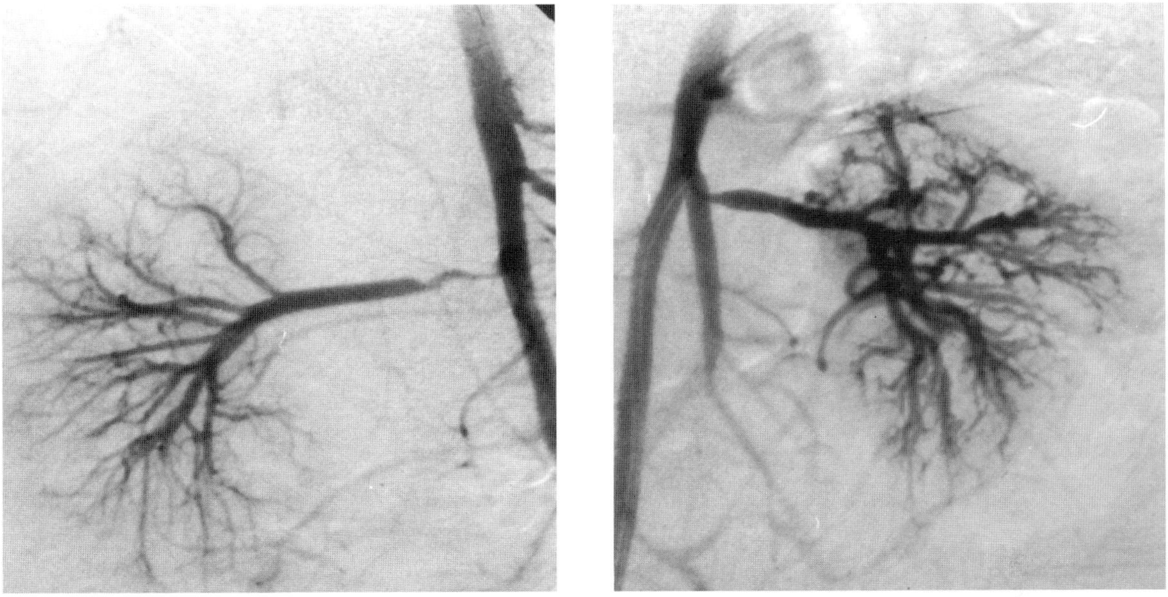

(a) (b)

Figure 18.3. Bilateral main renal artery stenosis. (a) Right selective renal angiogram. (b) Left selective renal angiogram with abnormalities in addition in the small intrarenal arteries.

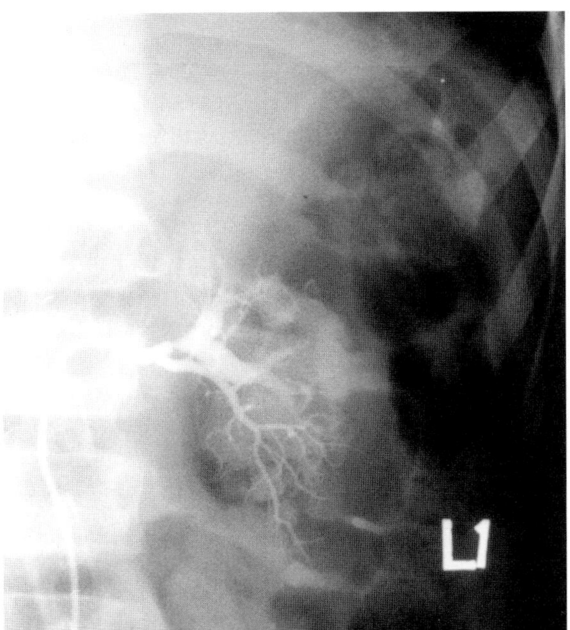

Figure 18.4. Major branch artery stenosis shown in left selective renal angiogram.

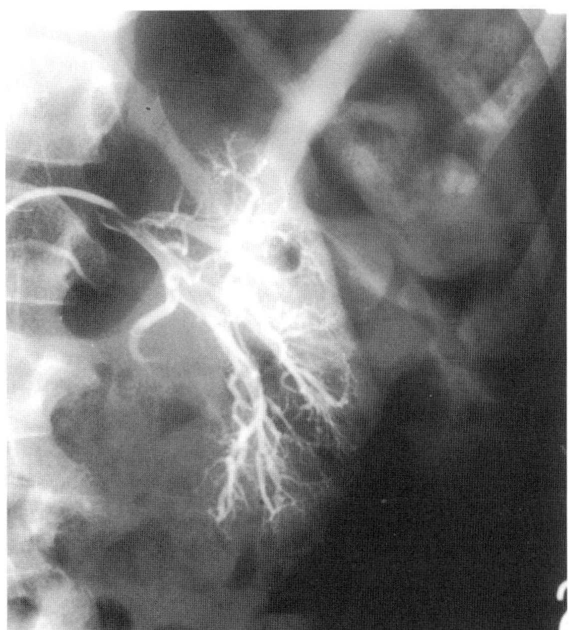

Figure 18.5. Extensive peripheral renal arterial abnormalities in a child with Feuerstein–Mims syndrome.

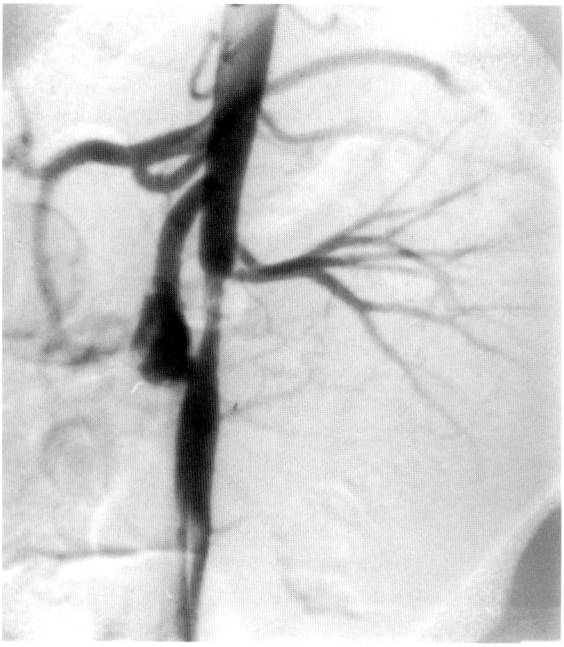

Figure 18.6. Mid-aortic coarctation plus proximal left renal artery stenosis in a child who had already undergone a right sapherous vein by-pass graft of a right sided renal artery stenosis.

Clinical presentation

The clinical presentation of children with renovascular hypertension is variable. In some series a proportion of patients are asymptomatic on presentation and indeed 9 of 17 patients described by Watson *et al.*[1] and 22 of 27 patients described by Daniels *et al.*[36] would come into this category. In the series from Great Ormond Street[6] 14 patients out of the 54 were found to be hypertensive during routine clinical examination, but of those with symptoms the most common were headache in 27 of 54 patients, and lethargy in 21 of 54 patients and this was particularly noticeable in older children. Younger children most often presented with failure to thrive. Twenty-six patients (48%) had accelerated hypertension (severely elevated blood pressure with evidence of end organ damage); of these, seven had convulsions and five presented with a hemiplegia. There were seven children also who presented with lower motor neuron facial palsy, which is a well-recognized presentation of severe hypertension in children. No

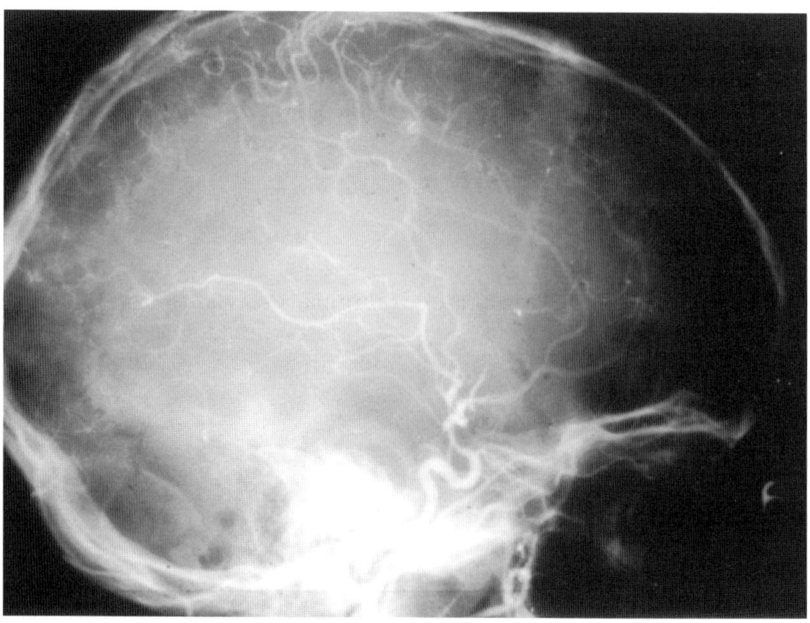

Figure 18.7. Carotid arteriogram showing narrowing in region of carotid syphon in a child with renovascular and cerebrovascular disease presenting with hypertension.

symptoms were pathognomonic of renovascular disease, but clearly associated findings on examination might be suggestive. Clinical findings of relevance, in this context, would be the association of hypertension with features of syndromes that are known to be associated with renovascular disease. Furthermore, the presence of an abdominal bruit may be helpful in defining the presence of renovascular disease, but there are limits to the clinical value of this observation with both false positive and false negative findings reported.[37] The presence of evident vascular disease at other sites than within the renal vasculature may also prove helpful and it would be worth considering a renovascular etiology for a high blood pressure in the presence of coarctation of the aorta and also if there was evidence of cerebrovascular disease, perhaps clinically defined by an audible bruit over the carotid arteries, the parietal area of the skull or the orbits.[35]

Diagnostic tests

There are recommended investigative procedures that have been published for the evaluation of children found to be hypertensive[3, 38] and these are likely to include a routine measurement of plasma electrolytes and renal function, urine analysis and some measure of end organ effect such as a 2D echocardiogram. An abdominal ultrasound and a ^{99m}technetium dimercaptosuccinic acid (DMSA) scan would give both structural and functional information concerning the kidneys. A peripheral plasma renin activity measurement and some measure of catecholamine excess, possibly a plasma catecholamine concentration, or alternatively a 24-h urine VMA analysis would complete this preliminary screening. Supplementary investigations would follow this according to the category of disease in which the hypertensive child would appear to fall according to these preliminary results. In children suspected of having renovascular disease there may be some degree of hypokalemia due to the secondary hyperaldosteronism, but renal function may or may not be impaired and this would depend on the severity of renal artery disease, as well as the possible effects of accelerated hypertension on glomerular filtration. It is likely that peripheral plasma renin activity levels will be high and the renal imaging in terms of ultrasonography and DMSA scanning will show kidneys that may be entirely normal in size and function or with evidence of renal asymmetry or of patchy decrease in isotope uptake within the renal parenchyma in severe renovascular disease.

Further investigations for renovascular disease would be justified if there was no evidence of an alternative explanation for the hypertension, or if the investigative findings were compatible with a renin-dependent hypertensive state without obvious cause. Additional investigative procedures might include Doppler ultrasonography to demonstrate changes in flow due to stenotic lesions[39, 40] or further radionuclide imaging, particularly utilizing angiotensin converting enzyme inhibitor sensitization, to unmask main renal artery or major branch artery stenosis.[41–48] Such techniques have mainly been utilized in adults but have also been evaluated in children and Gordon *et al.*[43] showed that compared with renal angiography captopril-primed DMSA scans gave a sensitivity of 80% and a specificity of 89% of the renal pathology being due to renovascular disease.

Other techniques have included the use of angiotensin converting enzyme inhibitors to identify children with hypertension associated with hyperreninemia by recording the magnitude of the hypotensive response to administered captropril.[44] However, interpreting the renin responsiveness to captopril as a means of diagnosing the nature of the underlying renal pathology causing hypertension or the potential for surgical cure is associated with uncertainties in children and adolescents.[49, 50] Some would argue that if a good plasma renin activity assay is available from a reliable laboratory it may not be necessary to embark on these indirect tests of the presence or absence of hyperreninemia and it may also be rather surprising to imagine that such techniques would be specifically helpful in terms of precise diagnostic categorization or, for that matter, of predictive value in terms of satisfactory response to surgical intervention.

On the other hand, selective main and segmental renal vein renin sampling [1, 6, 51–53] have proved valuable in lateralizing the kidney from which renin release is occurring and identifying from the segmenal veins where, within the renal parenchyma, local sources of renin release are situated.

Such investigative procedures are usually coupled with selective renal angiography[40, 51] and utilizing these techniques it is possible to demonstrate in children the frequency of bilateral renal artery disease and intrarenal arterial disease, which in the Great Ormond Street series came to 70 and 76% of the total respectively.[6] It is critically important when selective renal arterial injections are being undertaken that both posterior and oblique views are obtained to demonstrate these small intrarenal vessel abnormalities.[40]

The role of magnetic resonance angiography in childhood renovascular disease awaits evaluation, since currently it only seems to be valuable in detecting pathology in the main renal artery or its major branches.[54] This is, therefore, less attractive an investigative tool in pediatric practice when so frequently intrarenal and small artery involvement is present.

In view of the association with extrarenal arterial disease, cerebral angiography is at times required, especially in relation to children in whom there have been cerebral symptoms or suggestive features of cerebral arterial involvement, such as cranial bruits. More than 50% of children with renovascular disease and neurological features who underwent cerebral angiography in the Hospital for Sick Children series had intracranial arterial disease as well.[6, 35] Occasionally indirect information concerning cerebral arterial pathology can be obtained by undertaking functional studies of cerebral blood flow, for example using ^{99m}Tc hexamethylpropyleneamine oxine (HMPAO), which may provide evidence of relative cerebral ischemia in the presence of intracranial arterial disease.

Treatment

Management initially would involve antihypertensive drug therapy and only after stabilization would surgical or transluminal angioplasty treatment be considered if feasible. The range of hypotensive agents that can be utilized in managing children with hypertensive disease has been reviewed[55, 56] and in Fig. 18.8 a flowchart of treatment is illustrated. The nature of the pharmacological agents used depends upon the severity of the hypertension being treated, but in childhood the most appropriate drugs to use are often those that have been found to be safe and effective in the hands of the clinicians treating the child, rather than the newest hypotensive agents that have not been fully evaluated in younger patients.

It is clear that there has to be some care exercised if it is suspected that renovascular disease is on the agenda. For example, hypotensive agents such as angiotensin converting enzyme inhibitors may be contraindicated, at least in the first instance, because of the risks of causing severe reduction in renal perfusion. There is certainly evidence that renal functional deterioration can occur due to deleterious effects on glomerular hemodynamics distal to stenotic lesions after administration of such agents[57, 58] and this is particularly relevant in patients with critical main renal artery stenosis. In the absence of clear information as to the nature of the renovascular disease or its severity, a combination of β-blocker and either a vasodilator or a calcium channel inhibitor may be the safest option in the first instance with diuretics being reserved only for patients with clear evidence of salt and water overload. Most children with severe renovascular hypertension are salt and water depleted unless renal impairment is present.

As far as surgical management is concerned, this might be considered under the headings of nephrectomy, partial nephrectomy, revascularization by reconstructive vascular surgery, or autotransplantation. The development of interventional radiology has also allowed intraluminal dilatation or angioplasty to be undertaken. Decisions concerning surgical feasibility and the likely outcome in terms of cure of hypertension require much care and the information provided by the refined investigative procedures already described.

The ideal lesion for revascularization surgery or intraluminal angioplasty is a unilateral short segment main renal artery stenosis with no evidence of intrarenal or contralateral renal artery disease and clear lateralization of renin release to

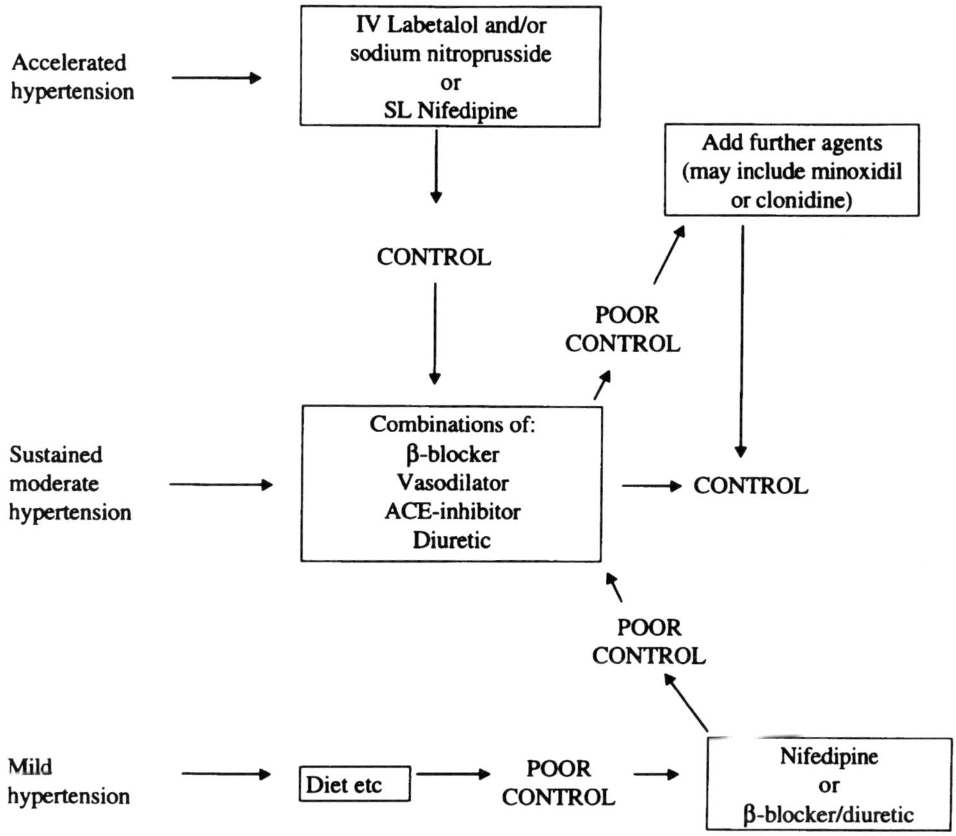

Figure 18.8. Flow chart of medical treatment of hypertension.

the affected side. Bilateral main renal artery stenosis and also intrarenal segmental artery stenosis are amenable to revascularization or angioplastic techniques, but preoperative anatomical or functional localization is essential before proceeding. For segmental lesions, heminephrectomy may prove to be the procedure of choice. Surgical techniques include saphenous vein bypass procedures or other reconstructive techniques including splenorenal, hepatorenal, internal iliac-renal astomoses, and the use of Dacron grafts and autotransplantation.[6,7,12,21,59–62]

Cure rates of 59–86% have been seen in children;[63] but again these were highly selected patients, and other centers have found that surgical intervention is often not technically feasible in many cases of renovascular disease in children. Of the 27 children reviewed by Daniels *et al.*,[36] 14 (52%) were treated surgically, 12 were revascularized and 2 underwent unilateral nephrectomy, but the cure rate was only 36%. In the Great Ormond Street series only ten (18%) of the patients were considered suitable for a revascularization procedure, because of the extensive nature of their renovascular disease.[6] Nephrectomy or heminephrectomy, although successful in curing five of the cases and improving the clinical situation in six other children, may obviously be an appropriate therapeutic step, but caution needs to be exercised since the associated reduction in renal mass may have important potential long-term consequences. Nephrectomy might be seriously considered if renal function in the affected kidney is poor or absent, if there has been vascular occlusion following an attempted revascularization, or if there is uncontrollable hypertension and no alternative therapy is available.

Success rates of percutaneous angioplasty in children have varied between 38 and 90%.[64–67] However, the majority of these describe reports on selected patients with unilateral or limited disease who are not representative of the usual spectrum of renal artery disease seen in children. Of the 32 cases reviewed by Chevalier *et al.*[65] who were treated by percutaneous transluminal angioplasty, 19 were successful, but only 4 of these children had bilateral lesions. Cases suitable for angioplasty must be carefully selected; children with fibromuscular dysplasia who have unilateral main artery or main branch lesions that are accessible and those without ostial lesions have the greatest reported success rates.[67]

Patients with renovascular disease may, as has also been mentioned, have significant arterial abnormalities involving extrarenal arteries and those affecting the cerebral vascalature are the most important in view of the risks involved in both controlling the blood pressure and undertaking surgery on the renal vessels. Should the risk of sudden hypotension during surgical revascularization procedures be such that severe brain ischemia would result then either a non-interventional control of blood pressure or preliminary revascularization of the brain by extra-intracranial arterial anastomosis may be worth considering.[35]

Conclusion

Childhood renovascular disease, although comprising only 10% of children with severe hypertension requiring treatment, is an important group since there is the potential for surgical care in selected cases. There is, therefore, a need for an awareness that this type of hypertensive disease can and does occur in childhood, but that investigations must be undertaken in centers with facilities to define the full extent of the underlying pathology so that rational decisions can be taken concerning appropriate therapy. It is also important to appreciate that the renal arteries may not be the only ones affected in the disease process and that renovascular disease can be a part of a number of syndromes with their own additional features and long-term implications.

References

1 Watson AR, Balfe, JW, Hardy BE. Renovascular hypertension in childhood: a changing perspective in management. *J Pediatr* 1985; **106:** 366–72.
2 Berglund G, Andersson O, Wilhelmsen L. Prevalence of primary and secondary hypertension: studies in a random population sample. *Br Med J* 1976; **2:** 554–6.
3 Dillon MJ. Investigation and management of hypertension in children. *Pediatr Nephrol* 1987; **1:** 59–68.
4 Liebermann E. Hypertension in childhood and adolescence. In Kaplan NM (ed.) *Clinical Hypertension*, pp. 407–33. Baltimore: Williams and Wilkins, 1990.
5 Loirat C, Pillion G, Blum C. Hypertension in chidren: present data and problems. *Adv Nephrol* 1982; **11:** 65–98.
6 Deal JE, Snell ME, Barratt TM, Dillon MJ. Renovascular disease in childhood. *J Pediatr* 1992; **25:** 55–65.
7 Fry WJ, Ernst CB, Stanley JC, Brinnk B. Renovascular hypertension in the pediatric patient. *Arch Surg* 1973; **107:** 692–8.
8 Stanley JC. Surgical intervention in pediatric renovascular hypertension. *Clin Nephrol Urol* 1992; **12:** 167–76.
9 Leadbetter WF, Burkland CE. Hypertension in unilateral renal disease. *J Urol* 1938; **39:** 611.
10 Fry WJ, Daniells SR. Renovascular hypertension in the pediatric age group. In Loggie JMH (ed.) *Pediatric and Adolescent Hypertension*, pp. 252–63. Oxford: Blackwell Scientific, 1992.
11 Hiner LB, Falkner B. Renovascular hypertension in children. *Pediatr Clin North Am* 1993; **40:** 123–40.
12 Lawson JB, Boerth R, Foster JH, Dean RH. Diagnosis and management of renovascular hypertension in children. *Arch Surg* 1977; **122:** 1307–16.
13 Stanley P, Gyepes MT, Olsen DL, Gates GF. Renovascular hypertension in children and adolescents. *Radiology* 1978; **129:** 123–131.
14 Makker SP, Moorthy B. Fibromuscular dysplasia of renal arteries. An important cause of renovascular hypertension in children. *J Pediatr* 1979; **95:** 940–5.
15 Wise KL, McCann RL, Dunnick NR, Paulson DF. Renovascular hypertension. *J Urol* 1988; **140:** 911–24.
16 Leumann EP. Blood pressure and hypertension in childhood and adolescence. *Ergeb Inn Med Kinderheilk* 1979; **43:** 109–83.
17 Halpern M, Currarino G. Vascular lesions causing hypertension in neurofibromatosis. *N Engl Med* 1965; **273:** 248–52.
18 Mena E, Bookstein JJ, Holt JF, Fry WJ.

Neurofibromatosis and renovascular hypertension in children. *Am J Roentgenol* 1973; **118:** 39–45.

19 Green JF, Fitzwater JE, Burgess J. Arterial lesions associated with neurofibromatosis. *Am J Clin Pathol* 1974; **62:** 481–7.

20 Muller Wiefel DE. Renovasculare hypertension bei neurofibromatose von Recklinghausen. *Monatsschr Kinderheilk* 1978; **126:** 113–18.

21 Kaufmann JJ, Goodwin WE, Waisman J, Gyepes MT. Renovascular hypertension in children. Report of seven cases treated surgically including two cases of renal auto transplantation. *Am J Surg* 1972; **124:** 149–57.

22 Wiltese HE, Goldbloom RB, Asuquo AU *et al.* Infantile hypercalcaemia syndrome in twins. *N Engl J Med* 1966; **275:** 1157–60.

23 Loughridge LW. Renal abnormalities in the Marfan syndrome. *Quart J Med* 1959; 531–44.

24 Menser MA, Dorman DC, Reye RDK, Reid RR. Renal artery stenosis in the rubella syndrome. *Lancet* 1966; **1:** 790–2.

25 Wiggelinkhuizen J, Cremin BJ. Takayasu arteritis and renovascular hypertension in childhood. *Pediatrics* 1978; **62:** 209–17.

26 Proesmans W. Syndrome de Klippel-Trenaunay avec hypertension arterielle et insuffisance renale chronique. *Ann Pediatr* 1982; **29:** 671–4.

27 Palmer JM, Connolly JE. Intrarenal arteriovenous fistula; surgical excision under selective renal hypothermia with kidney survival. *J Urol* 1966; **96:** 599–605.

28 Adelman RD. Neonatal hypertension. *Pediatr Clin North Am* 1978; **25:** 99–110.

29 O'Malley B, D'Angio GJ, Vawter GF. Late effects of roentgen therapy given in infancy. *Am J Roentgenol* 1963; **89:** 1067–74.

30 Koskimies Ø. Arterial hypertension developing 10 years after radiotherapy for Wilms' tumour. *Br Med J* 1988; **285:** 996–8.

31 Alvestrand A, Bergstroem J, Wehle B. Pheochromocytoma and renovascular hypertension. A case report and review of the literature. *Acta Med Scand* 1977; **202:** 231–6.

32 Spahr J, Demers LM, Shochat SJ. Renin producing Wilms' tumour. *J Pediatr Surg* 1981; **16:** 32–4.

33 Inglefinger JR. Renovascular disease in children. *Kidney Int* 1993; **43:** 493–505.

34 Sumboonnanonda A, Robinson BL, Gedroye WMW *et al.* Middle aortic syndrome: clinical and radiological findings. *Arch Dis Child* 1992; **67:** 501–5.

35 Daman Willems CD, Salisbury DM, Lumley JSP, Dillon MJ. Brain revascularisation in hypertension. *Arch Dis Child* 1985; **60:** 1177– 9.

36 Daniels SR, Loggie JMH, McEnery PT, Towbin RB. Clinical spectrum of intrinsic renovascular hypertension in children. *Pediatrics* 1986; **80:** 698–704.

37 Korobkin M, Perloff DL, Palobinskas AJ. Renal arteriography and the evaluation of unexplained hypertension in children and adolescents. *J Pediatr* 1976; **88:** 388–93.

38 Inglefinger JR, Dillon MJ. Evaluation of secondary hypertension. In Holliday MA, Barratt TM, Avner ED (eds) *Pediatric Nephrology*, 3rd edn, pp. 1146–64. Baltimore: Williams and Wilkins, 1994.

39 Tapper D, Brand T, Hickman R. Early diagnosis and management of renovascular hypertension. *Am J Med* 1987; **153:** 495–500.

40 Siegel MJ, Amour TES, Siegel BA. Imaging techniques in the evaluation of pediatric hypertension. *Pediatr Nephrol* 1987; **1:** 76–88.

41 Sfakianakis GN, Bourgoigne JJ, Jaffee D *et al.* Single dose captopril scintigraphy in the diagnosis of renovascular hypertension. *J Nucl Med* 1987; **28:** 1383–92.

42 Meier GH, Sumpio B, Black HR, Gusberg RJ. Captopril renal scintigraphy – an advance in the detection and treatment of renovascular hypertension. *J Vasc Surg* 1990; **11:** 770–7.

43 Gordon I, Lythgoe M, Minty I, Dillon MJ. Diagnosis of renovascular hypertension: improved specificity of ^{Tc99m} DMSA using captopril. *Pediatr Nephrol* 1993; **7:** C36.

44 Daman Willems CD, Shah V, Uchiyama M, Dillon MJ. The captopril test; an aid to investigation of hypertension. *Arch Dis Child* 1989; **4:** 229–34.

45 Frommei E, Bellina R, Bertelli P, Gazzetti P *et al.* Interactive functional imaging of renal scientigraphy after captopril in the detection of global or segmental hypoperfusion. *Contrib Nephrol* 1987; **56:** 111–16.

46 Fommei E, Mezzasalma L, Ghione S *et al.* European captopril radionuclide test multicentre study. Preliminary results. Inspective renographic analysis. *Am J Hypertension* 1991; **4:** 690S-697S.

47 McLean AG, Hilson AJ, Scoble JE *et al.* Screening for renovascular disease with captopril enhanced renography. *Nephrol Dial Transplant* 1992; **7:** 211–15.

48 Dondi M. Captopril renal scintigraphy with 99mTc mercaptoacetyl triglycine (^{99m}Tc-MAG3) for detecting renal artery stenosis. *Am J Hypertension* 1991; **4:** 737S-740S.

49 Hamed RMA, Balfe JW, Ellis G. The use of the captopril test to assess renin responsiveness in children with hypertension and renal disease. *Child Nephrol Urol* 1990; **10:** 181–5.

50 Gauthier B, Trachtman H, Frank R, Pillari G. Inadequacy of captopril challenge tests for diagnosing renovascular hypertension in children and adolescents. *Pediatr Nephrol* 1991; **5:** 42–4.

51 Stringer DA, de Bruyn R, Dillon MJ, Gordon I. Comparison of aortography, renal vein renin sampling, radionuclide scans, ultrasound and the IVU in the investigation of childhood renovascular hypertension. *Br J Radiol* 1984; **57:** 111–21.

52 Godard C. Predictive value of renal-vein renin measurements in children with various forms of renal hypertension: an international study. *Helv Paediatr Acta* 1977; **32:** 49–57.
53 Dillon MJ, Shah V, Barratt TM. Renal vein renin measurements in children with hypertension. *Br Med J* 1973; **2:** 168–70.
54 Stark DD, Bradley WG. *Magnetic Resonance Imaging*, 2nd edn. St Louis: CV Mosby, 1991.
55 Houtman PN, Dillon MJ. Medical management of hypertension in childhood. *Child Nephrol Urol* 1992, **12:** 154–61.
56 Dillon MJ, Ingelfinger JR. Pharmacological treatment of hypertension. In Holliday MA, Barratt TM, Avner ED (eds) *Pediatric Nephrology*, 3rd edn, pp. 1165–74. Baltimore: Williams and Wilkins, 1994.
57 Hrieik DE, Browning PJ. Kopelman R *et al.* Captopril induced functional renal insufficiency in patients with bilateral renal artery stenosis or renal artery stenosis in a solitary kidney. *N Engl J Med* 1983; **308:** 373–6.
58 Brogden RN, Todd PA, Sorkin EM. Captopril: an update of its pharmacodynamic and pharmacokinetic properties, and therapeutic use in hypertension and congestive cardiac failure. *Drugs* 1988; **36:** 540–600.
59 Stoney RJ, Cooke PA, Stoney ST. Surgical treatment of renovascular hypertension in children. *J Pediatr Surg* 1975; **10:** 631–9.
60 Novick AC, Straffon RA, Stewart BH, Benjamin S. Surgical treatment of renovascular hypertension in the pediatric patient. *J Urol* 1978; **119:** 794–805.
61 Berkowitz HD, O'Neill JA. Renovascular hypertension in children. Surgical repair with special reference to the use of reinforced grafts. *J Vasc Surg* 1989; **9:** 46–55.
62 Sinaiko A, Najarian J, Michael AF, Mirkin BL. Renal autotransplantation in the treatment of bilateral renal artery stenosis. Relief of hypertension in an eight year old boy. *J Pediatr* 1973; **83:** 409–13.
63 Stanley JC. Surgical intervention in pediatric renovascular hypertension. *Child Nephrol Urol* 1993; **12:** 167–74.
64 McCook TA, Mills SR, Kirks DR *et al.* Percutaneous transluminal renal artery angioplasty in a 3½ year old hypertensive girl. *J Pediatr* 1980; **97:** 958–60.
65 Chevalier RL, Tegtmeyer CG, Gomez RA. Percutaneous transluminal angioplasty for renovascular hypertension in children. *Pediatr Nephrol* 1987; **1:** 89–98.
66 Goertz KK, Linshaw MA, Lee KA *et al.* Transluminal arterial dilatation of a post surgical stenosis of renal artery implant in a child with recurrent hypertension. *Pediatrics* 1982; **69:** 489–91.
67 Norling LL, Chevalier RL, Gomez RA, Tegtmeyer CJ. Uses of interventional radiology for hypertension due to renal artery stenosis in children. *Child Nephrol Urol* 1992; **12:** 162–6.

19

Therapeutic decision making in renal vascular hypertension

JEFFREY M RIMMER, DENNIS A PLANTE, NICOLAOS E MADIAS

Introduction

Medical decisions evolve as the clinician weighs many variables. Among these are the probability of a certain disease being present, its natural history, the accuracy of available tests, the chances of favorable and unfavorable outcomes when diagnostic and therapeutic maneuvers are undertaken, and the desires of the patient. In the modern era, the expense of alternative management pathways has been the subject of increasing societal concern. Indeed, the issue of minimizing cost now often enters the individual clinician–patient relationship. When the clinical problem is simple, the point where these considerations balance can be intuitively obvious. With more complex problems, however, as is the diagnosis and management of renovascular hypertension, determination of the most appropriate approach can be more challenging.

Clinical decision analysis is a method that allows the quantitative examination of clinical problems.[1, 2] In a common form of this discipline, a decision tree is created that maps the possible outcomes of alternative diagnostic and therapeutic strategies. Branch points within the tree, or nodes, represent places where clinical choices or chance outcomes will occur. Probabilities are assigned to chance outcomes, as gleaned from the medical literature and clinical experience. These probabilities allow calculation of the likelihood of arriving at various possible endpoints. A measure of utility is then calculated for each endpoint, such as years of survival or cost, thus permitting mathematical comparison of the desirability of the mapped strategies. As a result of this analysis, the component parts of clinical decisions can be examined in an organized fashion and their relative importance estimated.

Although decision analysis has been applied to the problem of renovascular hypertension on several occasions in the past 20 years, those analyses have utilized older data or have been limited to specific aspects of the entity.[3, 4, 5] For these reasons a new model is discussed in this chapter. It revolves around a number of the possible diagnostic and therapeutic strategies that may be chosen in the management of a hypertensive population where atherosclerotic renovascular disease is being considered as an etiology. We chose to model atherosclerotic disease because patients with this process are generally more fragile, and tend to respond to intervention less satisfactorily than patients with renal artery stenosis secondary to fibromuscular dysplasia. These considerations augment the uncertainty of decisions in the patient with suspected atherosclerotic renovascular hypertension. It should be emphasized that the model is not intended to function as a management tool for individual patients, but rather as a theoretical and operational framework. It serves to demonstrate relationships and trends which should enhance the readers' ability to integrate the state-of-the-art information contained in this volume with their current knowledge and experience as well as the particular characteristics of their own practice. In this way, the model offers the opportunity to consider how local variations in diagnostic and therapeutic skills, as well as the patient populations encountered can alter the 'appropriate' approach when entertaining the diagnosis of renovascular hypertension.

The model

The general structure of the model is as follows (for details see Appendix, Figs 19.11–19.13).

One of eight choices may be made when a patient presents with hypertension and consideration is given to renal artery stenosis as a possible etiology. In the first choice (Angio), angiography is performed immediately and can lead to associated adverse consequences as well as the determination of whether renal artery stenosis is present. Those with stenosis immediately undergo percutaneous transluminal renal angioplasty (PTRA), whereas the remainder start medical therapy. Those who survive angioplasty without developing chronic renal failure, but remain hypertensive, are entered into a surgical branch (Appendix, Fig. 19.12). Patients who survive surgery then enter terminal pathways where they are modeled for the possibility and effects of adequate blood pressure control, persistent hypertension, or the onset of chronic renal failure (CRF) requiring dialysis (Appendix, Fig. 19.13). Choice two (Ang/RVR) is similar to the first, except that renal vein renins are used to determine who will receive non-medical intervention. If stenosis is present, but lateralization of renin activity cannot be demonstrated, the patient is entered into medical therapy. The third choice (Test) models the use of a hypothetical non-invasive test. A positive test leads to angiography, while a negative test initiates medical therapy without the possibility of further investigation for renal artery stenosis. Pathway four (Test-Ang) also screens using a non-invasive test, with a positive test going to angiography and a negative test directing to medical therapy, but in contrast to choice three (Test), poor medical control of blood pressure returns the patient to the angiography branch. The fifth pathway (Test-Ang/RVR) is similar to the fourth except that renal vein renins are used to determine whether repair of a stenosis will be attempted. In the sixth choice (MedRx), medical therapy of hypertension is attempted but no further investigation is undertaken regardless of the response to therapy. Choice seven (Med-Ang) starts with medical therapy but patients whose blood pressure remains uncontrolled are returned to the angiography branch. The eighth and final possible choice (Med-Ang/RVR) is similar to choice seven (Med-Ang) except that renal vein renins are used to determine whether a stenosis should be repaired.

After a choice is made, the probability of patient survival is calculated using observed outcomes that have been obtained from the renovascular hypertension literature or probabilities assigned for the purposes of analysis. Where possible, the probability and outcome data are obtained from groups with atherosclerotic renovascular hypertension alone, devoid of other complications of renal artery stenosis. Simplifying assumptions include omitting the effects of restenosis and the possibility of developing recurrent hypertension in patients cured of renovascular hypertension. It was also elected to assume that the initial approach to revascularization would always be PTRA in a population presenting with hypertension as the only manifestation of disease. When ranges of probabilities are available, an effort has been made to err on the side of biasing the model against invasive intervention. Table 19.4 of the Appendix lists the variables, the range of values with their bibliographic support and the baseline values used in the model. The dominant measure of estimated utility is predicted patient survival, unadjusted for quality of life or cost. These assumptions are applied to a population with an age range that would have an average expected survival of 25 years.

Because survival is the primary measure of utility, factors that minimize the risk of death will determine the relative value of various choices. The immediate mortality of procedures is important, but the cumulative mortality of uncontrolled hypertension and the future high mortality of dialysis associated with hypertension may ultimately have a dominant influence on which choice is considered most beneficial, by increasing late deaths. It should be kept in mind that in most of the analyses the majority of patients entering a strategy do not have renovascular hypertension (i.e. when the prevalence of renovascular hypertension is set at 20%, 80% of those entering the pathway are assumed to have essential hypertension). Obviously, this preponderance of patients with essential rather than renovascular hypertension importantly influences the estimated survival rates.

Effect of prevalence of renovascular hypertension

The prevalence of a disorder has a profound influence on the utility of attempting to detect it within a large population. When survival is used as a measure of utility, the magnitude of the effect of prevalence will largely depend upon death rates secondary to diagnostic testing and therapeutic maneuvers as well as the difference between the mortality rates of undiscovered and discovered disease. If a disease is very uncommon and there is significant risk associated with diagnostic testing, then the harm to a population may be greater than the benefit. On the other hand, if mortality is greatly reduced by making a correct diagnosis and initiating specific treatment, the resultant benefit may outweigh the risk of testing.

Figure 19.1 demonstrates the expected utility of each of the clinical choices employed in the model as the probability of renovascular hypertension increases. The eight strategies are graphed over the entire range of likelihood of renovascular hypertension from 0 to 100%. Several of the approaches cluster, making it difficult to identify individual lines, but a general pattern is discernible at almost all prevalences of renovascular hypertension. The five choices with the greatest calculated utility are all testing options. Three strategies that directly search for renovascular disease (Angio, Test-Ang, Test) comprise the uppermost lines. Two approaches with immediate testing, which includes renal vein renin measurements (Ang/RVR, Test-Ang/RVR) fall slightly below these. The two strategies featuring medical therapy first, followed by investigation if hypertension is not controlled (Med-Ang, Med-Ang/RVR), come next. Finally, for most prevalences of renovascular hypertension, medical therapy with no possibility of further investigation (MedRx) has the lowest utility.

Several of the baseline probabilities used in the model force the segregation of strategies. Included among these is the assumption that 70% of patients with renovascular hypertension

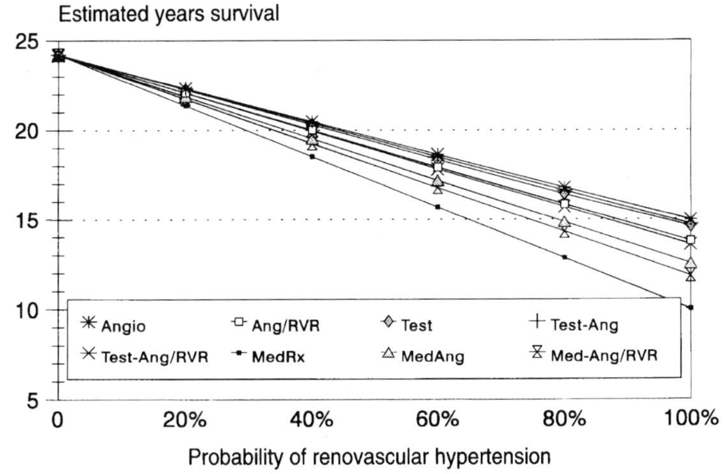

Figure 19.1. Calculated utilities (reported as estimated years survival) determined for all eight management strategies over the entire possible range of prevalence of renovascular hypertension.

will have their blood pressure controlled by medication. This assumption is important because patients with controlled hypertension, but underlying renovascular disease, will escape detection in those pathways that include either no early investigation for renal artery stenosis or investigation only when blood pressure remains uncontrolled. In the model, a penalty is imposed not only for uncontrolled hypertension but also for undetected renovascular disease, even if the blood pressure is medically normalized. This penalty includes an increased mortality rate associated with atherosclerotic renovascular disease as well as an increased chance of end-stage renal disease with its additional increase in the risk of death. Just like much of the information about renovascular disease, these assumptions are merely patterns that emerge from uncontrolled series of patients; consequently, their validity can be debated. There are as yet no results reported from long-term controlled comparisons of outcomes in patients with medically treated renovascular hypertension vs those who have undergone renal revascularization.

Closer examination of utilities shows that at very low probabilities of renovascular hypertension, immediate angiography is not the favored strategy. Figure 19.2 is an expanded view of the utility of three approaches, medical therapy alone (MedRx), a non-invasive test that is followed by angiography if the test is positive or if hypertension cannot be controlled (Test-Ang) and immediate angiography (Angio). The utility of these three approaches is graphed as the prevalence of renovascular hypertension is varied from 0 to 20%, a range likely to be representative of most populations presenting with hypertension alone. Among the eight original strategies, medical therapy alone is actually the preferred approach when renovascular hypertension is highly unlikely. The non-invasive testing strategy, Test-Ang, then replaces this approach as the most useful strategy when the probability of renovascular hypertension is intermediate. Finally, when renovascular hypertension becomes more common, immediate angiography is calculated to be the best plan. The threshold probability of renovascular hypertension (i.e. the point where the utilities of two options cross on the graph) for the MedRx and Test-Ang options is 0.13%. The threshold for the Test-Ang and Angio options is 13.5%. This means that Test-Ang becomes preferable to MedRx when the prevalence of renovascular hypertension is above 0.13%, and that the Angio strategy surpasses Test-Ang when the prevalence is above 13.5%.

These findings can be explained by examining the structure of the model. There is some risk associated with undergoing angiography. At low prevalences of renovascular hypertension, the population obtains little benefit from angiography, yet all patients acquire the risk of an

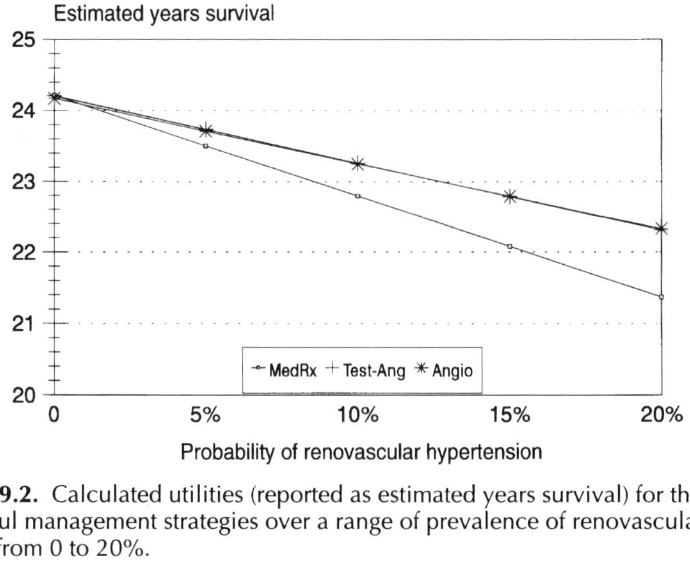

Figure 19.2. Calculated utilities (reported as estimated years survival) for three most successful management strategies over a range of prevalence of renovascular hypertension from 0 to 20%.

invasive procedure. Therefore, when it is very unlikely that renal artery stenosis will be discovered, medical therapy alone is the best approach. As the prevalence of disease increases, the penalty imposed by the model for missing renovascular hypertension increases. A screening strategy increases the probability that patients who undergo angiography actually have renovascular disease and therefore may benefit from invasive examination. It also reduces the risk that patients who may benefit from renal revascularization will remain undetected. These considerations favor a screening strategy because it improves the risk/benefit ratio of performing angiography as it reduces the number of undiagnosed cases. The sensitivity and specificity of the screening procedure will also influence its value in the decision model. Because the model assumes that our hypothetical screening test is not as effective as angiography, as the prevalence of renovascular disease increases, the screening test strategy will result in a growing fraction of the hypertensive population having undiscovered renovascular hypertension. The survival benefit assigned to revascularization is high enough that at some prevalence of renovascular disease (e.g. in this model, >13.5%), the risk of angiography imposed on the hypertensive population is exceeded by the risk created by missing the diagnosis with a screening test. At this point, the immediate angiography strategy becomes preferable. These observations suggest that for a clinician to choose among these three options (medical therapy only, screening for renovascular disease and immediate angiography) in the management of a given patient, the prevalence of the disease, the risk of testing, the characteristics of the test and the survival benefit of intervention should be known. Although the true prevalence of renovascular hypertension will be unknown, it can be estimated from the individual characteristics of the patient. The risk, the sensitivity and the specificity of most tests have been reasonably well demonstrated. It is the uncertainty as to the existence and magnitude of a survival benefit conferred by renal revascularization that continues to cause debate about when it is appropriate to pursue the diagnosis of renovascular hypertension. A final point should be made about the comparison of the immediate angiography vs Test-Ang algorithms as potential management plans. Although the strategy of immediate angiography has a higher utility than initial screening when the prevalence of renovascular hypertension is above 13.5%, its slope does not differ perceptibly from that of the Test-Ang strategy. This similarity of slopes reflects the fact that the latter choice potentially contains consecutive tests. A patient with renovascular hypertension who has had a negative screening test will be returned to angiography if medical therapy fails. This design results in an estimated utility of 22.31 and 22.32 years' survival for the Test-Ang and immediate angiography strategies, respectively, when the prevalence of renovascular hypertension is set at 20%. At lower prevalences of renovascular hypertension, the difference in calculated lifespan is even smaller. Indeed, if immediate angiography has substantially higher financial costs or morbidity, these factors essentially negate the small survival advantage this approach has when compared with the Test-Ang strategy.

Sensitivity and specificity of screening tests

Given the foregoing discussion about prevalence, it might be anticipated that changes in the sensitivity and specificity of the hypothetical screening test would have a major impact on the expected utility of the screening strategy, Test-Ang. As detailed elsewhere in this volume, much effort has been directed toward developing highly sensitive and specific non-invasive screening tests for detecting renovascular hypertension. The effect of altering the sensitivity and specificity of the screening test is demonstrated by assessing the expected utility of the Test-Ang strategy using screening tests that are assigned different values. Utilities are initially calculated with a test assumed to have a sensitivity of 80% and a specificity of 85%. These values are simultaneously increased by 5% until the final calculations are performed with a sensitivity and a specificity of 95% and 100%, respectively. The threshold values are listed in Table 19.1 and the utilities are graphed in Fig. 19.3. Threshold

Table 19.1. The effect of varying the sensitivity/specificity of a hypothetical screening test on the prevalence of renovascular hypertension at which the utility of a new management strategy surpasses the previously favored approach (the threshold)

Sensitivity/ specificity	MedRx vs Test-Ang threshold (%)	Test-Ang vs Angio threshold (%)
0.80/0.85	0.23	6.46
0.85/0.90	0.17	8.89
0.90/0.95	0.12	13.38
0.95/1.0	0.08	24.53

This table contains the thresholds at which the utility of the Test-Ang strategy surpasses the MedRx strategy and those at which the Angio strategy is better than the Test-Ang Strategy using tests assigned different degrees of accuracy.

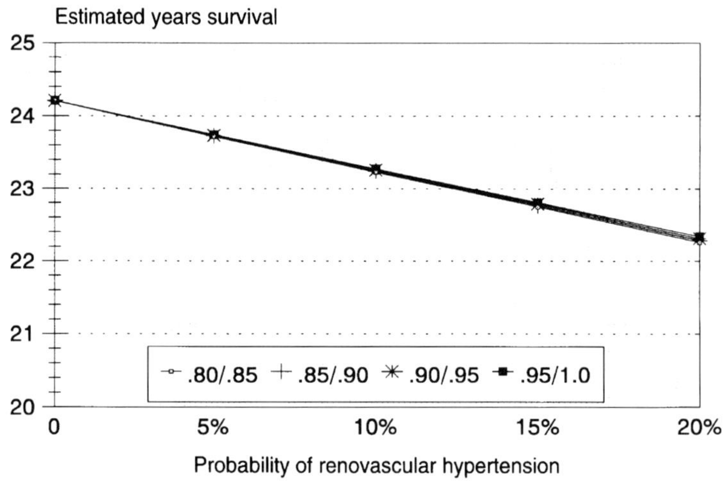

Figure 19.3. The effect of varying the sensitivity/specificity of a hypothetical screening test on calculated utilities of the most successful screening strategy (Test-Ang) in populations with the prevalence of renovascular hypertension varied from 0 to 20%.

analysis shows what appears to be the predicted effect. The prevalence of renovascular hypertension at which the utility of the screening strategy exceeds that of medical therapy alone decreases by almost 65% from the test of lowest sensitivity and specificity to that with the highest. Likewise, the prevalence at which the value of initial angiography exceeds that of the screening approach almost quadruples between the least and most discriminating values, increasing from approximately 6.5 to 24.5% (Table 19.1). These changes in thresholds suggest that incremental improvements in sensitivity and specificity appear to be of considerable benefit by expanding the fraction of the population in which the Test-Ang strategy has the highest calculated utility. When absolute values of expected utilities are examined, however, the practical aspects of this conclusion can be questioned. As noted earlier (Fig. 19.2), the slopes for the angiography and Test-Ang lines are very similar and a small change in the slope of one line can markedly change the prevalence at which they intersect (i.e. the threshold). Despite this, there is only a trivial change in the distance between the two lines, the difference in calculated survival. This is emphasized in Fig. 19.3, where there is little difference in estimated utilities among the four possible screening tests. Indeed, when the prevalence of renovascular hypertension is assumed to be 20%, the actual calculated survival difference is only 0.08 years using the least vs the most effective screening test.

Efficacy of angioplasty

Efficacy of transluminal angioplasty is the product of the probabilities that the artery will be successfully dilated and that dilatation will result in control of hypertension, with or without medications. The importance of this variable is modeled by varying its value from 50 to 90% in 20% increments and performing threshold and utility analyses. The expected utilities for immediate angiography, the clinical strategy most sensitive to this change, are graphed in Fig. 19.4, which demonstrates little change in utility as efficacy of angioplasty declines. The structure of the modeled approach reduces the impact of failed angioplasty by diverting the PTRA failures to a surgical treatment branch. As long as the efficacy of surgery is high and surgical mortality is low, unsuccessful angioplasty will not markedly lower survival. Threshold calculations demonstrate that as the efficacy of PTRA declines from 90 to 50% the prevalence at which the utility of MedRx exceeds Test-Ang rises only from 0.12 to 0.14%. As angioplasty becomes less effective, the risk/benefit ratio of performing angiography gradually increases. Consequently, the threshold for initial angiography being superior to a screening strategy shifts upwards from a prevalence level of 12.4 to 15.1% as the efficacy of PTRA declines from 90 to 50%.

Mortality of angioplasty

As the death rate secondary to percutaneous angioplasty increases, the expected utility of any choice that contains an angiography branch will decline. The magnitude of this effect is demonstrated by calculating the expected utility of choices while varying the procedure mortality rate assigned to PTRA. Changes for threshold values are listed in Table 19.2. The threshold for favoring immediate angiography, rather than a non-invasive testing strategy, increases from a prevalence of renovascular hypertension of approximately 13.4 to 20.8% as the mortality rate of PTRA is increased from 0.5 to 10%.

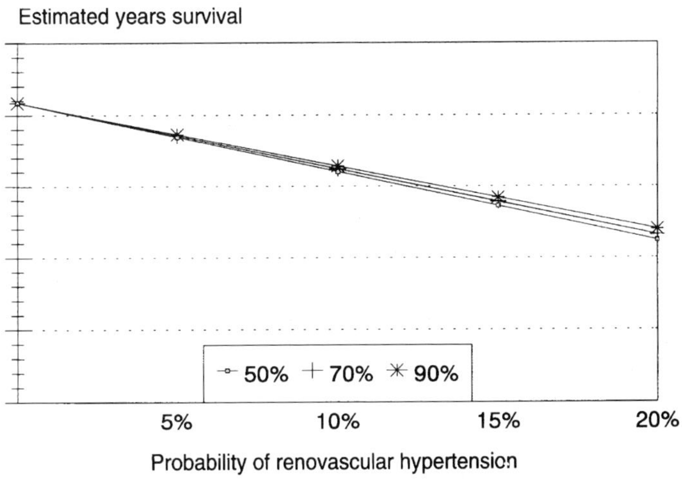

Figure 19.4. The effect of varying the percentage of PTRA procedures which result in a dilated artery and control of hypertension on calculated utilities for the Angio strategy in populations with the prevalence of renovascular hypertension varied from 0 to 20%.

Table 19.2. The effect of increasing the probability of death during PTRA on the prevalences of renovascular hypertension at which the Test-Ang strategy becomes favored over MedRx, and prevalences at which the Angio strategy is considered better than Test-Ang.

Probability of PTRA death (%)	MedRX vs Test-Ang threshold (%)	Test-Ang vs Angio threshold (%)
0.5	0.12	13.38
1.0	0.12	13.63
5.0	0.14	16.09
10.0	0.17	20.79

As the risk of angioplasty rises it requires a greater prevalence of renovascular hypertension for the more aggressive strategies to be favored.

Again, although this appears to be a major change, the actual decrease in expected survival is small. For the angiography branch of the model (Fig. 19.5), the calculated survival at a prevalence of renovascular hypertension of 20% only declines from 22.33 years to 22.04 years as the mortality rate assigned to angioplasty is increased from 0.5 to 10%. The survival rate for the Test-Ang approach is very similar to that calculated for immediate angiography, as the former strategy results in almost as many hypertensive patients being exposed to angioplasty. By virtue of the baseline assumptions made in the model, the negative consequences of not attempting to reperfuse an ischemic kidney are quite powerful. At a likelihood of renovascular hypertension of 20%, the mortality rate for PTRA must exceed 23.5% for the test first strategies to be replaced by one of the medical therapy first strategies. In point of fact, for medical therapy alone (with no workup for renovascular hypertension) to become the favored strategy, the mortality rate for PTRA must exceed 56.0% when the prevalence of renovascular hypertension is set at 20%. These calculations again point out the substantial reduction in long-term mortality that the model attributes to repair of renal artery stenosis.

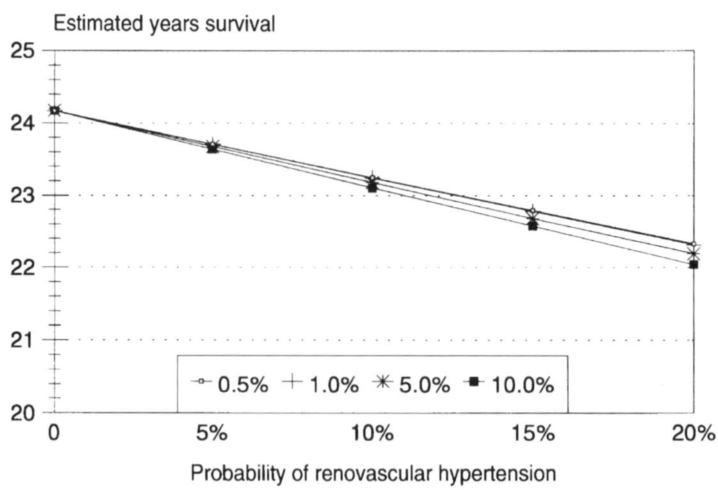

Figure 19.5. The effect of varying the percentage of times the PTRA procedure results in death on calculated utilities for the Angio strategy in populations with the prevalence of renovascular hypertension varied from 0 to 20%.

Determination of renal vein renin activity

Measurement of renin activity in renal vein effluent is a test commonly used to infer that renal artery stenosis is contributing to hypertension. The model predicts that renal vein renin measurements infrequently add to the utility of management strategies. This lack of an effect results from the probabilities used in the simulation, specifically the fact that repair of renal artery stenosis improves patient outcome, regardless of whether control of hypertension is simultaneously attained. The improved prediction of blood pressure response to dilatation of a stenosis afforded by lateralization of renin activity seldom outweighs the negative consequences assigned to not repairing a stenosis even when this test is negative. A strategy that contains renal vein renin measurements emerges as having the highest expected utility over a narrow range of incremental risk of death from PTRA when the prevalence of renovascular hypertension is set at 10%. In this context, the Med-Ang/RVR strategy replaces Med-Ang as the favored therapeutic approach when the risk of PTRA-induced death reaches 53% and then, in turn, it is replaced by the MedRx approach as the risk of death exceeds 56%. In this very restricted situation, the additional survival value added by a higher probability of control of hypertension is able to counteract the increasing mortality risk of angioplasty. When the risk of death from angioplasty reaches 56%, however, the survival advantage of any of the intervention strategies is overwhelmed, thus rendering medical therapy alone the most appropriate approach.

Mortality of surgery

The effect of surgical mortality on the utility of strategies that attempt to detect renovascular hypertension is very small within the model. This limited effect is a product of the design, as surgery is not used as a primary therapy for renovascular hypertension. When the probability of renovascular hypertension is set within a realistic range and the efficacy of angioplasty is assumed to be reasonably high, only a small fraction of patients with hypertension will ultimately undergo surgery. Although the operative risk faced by a patient who actually requires surgery may be high, surgery imposes a relatively small risk on the patient who is being investigated for renovascular hypertension, as the odds of eventually needing surgery are quite low. This conclusion is graphically represented in Fig. 19.6, which shows the effect of increasing the surgical mortality rate on the expected

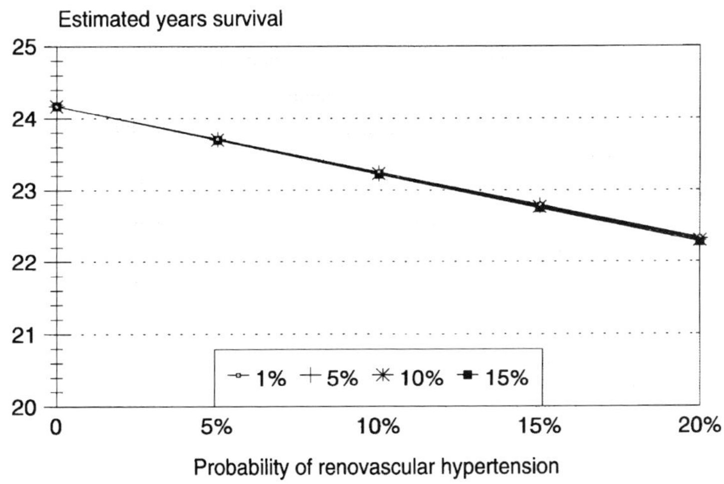

Figure 19.6. The effect of varying the percentage of times the surgical procedure results in death on calculated utilities for the Angio strategy in populations with the prevalence of renovascular hypertension varied from 0 to 20%.

utility of the immediate angiography strategy. This branch of the decision tree has the highest probability of directing a patient to surgery, and therefore its expected utility will be most sensitive to increases in surgical mortality. When the probability of renovascular hypertension is assumed to be 20%, the calculated survival in the immediate angiography strategy is 22.33 years with surgical mortality set at 1% and decreases to only 22.27 years as the surgical mortality is increased to 15%.

Probability of developing chronic renal failure

The mortality associated with requiring dialysis is an important determinant of the utility of the various strategies. If a therapy allows renovascular disease to progress until renal failure ensues, the odds of staying alive must be reduced. This effect is demonstrated in Fig. 19.7, which shows the expected years of survival in populations with different prevalences of renovascular hypertension that are treated with the medical therapy alone strategy while the probability of developing chronic renal failure is varied. If the likelihood of patients with renovascular hypertension to develop chronic renal failure within 1 year is increased from 1 to 25% in a population with a 20% chance of underlying renovascular hypertension, the expected utility of the medical therapy alone strategy loses three-quarters of a year of expected life. This scenario assumes that deterioration in renal function will remain uninvestigated. If medical therapy alone is compared with immediate angiography, in which the rate of progression to renal failure is assumed to be reduced by revascularization, there is a 1.8-year predicted survival advantage for the latter approach.

In addition to the natural history of untreated atherosclerotic renal artery stenosis, end-stage renal disease may develop as a consequence of attempted angioplasty. This possibility decreases the calculated utility of any therapeutic pathway that contains angioplasty as a possibility. The effect of increasing the risk of procedure-induced renal failure is shown in Fig. 19.8. The probability of inducing chronic renal failure with angioplasty is varied between 0.5 and 20% and the estimated survival values for the immediate angiography strategy are calculated. As expected, the calculated utilities decrease as the risk of precipitating chronic renal failure is increased. In a population that has a 20% prevalence of renovascular hypertension, the estimated survival

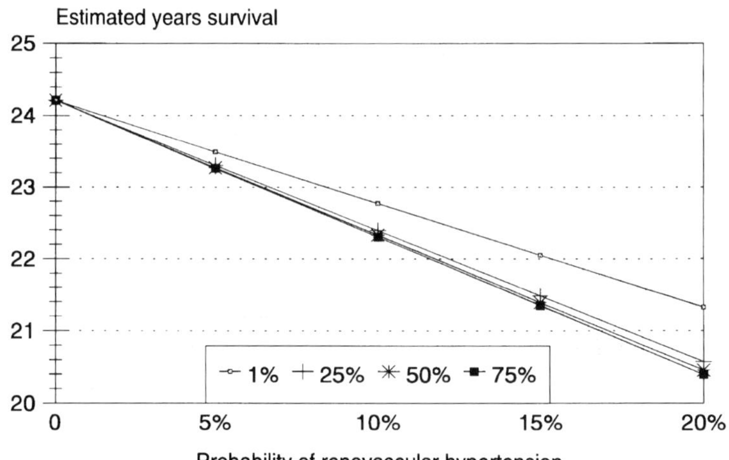

Figure 19.7. The effect of varying the percentage of patients with renovascular hypertension who will progress to needing dialysis within 1 year on the calculated utility of the medical therapy only strategy in populations with the prevalence of renovascular hypertension varied from 0 to 20%.

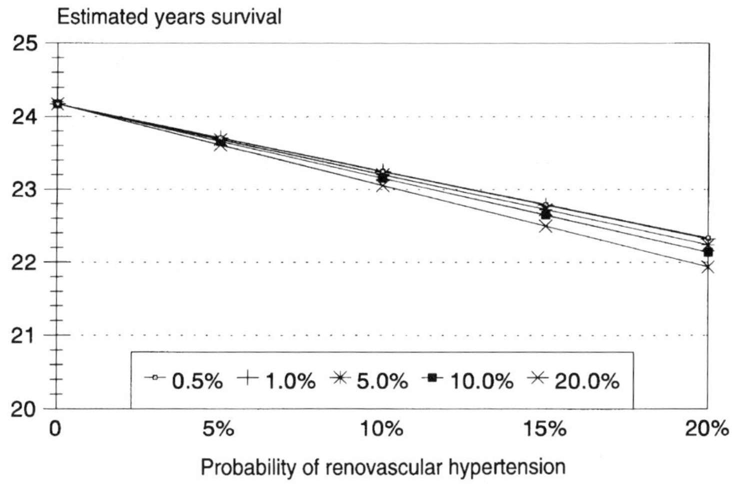

Figure 19.8. The effect of varying the percentage of PTRA procedures which will result in patients requiring chronic dialysis on the calculated utility of the Angio strategy in populations with the prevalence of renovascular hypertension varied from 0 to 20%.

decreases about 0.4 years as the risk of requiring chronic dialysis increases from 0.5 to 20%.

Varying the probability of progression to chronic renal failure also demonstrates the potential benefit of having a predictive test. The value of a test, such as a genetic marker or a cluster of clinical characteristics that anticipates progression to chronic renal failure, can be simulated by increasing the probability of chronic renal failure to 95%. This test would likely be applied only to those known to have renovascular hypertension, thus making it equivalent to setting the prevalence of renovascular hypertension at a very high level. Calculating survival utilities for a prevalence of 100% and a probability of progression to chronic renal failure of 95% gives a 9.5 years' survival advantage to the immediate angiography strategy when compared with using medical therapy alone. As expected, the ability to predict progression of vascular disease would be an important indicator for deciding who would benefit from revascularization.

Characteristics of medical therapy

It is likely that different medical therapies have differing effects on the various risks associated with renovascular hypertension. For example, angiotensin converting enzyme (ACE) inhibitors are particularly effective in controlling hypertension in patients with renal artery stenosis.[6] Also, they have been demonstrated to be effective in prolonging survival in patients with heart failure.[7] The reported positive correlation between increased activity of the renin–angiotensin system and the probability of myocardial infarction[8] has also raised the prospect that ACE inhibitors may decrease the risk of coronary artery disease in some populations. These observations suggest that there may be a particular survival advantage if this category of antihypertensive agents is used. On the other hand, it has been shown that the use of ACE inhibitors in certain patients with renovascular disease increases the risk of acute renal failure.[9] In addition, animal models of renal artery stenosis have also suggested the possibility that these drugs may also contribute to chronic renal failure.[10]

Altering the probabilities used in the model offers the opportunity to estimate the magnitude of changes in outcome, which might be expected with treatments that have different characteristics. To simulate the hypothetical advantages and disadvantages of ACE inhibitors, two additional medical therapies are tested that feature assumptions different from those in the baseline model. In Therapy 1, the efficacy of medical therapy is increased from 70 to 95%, whereas the excess mortality associated with having renovascular disease is decreased by 10%. In addition, Therapy 1 doubles the risk of developing end-stage renal disease regardless of whether control of hypertension is attained. In Therapy 2, the same assumptions are made about blood pressure control and changes in mortality risk, but the risk of developing chronic renal failure is not increased. In a population with a 10% prevalence of renovascular hypertension, the expected survival for medical therapy with the baseline assumptions is 22.79 years, whereas it is 22.91 years for Therapy 1 and 22.98 years for Therapy 2. When the assumptions are applied to a patient known to have renovascular hypertension (i.e. prevalence of 100%), the calculated survival for the baseline medical therapy is 10.00 years, whereas those calculated for Therapies 1 and 2 are 11.09 years and 11.81 years, respectively. The decision model suggests a difference in outcome that is large enough to justify the comparison of different medical therapies in patients with renovascular hypertension.

Comparative costs of strategies

As noted previously, if the actual survival difference among therapies is small or non-existent, differences in the cost of approaches argue for the strategy that is less expensive. The potential costs of the strategies modeled in this chapter can be estimated by applying the charges for the corresponding procedures at the Medical Center Hospital of Vermont (see Appendix, Table 19.5). The model assumes that if end-stage renal disease develops, dialysis will be used as a supportive therapy. These assessments probably underestimate costs at many other institutions, but the relative relationship between charges is instructive. The analysis only models for the direct estimated costs of procedures used to treat renovascular hypertension and renal failure, and does not account for possible changes in patterns of cost for other medical and supportive care or changes in the earnings potential of patients and their families.

Cost analyses may be reported in a number of different forms. These include the total cost of a strategy calculated for the entire estimated lifespan; the average cost per year of survival; and, more commonly, the additional cost per extra year of life offered by a superior strategy when

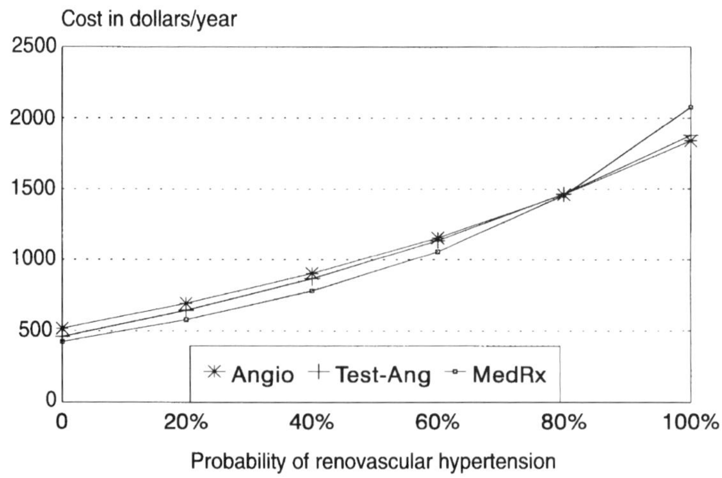

Figure 19.9. The estimated average cost of a year of life for the three most successful management strategies calculated for the entire possible range of prevalence of renovascular hypertension.

compared with a less expensive, but less effective, option (this latter type of analysis is referred to as marginal cost effectiveness). Figure 19.9 graphs the average yearly costs for the three therapies that have been identified previously as providing the greatest survival advantage. The average yearly cost for medical therapy alone compared with immediate angiography or Test-Ang remains the lowest until the prevalence of renovascular hypertension reaches about 80%. At that point, the financial penalty imposed by missing a potentially reversible cause of chronic renal failure, which requires dialysis, begins to be greater than the cost of attempting to identify and treat renovascular hypertension. An additional disadvantage of choosing medical therapy alone is a loss of about 2.5 years' survival when the prevalence of renovascular hypertension is 40% and 5 years when the prevalence reaches 100%. Analyses that calculate the cost of this additional survival time are often more meaningful. Table 19.3 lists and Fig. 19.10 graphs the marginal costs of additional years of survival when the prevalence of renovascular hypertension is varied over a realistic clinical range of between 5 and 20%. Immediate angiography carries a high marginal cost for a relatively short increase in lifespan, when the prevalence of renovascular

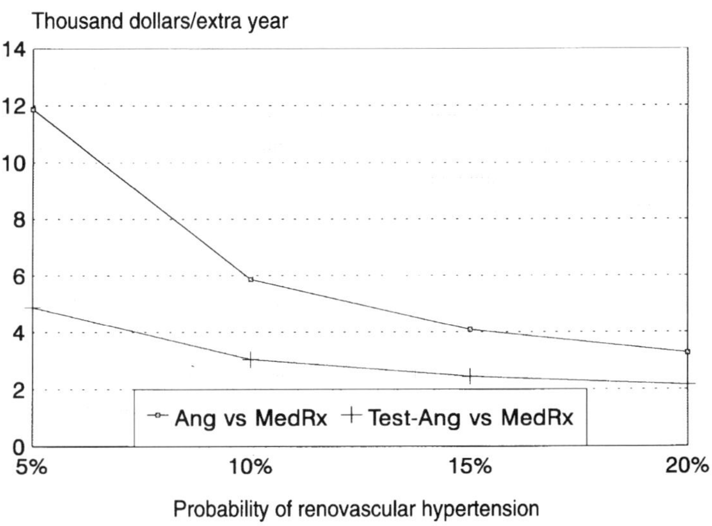

Figure 19.10. The marginal cost effectiveness graphed as the dollar cost per extra year of life of the more successful Angio and Test-Ang strategies compared with the less expensive MedRx strategy.

Table 19.3. A cost comparison of the Angio vs MedRx strategies and the Test-Ang vs MedRx strategies

Probability of renovascular hypertension (%)	Strategy comparison	Marginal survival (years)	Marginal cost (dollars)	Marginal cost effectiveness (dollars/extra year)
5	Angio vs MedRx	0.207	2457	11 870
	Test-Ang vs MedRx	0.230	1122	4879
10	Angio vs MedRx	0.457	2683	5870
	Test-Ang vs MedRx	0.467	1423	3047
15	Angio vs MedRx	0.711	2909	4091
	Test-Ang vs MedRx	0.703	1723	2450
20	Angio vs MedRx	0.958	3136	3273
	Test-Ang MedRx	0.939	2025	2157

The table demonstrates the excess life provided by the favored strategies, the cost of that increase in lifespan, and the marginal cost effectiveness (the dollar cost per extra year of life).

hypertension is 5% or less. Although the strategy Test-Ang provides a similar small increase in estimated survival, it does this at a much lower cost than starting with angiography. This is accomplished by using the less expensive screening option to target a smaller group with a higher prevalence of renovascular hypertension that will be subjected to the more costly test, angiography. As the prevalence of renovascular hypertension increases, the model predicts a decreasing cost for additional calculated years of survival, when strategies that test for renovascular hypertension are used. This result stems predominantly from a progressive increase in estimated survival. Relatively stable diagnostic costs are spread over this longer lifespan, reducing the marginal cost per extra year of life. Because more patients have renovascular hypertension, aggressive diagnostic strategies also generate savings by reducing medication costs and decreasing the number of patients who ultimately require dialysis.

Summary

Making the decision to pursue the diagnosis of renovascular hypertension is often difficult. This difficulty stems in large part from the requisite process of balancing the potential harmful and beneficial aspects of tests and therapeutic procedures. The dilemma is magnified in patients suspected of having atherosclerotic renovascular disease because of the perception that this population is particularly vulnerable to the complications of interventions. Decision analysis offers a method for assessing the importance of the variables that will determine the outcomes of differing approaches to renovascular hypertension. This technique is particularly powerful and revealing, as it can examine the influence of a single variable on outcome within the context of the entire chain of events comprising the diagnosis and management of the disease. Given this perspective, the effect on expected outcome is often surprisingly small, even with substantial changes in an apparently important aspect of diagnosis or management. Nonetheless, these small changes in outcome should not be dismissed as clinically irrelevant. They are probably best viewed as analogous to outcomes in clinical trials, in which a 5 or 10% difference between groups is often of great importance, particularly if the disease under consideration is common.

Analysis using a classic decision tree suggests that reasonable management progresses from medical therapy alone to a screening strategy and finally to immediate angiography as the prevalence of atherosclerotic renovascular disease increases. This hierarchy of strategies is not surprising, and in fact it may have been predicted by the thoughtful physician without resorting to the trouble of modeling. Of more interest is the quantification of the utility of various approaches as the characteristics of different elements of clinical choices are varied.

Before considering these findings, it should be remembered that these conclusions are made using changes in estimated lifespan as the dominant measure of value. Other measures of value can give different results. For example, when the model is run using estimates that predict the fewer extra deaths and the very low probability of progressive renal failure likely to occur in fibromuscular dysplasia, the strategy of medical therapy followed by angiography only if hypertension persists, Med-Ang, has the highest calculated utility at all prevalences of renovascular hypertension. Despite this, a clinician who suspects fibromuscular dysplasia in a young patient might well elect to pursue the diagnosis of renal artery stenosis, even if hypertension is controlled by medical means, in order to avoid the negative impact on quality of life produced by lifelong antihypertensive therapy.

In spite of its limitations, the model offers insight into the decisions that surround the diagnosis and management of atherosclerotic renovascular hypertension. The prevalence of renovascular hypertension at which medical therapy alone is the favored approach is under 0.13% using baseline assumptions. This implies that the risk of death is not a strong argument against attempts to detect renovascular hypertension in most cases. It is the high marginal cost of attempted diagnosis at low prevalences, which makes this approach a questionable financial investment in a population in which atherosclerotic renovascular hypertension is unlikely to be found. As the prevalence of renovascular hypertension rises to 10%, it is estimated that almost half a year of life is added by aggressive investigation and intervention. Increases in survival of this magnitude are sufficient to be considered of practical importance by many clinicians. Of interest, the model suggests that the major variable which influences outcome is simply the decision to investigate for the presence of renovascular hypertension. Sizable variations in the characteristics of tests and therapeutic interventions result in fairly minor changes in outcome when the model is applied to populations in which the prevalence of renovascular hypertension approximates what is likely to be found in clinical practice. Further, the analysis predicts that attempts to identify and repair renal artery stenosis as a cause of hypertension are appropriate, even when diagnostic and reparative procedures do not have optimal results. However, this should not be taken to mean that efforts to increase the accuracy of testing and the success of renal revascularization are without value. Indeed, the simulation does suggest that a method that accurately predicts progression to renal failure would be very useful in the management of renovascular hypertension.

Finally, all of these conclusions are driven by the assumption that renal revascularization provides a survival advantage that is largely derived from the prevention of chronic renal failure and other factors that reduce the risk of death. These factors are only partially dependent on blood pressure control. How renal revascularization would enhance survival beyond its effect on hypertension is unclear, but it is not unreasonable to consider the possibility that such an additional benefit might be derived from suppression of the renin–angiotensin system. Maximum inhibition of this system might reduce stimulation of vascular smooth muscle growth thereby retarding the development of ventricular hypertrophy, atherosclerosis and glomerulosclerosis. Because this supposition is only implied by available clinical reports, informed decision making in renovascular hypertension will remain elusive until this and other assumptions employed in this model are subjected to formal testing.

Appendix

Clinical decision analysis is a quantitative, probabilistic technique that is used to examine decisions under conditions of uncertainty. By creating an explicit, mathematical representation of the problem being evaluated, decision analysis can provide the clinician with a preferred management plan. The steps involved in creating a decision analysis model include:

1. Structuring (focusing) the clinical problem to be analyzed.
2. Assigning probability values to all chance events.
3. Assigning a utility (i.e. some value measure) to all outcome states.
4. Analyzing the baseline decision model.
5. Performing sensitivity analyses (i.e. repeating the analysis with changed probability or utility values, or with changed model structure).

The decision model

Figure 19.11 illustrates the main decision tree used in the analysis of choices that are made in the process of detecting and treating renovascular hypertension. The square symbol represents a decision node (where the clinician decides which strategies or options to consider for evaluation). The small circular symbols represent chance nodes that may follow a particular decision. The branches at the decision node are under the control of the 'decision maker' – only those options to be considered are represented. The branches at a chance node, however, are out of the control of the 'decision maker' – they occur based upon the probabilistic data relevant to the situation. The rectangular boxes represent the terminal branches or outcome states for each decision pathway.

The decision node at the far left of the tree contains the eight options being considered. The top choice (Angio) is to perform immediate angiography. If angiography is performed, there is a risk of dying from the procedure or developing chronic renal failure (CRF) requiring dialysis. Fortunately, most patients will survive angiography, at which point the presence or absence of renovascular disease (RVD) will be known. If RVD is present, then the strategy moves on to the percutaneous transluminal renal angioplasty (PTRA) part of the decision model (or subtree), depicted in Fig. 19.12. If RVD is not found, the patient will be treated with medical therapy. The second option (Ang/RVR) is identical to the Angio choice, except that renal vein renins are measured in patients with RVD to determine if PTRA will be performed. If the renal vein renin values lateralize, then PTRA is performed; if no lateralization is found, then the patient will be treated with medical therapy alone. This option differs from the Angio option in that the efficacy of PTRA is set higher when lateralization is present.

The next three options model the various non-invasive screening strategies. In the Test option, the results of the test determine the next approach: 'positive' results proceed to angiography, 'negative' results proceed to medical therapy. The likelihoods of 'positive' and 'negative' results are based on the sensitivity and the specificity of the test and the prevalence of RVD. The probability of a 'positive' result equals the sensitivity times the probability of RVD plus the false

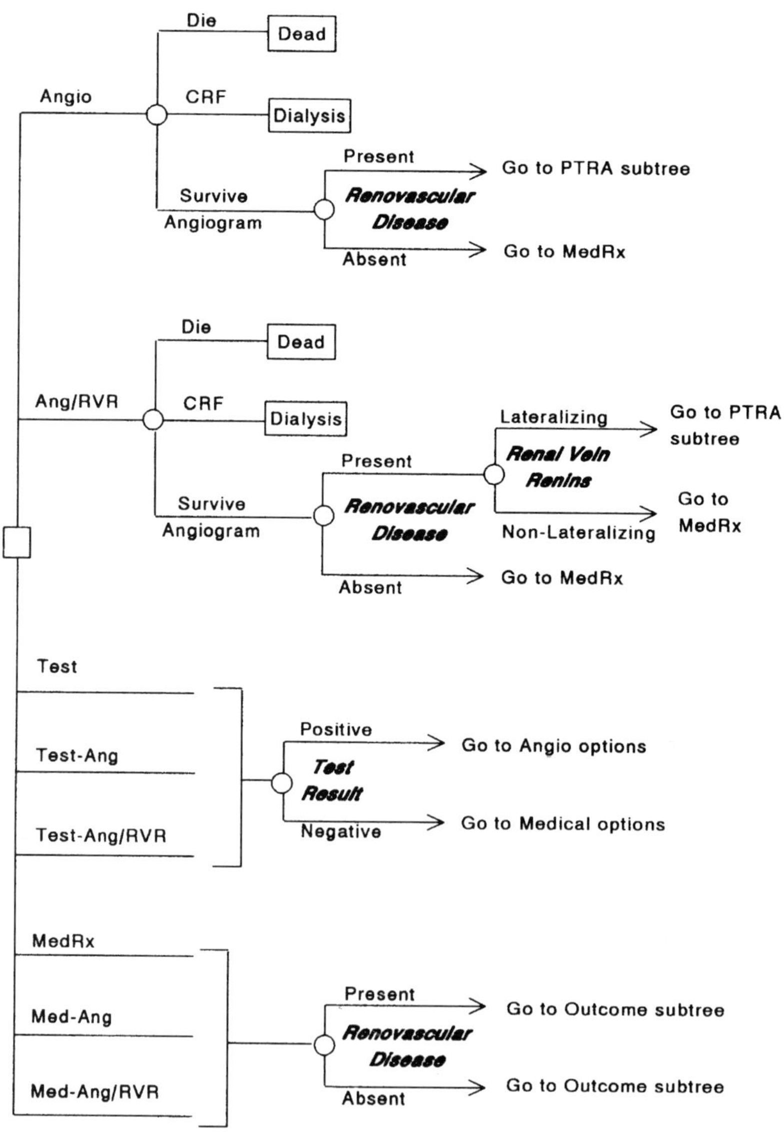

Figure 19.11. Master decision tree with the choice node demonstrating the eight possible management choices and the first chance nodes which follow the choice. Ultimately hypothetical surviving patients may cycle through to the PTRA subtree and the Outcome subtree.

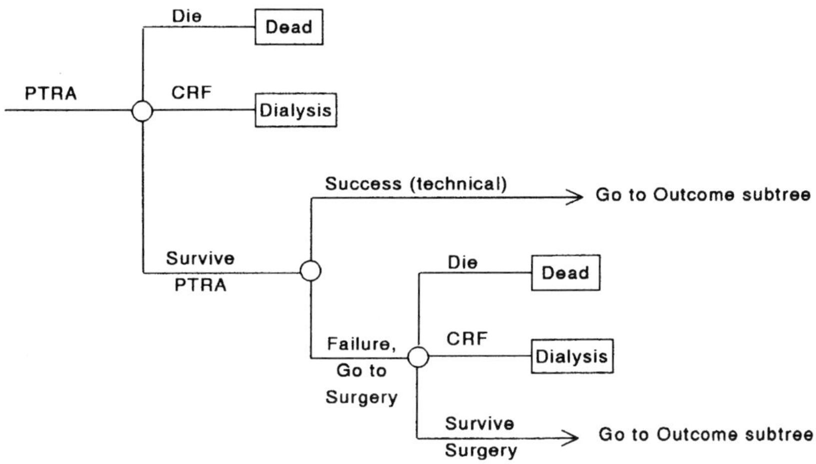

Figure 19.12. The PTRA subtree diagrams the flow of chance events that may occur following the PTRA procedure.

positive rate (one minus the specificity) times the probability of no RVD. The probability of a 'negative' result is simply modeled as one minus the likelihood of a 'positive' result. With the Test-Ang option, a 'positive' result will proceed to the Angio option, whereas a 'negative' result will proceed to medical therapy with the Angio option available as a 'bailout' if the hypertension continues to be difficult to control. With the Test-Ang/RVR option, a 'positive' result will proceed to the Ang/RVR option, and a 'negative' result will proceed to medical therapy with the Ang/RVR option available as a 'bailout' if the hypertension continues to be difficult to control. In the testing options, the actual probability of RVD following a test result is based upon the reported frequency of correct classification of disease status by the test (i.e. the positive or negative predictive value of the test).

The last three strategies model the various medical options being considered. In the MedRx choice, the patient is treated with medical therapy regardless of the likelihood of renovascular hypertension. In the Med-Ang strategy, the patient will go on to angiography as a 'bailout' if the hypertension continues to be difficult to control. In the Med-Ang/RVR choice, the patient will go on to angiography with renal vein renin determination if the hypertension continues to be difficult to control. These events are modeled in the Outcome subtree (Fig 19.13).

Figure 19.13 represents the events modeled in the PTRA subtree. Following PTRA, the patient may die, develop CRF requiring dialysis, or may survive the procedure. The next chance event is the likelihood of technical success or failure. If the procedure is successful, then the strategy proceeds on to the Outcome subtree. If the procedure fails, then surgical revascularization is performed. If the patient survives surgery without chronic renal failure, the strategy proceeds to the Outcome subtree.

The Outcome subtree (Fig. 19.13) represents both the short-term likelihood of successful control of hypertension (Controlled BP vs Still HBP) and the long-term events contained in the Markov cycle trees denoted by the linked circular symbols. As described later, it is iterations of these Markov cycles that will determine the long-term utility (survival) assigned to the various choices. The control of hypertension is modeled as the efficacy of the various treatments preceding the Outcome subtree. If the blood pressure is still high (Still HBP), then the patient may go on to the Angio or Ang/RVR strategies if these are active options (i.e. if the 'bailout' options are being allowed for the pertinent testing or medical therapy choices and angiography has not already been performed). The triangular symbols mark 'switch' nodes at which the tree will be preset to proceed in one of two directions (i.e. at Still HBP, patients will be directed to either the Angio or the No Angio, HBP Rx options and at Angio, they will be directed to the RVR or no RVR branch). In each of these 'bailout' situations, the probability of RVD at angiography is reset at either 100 or 0% in accordance with whether RVD was defined as present or absent prior to the Outcome subtree.

The final events of this decision tree are modeled in the two Markov cycle trees. It is these iterations that will calculate the long-term survival of those patients who have survived the early diagnostic and therapeutic procedures. The upper Markov cycle tree models events if the patient has normal blood pressure (Controlled

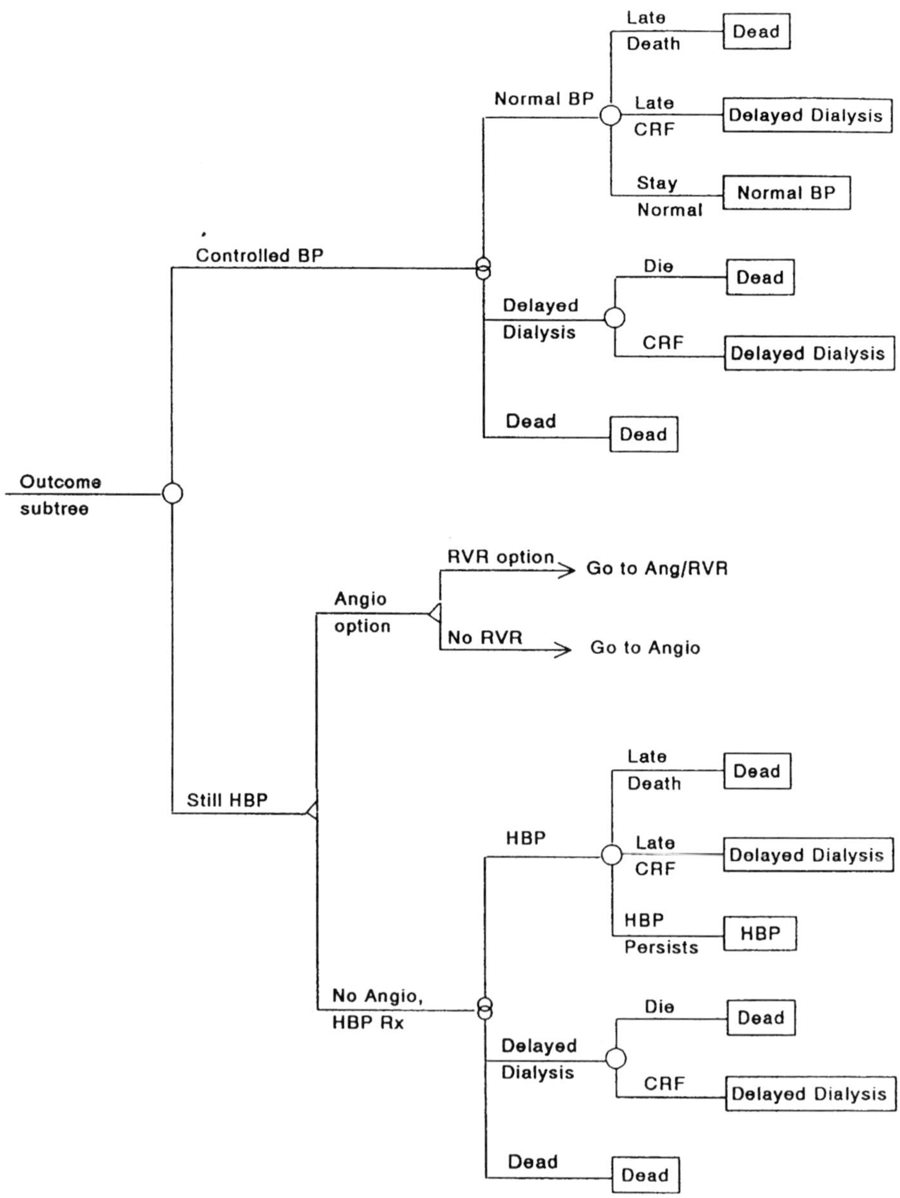

Figure 19.13. The Outcome subtree diagrams the terminal chance events encountered by the hypothetical patients. The pattern of flow is conditioned by assumptions made about the initial management choice and probabilities assigned in preceding elements of the decision tree. These details are described in the text of the Appendix.

BP); the lower Markov cycle tree models events for persistent hypertension (HBP). The initial branches of a Markov cycle tree represent the various states of health that a patient may end up in over time. The chance events in a Markov cycle tree represent the likelihoods of changing from one state to another state during some unit of time (typically a year). Although the ultimate likelihood of ending up in a state such as CRF requiring dialysis may be high over a person's lifetime, the annual risk (i.e. transition probability) will be much smaller. The 'terminal' nodes in a Markov cycle tree refer to the 'state' that a patient ends up in at the end of the cycle. A measure of utility is then calculated for the different outcome states and the sum of these utilities determines the incremental value of the cycle. Cycles are repeated until the incremental value of the next cycle is very small (i.e. essentially everyone is in the Dead state where no incre-

Table 19.4. Range of values, baseline values and pertinent reference for the variables used in the decision model

Variable	Range of values	Baseline values	References
Baseline life expectancy		25 years	
Efficacy of medical therapy of essential hypertension	53–95.8%	90%	11, 12, 13
Efficacy of medical therapy of renovascular hypertension	36–99%	70%	14, 15, 16
Efficacy of PTRA	38–99%	73%	17, 18, 19
Efficacy of PTRA with lateralizing renal vein renins	100%	95%	20, 21
Efficacy of surgery	80–89%	80%	22, 23, 24
Efficacy of surgery with lateralizing renal vein renins	89–95%	90%	24, 25
Excess mortality of chronic renal failure	20–30%/year	20%/year	26, 27, 28
Excess mortality of uncontrolled essential hypertension	0.4–0.6%/year	0.5%/year	29
Excess mortality of uncontrolled renovascular hypertension	10%/year	10%/year	30
Excess mortality of uncontrolled hypertension following angioplasty	1.4–10%/year	3%/year	18, 19, 31, 32
Excess mortality of uncontrolled hypertension following surgery	3.5%–15%/year	4%/year	23, 33, 34
Excess mortality of controlled essential hypertension	0–0.25%/year	0%/year	35
Excess mortality of controlled renovascular hypertension	4%/year	4%/year	30
Excess mortality of controlled hypertension following angioplasty	0.2–3.0%/year	2%/year	18, 19
Excess mortality of controlled hypertension following surgery	1.0–3.5%/year	2%/year	23, 33, 36
Probability of chronic renal failure following angiography	No clear range	0.10%	5, 37
Probability of death from angiography	No clear range	0.10%	38, 39
Probability of chronic renal failure from uncontrolled essential hypertension	0–0.06%/year	0.012%/year	40, 41, 42, 43
Probability of chronic renal failure from uncontrolled renovascular hypertension	0.3–3.0%/year	0.7%/year	15, 30, 44
Probability of chronic renal failure with hypertension following angioplasty	0–1.4%/year	0.25%/year	18, 19, 24, 31, 45
Probability of chronic renal failure with hypertension following sugery	0–0.25%/year	0.125%/year	5, 24, 32, 45, 46, 47
Probability of chronic renal failure with controlled essential hypertension	No clear range	0%/year	40, 41, 42, 43
Probability of chronic renal failure with medical control of Renovascular hypertension	No clear range	0.6%/year	15, 30, 44
Probability of chronic renal failure with controlled hypertension following angioplasty	No clear range	0.20%	18, 19, 14, 21, 36
Probability of chronic renal failure with controlled hypertension following sugery	No clear range	0.12%	15, 24, 32, 45, 46, 47
Probability of lateralization of renal vein renins in unilateral renal artery stenosis	No clear range	69%	25
Probability of PTRA-induced chronic renal failure	0.1–1%	0.50%	18, 19, 21, 24, 45
Probability of PTRA-induced death	0.1–1%	0.50%	18, 19, 21, 24, 31, 45, 48
Probability of PTRA-technical success	60–90%	85%	18, 19, 24, 31, 45, 48
Probability of renovascular hypertension	1.0–38%	Vary	49, 50, 51
Probability of surgery-induced chronic renal failure	0.1–1.0%	50%	22, 32, 47, 52, 53
Probability of surgical death	1.0–10.0%	2.00%	22, 23, 24, 46, 52, 53
Sensitivity of non-invasive test	80–95%	90%	54, 55, 56
Specificity of non-invasive test	80–100%	95%	54, 55, 56

Values utilized in the model are tabulated under baseline values, unless otherwise specified.

mental value accrues). The expected utility of a Markov cycle tree is thus the cumulative value of the various cycle iterations.

An important simplifying assumption is that hypertension does not develop in the Normal BP Markov cycle tree, and adequate control of hypertension is never achieved in the HBP Markov cycle tree. The model also assumes that an unselected individual of the same age as those being evaluated for hypertension would have a 25-year life expectancy.

Probability, outcome and costs data

Table 19.4 records the data used for the variables in this decision model. The range of values found in the literature, along with the baseline values used in the model, and the pertinent references are listed. The cost data are listed in Table 19.5, and are based on direct charges at the Medical Center Hospital of Vermont. Only the direct costs associated with investigation and treatment of hypertension and with dialysis are considered.

Table 19.5. Approximate charges for procedures other than dialysis at the Medical Center Hospital of Vermont in 1994

Procedure	Charge ($)
Angiography	2000
Angioplasty	6000
ESRD/year	50 000
Medication	350
Renal vein renin	1500
Surgery	17 500
Test	500

The cost for 1 year of care for a dialysis patient with the primary diagnosis of renovascular disease was estimated at $50 000.

References

1 Pauker SD, Kassirer JP. Decision analysis. *N Engl J Med* 1987; **316:** 250–8.
2 Kassirer JP, Moskowitz AJ, Lau J, Pauker SD. Decision analysis: a progress report. *Ann Int Med* 1987; **106:** 279–91.
3 McNeil BJ, Varady PD, Burrows BA, Adelstein SJ. Cost-effectiveness calculations in the diagnosis and treatment of hypertensive renovascular disease. *N Engl J Med* 1975; **293:** 216–21.
4 McNeil BJ, Adelstein SJ. The value of case finding in hypertensive renovascular disease. *N Engl J Med* 1975; **293:** 221–6.
5 Kopelman RI, McNutt RA, Pauker SG. Use of decision analysis in a complicated case of renovascular hypertension. *Hypertension* 1988; **12:** 611–19.
6 Hollenberg NK. Medical therapy for renovascular hypertension: a review. *Am J Hypertension* 1987; **1:** 338S–343S.
7 The Consensus Trial Study Group. Results of enalapril on mortality in severe congestive heart failure: result of the cooperative north scandinavian enalapril survival study. *N Engl J Med* 1987; **316:** 1429–35.
8 Alderman MH, Madhavan D, Ooi WL *et al.* Association of the renin–sodium profile with the risk of myocardial infarction in patients with hypertension. *N Engl J Med* 1991; **324:** 1098–104.
9 Hricik DE, Browning PJ, Kopelman R *et al.* Captopril-induced functional renal insufficiency in patients with bilateral renal-artery stenoses or renal-artery stenosis in a solitary kidney. *N Engl J Med* 1983; **308:** 373–6.
10 Hricik DE, Dunn MJ. Angiotensin-converting enzyme inhibitor-induced renal failure: causes, consequences and diagnostic uses. *J Am Soc Nephrol* 1990; **1:** 845–58.
11 Hypertension Detection and Follow-up Program Cooperative Group. Five-year Findings of the Hypertension Detection and Follow-up Program I. Reduction in mortality of persons with high blood pressure, including mild hypertension. *JAMA* 1979; **242:** 2562–671.
12 Alderman MH, Bunder N, Cohen H *et al.* Prevalence of drug resistant hypertension. *Hypertension* 1988; **11:** (Suppl. II) 71–5.
13 Isaksson H, Danielson M, Rosenhamer G *et al.* Characteristics of patients resistant to antihypertensive drug therapy. *J Inter Med* 1991; **229:** 421–6.
14 Rosenthal T. Drug therapy of renovascular hypertension. *Drugs* 1993; **45:** 895–909.

15 Hunt JC, Strong CG. Renovascular hypertension mechanisms, natural history and treatment. *Am J Cardiol* 1973; **32:** 562–74.
16 Hollenberg NK. Medical therapy of renovascular hypertension: efficacy and safety of captopril in 269 patients. *Cardiovasc Rev Rep* 1985; **4:** 852–78.
17 Ram VS. Southwestern internal medicine conference: current concepts in renovascular hypertension. *Am J Med Sci* 1992; **304:** 53–71.
18 Losinno F, Zuccala A, Busato F, Zucchelli P. Renal artery angioplasty for renovascular hypertension and preservation of renal function: long-term angiographic and clinical follow-up. *Am J Roentgenol* 1994; **162:** 853–7.
19 Weibull H, Bergquist D, Jonsson K *et al.* Long-term results after percutaneous transluminal angioplasty of atherosclerotic renal artery stenosis – the importance of intensive follow-up *Eur J Vasc Surg* 1991; **5:** 291–301.
20 Pickering TG, Sos TA, Vaughn DA *et al.* Predictive value and changes of renin secretion in hypertensive patients with unilateral renovascular disease undergoing successful renal angioplasty. *Am J Med* 1984; **76:** 398–403.
21 Mahler F, Probst P, Haertel M *et al.* (Lasting improvement of renovascular hypertension by transluminal dilation of atherosclerotic and nonatherosclerotic renal artery stenosis. A follow-up study. *Circulation* 1981; **65:** 611–17.
22 Hansen KJ, Starr SM, Sands *et al.* Contemporary surgical management of renovascular disease. *J Vasc Surg* 1992; **16:** 319–31.
23 Novick AC, Ziegelbaum MD, Vidt DG *et al.* Trends in surgical revascularization for renal artery disease ten years' experience. *JAMA* 1987; **257:** 498–501.
24 Weiball H, Bergquist D, Bergentz SE *et al.* Percutaneous transluminal renal angioplasty versus surgical reconstruction of atherosclerotic renal artery stenosis: a prospective randomized study. *J Vasc Surg* 1993; **18:** 841–52.
25 Marks LS, Maxwell MH. Renal vein renin value and limitations in the prediction of operative results. *Urol Clin North Am* 1975; **2:** 311–25.
26 Mailloux LU. Atherosclerotic renovascular disease causing end-stage renal disease: the case for earlier diagnosis and therapy. *J Vasc Med Biol* 1993; **4:** 277–84.
27 Byrne C, Vernon P, Cohen JJ. Effect of age and diagnosis on survival of older patients beginning chronic dialysis. *JAMA* 1994; **271:** 34–6.
28 Churchill DN, Taylor DW, Cook RJ *et al.* Canadian hemodialysis morbidity study. *Am J Kidney Dis* 1992; **19:** 214–34.
29 The Society of Actuaries and Association of Life Insurance Medical Directors of America. *Blood Pressure Study 1979*. Boston, 1980.
30 Wollenweber J, Sheps SG, Davis GD. Clinical course of atherosclerotic renovascular disease. *Am J Cardiol* 1968; **21:** 60–71.
31 Klinge J, Mali WPTM, Puijlaert CBAJ *et al.* Percutaneous transluminal renal angioplasty: initial and long-term results. *Radiology* 1989; **171:** 501–6.
32 Olin JW, Vidt DG, Gifford RW, Novick AC. Renovascular disease in the elderly: an analysis of 50 patients. *J Am Coll Cardiol* 1985; **5:** 1232–8.
33 Dean RH. Late results of aortorenal bypass. *Urol Clin North Am* 1984; **11:** 425–34.
34 Hallett JW, Fowl R, O'Brien PC *et al.* Renovascular operations in patients with chronic renal insufficiency: do the benefits justify the risks? *J Vasc Surg* 1987; **5:** 622–7.
35 Lew EA. Hypertension and longevity. In Laragh JH, Brenner BM (eds) *Hypertension Pathophysiology, Diagnosis and Management*, pp. 175–190. New York: Raven Press, 1990.
36 Novick AC, Texter SC, Bodie B, Kauli RB. Revascularization to preserve renal function in patients with atherosclerotic renovascular disease. *Urol Clin North Am* 1984; **11:** 477–80.
37 Berns JS, Rudnick MR. Radiocontrast media associated nephrotoxicity. *Kidney* 1992; **24:** 1–5.
38 Ansell G. An epidemiologic report on adverse reactions in urography: ionic and nonionic media. *Diagn Imaging* 1987; (May suppl.): 6–10.
39 Kadir S. *Diagnostic Angiography*, pp. 679. Philadelphia: WB Saunders, 1986.
40 Raine AEG. Hypertension and the kidney. *Br Med Bull* 1994; **50:** 322–41.
41 Walker WG, Neaton JI, Cutler *et al.* Renal function change in hypertensive members of the multiple risk factor intervention trial. *JAMA* 1992; **268:** 3085–91.
42 Perneger TV, Nieto J, Whelton PK, *et al.* A prospective study of blood pressure and serum creatinine. *JAMA* 1993; **269:** 488–93.
43 Brown MA, Whitworth JA. Hypertension in human renal disease. *J Hypertension* 1992; **10:** 701–12.
44 Dean RH, Kieffer RW, Smith BM *et al.* Renovascular hypertension anatomic and renal functional changes during drug therapy. *Arch Surg* 1981; **116:** 1408–1415.
45 Canzanello VJ, Millan VG, Spiegel JE *et al* Percutaneous transluminal renal angioplasty in management of atherosclerotic renovascular hypertension: results in 100 patients. *Hypertension* 1989; **13:** 163–72.
46 Hansen KJ, Ditesheim JA, Metropol SH *et al.* Management of renovascular disease in the elderly population. *J Vasc Surg* 1989; **10:** 266–73.
47 Isles C, Main J, O'Connell J, Brown I *et al.* Survival associated with renovascular disease in Glasgow and Newcastle: a collaborative study. *Scot Med J* 1990 **35:** 70–3.
48 Englund R, Brown MA. 1991, Renal angioplasty for renovascular disease: a reappraisal. *J Cardiovasc Surg* **32:** 76–80.

49 Gifford RW Jr. Evaluation of the hypertensive patient. Emphasis on detecting curable causes. *Milbank Mem Fund Q* 1969; **37:** 170–86.
50 Anderson GH, Blakeman N, Streeter DHP. Prediction of renovascular hypertension: comparison of clinical diagnostic indices. *Am J Hypertension* 1988; **1:** 301–4.
51 Davis BA, Crook JE, Vestal RE, Oates JA. Prevalence of renovascular hypertension in patients with grade III or IV hypertensive retinopathy. *N Engl J Med* 1989; **301**: 1273–6.
52 Torsello G, Sacks M, Kniemeyer H *et al.* Results of surgical treatment for atherosclerotic renovascular occlusive disease. *Eur J Vasc Surg* 1990; **4:** 472–82.
53 Bredenberg CE, Sampson LN, Ferris SR *et al.*. Changing patterns in surgery for chronic renal artery occlusive diseases. *J Vasc Surg* 1992; **15:** 1018–24.
54 Mann SJ, Pickering TG. Detection of renovascular hypertension state of the art: 1992. *Ann Int Med* 1992; **117:** 845–53.
55 Davidson RA, Wilcox CS. Newer tests for the diagnosis of renovascular disease. *JAMA* 1992; **268:** 3353–8.
56 Nally JV, Olin JW, Lammert GK. Advances in noninvasive screening for renovascular disease. *Cleve Clin J Med* 1994; **61:** 328–36.

20

Renal vascular hypertension in the transplant patient

MARK L JORDAN, JEAN L HOLLEY, ALBERT B ZAJKO

Introduction

Renal transplantation is now the preferred form of therapy for end-stage renal disease. Although renal transplantation provides the obvious benefit of re-establishing renal function and eliminating the need for dialysis, one of the most common complications of transplantation and one that leads to potential morbidity and mortality in approximately 50–80% of renal transplant patients is persistent hypertension.[1–5] Since hypertension is one of the most important risk factors for cardiovascular morbidity and mortality after transplantation[2, 4, 5] it is imperative for the transplant surgeon to be able to identify, investigate and treat all potentially correctable causes of hypertension in the transplant recipient. Post-transplant hypertension is often multifactorial but can be broadly classified as (1) resulting from impaired allograft function, usually due to chronic rejection or recurrent disease, (2) secondary to the drugs used for immunosuppressive therapy, (3) persistent essential hypertension and (4) renal vascular hypertension, as a consequence of disease either in the native kidneys or transplant renal artery.

The purpose of this chapter is to discuss the pathophysiology, etiology, clinical features, diagnosis and treatment of renal vascular hypertension in the transplant recipient. Because true renal vascular hypertension in the transplant recipient cannot always be clearly distinguished from the other causes described above, a brief discussion of non-renovascular causes of post-transplant hypertension will first be provided, followed by a more in-depth review of renovascular hypertension in the transplant patient.

Etiology of post-transplant hypertension

Allograft dysfunction

The most common cause of hypertension in renal transplant recipients is chronic rejection.[2, 4, 6] Chronic allograft damage produces renal parenchymal disease resulting in narrowing of small vessels with chronic transplant glomerulopathy.[2] This form of chronic renal damage may closely resemble chronic native kidney disease with decreased renal blood flow and elevated plasma renin. Therefore, although chronic rejection is not specifically a renal vascular disorder *per se*, hyperreninemia may play an etiologic role in the pathogenesis of hypertension associated with chronic rejection.[6]

Other causes of renal allograft dysfunction must also be considered in a patient with post-transplant hypertension, including recurrence of the original kidney disease. The most common recurrent disease causing hypertension in this setting is focal segmental glomerulosclerosis.[7] However, the original cause of end-stage renal disease does not necessarily predict if hypertension will recur after transplantation. It has been shown by several investigators that recipient sex, race, age and family history of hypertension do not affect the prevalence of post-transplant hypertension.[8, 9] It has likewise been shown that post-transplant hypertension may be associated with the use of cadaver donors, impaired allograft function, the presence of native kidneys, and the use of cyclosporin (CyA).[2]

The presence of hypertension post-transplantation does adversely affect allograft survival. Hypertensive recipients are more likely to lose their allografts during the first 3 months after transplantation than normotensive recipients.[2, 8, 10] These patients also experience a higher rate of cardiovascular complications. Several animal studies have been performed in order to clarify the pathophysiology of post-transplant hypertension. It has been shown that transplantation of kidneys from spontaneously hypertensive rats into nephrectomized non-hypertensive rats reproduces hypertension in the recipient.[11] In contrast, transplantation from normotensive rats into spontaneously hypertensive rats that have been nephrectomized yields normotension in the recipient rat.[11] This has led to the hypothesis that the transplanted kidney itself may somehow be responsible for mediating blood pressure regulation in the recipient. None of the animal models however can completely mimic the human situation because of the inherent lack of chronic native kidney damage in these models.

Immunosuppressive drugs and post-transplant hypertension

In the pre-CyA era, it was thought that chronic prednisone therapy played an important etiologic role in post-transplant hypertension.[9] However, most studies failed to demonstrate a definite correlation between the dose of maintenance prednisone and the resultant incidence of recipient hypertension.[1, 8] Although high dose steroid therapy probably does contribute to elevated blood pressure because of fluid retention as well as potential mineralocorticoid effects,[2] this initial post-transplant hypertension generally resolves as steroid doses are tapered. This, in conjunction with improving allograft function (which of itself may lead to improvement in blood pressure), makes it difficult to implicate steroids as an important cause of post-transplant hypertension. Some studies have suggested that alternate-day steroid therapy may be preferable to daily steroid therapy in ameliorating blood pressure control,[12] however this has not been confirmed by others.[13] It is likely that chronic steroid therapy does contribute to some degree to post-transplant hypertension, however neither increased sodium retention nor increased sensitivity of the renin–angiotension system has been proven as a result of steroid therapy.[1] As refinements in new immunosuppressive drugs are developed, steroid tapering and elimination of steroid therapy will become more commonplace and the role of steroids in causing post-transplant hypertension will likely become less important.

The introduction of CyA in the early 1980s led to marked improvements in graft survival in renal transplantation.[14] However, one of the disadvantages of CyA, in addition to its nephrotoxicity, has been an increased incidence of hypertension post-transplantation.[14–17] There is little doubt that CyA does cause changes in the transplant kidney that may be responsible for post-transplant hypertension.[2, 18, 19] It is unclear whether these changes are renin mediated.[20] Cyclosporin-induced renovascular constriction has been shown in several animal models[21] but CyA-induced hypertension is not sensitive to converting enzyme inhibition.[22] After chronic CyA administration, thickening of the afferent arterial wall may resemble that seen in essential hypertension.[23, 24] Other factors that have been implicated in CyA-induced hypertension include increased glomerular surface area resulting in compensatory hyperfiltration of the remaining glomeruli, interstitial fibrosis and direct cellular toxicity.[18–24] In addition, CyA has been shown to cause changes in intrarenal arachidonic acid metabolism, with inhibition of vasodilatory prostaglandin products with sparing of vasoconstricting thromboxane metabolites.[25, 26] Finally, CyA appears to impair salt and water excretion and leads to a blunted natriuresis when the patient has an expanded extracellular fluid volume.[2, 5, 23, 24] Many of these changes are reversible even up to a year after therapy has begun and usually respond to lowering of the

CyA dosing. Cyclosporin has also been found to cause an increase in mean arterial pressure and renal vascular resistance along with decreased renal blood flow and glomerular filtration.[4] In the non-transplant population, CyA also causes similar changes in intrarenal vascular tone. Since hypertension associated with CyA is unresponsive to converting enzyme inhibitors and plasma renin activity is usually normal, this usually represents a non-renin dependent form of hypertension.[27] More recently, endothelin, which is a potent renal vasoconstrictor, has been implicated in the mediation of CyA-induced hypertension. It has been demonstrated that CyA can stimulate endothelin production in cultured endothelial cells.[28] Furthermore, Kon has shown that circulating levels of endothelin are elevated in animal models after CyA administration and antiendothelin antibody reverses these effects.[29] It remains to be seen whether the newer immunosuppressive macrolide derivatives, such as tacrolimus (Prograf[R]), which has been proven efficacious in early trials of renal transplantation,[30] produce similar renal hemodynamic changes. Early clinical trials with tacrolimus have revealed a lower incidence of post-transplant hypertension and reduced requirement for antihypertensive drugs post-transplant, suggesting that some of these mechanisms may not be operative with this drug.[30, 31] However, this will need to be studied further before any definite conclusions can be drawn.

Other causes of post-transplant hypertension

In addition to chronic renal dysfunction and drug toxicity, several other factors may contribute to the incidence of post-transplant hypertension which is unrelated to renovascular causes. For example, it has been shown that renal transplant recipients may have increased aldosterone secretion rates, although others have also demonstrated increased aldosterone secretion rates in normotensive transplant patients.[1] Cooke concluded that aldosterone regulation was normal but that steroid therapy altered the circadian rhythm of aldosterone secretion.[32] Most studies have concluded that the effects on aldosterone, if present, are likely a consequence of the administration of steroids.[1]

Several studies have also suggested that decreased secretion of kallikrein in renal transplant patients may be responsible for post-transplant hypertension. Kallikrein is a vasodilator secreted by the kidneys which may be under neuroregulation.[1] It has been hypothesized that the denervated transplant kidney may therefore lack the ability to secrete kallikrein.[1] Some reports have documented the initial production of kallikrein by the transplanted kidney which then decreases with time in hypertensive patients but remains at initial levels in normotensive transplant patients.[1, 33] Since kallikrein production is influenced by renal plasma flow, these observations may have been secondary to the decreased renal plasma flow seen with hypertension.

Another potential cause of post-transplant hypertension may be abnormal electrolyte handling by the transplant kidney. Kornerup extensively studied sodium metabolism in hypertensive transplant patients and concluded that sodium retention was inappropriately increased in these patients.[34] This is what would be expected in a single-kidney Goldblatt model where the hypertension is secondary to volume expansion.

Hypercalcemia associated with persistent hyperparathyroisism is also associated with post-transplant hypertension.[1, 6] The increased blood pressure seen with hypercalcemia is thought to be mediated though changes in cardiac output and peripheral vascular resistance or possibly through alternative release or action of pressor substances including renin and catecholamines.[35]

Renovascular hypertension after renal transplantation: etiology and pathophysiology

A renovascular etiology for hypertension in the post-transplant period should be suspected when the hypertension is severe, resistant to multiple drug administration and is associated with relatively preserved renal transplant function. In addition, other causes of transplant dysfunction, such as acute or chronic rejection, urinary obstruction, and drug toxicity must be considered before establishing a renovascular etiology (see above). For this reason, baseline studies of the kidney including serum creatinine, creatinine clearance, allograft biopsy, and ultrasound examination should be performed to rule out these entities. The next step is to distinguish whether the potential exists for renovascular hypertension from either the native kidneys or from the renal transplant. A definite role for the native kidneys in the pathogenesis of post-transplant hypertension has been demonstrated in several studies. De Strihou[8] and Pollini[36] found that patients having had native nephrectomy prior to transplantation have a lower incidence of post-transplant hypertension than those with retained native kidneys. Furthermore, hypertension can be improved post-transplant after native nephrectomy.[23] Unfortunately, determining the contribution of the native kidneys by measuring native renal vein renin secretion or plasma renin activity has not been reliable, probably because of the global decrease in renal blood flow and renin secretion in the diseased native kidneys.[1, 8, 23, 36] Despite these caveats, Grunfeld *et al.* showed excess renin secretion by the native kidneys in 10 of 14 cases.[37] However, blood pressure decreased in all 14 patients after native nephrectomy.[37] Proper identification of those transplant patients in whom the hypertension is secondary to retained native kidneys or due to transplant renal artery disease can be a challenging problem. The administration of captopril has been shown to be helpful in distinguishing between these two entities. With native kidney-induced hypertension, the administration of captopril results in improvement in the hypertension with no change in transplant allograft function and improved renal plasma flow in the transplant kidney.[1, 20] In the case of transplant renal artery stenosis, which resembles a one-kidney, one-clip Goldblatt model, glomerular filtration rate (GFR) is maintained by constriction of the efferent arteriole with local autoregulation by the renin–angiotension system. In this case, the hypertension is volume mediated and after captopril administration, the efferent arterial vasoconstriction is now inhibited, resulting in a decreased effective filtration fraction and decreased GFR. As a result, renal function is reversibly impaired within 12–24 h of captopril administration, but the hypertension is unaffected because the diseased kidney is unable to excrete the additional volume which is mediating the hypertension. Thus, captopril administration may be useful in distinguishing whether renovascular hypertension is originating from the native kidneys or from the transplant kidney. Unfortunately, with the use of CyA, these tests are not as clear-cut because CyA itself causes renal vasoconstriction and results in fluid retention, and the usual response to captopril in native kidney-mediated hypertension in CyA-treated patients is masked.[4, 38]

Clinical features of renovascular hypertension in the transplant patient

As outlined above, hypertension occurs in up to 80% of renal transplant recipients[1–3, 36] and can be related to multiple factors, including allograft dysfunction, immunosuppression (particularly CyA), acute and chronic allograft rejection, native kidney hypertension and renal artery stenosis. Because transplant renal artery stenosis can cause allograft dysfunction and is potentially remediable, it is important to distinguish it from other forms of hypertension in transplant recipients. The clinical features of transplant renal artery stenosis are non-specific, therefore requiring an index of clinical suspicion to consider the diagnosis. The new onset of hypertension, intractable hypertension unresponsive to antihypertensive therapy, and an unexplained decline in allograft function should prompt consideration of renal artery stenosis in the transplant patient.[2, 39] A systolic bruit heard over the allograft may be an additional clue to the presence of renal artery stenosis[2, 40, 41] but is not always present.[42] Additionally, the disappearance of a previously noted bruit over the allograft may herald the development of renal artery stenosis, particularly in allografts with end-to-end anastomoses.[43, 44] All of these signs are non-specific, easily obscured by pre-existing hypertension and/or atherosclerosis, and are of little diagnostic value. The prevalence of renal artery stenosis in kidney transplant programs varies, at least in part because of the readiness of some programs to perform angiography for suspected renal artery stenosis in the absence of specific clinical features.[1] The incidence of transplant renal artery stenosis is reported to be 2–25% in various series.[42, 45–53]

As discussed previously, angiotensin converting enzyme (ACE) inhibitors can provide another clinical clue to the diagnosis of renal artery stenosis through their effects on efferent arteriolar constriction that occurs with renal autoregulation.[54] Early reports[55, 56] of reversible renal dysfunction in kidney transplant patients given captopril for blood pressure control were subsequently validated and explained pathophysiologically.[20, 57] Thus, a rise in serum creatinine after the administration of ACE inhibitors can be an additional clue to the diagnosis of functionally significant renal artery stenosis in a transplant patient.[2, 20, 58] However, ACE inhibitors do not always cause acute deterioration of renal function in the presence of renal artery stenosis.[59, 60] The functional significance of the stenosis and the patient's volume status (volume depletion enhances ACE inhibitor effects) may also contribute to ACE inhibitor-mediated renal dysfunction in the setting of renal artery stenosis.[2, 57, 60] Renal dysfunction unrelated to renal artery stenosis may also occur with ACE inhibition.[2] Acute renal failure induced by ACE inhibitors in a transplant patient is therefore suggestive, but not diagnostic of renal artery stenosis. Nevertheless, renal function should be monitored closely in transplant patients who are given an ACE inhibitor.[2, 20]

Renal artery stenosis

Renal artery stenosis in the transplant patient may occur secondary to technical problems with either the recipient or donor artery or at the anastomotic site; rejection may also contribute to renal artery stenosis in some cases.[42, 46–51, 53] Most renal artery stenoses in transplant patients are due to technical problems[42, 61] and occur either at or distal to the anastomosis.[48, 61, 62] Stenosis of the donor renal artery can be caused by arterial injury from perfusion of the organ, vessel injury during donor nephrectomy, torsion, kinking or angulation of the vessel due to excessive post-anastomotic length, and turbulent blood flow caused in part by angulation of the artery.[41, 46, 48, 61] In one study 70% of the stenotic lesions were due to either torsion or kinking of the donor artery or postanastomotic stenosis from perfusion damage.[61] Anastomotic stenosis can result from intimal disruption from perfusion injury but is most commonly caused by faulty suture technique with incomplete intimal approximation.[46, 48, 50, 53] Suture errors may be common in end-to-end anastomoses due to the differences in vessel texture and caliber.[46, 48] Pre-existing atheroma of the recipient artery may also result in stenosis[48] as may clamp or traction injury of the recipient vessel at the time of transplantation.[2, 48]

In addition to technical problems with the vessels, an immune-mediated etiology is believed to cause some cases of transplant renal artery stenosis.[2, 48, 53] Renal artery stenosis associated with chronic rejection typically results in stenosis of multiple intrarenal vessels.[2, 48, 62] Early pathologic study of such lesions suggested an immune mechanism because the subintimal fibrosis and intimal proliferation in the stenosed arteries resembled the vascular lesions of allograft rejection. Moreover, in some cases the vascular lesions affected the entire arterial tree of an allograft, from the main renal artery to renal capillaries.[48] It was postulated that fibrin and platelet deposition on the endothelium of the vessel led to endothelial proliferation and intimal fibrosis, resulting in multiple areas of stenosis.[48, 50] The presence of IgM and C3 staining in a fibrotic segment of a donor renal artery[51] and the occurrence of renal artery stenosis more commonly in cadaveric than living related donors[2, 42, 48] provide additional indirect support for an immunological etiology of renal artery stenosis. However, histologic evidence supportive of chronic rejection in cases of renal artery stenosis is not invariably present[46] and additional study in this area is needed.

Although some claim that hyperreninemia is a feature of transplant renal artery stenosis in transplant patients,[61, 63, 64] pathophysiologic lessons from the Goldblatt models of hypertension contradict that assertion. In the chronic phase of the one-kidney, one-clip Goldblatt model (assumed to be analogous to a renal transplant), hypertension is primarily sodium (volume) mediated rather than renin mediated.[1] In such circumstances, peripheral plasma renin activity would be depressed and unresponsive to ACE inhibitors. A series of autotransplantation dog studies[65] and a study of renin secretion in renal transplant patients with multiple kidneys[66] support this hypothesis. A study of nine hypertensive transplant patients with transplant renal artery stenosis showed that preoperative plasma renin levels did not predict the response of hypertension to surgical repair of the stenosis, further suggesting that sodium retention counterbalanced the increased renin activity.[67] These findings support the predictions of the one-kidney, one-clip Goldblatt model and suggest that high renin levels in transplant patients with renal artery stenosis likely occur primarily in patients who receive diuretics and thus are hyperreninemic as a result of volume depletion.[1, 36] Peripheral renin levels are therefore seldom helpful in diagnosing transplant renal artery stenosis.[1] Moreover, since a renal allograft is classically a solitary kidney, measurement of renal vein renin levels is seldom helpful because there is no contralateral kidney with which to compare levels of renin secretion. For these reasons, peripheral and renal vein renin levels are rarely useful in diagnosing renal artery stenosis in transplant patients[1, 2, 68, 69] or in predicting blood pressure response to repair of stenoses.[67, 70]

As discussed earlier, lessons from the Goldblatt model of hypertension are also helpful in explaining the rise in serum creatinine that occurs when a transplant patient with a functionally significant renal artery stenosis is given an ACE inhibitor. In such cases, there is baseline efferent arteriolar constriction as part of renal autoregulation to maintain filtration fraction and GFR[54] in the face of reduced perfusion due to the stenosis. With the introduction of an ACE inhibitor, efferent vasodilation occurs with a concomitant fall in hydrostatic filtration pressure and, consequently, a reduction in the GFR.[54] As noted earlier, a rise in serum creatinine with administration of ACE inhibitors can therefore be used as a clue to the presence of a functionally significant renal artery stenosis.[2, 20, 58, 62] Interestingly, because a pediatric en bloc allograft is essentially a two-kidney, rather than a single-kidney model, stenosis of one of the en bloc allografts (two-kidney, one-clip Goldblatt model) would not be expected to cause renal functional impairment in the setting of ACE inhibitor administration.[71] A case report in which renal artery stenosis of one renal artery in a pediatric en bloc transplant was diagnosed by captopril-enhanced renal scintigraphy supports this theory.[72]

Other causes of post-transplant renovascular hypertension

In addition to transplant renal artery stenosis, there are several other specific entities which may produce post-transplant renovascular hypertension. Arteriovenous (AV) fistula has been reported to present with hypertension in the renal transplant recipient.[73, 74] Although small AV fistulas may be caused by percutaneous allograft biopsy, these usually resolve spontaneously and rarely cause hypertension.[75] However, the complex vascular reconstruction which is occasionally required for multiple transplant renal arteries which have been transected or injured during organ recovery may sometimes result in AV fistula formation and may result in hypertension. Arteriovenous fistulas are visible on angiography (Fig. 20.1) and may also be seen with color-aided duplex Doppler.

It has been reported[76] that fibromuscular dyplasia originating in the donor kidneys may lead to hypertension in the transplant recipient. In most cases, however, significant arterial abnormalities in the donor kidney should be obvious at the time of transplantation and the abnormal area of renal artery can be excised or repaired. However, since fibromuscular dysplasia is a progressive disease, unrecognized branch lesions at the time of transplantation may progress to the extent where renovascular hypertension may occur. Since pre-transplant arteriography is employed routinely only in living-related transplantation, it is conceivable that this entity may be more common in cadaver transplantation than with living-related donors.

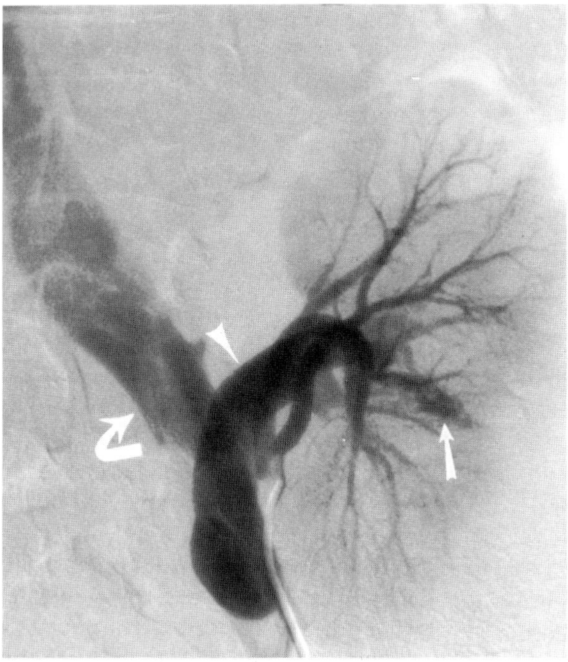

Figure 20.1. Intrarenal arteriovenous fistula (arrow) demonstrated on selective allograft renal arteriogram in a patient with hematuria following percutaneous biopsy. Note early filling of the renal vein (arrowhead) draining into the iliac vein (curved arrow).

Aneurysms of the renal transplant artery or iliac artery may cause turbulent blood flow resulting in relative ischemia to the transplant kidney.[77–80] It is important to distinguish between true aneurysms of the transplant renal artery and mycotic pseudo-aneurysms.[80] True renal artery aneurysms involve the entire thickness of the renal artery, are not associated with infection but may accompany technical complications and rejection.[80] Mycotic pseudo-aneurysms are more common than true renal artery aneurysms and are by definition associated with infection, often resulting from intraoperative contamination or from the organ preservation solution. In contrast to true renal artery aneurysms, mycotic pseudo-aneurysms consist of a complete rupture of the entire thickness of the arterial wall with formation of a sac consisting only of periarterial tissue.[80, 81] Mycotic pseudo-aneurysms represent a life-threatening complication because of their propensity to rupture. Treatment for mycotic pseudo-aneurysms is generally ligation of the artery above the aneurysm with removal of the allograft. With true renal artery aneurysm, it is possible to repair the aneurysm by excision and patch angioplasty, depending upon the site and nature of the aneurysm. Figure 20.2 demonstrates a pseudo-aneurysm arising from the proximal allograft renal artery anastomosis with compression of the iliac artery from the aneurysm. In this case, the patient developed hypertension as a result of impaired arterial inflow to the allograft. Figure 20.3 shows a mycotic pseudo-aneurysm arising from an extension graft anastomosis of a pediatric en bloc transplant. This patient underwent surgical repair of the aneurysm by excising the aneurymal sac and oversewing the healthy vessel with a patch angioplasty using saphenous vein.

Diagnostic tests for renal artery stenosis in the transplant patient

Although many non-invasive tests for renal artery stenosis in transplant patients are available, inadequacies in the predictive value of such tests limit

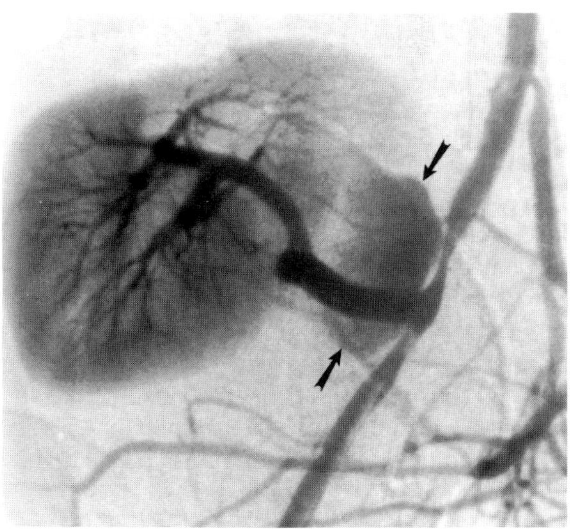

Figure 20.2. Large pseudo-aneurysm (arrows) arising from the proximal renal allograft artery anastomosis demonstrated on external iliac artery arteriogram. Also note the stenosis in the iliac artery due to compression by the aneurysm.

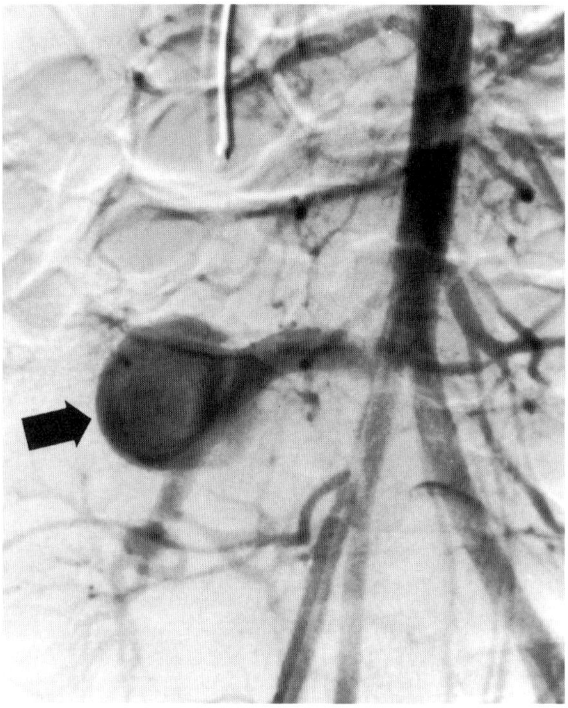

Figure 20.3. Large mycotic pseudo-aneurysm (arrow) arising from an extension graft anastomosis of a pediatric en bloc transplant demonstrated on abdominal aortogram.

their usefulness.[82] Thus, angiography remains the standard for diagnosing renal artery stenosis.[2, 82] The potential complications of angiography include vessel dissection, thrombosis and contrast-induced acute renal failure and have spurred the search for effective non-invasive procedures.[83] Such tests or procedures are generally based on screening (duplex Doppler ultrasonography, magnetic resonance imaging) or ascertainment of functional significance using an ACE inhibitor such as captopril. A review of the available tests for renal artery stenosis in the transplant patient follows. It should be borne in mind that the usefulness of many of these procedures vary among the reported studies, in part because they tend to be highly operator dependent.

Duplex ultrasonography

Duplex Doppler ultrasonography is the combination of ultrasonographic imaging of the renal artery and Doppler techniques to measure blood flow velocity in the vessel.[83–88] An abnormal result is indicated by changes in acceleration time or peak frequency or comparison of blood flow velocities in the renal artery and aorta (Fig. 20.4). Images may be also be color coded (Colour plate 2). Most report a high sensitivity for the detection of renal artery stenosis using duplex Doppler ultrasonography in the transplant population[82, 84] but one study reported only 58% sensitivity in 13 patients.[88] The observer dependence and the lack of standard criteria for stenosis using this technique probably contribute to differences in predictive value of duplex Doppler ultrasonography among different studies.[82, 88] A prospective study comparing non-invasive screening tests for renal artery stenosis in transplant patients found only duplex Doppler ultrasonography acceptable; the other techniques examined (captopril-stimulated renin levels, renography with technetium-99m diethylenetriaminepentaacetic acid [DTPA] before and after administration of the ACE inhibitor with measurement of GFR and effective renal plasma flow) all had sensitivities less than 100%.[82] However, the specificity of duplex Doppler ultrasonography (as verified by angiography) was 75%.[82]

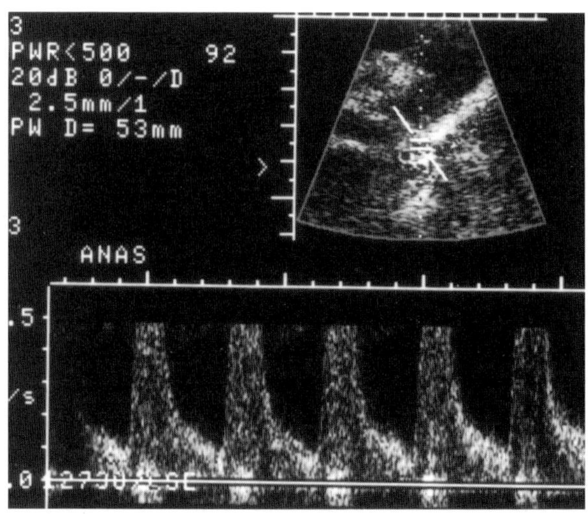

Figure 20.4. Duplex Doppler showing focal high velocity flow (> 150 cm/s) at stenosis of main renal artery anastomosis.

Digital subtraction and angiography

Digital subtraction angiography (DSA) has certain advantages over standard angiography.[52, 53] These include the limited amount of contrast material necessary, as well as the use of a smaller catheter than that used for conventional angiography.[89] Intra-arterial DSA has the advantage over intravenous DSA which is of relatively limited value because the latter approach often produces inadequate contrast enhancement and motion artifacts from the gastrointestinal tract, and boney structures impair visualization.[90] In a study by Duda *et al.*,[89] color-aided duplex Doppler sonography was compared with intra-arterial DSA. Color Doppler provided a sensitivity of 100% with a specificity of 86% and was concluded to be a very useful screening test for confirmation of transplant renal artery stenosis verified angiographically.

Captopril renography/scintigraphy

In the two-kidney, one-clip Goldblatt model, the GFR falls after ACE inhibition in the kidney with a partial vascular obstruction while the GFR in the unobstructed, contralateral kidney is preserved.[71] Because DTPA is filtered by the glomerulus and not absorbed, it can serve as a marker for GFR in renal scintigraphy, with the poststenotic kidney displaying reduced GFR.[83] As previously discussed, in the non-transplant population, the utility of this technique is usually based upon comparison of diseased and normal kidneys, a situation non-existent in the usual transplant patient due to the lack of a normal contralateral kidney. Additionally, the ACE inhibitor-induced scintigraphic pattern in patients with a hemodynamically significant renal artery stenosis may be identical to the pattern of acute rejection,[91] further compromising the utility of this technique in the diagnosis of transplant renal artery stenosis. Thus, despite some encouraging results with captopril renography in the diagnosis of transplant renal artery stenosis,[88, 91] additional experience with this technique is needed before widespread use can be advocated.

Conventional angiography

Although color-aided duplex Doppler and captopril renography have been used with increasing success for initial screening of transplant renal artery disease, the gold standard for imaging of the transplant renal artery remains conventional angiography. Although DSA may be sufficient for screening in most cases, intra-arterial DSA may not be sufficient to image small branch renal arteries which are only visible on conventional angiography. Any contemplated surgical repair or angioplasty of transplant renal artery stenosis should always be preceded or accompanied by conventional angiography.

Magnetic resonance imaging and spiral computed tomography

Although initial results using magnetic resonance imaging (MRI) to diagnose renal artery stenosis in the general population have been encouraging,[83] there is little information about this technique in the kidney transplant population. Advantages of MRI include the potential ability to obtain satisfactory images without vessel puncture and contrast exposure. There is currently little experience using MRI in transplant patients, in whom careful interpretation is required to avoid misdiagnosis.[92] Additional experience with this new imaging technique in the transplant population is needed. Similarly, spiral computed tomographic angiography (CTA), a new vascular imaging modality, was recently used to diagnose transplant renal artery stenosis[93] but the lack of clinical experience with this new technique precludes its endorsement. Potential advantages of CTA over standard angiography include the ability to construct images from any angle, lower cost and the lower volume of contrast required.[93] However, for the present, conventional angiography remains the standard for diagnosing transplant renal artery stenosis.

Renovascular hypertension after pediatric en bloc transplantation

Renovascular hypertension may also occur in pediatric en bloc renal transplants.[87, 94] These kid-

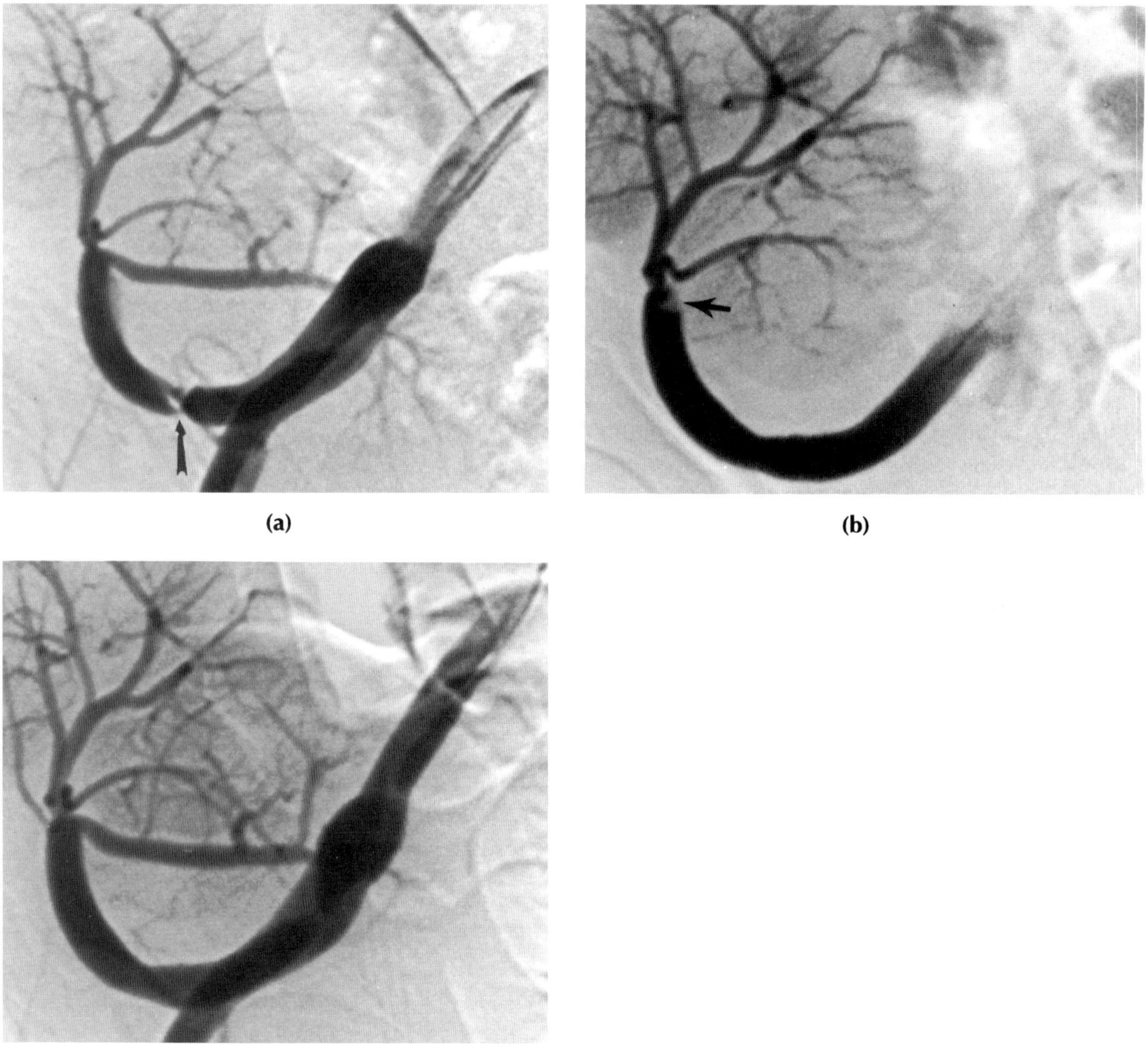

(a) (b) (c)

Figure 20.5. (a) Severe stenosis (arrow) at the anastomosis of an extension graft from the external iliac artery to the donor aorta of a pediatric en bloc transplant demonstrated on external iliac arteriogram. The anastomosis to the external iliac artery is normal. (b) Widely patent anastomosis demonstrated on selective renal arteriogram following balloon angioplasty. The procedure was complicated by occlusion of the inferomedial allograft due to a thrombus at the origin of the renal artery (arrow). An infusion of urokinase at 250 000 units per hour was started immediately. (c) Lysis of the clot in the main renal artery to the inferomedial graft demonstrated on selective arteriogram following 1 h of thrombolytic therapy.

neys are utilized from pediatric donors (usually under age 3 years) using the entire vena cava and aorta as conduits to the external iliac vein and artery, respectively.[80, 94] Because of the complex vascular reconstruction required, these unique grafts are more prone to technical complications than single adult kidneys.[94] Interestingly, in a large series of pediatric en bloc transplants renal artery stenosis was detected less frequently than in most adult series.[87] Since the renal arteries themselves are not involved in the vascular anastomoses, hypertension may result from turbulent flow in the cul-de-sac of the oversewn aorta, or in the case of an extension graft to the great vessels

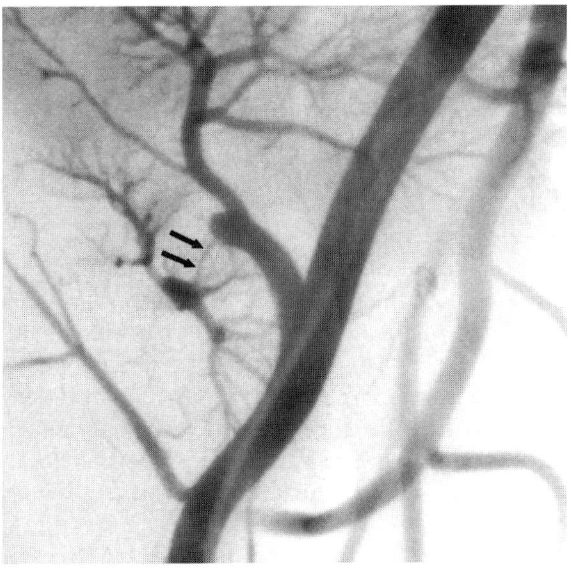

Figure 20.6. Marked stenosis of the main renal artery (arrows) to the inferior moiety of a pediatric en bloc transplant demonstrated on external iliac arteriogram. The superior moiety is normal.

of the donor, from stenosis of these anastomoses (Fig. 20.5). However, stenosis of the individual renal arteries in a pediatric en bloc transplant may also occur (Fig. 20.6). In the case of pediatric en bloc transplants, in which only one of the two renal arteries is stenotic, the two-kidney Goldblatt model would obtain, unlike most single adult kidney transplants which represents a single-kidney Goldblatt model. In a report by Nguyen,[72] captopril renal scintigraphy of a pediatric en bloc transplant in which the right renal artery was stenotic showed significant deterioration of flow and function post-captopril in the right moiety with normal flow and function in the left moiety. The patient was treated with percutaneous transluminal angioplasty (PTA) which cured the hypertension. Although this case represents an unusual complication in a pediatric en bloc transplant, it illustrates the potential utility of captopril testing and the fact that the two-kidney Goldblatt model pertains in this situation. With the increasing shortage of donor organs, many centers are turning to the use of pediatric en bloc kidneys for transplantation and a thorough knowledge of the anatomy and potential complications resulting from the use of these organs is necessary for the transplant surgeon to be able to deal with complications which may result.

Treatment options for renovascular hypertension in the transplant patient

Before deciding on specific treatment options for renovascular hypertension in the transplant patient, it is important to be able to evaluate correctly the cause of the renovascular hypertension and to develop an approach to the patient with persistent post-transplant hypertension. There are several questions which need to be considered during the evaluation of the hypertensive renal transplant recipient which will determine the treatment plan. First, if the hypertension is shown to be secondary to the native kidneys or due to transplant renal artery stenosis, is clinical intervention appropriate? Second, does the renal allograft itself possess sufficient preservation of function such that intervention to treat the hypertension will be successful or is it likely that the hypertension will persist because of allograft dysfunction? Finally, what is the likelihood of successful intervention leading to resolution or improvement of the hypertension?

In order to answer the first question, one must establish the degree of risk of any surgical or radiologic intervention vs the severity of the patient's hypertension and its ability to respond to medical therapy. In a young patient on multiple drug therapy with excellent allograft function, the answer to the question should be obvious, however in the older patient with multifactorial hypertension who has borderline renal function, such intervention may not be indicated. Curtis *et al.*[1] reported that interventional procedures, including native nephrectomy, have no benefit if the allograft possesses significant intrinsic disease. It has been suggested that a patient who is 1 year or more post-transplant with at least 6 months' stable serum creatinine levels with 24-h urine protein less than 500 mg and a creatinine clearance greater than 65 ml/min is unlikely to have sufficient intrinsic allograft damage to account for severe hypertension.[1] Any patient investigated for renovascular hypertension should have a percutaneous allograft biopsy to determine the degree of chronic renal injury, if any. What is the likelihood that the post-transplant hypertension will be persistent or will resolve? This is an important question to answer in determining whether interventional therapy should be undertaken. It has been postulated that native kidney renin production decreases with time after transplantation, but in some reports[1, 2] continued renin production may occur for several years. Probably the most important determinant of whether intervention will prove successful is whether the patient is responsive to captopril testing. Curtis *et al.* have noted a marked increase in allograft renal plasma flow and normalization of blood pressure with captopril and diuretic testing in those patients who have had beneficial response to native kidney nephrectomy.[1] In the case of transplant renal artery stenosis, it is imperative to determine if the renal artery stenosis is functional before any intervention is carried out. Although it is generally accepted that at least a 70% narrowing in vessel diameter is required before significant impairment of renal blood flow occurs, angiography alone is not necessarily sufficient to establish whether this degree of stenosis is functionally important. Again, lack of blood pressure response to captopril with a fall in allograft renal plasma flow and the onset of reversible renal failure post-captopril appears to be the most sensitive indicator of treatable transplant renal artery stenosis.

Treatment options

Native kidney-induced hypertension

Traditionally, bilateral native nephrectomy has been the treatment of choice when all other forms of hypertension have been ruled out and captopril testing has indicated that the native kidneys are the source of hypertension.[1, 95] Native renal artery embolization with ethanol has also been utilized to ablate the native kidneys.[96, 97] The disadvantages of embolization include the lack of certainty of ablation of all functioning renal tissue as well as potential morbidity from septic complications.[98]

Transplant renal artery stenosis

The incidence of renovascular hypertension due to stenosis of the transplant renal artery has been estimated in various series to be between 2 and 25%.[1–6, 42, 45–53] This incidence of course depends upon the index of suspicion for renal artery stenosis as well as the frequency with which these patients are investigated with arteriography. Most investigators report an overall incidence of renal artery stenosis of 5–10%.[42, 45–53] Stenosis of the transplant renal artery may occur at one of four major sites: at the anastomosis (Fig. 20.7), in the donor renal artery, in the recipient vessel, or as multiple stenotic lesions (Fig. 20.8) in the involved vessels.[46, 48] Stenosis in the donor vessel (preanastomotic) can result from kinking or rotation of the donor vessel, recovery injury from excessive traction on the vessel, allograft malposition or redundant vessel

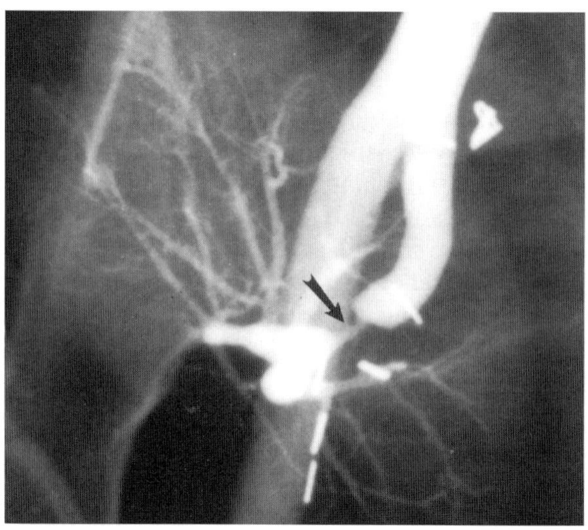

Figure 20.7. Severe stenosis (arrow) of the end-to-end anastomosis of the allograft renal artery to the hypogastric artery demonstrated on common iliac artery arteriogram.

length.[46–53] Stenosis at the anastomosis is usually due to faulty surgical technique at the time of anastomosis. Poor intimal approximation may lead to subintimal dissection with subsequent fibrosis. Poor approximation of the adventitia of the vessel may predispose to fibrin and platelet aggregration with resultant fibrosis and stenosis. In most series, the most common location of transplant renal artery stenois is postanastomotic.[46–53] This lesion may be due to chronic rejection as demonstrated by deposition of IgM and the third component of complement.[51] This type of stenosis usually begins at the anastomosis and extends distally into the transplant renal artery.

The treatment of transplant renal artery stenosis has undergone evolution over the past 10 years with the advent of PTA[99, 100] (Fig. 20.8). Before the availability of this modality, surgical repair of transplant renal artery stenosis was the only available option, other than medical therapy.[1, 2, 50, 51, 61] The specific techniques for renal revascularization for transplant renal artery stenosis are beyond the scope of this chapter and will be discussed elsewhere in this volume. What follows is a summary of the current results of surgery and PTA for the treatment of transplant renal artery stenosis.

Ricotta *et al.* described a series of 16 patients with transplant renal artery stenosis which represented an overall incidence of 5% in their transplant population.[61] Surgical correction was undertaken in 12 of these patients. With a reported mean follow-up of 24 months, 3 of 12 grafts were lost, and 8 patients were normotensive, 5 requiring no medication and 3 requiring two medications. There was one patient death for a mortality rate of 3%. Tilney *et al.*[42] reported on 25 patients with transplant renal artery stenosis at a median onset of 12 months after transplantation. Successful surgical repair was obtained in 14 of 21 patients (67%) in whom repair was attempted. There was a relatively high complication rate (7%), but no mortality. Five patients underwent attempted PTA in this series resulting in three complications, including femoral artery pseudo-aneurysm in one, an intimal flap in a second patient, and

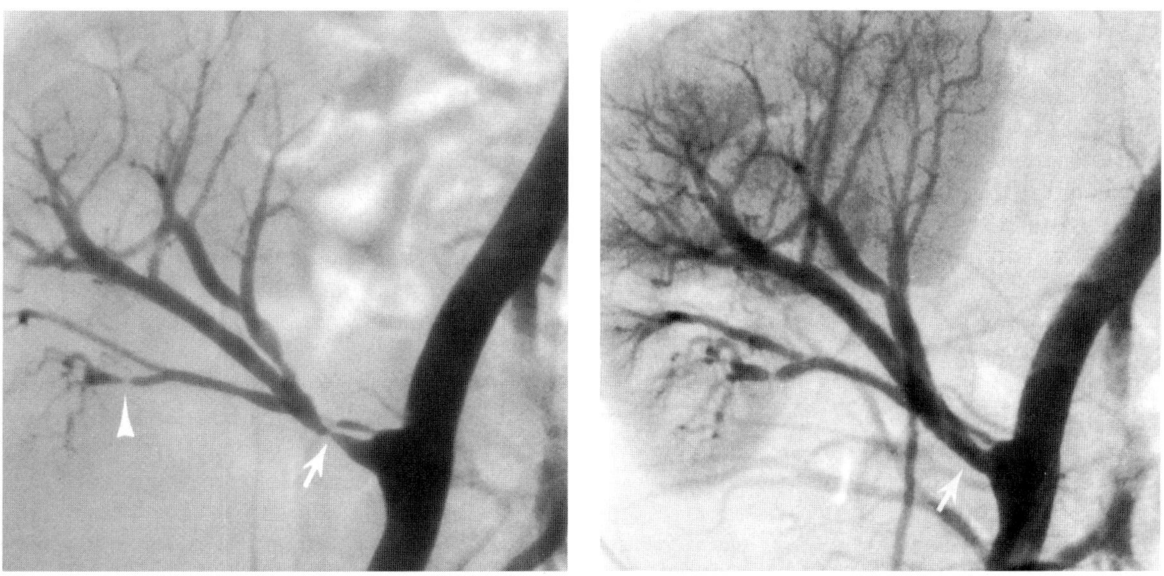

(a) (b)

Figure 20.8. (a) Severe stenosis of the proximal allograft renal artery (arrow) demonstrated on external iliac arteriogram. The end-to-side Carrell patch anastomosis with the external iliac artery is widely patent. Also note marked stenosis in lower pole intrarenal branch artery (arrowhead). (b) Following balloon angioplasty, the proximal renal artery is widely patent (arrow).

intimal dissection of the hypogastric artery in the third. Two of these complications required operative therapy. Based on these results, the authors felt that despite its potential risk, surgical repair should be offered initially to patients with documented renal artery stenosis with unmanageable hypertension. Other investigators have reported success rates ranging from 50 to 80% with surgical therapy.[46, 48–50, 53] In an earlier series, we found that renal artery stenosis was noted to be more common following end-to-end anastomosis compared with end-to-side anastomosis.[46]

Percutaneous transluminal angioplasty for renal artery stenosis was first described by Gruntzig in 1978.[99] This approach was initially used for native renal artery disease but was rapidly adopted for transplant renal artery stenosis. Sniderman *et al.*[100] reported on 12 patients who underwent angioplasty for transplant renal artery stenosis. Two patients required repeat angioplasty for recurrent stenosis and hypertension. The overall success rate was 78% in this series, including the two patients that required repeat angioplasty, however in this early report follow-up was relatively short (average 9 months). Grossman *et al.*[45] reported the results of angioplasty in 17 patients with transplant renal artery stenosis. Although 15 of 17 procedures were deemed successful by angiographic criteria, only 13 had long-term allograft survival and sustained decrease in blood pressure. The majority of patients in this series continued to require antihypertensive drugs postangioplasty. There was no mortality in this series and the morbidity was low. Although follow-up was relatively short, repeat angiograms were performed in nine patients an average of 61 weeks after angioplasty with no recurrent disease demonstrated. In a more recent series by Greenstein *et al.*,[101] angioplasty was successful in 76% (28 of 39 patients) in which this was attempted, with a mean follow-up of 30 months. The authors concluded that angioplasty was a safer and more effective procedure for the initial treatment of transplant renal artery stenosis than surgery. Fauchald *et al.*[102] reported on a large group of patients undergoing PTA. Of 25 patients treated, immediate success occurred in 88% but with a median follow-up of 3 months was only present in 63%. Only 1 patient of the 25 required subsequent surgical repair although 8 patients required repeat angioplasty. Complications occurred in five cases. In this series, nine patients without hypertension underwent angioplasty, and since renal biopsies were not done prior to angioplasty, the reasons for the impaired graft function in these patients preangioplasty were unclear. Despite these reports of success with angioplasty, as recently as 1989 Roberts *et al.* reported very poor results of angioplasty in 31 patients with transplant renal artery stenosis.[62] A total of 43 procedures were performed. Twenty of 43 procedures resulted in a poor result or failure, usually due to recurrent stenosis or arterial injury (which resulted in graft loss in four patients), and emergent surgery was required in three cases. Surgery was performed in 18 patients with 13 patients cured or improved. Since the majority (24/31) of the stenoses in this series were anastomotic, the authors concluded that angioplasty was not the procedure of choice for treating anastomotic stenoses. The authors also speculated that the reason for their inferior results was that angiography may have revealed false positive results in which the stenosis was not responsible for the hypertension. As a result they speculated that PTA was sometimes performed unnecessarily resulting in a falsely high failure rate.[62] With the availability of captopril testing, however, the incidence of false positive angiograms should be minimal and indicates once again that these patients must be very carefully screened before any attempt at intervention is made. Most recent reports have demonstrated excellent initial success rates with angioplasty with relatively long-term follow-up. Benoit *et al.*[103] performed a retrospective chart review of 1200 patients of whom 138 were identified with transplant renal artery stenosis (an incidence of 11.5%). Of these 138 patients, 88 underwent interventional therapy for renal artery stenosis. Forty-nine patients underwent angioplasty and 39 surgical repair. The immediate success rates were 92% for surgery and 69% for angioplasty with long-term success of 82% in the surgical group (57 months' mean follow-up) and 41% in the angioplasty group (32 months' mean follow-up). Despite these results, which apparently favored surgical therapy, the authors recommended angioplasty as the best first-line intervention if renal artery stenosis was of recent onset, linear and distal. Surgical therapy was favored for proximal renal artery stenosis and for those lesions which were felt to be due to torsion and kinking.

Transplant renal artery stenosis in children presents a more complex problem because of the potential long-term effects of antihypertensive medication in children. McMullin *et al.*[104] identified transplant renal artery stenosis in 30 of 262 children undergoing transplantation between 1967 and 1989. Angioplasty was performed in 21 patients with 9 angiographically improved and 7 clinically improved. Five patients required surgical therapy, four after a failed attempt at angioplasty. In another pediatric series reported by Fontaine *et al.*,[105] renal artery stenosis was identified in 69 of 715 pediatric transplants (incidence 9.8%). The patients were divided into three groups: medical therapy was used in 40 patients, angioplasty in 23 and surgical repair in 11 (5 of whom had failed angioplasty). In this series, angioplasty was successful in only 57% of the cases with surgery yielding an 82% success rate. Spijkerboer *et al.*[106] treated six patients with angioplasty with a 66% success rate, however two patients required repeat dilatation and all patients required ongoing antihypertensive drugs.

Most investigators now believe that angioplasty is the preferred initial therapy for the treatment of transplant renal artery stenosis. However, there have been no randomized trials comparing angioplasty with surgical repair and most series still report a relatively short follow-up for patients treated with angioplasty. The success rates in pediatric patients are generally inferior to those seen in adult patients, however angioplasty is also recommended as first-line therapy in the pediatric population.

Summary

Post-transplant hypertension is an important cause of morbidity occuring in the majority of patients after transplantation. It is important for the clinician to recognize the signs associated with a renovascular origin for post-transplant hypertension. These include, but are not limited to, severe hypertension which is resistant to medical therapy associated with relatively preserved renal function in patients in whom parenchymal allograft dysfunction is ruled out. Captopril appears to be an excellent initial screening tool to distinguish native kidney-mediated hypertension from allograft-mediated hypertension. In those patients so selected, a decision must be made whether to continue ongoing medical therapy or to proceed with interventional techniques. This decision is dependent in large part on the functional status of the renal allograft as well as the overall medical risk of the patient. Newer non-invasive diagnostic techniques for the detection of transplant renal artery stenosis appear to be promising, including MRI and spiral angiography. Nevertheless, the gold standard remains conventional angiography, which is also necessary in all cases planned for either angioplasty or surgical repair. The preferred initial treatment for proven transplant renal artery stenosis which is functionally significant should be PTA. Percutaneous transluminal angioplasty currently carries an initial success rate approaching 90% in most cases, with adequate sustained success at least for the first 12–24 months after therapy. Repeat angioplasty may be performed if necessary and surgical correction remains an option even after angioplasty failure. With the ever increasing shortage of donor organs, many transplant centers are ultilizing kidneys previously felt to be ‘marginal’, including kidneys with multiple renal vessels, pediatric kidneys either as single units or en bloc, and kidneys from older donors, which may have an increased incidence of glomerulosclerosis and interstitial fibrosis which may produce hypertension in the recipient. As a result, transplant surgeons may begin to see an increased incidence of technical complications from the use of these less than optimal donors, including renovascular hypertension due to transplant renal artery stenosis as well as hypertension due to impaired allograft function. A thorough familiarization with the recognition, diagnosis and treatment of post-transplant renovascular hypertension is essential for the transplant clinician to be able to deal effectively with this complication.

References

1 Curtis JJ. Hypertension and kidney transplantation. *Am J Kidney Dis* 1986; **VII:** 181–96.
2 Luke RG. Hypertension in renal transplant recipients. *Kidney Int* 1987; **31:** 1024–37.
3 Bachy C, Alexendre GPJ, van Ypersele de Strihou C. Hypertension after renal transplantation. *Br Med J* 1976; **2:** 1287–9.
4 Laskow DA, Curtis JJ. Post-transplant hypertension. *Am J Hypertension* 1990; **3:** 721–5.
5 Ponticelli C, Montagnino G, Arnoldi A *et al.* Hypertension after renal transplantation. *Am J Kidney Dis* 1993; **21:** (Suppl. 2) 73–8.
6 Waltzer WC, Turner S, Frohnert P, Rapaport FT. Etiology and pathogenesis of hypertension following renal transplantation. *Nephron* 1986; **42:** 102–9.
7 Cameron JS. Effect of the recipient's disease on the results of transplantation. *Kidney Int* 1983; **23:** 524–33.
8 De Strihou CuY, Vereerstraeten P, Wauthier M *et al.* Prevalence, etiology, and treatment of late post-transplant hypertension. In Hamburger J, Crosnier J, Grunfeld J-P and Maxwell MH (eds) *Advances in Nephrology*, pp. 41–60. Chicago: Year Book Medical, 1983.
9 Jacquot C, Idatte JM, Bedrossian J *et al.* Long-term blood pressure changes in renal transplantation. *Arch Int Med* 1978; **138:** 233–6.
10 Luke RG, Curtis JJ, Jones P *et al.* Mechanisms of post-transplant hypertension. *Am J Kidney Dis* 1985; **5:** A79–A84.
11 Rettig R, Folberth CG, Graf C *et al.* Are renal mechanisms involved in primary hypertension? Evidence from kidney transplantation studies in rats. *Klin Wochenschr* 1991; **69:** 597–602.
12 McDonald FD, Horenten ML, Mayor GB *et al.* Effect of alternate-day steroids on renal transplant function. A controlled study. *Nephron* 1976; **17:** 415–29.
13 Curtis JJ, Galla JH, Woodford SY *et al.* Comparison of daily and alternate-day prednisone during chronic maintenance therapy: a controlled crossover study. *Am J Kidney Dis* 1981; **1:** 166–71.
14 The Canadian Multicenter Transplant Study Group. A randomized clinical trial of cyclosporine in cadaveric renal transplantation. *N Engl J Med* 1983; **309:** 809–15.
15 Bennett WM, Porter GA. Cyclosporine-associated hypertension. *Am J Med* 1988; **85:** 131–3.
16 First WH, Oyer PE, Shumway NE. Long-term Renodynamic results after cardiac transplantation. *J Thoracic Cardiovasc Surg* 1987; **94:** 685–93.
17 Sherrer U, Vissing SF, Morgan BJ *et al.* Cyclosporine-induced sympathetic activity of hypertension after heart transplantation. *N Engl J Med* 1990; **323:** 693–9.
18 Curtis JJ, Luke RG, Dubousky E *et al.* Cyclosporine in therapeutic doses increases renal allograft vascular resistance. *Lancet* 1986; **2:** 477–9.
19 Luke RG. Mechanism of cyclosporine-induced hypertension. *Am J Hypertension* 1991; **4:** 468–71.
20 Curtis JJ, Luke RG, Whelchel JD *et al.* Inhibition of angiotensin-converting enzyme in renal transplant recipients with hypertension. *N Engl J Med* 1983; **308:** 377–81.
21 Murray BM, Paller MS, Ferris TE. Effect of cyclosporine administration on renal hemodynamics in conscious rat. *Kidney Int* 1985; **28:** 767–74.
22 Curtis JJ, Luke RG, Jones PA, Diethelm AG. Hypertension in cyclosporine-treated renal transplant patients in sodium dependent. *Am J Med* 1988; **85:** 134–8.
23 Mimran A, Mourad G, Ribstein J. Is renal transplantation useful for the understanding of the pathogenesis of hypertension? *Adv Nephrol* 1990; **19:** 53–68.
24 Myers BC, Ross J, Newton L *et al.* Cyclosporine-associated chronic nephropathy. *N Engl J Med* 1984; **311:** 699–705.
25 Makowka L, Lopatin W, Gilas T *et al.* Prevention of cyclosporine (CyA) nephrotoxicity by synthetic prostaglandins. *Clin Nephrol* 1986; **25:** (Suppl. 1) S89–S94.
26 Kawaguchi A, Goldman MN, Shapiro R *et al.* Increase in urinary thromboxane B2 in rats caused by cyclosporine. *Transplantation* 1985; **40:** 214.
27 Schachter M. Cyclosporine A and hypertension. *J Hypertension* 1988; **6:** 511–16.
28 Bunchman TE, Brookshire CA. Cyclosporine-induced synthesis of endothelin by cultured human endothelial cells. *J Clin Invest* 1991; **88:** 310–14.
29 Kon V, Sugiura M, Inagami T *et al.* Role of endothelin in cyclosporine-induced glomerular dysfunction. *Kidney Int* 1990; **37:** 1487–91.
30 Starzl TE, Fung J, Jordan M *et al* Kidney transplantation under FK 506. *JAMA* 1990 **264:** 63–7.
31 Jordan ML, Shapiro R, Vivas CA *et al.* FK 506 'rescue' for resistant rejection of renal allografts under primary cyclosporine immunosuppression. *Transplantation* 1994; **57:** 860–5.
32 Cooke CR, Ruiz-Maza F, Kawarski A *et al.* Regulation of plasma aldosterone concentration in anephric man and renal transplant recipients. *Kidney Int* 1973; **3:** 160–6.
33 Miyashita A, Sakai A, Butt KMH. Urinary kallikrein activity (esterase activity), plasma renin activity, and urinary aldosterone excretion in kidney transplantation patients. *Transplant Proc* 1983; **15:** 2136–8.
34 Kornerup HJ. The patterns of peripheral plasma

renin concentration in the early post-renal-transplant period. *Scand J Urol Nephrol* 1979; **13:** 185–9.
35 Weidmann P, Massry SG, Coburn JW *et al.* Blood pressure effects of acute hypercalcemia-studies in patients with chronic renal failure. *Ann Int Med* 1972; **60:** 447–61.
36 Pollini J, Guttman RD, Beadoin JG *et al.* Late hypertension following renal allotransplantation. *Clin Nephrol* 1979; **11:** 202–12.
37 Grunfeld JP, Kleinknecht D, Moreau JF. Permanent hypertension after renal homotransplantation in man. *Clin Sci Mol Med* 1975; **48:** 391–403.
39 Curtis J. Hypertension following kidney transplantation. *Am J Kidney Dis* 1994; **23:** 471–5.
39 Kasiske BL. Possible causes and consequences of hypertension in stable renal transplant patients. *Transplantation* 1987; **44:** 639–43.
40 Mell MW, Alfrey EJ, Rubin GD *et al.* Use of spiral computed tomography in the diagnosis of transplant renal artery stenosis. *Transplantation* 1994; **57:** 746–8.
41 Smellie WAB, Vinik M, Hume DM. Angiographic investigation of hypertension complicating human renal transplantation. *Surg Gynecol Obstet* 1969; **128:** 963–8.
42 Tilney NL, Rocha A, Strom TB, Kirkman RL. Renal artery stenosis in transplant patients. *Ann Surg* 1984; **199:** 454–60.
43 Anderson CF, Woods JE, Frohrert PP *et al.* Renal allograft bruit: an encouraging finding. *Mayo Clin Proc* 1973; **48:** 13–17.
44 Braun WE. The renal-allograft bruit as an indicator of good function. *N Engl J Med* 1972; **286:** 1350–2.
45 Grossman RA, Dafoe DC, Shoenfeld RB *et al.* Percutaneous transluminal angioplasty treatment of renal transplant artery stenosis. *Transplantation* 1982; **34:** 339–43.
46 Jordan ML, Cook GT, Cardella CJ. Ten years of experience with vascular complications in renal transplantation. *J Urol* 1982; **128:** 689–92.
47 Merkus JWS, Huysmans FTM, Hoitsma AJ *et al.* Renal allograft artery stenosis: results of medical treatment and intervention, A retrospective analysis. *Transplant Int* 1993; **6:** 111–15.
48 Lacombe M. Arterial stenosis complicatin renal transplantation in man: a study of 38 cases. *An Surg* 1973; **181:** 283–8.
49 Margules RM, Belzer FO, Kountz SL. Surgical correction of renovascular hypertension following renal allotransplantation. *Arch Surg* 1973; **106:** 13–16.
50 Palleschi J, Novick AC, Braun WE, Magnusson MO. Vascular complications of renal transplantation. *Urology* 1980; **16:** 61–7.
51 Smith RB, Ehrlich RM. The surgical complications of renal transplantation. *Urol Clin North Am* 1976; **3:** 621–46.
52 Flechner SM, Sandler CM, Childs T *et al.* Screening for transplant renal artery stenosis in hypertensive recipients using digital subtraction angiography. *J Urol* 1983; **130:** 440–4.
53 Sagalowsky AI, Peters PC. Revovascular hypertension following renal transplantation. *Urol Clin North Am* 1984; **11:** 491–502.
54 Hall JE, Guyton AC, Jackson TE *et al.* Control of glomerular filtration rate by renin–angiotensin system. *Am J Physiol* 1977; **233:** F366–372.
55 Farrow PR, Wilkinson R. Reversible renal failure during treatment with captopril. *Br Med J* 1979; **1:** 1680.
56 Colleste P, Haglund K, Lundgren G *et al.* Reversible renal failure during treatment with captopril. *Br Med J* 1979; **2:** 612–13.
57 Hricik De, Browning PJ, Kopelman R *et al.* Captopril-induced functional renal insufficiency in patients with bilateral renal-artery stenosis or renal-artery stenosis in a solitary kidney. *N Engl J Med* 1983; **308:** 373–6.
58 Van deer Woude FJ, van Son WJ, Tegzess AM *et al.* Effect of catopril on blood pressure and renal function in patients with transplant renal artery stenosis. *Nephron* 1985; **39:** 184–8.
59 Trachtman H, Butt KMH, Gordon D, Tejani A. The use of captopril to control hypertension in post-transplant renal artery stenosis. *Clin Nephrol* 1985; **23:** 203–6.
60 Gagnadoux HF, Niaudet P, Bacri JL *et al.* Captopril and transplant artery stenosis in children. *Transplant Proc* 1985; **17:** 187–8.
61 Ricotta JJ, Schaff HV, Williams GM *et al.* Renal artery stenosis following transplantation: etiology, diagnosis and prevention. *Surgery* 1978; **84:** 595–602.
62 Roberts JP, Ascher NL, Fryd DS *et al.* Transplant renal artery stenosis. *Transplantation* 1989; **48:** 580–3.
63 Hsu AC, Balfe JW, Olley PM *et al.* Allograft renal artery stenosis: increased peripheral plasma renin activity as an early indicator of uncontrollable hypertension. *Clin Nephrol* 1978; **10:** 232–8.
64 Whelton PK, Russell RP, Harrington DP *et al.* Hypertension following renal transplantation: causative factors and therapeutic implications. *JAMA* 1979; **241:** 1128–31.
65 Sankari BP, Stowe NT, Nally JV *et al.* Transplant renal artery stenosis in a canine model: evaluation of hemodynamic changes, renal function, and captopril renography. *J Urol* 1992; **147:** 723–6.
66 Linas SL, Miller PD, McDonald KM *et al.* Role of the renin—angiotensin system in post-transplantation hypertension in patients with multiple kidneys. *N Engl J Med* 1978 **298;** 1440–4.
67 Kornerup HJ, Pedersen EB, Fjeldborg O. Kidney transplant artery stenosis. *Proc Eur Dial Transplant Assoc* 1977; **14:** 377–85.

68 Rao TKS, Gupta SK, Butt KMH *et al.* Relationship of renal transplantation to hypertension in end-stage renal failure. *Arch Int Med* 1978; **138:** 1236–44.
69 Ladefoged J, Nerstrom B, Nielson I The possible significance of renin determination in selection of kidney transplanted patients for bilateral nephrectomy in treatment of hypertension. *Scand J Urol Nephrol* 1974; **8:** 240–1.
70 Casteneda MA, Garvin PJ, Codd JE, Carney K. Selective post-transplantation bilateral native nephrectomy. *Arch Surg* 1983; **118:** 1194–6.
71 Ploth DW. Angiotensin-dependent mechanisms in two-kidney, one clip renovascular, hypertension. *Am J Physiol* 1983; **245:** F131–141.
72 Nguyen BD, Adatepe MH. Renal artery stenosis in enbloc pediatric renal transplant: demonstration by captopril-enhanced renal scinigraphy. *J Nucl Med* 1992; **33:** 263–5.
73 Bennett WM, Strong D, Rosch J. Arteriovenous fistula complicating renal transplantation. *Urology* 1976; **8:** 254–7.
74 Pigott JP, Sharp WV. Arteriovenous fistula involving a transplant kidney. *Transplantation* 1987; **44:** 156–7.
75 Diaz-Buxo JA, Kopen DF, Donadio JV. Renal allograft arteriovenous fistula following percutaneous biopsy. *J Urol* 1974; **112:** 577–80.
76 Linder R, Billing H, Tibella T *et al.* Fibromuscular dysplasia in donor kidneys-experience with three cases. *Transplant Int* 1989; **2:** 228–31.
77 Goldman MH, Tilney NL, Vineyard GC *et al.* A twenty year survey of arterial complications of renal transplantation. *Surg Gynecol Obstet* 1975; **141:** 758–60.
78 Richardson AJ, Liddington M, Jaskowski A *et al.* Pregnancy in a renal transplant recipient complicated by rupture of a transplant renal artery aneurysm. *Br J Surg* 1990; **77:** 228–9.
79 Fleshner NE, Johnston KW. Repair of an autotransplant renal artery aneurysm: case report and literature review. *J Urol* 1992; **148:** 389–91.
80 Jordan ML. Mycotic aneurysm following kidney transplantation (Commentary). *Transplant Sci* 1992; **2:** 16–17.
81 Mulderije E, Berden J, Buskens FGM *et al.* False and true aneurysms of the renal artery after kidney transplantation. A report of two cases. *Br J Radiol* 1985; **58:** 896–9.
82 Erley CM, Duda SH, Wakat JP *et al.* Nonivasive procedures for diagnosis of renovascular hypertension in renal transplant recipients – a prospective analysis. *Transplantation* 1992; **54:** 863–7.
83 Davidson RA, Wilcox CS. Newer tests for the diagnosis of renovascular disease. *JAMA* 1992; **268:** 3353–8.
84 Plainfoose MC, Calonge VM, Beyloune-Mainardi C *et al.* Vascular complications in the adult kidney transplant recipient. *J Clin Ultrasound* 1992; **20:** 517–27.
85 Taylor KJW, Morse SS, Rigsby CM *et al.* Vascular complications in renal allografts: detection with duplex Doppler US. *Radiology* 1987; **162:** 31–8.
86 Dodd GD III, Tublin ME, Shah A, Zajko AB. Imaging of vascular complications associated with renal transplants. *Am J Radiol* 1991; **157:** 449–59.
87 Memel DS, Dodd GS III, Shah AN *et al.* Imaging of en bloc renal transplants: normal and abnormal postoperative findings. *Am J Radiol* 1993; **160:** 75–81.
88 Glicklich D, Tellis VA, Quinn T *et al.* Comparison of captopril and doppler ultrasonography as screening tests for transplant renal artery stenosis. *Transplantation* 1990; **49:** 217–19.
89 Duda SH, Erley CM, Wakat JP *et al.* Posttransplant renal artery stenosis-outpatient intraarterial DSA versus color aided duplex Doppler sonography. *Eur J Radiol* 1993; **16:** 95–101.
90 Svetkey LP, Dunnick NR, Coffman TM *et al.* Comparison of intravenous digital subtraction angiography and conventional arteriography in defining renal anatomy. *Transplantation* 1988; **45:** 56–8.
91 Dubovsky EV, Russell CS. Diagnosis of renovascular hypertension after renal transplantation. *Am J Hypertension* 1991; **4:** 724S–730S.
92 McCarty M, Gedroyc WMW. Surgical clip artifact mimicking arterial stenosis: a problem with magnetic resonance angiography. *Clin Radiol* 1993; **48:** 232–5.
93 Mell MW, Alfrey EJ, Rubin GD *et al.* Use of spiral computed tomography in the diagnosis of transplant renal artery stenosis. *Transplantation* 1994; **57:** 746–8.
94 Darras FS, Jordan ML, Shapiro R *et al.* Transplantation of pediatric en bloc kidneys under FK 506 immunosuppression. *Transplant Proc* 1991; **23:** 3089–90.
95 Curtis JJ, Diethelm AG, Luke RG *et al.* Benefits of removal of native kidneys in hypertension after renal transplantation. *Lancet* 1985; **11:** 739–42.
96 Thompson JF, Wood RFM, Taylor HM *et al.* Control of hypertension after renal transplantation by embolisation of host kidneys. *Lancet* 1984; **22:** 424–7.
97 Bonomini V, Campieri C, Mignani R *et al.* Long-term normalization of resistant renal hypertension after embolization of host kidneys in a transplanted patient – a case report. *Transplantation* 1987; **43:** 451.
98 Rodriguez-Perez JC, Maynar M, Palop L *et al.* Sepsis and death after embolization of host kidneys in a resistant renal hypertension transplanted patient. *Nephron* 1988: **50:** 75–6.
99 Gruntzig A, Vetter W, Meier B *et al.* Treatment

of renovascular hypertension with percutaneous transluminal dilatation of a renal-artery stenosis. *Lancet* 1978; **1:** 801–2.

100 Sniderman KW, Sprayregen S, Sos TA *et al.* Percutaneous transluminal dilation in renal transplant arterial stenosis. *Transplantation* 180; **30:** 440–4.

101 Greenstein SM, Verestandig A, McLean GK *et al.* Percutaneous transluminal angioplasty. The procedure of choice in the hypertensive renal allograft recipient with renal artery stenosis. *Transplantation* 1987; **43:** 29–32.

102 Fauchald P, Vatne K, Paulsen D *et al.* Long-term clinical results of percutaneous transluminal angioplasty in transplant renal artery stenosis. *Nephrol Dial Transplant* 1992; **7:** 256–9.

103 Benoit G, Moukarzel M, Hiesse C *et al.* Transplant renal artery stenosis: experience and comparative results between surgery and angioplasty. *Transplant Int* 1990; **3:** 137–40.

104 McMullin ND, Reidy JF, Koffman CG *et al.* The management of renal transplant artery stenosis in children by percutaneous transluminal angioplasty. *Transplantation* 1992; **53:** 559–63.

105 Fontaine E, Beurton D, Barthelemy Y *et al.* Renal artery stenosis following pediatric renal transplantation. *Transplant Proc* 1994; **26:** 293–4.

106 Spijkerboer AM, Mali WP, Donckerwolcke RAMG. Renal transplant artery stenosis in children: treatment with percutaneous transluminal angioplasty. *Pediatr Radiol* 1992; **22:** 519–21.

PART IV

Atherosclerotic Ischemic Renal Disease

21

Pathophysiology of renal failure in ischemic renal disease

STEPHEN C TEXTOR, LESLIE SMITH-POWELL

Introduction

'Ischemic nephropathy' is a term applied to gradual loss of kidney function caused by vascular occlusion. While the loss of blood supply represents an obvious threat to organ function, recognition that renovascular disease may be a reversible factor in progressive chronic renal failure is a comparatively recent concept. While renal artery stenosis has long been recognized as a cause of secondary hypertension, retrospective reviews suggest that between 5 and 15% of patients reaching end-stage renal disease (ESRD) may have a component related to vascular occlusion. Recent prospective studies confirm these suspicions.[1, 2] As discussed in this text and elsewhere, the prognosis of patients undergoing dialysis therapy with ischemic renal failure is poor.[3] Perhaps most importantly, clinical experience indicates that revascularization of a viable kidney sometimes leads to withdrawal from dialysis and long-term survival.[4] For these reasons, pressure is mounting to identify and define more precisely the pathogenesis of ischemic nephropathy on the basis of large vessel occlusive disease. It is hoped that improved understanding of this disorder may allow earlier and more effective identification, and perhaps prevention, of permanent injury to the kidney.

The most common form of this disorder is related to atherosclerotic vascular disease, which is found primarily in older patients. As both the longevity and median age of United States citizens increase, the number of patients with atherosclerotic disease affecting the kidney also is increasing. This is compounded by the diminished mortality from other diseases, including coronary and cerebral vascular events.[5] Hence, clinicians will encounter more frequently than before the need to establish whether vascular disease accounts for deteriorating renal function in such patients.

This chapter examines the current understanding of pathophysiologic events leading to renal dysfunction associated with chronic renovascular disease. Implicit in this discussion is the principle that identification of critical levels of vascular compromise will allow restoration of flow and recovery, or at least stabilization, of renal function. It should be understood that few studies have examined these issues directly. Hence, large conceptual gaps remain between steps in the proposed sequence of progressive renal injury leading to ESRD. It should be understood further that paradigms applied to *acute renal ischemic injury* may have limited applicability to *chronic vascular injury*. Identification of those gaps may assist in focusing further studies in this problematic area.

Pathology and background

The potential for renal arterial occlusion to lead to renal death is well established. Renal atrophy beyond a totally occluded artery is not rare (Fig. 21.1). Clinical examples of *acute renal artery occlusion* provide a model for demonstrating glomerular collapse, tubular necrosis, interstitial fibrosis and eventual scar formation.[6] Occasional reports of vascular reconstruction soon after acute arterial occlusion indicate that restoration of blood supply can restore renal function.[7]

Review of pathologic material in human kidneys reveals numerous features attributed to 'ischemia'. These include collapse of glomeruli with evident reduplication of the basement membrane. Areas of glomerular sclerosis are usually detected. Hypercellularity of the juxtaglomerular apparatus is a common finding, which correlates with increased renin content and release.[8] A variety of other features are described which include loss of tubular integrity, epithelial cell disruption, mesangial expansion with inclusion of a variety of materials, interstitial fibrosis and localized areas of chronic inflammation.[6, 9] Most of these changes are not specific to vascular disease. Since atherosclerotic vascular disease often supervenes upon long-standing hypertension, these findings commonly are interspersed with vascular changes of nephrosclerosis. Both of these processes may be complicated by coexistent diabetes and/or changes of aging.

Recent studies using experimental renal artery lesions indicate that renal tubular atrophy and interstitial inflammation trigger increased synthesis of matrix proteins, such as vimentin, and alter the presentation of epithelial antigens similar to other forms of chronic interstitial nephritis.[10] While these studies are conducted using models with rapid, usually severe, vascular compromise, they nonetheless establish a mechanism linking vascular disease with chronic interstitial fibrosis.

It is less clear what pathologic events occur during *gradual* compromise of the renal circulation, which is central to the condition addressed

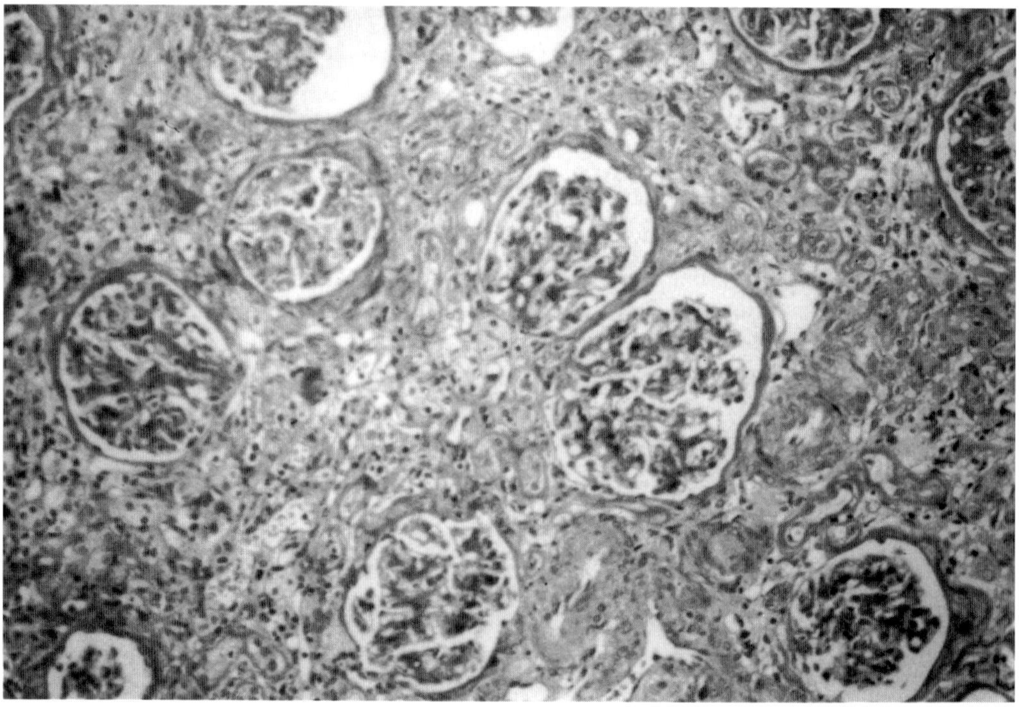

Figure 21.1. Pathologic specimen of kidney beyond an arterial occlusion: major features include glomerular collapse with loss of tuft volume, tubular atrophy and interstitial fibrosis. Loss of tubular structures and interstitial inflammation are consistent with irreversible loss of kidney viability. Reproduced courtesy of Dr K. Holley, Mayo Clinic.

here. Recent textbooks of renal pathology scarcely mention chronic vascular disease as a cause of chronic renal failure.[6] 'Ischemic nephropathy' is used by some authors to denote progressive renal failure caused by large vessel renal artery disease.[11, 12] It has been considered an 'overlooked' entity, because of its rarely being identified and reversed before reaching advanced levels.[11]

Several key elements are implicit in the paradigm connecting renal injury to ischemic nephropathy (Fig. 21.2).

Central to this concept is that a sufficiently severe vascular lesion reduces renal perfusion pressure below a 'critical perfusion pressure' required for continued function. When the kidney is perfused at these reduced arterial pressures, a series of changes develop including reduced blood flow and reduced filtration and tubular reabsorptive function. An important corollary is that these functional changes are reversible if perfusion can be restored by means of renal revascularization. It is clear, however, that restoration of function is limited, i.e. at some point loss of renal function becomes irreversible. The basis for this transition from a reversible phase to irreversible phase has not been examined or defined precisely. When irreversible changes affect the entire renal mass, i.e. when both kidneys or a solitary functional kidney are involved, clinical consequences of renal failure ensue.

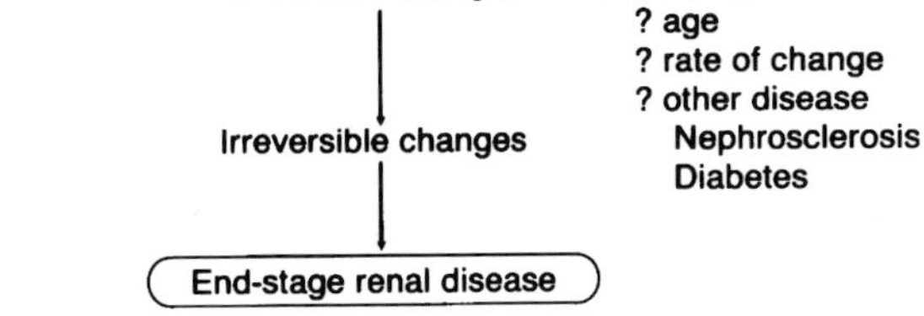

Figure 21.2. Theoretical scheme by which renal artery stenosis leads to end-stage renal disease. Central to this model is the concept that vascular compromise leads to intermediate events which injure the kidney. How these events change from 'reversible' to 'irreversible' tissue damage is a major issue remaining to be clarified (see text). From ref. 25 with permission.

Critical perfusion pressure

The renal capacities for autoregulation of blood flow[13, 14] and glomerular filtration[15] have been studied extensively (Fig. 21.3). Both are maintained over a wide range of renal perfusion pressures, but fall when mean renal pressures are reduced below 70–80 mmHg during short-term experiments.

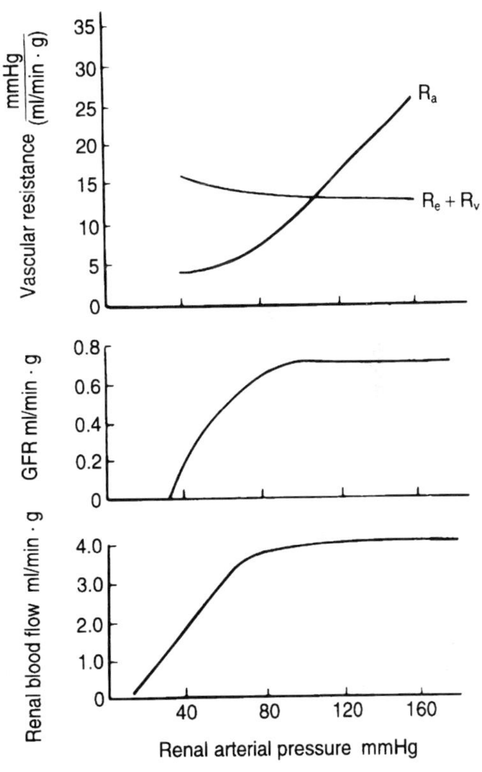

Figure 21.3. Autoregulation of blood flow in the kidney: both blood flow and glomerular filtration are regulated precisely to remain at nearly constant level when renal perfusion pressures are above 70–80 mmHg. GFR is limited by alterations in afferent renal arteriolar tone (Ra). As renal perfusion pressure falls below the lower limits of autoregulation, however, both blood flow and GFR fall rapidly. From ref. 53 with permission.

Few data are available regarding the long-term effects of pressure reduction upon cellular and structural elements of the kidney. Nonetheless, it is clear that if renal perfusion remains below the limits of autoregulation, renal function deteriorates. It follows that reduction of systemic blood pressure with antihypertensive therapy in patients with high grade renal artery lesions carries with it the potential of reducing borderline poststenotic perfusion pressures to below 'critical' levels and inducing acute renal insufficiency, a phenomenon we have employed to identify some patients at risk for progressive renal failure prior to renal revascularization.[16] Such pressure sensitivity of renal function can be reversed by successful renal revascularization.[17]

Early studies of arterial lesions in several vascular beds demonstrated that compromise of the arterial lumen must reach an advanced level, exceeding 80–85% cross-sectional obstruction, before hemodynamic changes are evident (Fig. 21.4).[18]

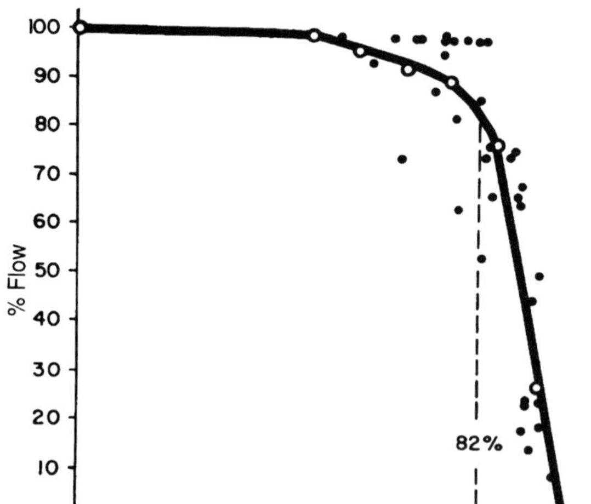

Figure 21.4. Hemodynamic effects of a stenotic lesion: cross-sectional area was determined precisely by measurement of postmortem latex casts from a blood vessel undergoing experimental occlusion in the leg. These studies demonstrate that both blood flow and pressure gradients induced by vascular stenosis are negligible until the lumen narrows to more than 70–80% of total occlusion. Further stenosis produces abrupt loss in blood flow. From ref. 18 with permission.

These observations form the basis of recognizing that arterial lesions of lesser degree offer no hemodynamic limit to flow or perfusion pressure and therefore are 'not significant' clinically. It is notoriously difficult to establish the true dimensions of a stenotic lesion from a two-dimensional arteriogram, however. Physiologic features may identify those lesions which are sufficient to induce acceleration of blood flow by the Venturi effect, however, leading to poststenotic dilation, flow acceleration and disturbed flow patterns measured by duplex ultrasonography.[19,20]

It is important to recognize that the hemodynamic effects of a stenotic lesion depend upon the flow characteristics present within the circulation at the moment of measurement.[21] Higher flows magnify the relative effects of moderate stenotic lesions. An important corollary of these data is that renal perfusion beyond the stenotic lesion may vary considerably under different conditions. In most instances, reduction of renal perfusion pressures initiates a rise in systemic arterial pressure which ultimately restores renal perfusion pressures close to normal (Figs. 21.5a and 21.5b).

Hence, despite severe renal stenosis, poststenotic blood flow may be near normal, unless systemic arterial pressures are reduced or the lesion progresses further.

It is also important to recognize that detection of hemodynamic effects related to vascular stenosis implies far advanced vascular lumen obstruction, as illustrated in Fig. 21.4. Hence, further obstruction presents the risk of imminent further loss of poststenotic perfusion and perhaps total arterial occlusion. The practical corollary to this observation is that identification of functional consequences of stenosis, such as reduced blood flow, reduced filtration or kidney size implies that further lumen compromise will have additional severe effects. Progression of arterial narrowing in such instances therefore poses the hazard of rapidly declining blood flow.

Intermediate mechanisms of poststenotic renal injury

Does gradual reduction in renal perfusion pressure in fact lead to renal ischemia? The answer

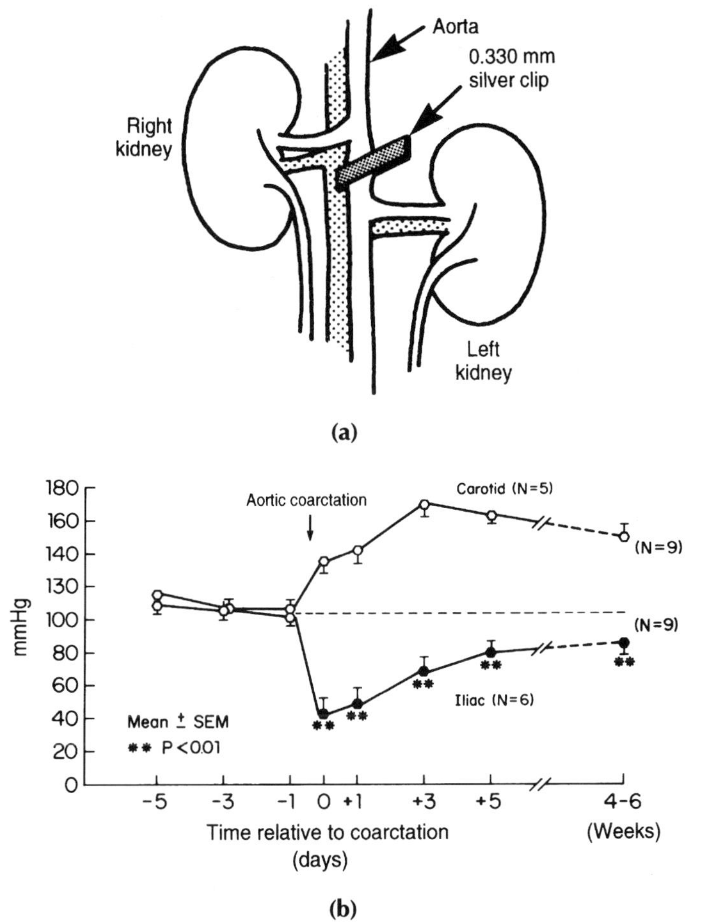

Figure 21.5. (a) Illustration of placement of a silver aortic clip between the renal arteries in the rat for the study of poststenotic hemodynamic characteristics in the conscious animal. This model allows measurement of systemic arterial pressures (via the carotid artery) or poststenotic renal perfusion pressures (via the iliac artery) in one-kidney (as shown) or two-kidney coarct models analagous to one-kidney and two-kidney Goldblatt experimental hypertension. (b) Arterial pressures before and after placement of the aortic coarct. Despite the development of a signficant pressure gradient across the lesion, systemic pressures rise leading to restoration of near normal perfusion pressures to the poststenotic kidney. Hence, renal blood flow is compromised beyond the stenosis primarily when systemic pressures are lowered or the lesion progresses further. When renal function deteriorates with further pressure reduction, the lesion is considered to have reached 'critical' renal artery stenosis. From ref. 26 with permission.

to this question is not known. Unlike brain or coronary circulations, which function continuously at high oxygen extraction, the kidney is oversupplied with oxygenated blood. This feature is consistent with its function as a filtering organ. Actual metabolic energy requirements in the kidney, and therefore need for oxygen as an energy source, for filtration, tubular reabsorption and metabolism are 10–15% of delivered oxygen.[13] Hence, oxygen saturation of renal venous blood remains above 80%.[22] Recent studies of renal venous oxygen levels from kidneys with proven renovascular hypertension indicate that oxygen saturation is *higher* in severely stenotic kidneys with reduced renal blood flow, rather than lower, as might be expected.[22] The authors propose that reduced filtration, and thereby reduced tubular reabsorptive work, diminish energy requirements in hypoperfused kidneys. These data are supported by other studies which detected no differences in renal venous erythropoeitin levels from stenotic vs non-stenotic kidneys, despite lateralization of renin secretion and asymmetric kidney size.[23, 24] Such observations cast doubt on the proposition that reduction in renal size and function in poststenotic kidneys reflects primarily failure of oxygenation, *per se*. The possibility of undetected, localized oxygen deficits within specific regions of the kidney, such as the medulla, cannot be excluded.

Poststenotic renal perfusion pressures

If not oxygen deprivation, then can reduced arterial pressure alone be sufficient to lead to glomerular collapse and permanent parenchymal renal injury? Recent studies in the rat suggest that perhaps more importantly than absolute renal pressure levels, the *rate of change* of arterial pressure may dictate structural injury.[25] This has been a difficult issue to address without suitable means of measuring poststenotic arterial pressures in the conscious subject or animal. We sought to develop a model using an aortic coarct placed between the two renal arteries of the rat, allowing study of two-kidney and one-kidney aortic coarct models analogous to Goldblatt (renal artery clip) models used elsewhere (Fig. 21.5).

An advantage of this model is that poststenotic arterial pressures can be measured precisely by means of an iliac artery catheter, as previously described.[26] When renal structure and function were studied in conscious animals after abrupt placement of an aortic coarct, which produced drastic immediate poststenotic pressure reduction which after 4 weeks stabilized at 62 ± 2 mmHg, permanent loss of glomerular size, function and tubular fibrosis ensued (Fig. 21.6).[25] Similar studies using a high grade renal ligature induced widespread interstitial inflammation, tubular collapse and fibrosis.[10]

When similar poststenotic pressures (mean = 50 ± 3 mmHg) developed over 4 weeks by means of pressure reduction using an angiotensin converting enzyme (ACE) inhibitor and low sodium diet, glomerular volumes were indeed reduced, but the integrity of renal structures was preserved, as reflected by morphometric histology and electron microscopy.[25] Furthermore, the integrity of renal function was

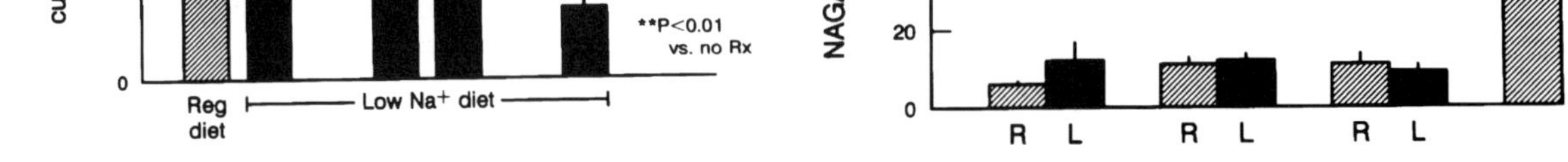

(a) (b)

Figure 21.6. (a) Glomerular tuft volume measured after *in situ* perfusion fixation in a variety of experimental stenotic models. Tuft volume declines as a function of poststenotic perfusion pressure. (b) Urinary excretion of a proximal tubular lysozyme (NAGA: N-acetyl-glucosaminidase) in the same groups. Remarkably, NAGA from coarct stenotic animals treated with ACE inhibition and with sustained poststenotic renal pressures between 50 and 60 mmHg did not undergo tubular necrosis and maintained appropriate sodium reabsorption. By contrast, those animals with a severe coarct alone with similar poststenotic pressures developed tubular necrosis, elevated NAGA excretion and non-functional kidneys. These results indicate that poststenotic pressures alone do not determine the viability of the kidney. From ref. 25 with permission.

preserved also, as reflected by appropriate fractional excretion of sodium and normal levels of urinary lysozyme excretion (N-acetyl-glucosaminidase). Grone *et al.* performed similar studies[27] in two-kidney, one-clip renovascular hypertensive rats treated with low sodium diet and enalapril. Although glomerular filtration rate (GFR) was impaired, these authors identified only modest tubular atrophy in the poststenotic kidney with normal appearing tubular brush borders. When kidneys were examined 9–15 days after discontinuing antihypertensive therapy, GFR had recovered and the histologic appearance was normal.

Taken together, these studies highlight some pitfalls in the study of poststenotic renal injury. They indicate that the severity of parenchymal injury may vary widely under different conditions. How such changes translate into irreversible renal structural and functional changes in humans is not yet established. It appears that pathologic changes depend upon many factors, including the rate and severity of perfusion decrements. In some models of reduced renal perfusion, such as experimental nephrotoxicity induced by cyclosporin A, high levels of angiotensin appear to stimulate tubulointerstitial fibrosis directly, which may be prevented by treatment with ACE inhibitors.[28] Whether this effect is present in human renovascular disease is unknown. In most clinical disease states, additional factors of age and associated diseases such as hypertensive nephrosclerosis and diabetes mellitus may be paramount. It is likely that additional factors, not yet fully elucidated, play important roles.

Mechanisms by which renal hypoperfusion injures the kidney

By what mechanisms does impaired renal circulation lead to irreversible kidney damage? A large body of work has accumulated regarding the mechanisms by which acute ischemic renal failure develops, some of which are summarized in recent reviews.[6, 29] It should be emphasized that conclusions from studies of acute renal failure may have limited relevance to the issues of chronic renal failure addressed here. While this literature is unlikely to translate directly to ischemic nephropathy, they do provide, nonetheless, a conceptual framework with which to consider the problem.

Abnormalities of the vasculature

Recent studies emphasize the potential for vascular endothelium and products of vascular smooth muscle to release materials with major effects upon organ structure and function.[30] This work indicates that potent vasoconstrictor substances, such as the peptide endothelin (ET), and vasodilator materials, such as prostacyclin and nitric oxide (NO, also referred to as endothelium-derived relaxing factor, EDRF), are released during vascular injury of many kinds. The hallmark of these systems is their role in directly modifying local vascular tone and function. It is recognized that alterations of both distending vessel pressures and shear stress to the arterial wall are capable of inducing major disturbances of the balance in these vasoactive substances (Fig. 21.7).

Endothelin is among the most potent vasoconstrictors known. It appears to be preferentially active within the renal vascular bed, affecting arteriolar constriction, glomerular and mesangial cell contraction and filtration properties, sodium reabsorption and interstitial cytokine release.[31–33] When released during aortic cross-clamping, ET has profound renal effects which can be blocked by receptor antagonists.[34] Endothelin appears to have many additional properties, including modulation of signal-transduction pathways and initiation of mitogenesis, which in principle might participate in the transition between vascular compromise and irreversible parenchymal tissue injury.[35] The degree to which ET participates in this regard awaits investigation and application of receptor antagonists in clinically relevant models.

It is equally possible that vascular injury compromises protective vasodilator mechanisms, such as those mediated by NO and prostacyclin. The capacity for vascular NO production appears to be regulated by shear stress affecting the blood vessel wall. Recent experimental studies in two-kidney, one-clip renovascular hypertensive rats demonstrate diminished NO release

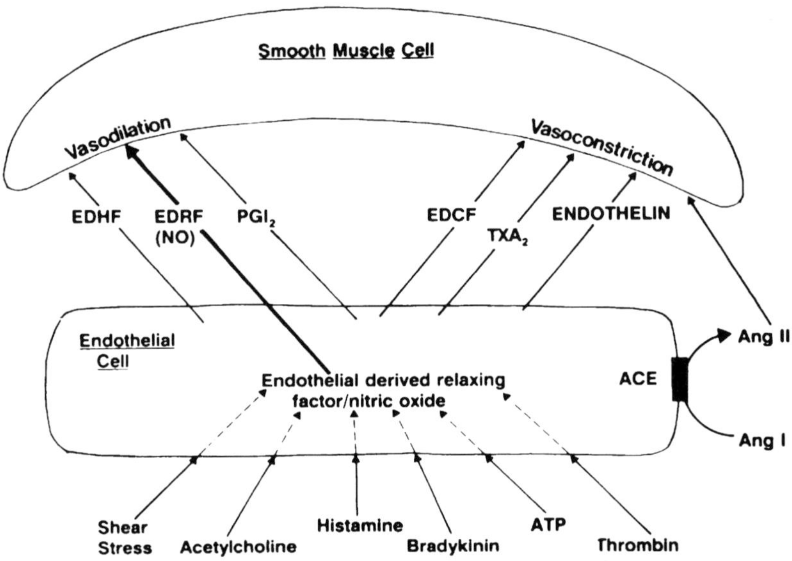

Figure 21.7. The endothelial surface of arterial vessels is recognized to be the source of multiple potent vasoactive materials. These include vasoconstrictors, such as endothelin and thromboxane (released from platelets upon wall contact) and vasodilators, such as prostacyclin (PGI2) and nitric oxide (NO), which appear to participate in determining basal vascular dimensions. These systems tend to interact and counter each other's effects under normal circumstances, but are disturbed in the presence of reduced arterial perfusion pressure and/or intrinsic disease of the vascular wall, such as atherosclerosis.

in the poststenotic kidney, whereas increased NO activity was demonstrated in the contralateral kidney exposed to higher arterial pressures.[36] Hence, NO vasodilatory activity may diminish in the stenotic kidney. It is known that both NO and prostacyclin oppose the vasoconstrictor effects of angiotensin II in the kidney. Loss or attenuation of these vasodilator mechanisms thereby exposes the poststenotic kidney to unopposed actions of vasoconstrictors, thereby amplifying the actions of endothelin and angiotensin II.

Both the renin–angiotensin and sympathetic adrenergic systems are activated within the kidney in response to compromised arterial pressures.[37] Within limits, these systems offer compensatory postglomerular vasoconstriction which serve to preserve glomerular filtration and reduce sodium excretion. When carried to extreme levels, however, vasoconstriction and perhaps additional effects, such as direct mitogenic stimulation by angiotensin II[38] offer the potential to damage the kidney and stimulate interstitial fibrosis. As noted above, blockade of the renin–angiotensin system in some experimental models attenuates glomerular injury beyond an arterial lesion when compared with antihypertensive therapy with other agents[39] and may restore endothelial vasodilatory function.[40] Whether these effects apply to human renovascular disease is unknown.

Depletion of parenchymal energy stores: adenosine triphosphate

During experimental tissue oxygen deprivation, cellular pools of high energy phosphate stores in the kidney are depleted rapidly. When adenosine triphosphate (ATP) is reduced, further metabolism to adenosine phosphate (AMP), then hypoxanthine and finally to uric acid can occur. It is important to recognize that loss of ATP exposes tissue to both requirements for alternate energy sources, such as glycolysis, and further exposes tissue to generation of free radicals during 'reperfusion' when oxygen combines with xanthine and hypoxanthine.[41]

Some investigators propose that prevention of free radical damage is central to preventing

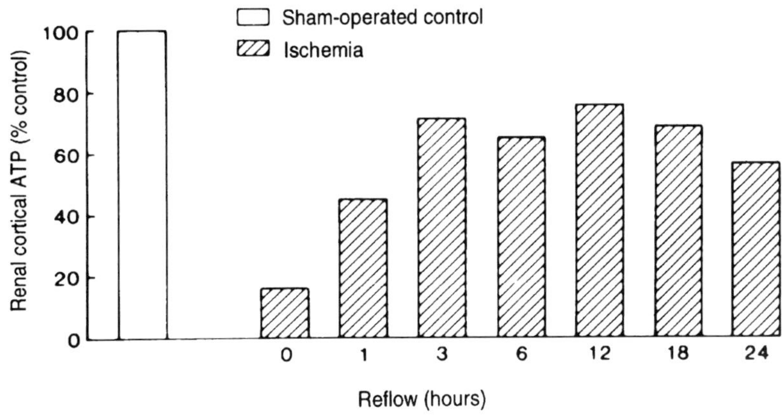

Figure 21.8. Adenosine triphosphate (ATP) levels in kidney cortex following total renal occlusion. Cortical levels gradually return to normal during restoration of blood flow. Consumption of ATP favors production of free radical intermediates, specifically peroxides, which are thought to mediate tissue injury. From ref. 54 with permission.

ischemic damage in some forms of experimental acute renal failure (see below). The relative importance of ATP depletion and xanthine metabolism depends greatly on both the severity and duration of the ischemic insult.

Recovery of renal function after ischemic insults, such as renal artery cross-clamping, develops in parallel with recovery of ATP levels (Fig. 21.8).[29] This process occurs rapidly, i.e. within minutes of vascular compromise and recovery, although it may take longer to reach completion. Whether chronic vascular occlusion produces intermittent or partial depletion of energy stores beyond a stenotic lesion is not known. Whole kidney studies suggest that oxygen deprivation itself is not a major component of most renal artery disease, as noted above. Nonetheless, intermittent or locally severe ischemia cannot be excluded and may lead to recurrent episodes of locally severe ATP depletion.

Transcellular ion gradients

Maintaining ion gradients for potassium, sodium and calcium are vital to sustained cellular integrity and function, in the kidney and elsewhere. Numerous transmembrane sodium pumps have been identified, some of which are linked to other cations, particularly calcium.

Ion gradients depend upon the availability of adequate energy and are therefore affected soon after reduction of ATP. Other factors have been identified which accelerate these changes in addition to altered energy availability. These include loss of functional transport proteins, often on the cell membrane, and loss of the epithelial polarity of transport enzymes.

The degree to which specific ion gradients participate in tissue injury, or participate as part of a multicomponent stress is not yet entirely clear. Efforts to prevent intracellular potassium depletion by means of extremely high extracellular potassium baths have reduced tissue injury, but only partially.[42]

Studies of acute renal injury have identified early interference with sodium–calcium extrusion (within 15 min), leading to *intracellular calcium overload* (Fig. 21.9).

It is recognized that many vital cell functions depend upon appropriate intracellular compartment localization of calcium. Removal of extracellular calcium, or prevention of calcium influx by means of bathing the kidney in calcium channel blocking agents have been applied to protecting kidneys harvested for transplantation[43] and have been studied as means to retard tissue injury in a variety of acute renal insults. Conversely, experimental addition of calcium ionophores which facilitate cytosolic calcium loading increase tissue injury[44] in several models. It should be emphasized that the sensitivity

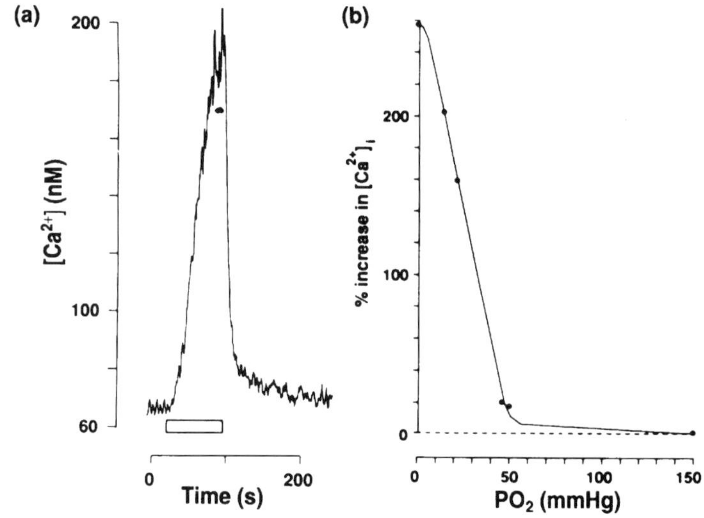

Figure 21.9. Rapid intracellular calcium accumulation following ischemic cellular injury. Several lines of study suggest that translocation of calcium and other cations are central to the development of disturbed intracellular processes and eventual cell death. From ref. 55 with permission.

of the kidney to calcium overload varies greatly with the degree of hypoxia and/or total renal ischemia induced. Other changes, such as intracellular acidosis and changed cellular membrane characteristics, may serve important roles to modify the degree of these effects.

Secondary effects of cell injury

Cellular injury leads to several consequences, such as changes in intracellular pH, release of intracellular enzymes and generation of oxygen free radicals. These changes in turn have the potential to modify further tissue injury.

Release of *intracellular enzymes*, including tubular lysozymes such as N-acetyl-glucosaminidase, or intermediate enzymes such as lactate dehydrogenase (LD) have been used as markers of cell injury. It is possible that these materials produce secondary effects, although the consequences of these effects under chronic conditions are poorly understood.

Some results indicate evidence that reduced *intracellular pH* during acute ischemic insults is protective to renal tubular cells, in part by retarding the accumulation of calcium.[45] The extent of this effect and its role in modifying intracellular calcium depends upon the severity and duration of the hypoxic insult. Whether such effects participate in intermittent hypoperfusion injury is not yet known.

Changes in cell *membrane composition* and phospholipase activity develop rapidly during hypoxic injury. Abrupt changes in free fatty acid release have been observed *in vitro*.[46] Some associated materials, such as phosphatidic acid, may function as calcium ionophores, and may act as cellular 'detergents', decreasing cell membrane integrity. Lipids released locally are further subject to peroxidation during generation of free radicals, which may accelerate tissue injury.

The role of *oxygen free radical generation* in renal injury is complex and not yet resolved. Experimental models using the rat demonstrate marked sensitivity to oxidative injury, which is not shared universally with other species, including the human.[29] Nonetheless, the potential for 'reperfusion' injury to occur during periods of intermittent arterial hypotension to the kidney beyond a critical vascular lesion is plausible, similar to that observed during reperfusion after warm ischemia after transplant organ harvesting. The fundamental assumption of this mechanism is that specific chemical entities, such as reduced adenosine, produced during oxygen deprivation, are liable to formation of toxic peroxides during restoration of oxygen delivery. Formation of these species is rapid and modified by the activity of intermediates, including glutathione and tissue-derived eicosanoids.[29, 41] It is of interest that the severity of renal injury may be magnified by intermittent reperfusion in studies of acute renal failure; this has been attributed to allowing washout of cellular glutathione stores.[47] It should be observed that disruption of cellular relationships, such as during endothelial cell swelling from free radical injury, exposes injured collagen surfaces to platelets and neutrophils. Experimental models which prevent free radical generation under these circumstances reveal markedly reduced cell adhesion and subsequent tissue injury.[48]

The effects of injury pathways may be modulated by local factors. Mesangial cells, for example, trap toxic activated neutrophils and platelets in some experimental models, magnifying their effects upon glomerular structures. Hence, the effects of vasoactive materials such as ET may be focused downstream, both injuring glomerular membranes and promoting fibrin deposition in efferent arterioles. Platelets are a rich source of the potent vasoconstrictor, thromboxane A2. Inhibition of thromboxane synthesis reduces injury in some models of ischemic renal failure.[29]

Recent studies indicate that *cytoskeletal characteristics* of renal parenchymal cells are altered fundamentally in response to hypoxic injury in a manner that may itself participate in cell destruction.[49] Distribution of membrane-bound enzymes, adherence at cellular tight junctions, and internalization of microvilli are easily and rapidly disturbed. Such changes impair normal protective functions of localized cell activity, exposing parts of the cell membrane to unusual stresses. It has been proposed that tight junctions protect areas of the cell from hypoxic injury. Breakdown of tight junctions with disintegration of apical filament structures has been demonstrated rapidly after ischemia. Changes within apical structures, including cellular 'blebs' may occur within minutes. Regulation of the processes that maintain regional integrity within renal cells is not yet well understood.

Disturbed cellular repair processes

Even less well understood are the complex processes by which acutely injured kidney tissue recovers normal structure and function after removal of the toxic insult. It is recognized that proximal tubular cells, especially, are capable of completely restoring and relining epithelial surfaces, perhaps in response to local cytokines and growth factors. Regeneration appears to involve expression of normally suppressed genes, some specific to the kidney.[50] Whether this requires a population of 'stem cells' from which new epithelial cells originate is not yet certain. It is of interest that adult renal tissue contains some genes not normally expressed which are capable of regulating ontogenic renal cellular differentiation. The ability of a healthy kidney to regenerate may determine the difference in renal injury beyond an arterial stenosis observed between younger and older individuals. It is recognized that older kidneys lack the capacity to express some of these genes.

The effects of associated disease states have yet to be ascertained. It is known that aging itself alters both tubular function and reactivity of vascular structures in the kidney.[51, 52] Whether these characteristics predispose to poststenotic kidney injury appears likely, but has not been established. Parenchymal atrophy and progressive renal failure appear primarily in older patients with atherosclerotic disease and are comparatively rare in younger patients with fibromuscular disease of the renal arteries, despite sufficient renal hypoperfusion to produce hypertension.

The role of repetitive hypoperfusion

As noted above, chronic ischemic renal injury beyond a stenotic lesion differs from acute ischemic injury in many respects. One of the most important of these is that vascular lesions likely induce varying degrees of relative renal hypoperfusion at different times. Factors affecting systemic arterial pressures, such as antihypertensive agents, diurnal variation and alterations in cardiac output and/or oxygenation, may lead to

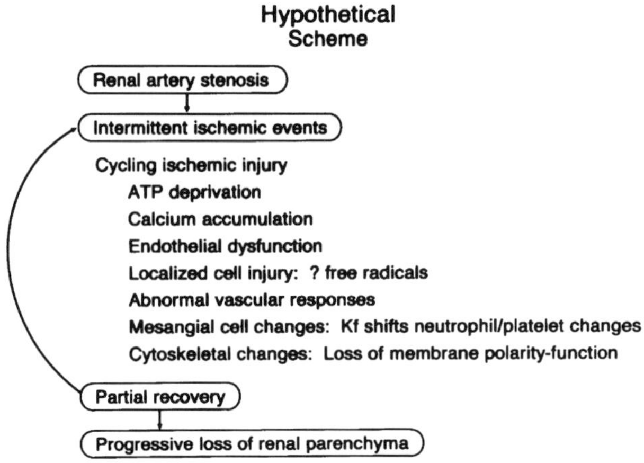

Figure 21.10. Proposed sequence of events by which repetitive episodes of of renal hypoperfusion might produce irreversible renal parenchymal injury beyond a stenotic arterial lesion. Data to support the role of each step have been obtained from models of acute ischemic renal failure (see text), although their role in chronic renovascular disease is not yet established. From ref. 25 with permission.

widely different renal perfusion states. Hence, we postulate one model of poststenotic renal injury based upon cycles of repetitive, partial reductions in arterial pressure (Fig. 21.10). Is it possible that chronic renal injury beyond a stenosis represents cyclic acute insults to the kidney, the effects of which are incompletely resolved at the time of the next insult?

While by no means the only model by which one can conceive the development of chronic renal failure, this model suggests that many of the intermediate mechanisms identified above may apply in repeated fashion.

Studies to define these issues more precisely are needed. While renal revascularization offers the potential to reverse the process of renal loss, this is not true for all poststenotic kidneys. It would be of enormous value to identify prospectively which kidneys are at true risk for progressive tissue injury, which are truly salvageable and which are beyond reasonable prospect of recovery. Such tools are not yet available. Furthermore, better understanding of the underlying mechanisms by which hypoperfusion leads to irreversible injury may allow intervention. Is it possible that carefully designed medical therapy may protect the poststenotic kidney from such injury until revascularization can be achieved or even indefinitely?

Summary

Poststenotic kidneys are subject to loss of glomerular volume and tubular atrophy, which may become irreversible if left untreated. The mechanisms by which permanent renal injury develops are complex and poorly understood. Current data indicate that neither ischemia itself nor absolute levels of poststenotic perfusion pressures explain the pathogenesis of renal failure in this setting. It is likely that repeated cycles of vascular underperfusion activate numerous pathways, which may include vascular endothelial factors, local energy depletion, free radical generation during reperfusion, disturbed intracellular ion gradients, cytoskeletal disruption and impaired cellular repair processes. Taken together, these processes lead to progressive renal injury if left untreated. Further studies should be directed at more precise understanding of these processes in order to identify salvageable kidneys and delay progression to irreversible renal failure.

Acknowledgement

Supported in part by the Steven Gallant Research Fellowship, City of Hope National Medical Center, Duarte, CA.

References

1 Scoble JE, Hamilton G. Atherosclerotic renovascular disease: remediable cause of renal failure in the elderly. *Br Med J* 1990; **300:** 1670–1.

2 O'Neil EA, Hansen KJ, Canzanello VJ *et al.* Prevalence of ischemic nephropathy in patients with renal insufficiency. *Ann Surg* 1992; **58:** 485–90.

3 Mailloux LU, Bellucci AG, Mossey RT *et al.* Predictors of survival in patients undergoing dialysis. *Am J Med* 1988; **84:** 855–62.

4 Kaylor WM, Novick AC, Ziegelbaum M, Vidtt DG. Reversal of end stage renal failure with surgical revascularization in patients with atherosclerotic renal artery occlusion. *J Urol* 1989; **141:** 486–8.

5 Joint National Committee on Detection The fifth report of the Joint National Committee on Detection, Evaluation and Treatment of High Blood Pressure (JNC V). *Arch Int Med* 1993; **153:** 154–84.

6 Wiggins RC, Fantone J, Phan SH. Mechanisms of vascular injury. In Tisher CC *et al.* (eds) *Renal Pathology with Clinical and Functional Correlations*, pp. 965–93. Philadelphia: JP Lippincott, 1989.

7 Morris GC, DeBakey NE, Cooley DA. Surgical Treatment of renal failure of renovascular origin. *JAMA* 1962; **182:** 609–12.

8 Brunner H, Desaulles PA, Regoli D, Gross F. Renin content and excretory function of the kidney in rats with experimental hypertension. *Am J Physiol* 1962; **202:** 795–9.

9 Rimmer JM, Gennari FJ. Atherosclerotic renovascular disease and progressive renal failure. *Ann Int Med* 1993; **118:** 712–19.

10 Truong LD, Farhood A, Tasby J, Gillum D. Experimental chronic renal ischemia: morphologic and immunologic studies. *Kidney Int* 1992; **41:** 1676–89.

11 Jacobson HR. Ischemic renal disease: an overlooked clinical entity. *Kidney Int* 1988; **34:** 729–43.

12 Dean RH, Tribble RW, Hansen KJ *et al.* Evolution of renal insufficiency in ischemic nephropathy. *Ann Surg* 1991; **213:** 446–55.

13 Ofstad J, Aukland K. Renal circulation. In Seldin DW *et al.* (eds) *The Kidney: Physiology and Pathophysiology*, pp. 471–96. New York: Raven Press, 1985.

14 Guyton AC. Dominant role of the kidneys in long-term regulation of arterial pressure and hypertension: the integrated system for pressure control. In Guyton AC (ed.) *Textbook of Medical Physiology*, pp. 205–20. Philadelphia: WB Saunders, 1991.

15 Hall JE, Guyton AC, Jackson TE *et al.* Control of glomerular filtration rate by renin-angiotensin system. *Am J Physiol* 1977; **233:** F366-F372.

16 Textor SC, Novick A, Tarazi RC *et al.* Critical perfusion pressure for renal function in patients with bilateral atherosclerotic renal vascular disease. *Ann Int Med* 1985; **102:** 309–14.

17 Textor SC, Novick AC, Steinmuller DR, Streem SB. Renal failure limiting antihypertensive therapy as an indication for renal revascularization. *Arch Int Med* 1983; **143:** 2208–11.

18 May AG, DeWeese JA, Rob CG. Hemodynamic effects of arterial stenosis. *Surgery* 1963; **53:** 513–24.

19 Hansen KJ, Tribble RW, Reavis SW *et al.* Renal duplex sonography: evaluation of clinical utility. *J Vasc Surg* 1990; **12:** 227–36.

20 Stavros AT, Parker SH, Yakes WF *et al.* Segmental stenosis of the renal artery: pattern recognition of tardus and parvus abnormalities with duplex sonography. *Radiology* 1992; **184:** 487–92.

21 Gould KL. Dynamic coronary stenosis. *Am J Cardiol* 1980; **45:** 286–92.

22 Nielsen K, Rehling M, Henriksen JH. Renal vein oxygen saturation in renal artery stenosis. *Clin Physiol* 1992; **12:** 179–84.

23 Wiecek A, Kokot F, Kuczera M *et al.* Plasma erythropoietin concentration in renal venous blood of patients with unilateral renovascular hypertension. *Nephrol Dial Transplant* 1992; **7:** 221–4.

24 Jensen G, Bjorck S, Nielsen OJ *et al.* Diagnostic use of renal vein erythropoietin measurements in patients with renal artery stenosis. *Nephrol Dial Transplant* 1992; **7:** 400–5.

25 Textor SC. Pathophysiology of renal failure in ischemic nephropathy. *Am J Kidney Dis* 1994; **24:** 642–21.

26 Textor SC, Smith-Powell L. Post-stenotic arterial pressure, renal haemodynamics and sodium excretion during graded pressure reduction in conscious rats with one- and two-kidney coarctation hypertension. *J Hypertension* 1988; **6:** 311–19.

27 Grone HJ, Helmchen U. Impairment and recovery of the clipped kidney in two kidney, one clip hypertensive rats during and after antihypertensive therapy. *Lab Invest* 1986; **54:** 645–55.

28 Elzinga LW, Rosen S, Bennett WM. Dissociation of glomerular filtration rate from tubulointerstitial fibrosis in experimental chronic cyclosporine nephropathy: role of sodium intake. *J Am Soc Nephrol* 1993; **4:** 214–21.

29 Burke TJ, Schrier RW. Pathophysiology of cell ischemia. In Schrier RW *et al.* (eds) *Diseases of*

the Kidney, pp. 1257–86. Boston: Little, Brown, 1993.
30 Vane JR, Anggard EE, Botting RM. Regulatory functions of the vascular endothelium. *N Engl J Med* 1990; **323:** 27–36.
31 Brenner BM, Troy JL, Ballermann BJ. Endothelium-dependent vascular responses. *J Clin Invest* 1989; **84:** 1373.
32 Badr KF, Murray JJ, Breyer MD *et al* Mesangial cell, glomerular and renal vascular responses to endothelin in the rat kidney. *J Clin Invest* 1989; **83:** 336–42.
33 Zeidel ML. Hormonal regulation of inner medullary collecting duct sodium transport. *Am J Physiol* 1993; **265:** F159-F173.
34 Singo AJ, Clavell AL., Aarhus L, Burnett JC. Biologic role for the endothelin-A receptor in aortic cross-clamping. *Hypertension* 1993; **22:** 62–6.
35 Marsden TA, Schramek H, Dunn MJ. Renal actions of endothelin: linking cellular signaling pathways to kidney disease. *Kidney Int* 1994; **45:** 336–44.
36 Sigmon DH, Beierwaltes WH. Renal nitric oxide and angiotensin II interaction in renovascular hypertension. *hypertension* 1993; **22:** 237–42.
37 Wyss JM, Oparil S, Sripairojthikoon W. Neuronal control of the kidney: contribution to hypertension. *Can J Physiol Pharmacol* 1992; **70:**759–69.
38 Daemen MJAP, Lombardi DM, Bosman FT, Schwartz SM. Angiotensin II induces smooth muscle cell proliferation in the normal and injured rat arterial wall. *Circ Res* 1991; **68:** 450–6.
39 Jackson B, Franze L, Sumithran E, Johnston CI. Pharmacologic nephrectomy with chronic angiotensin converting enzyme inhibitor treatment in renovascular hypertension in the rat. *J Lab Clin Med* 1990; **115:** 21–7.
40 Auch-Schwelkt W, Duske E, Hink U *et al.* Vasomotor responses in cyclosporine A treated rats after chronic angiotensin blockade. *Hypertension* 1994; **23**:832–7.
41 McCord JM. Oxygen-derived free radicals in postischemic tissue injury. *N Engl J Med* 1985; **312:** 159.
42 Weinberg JM, Davis JA, Abarzua M *et al.* Ouabain-induced lethal proximal tubule cell injury is prevented by glycine. *Am J Physiol* 1990; **258:** F346–999.
43 Cotterill LA, Gower JD, Fuller BJ, Green CJ. Oxidative damage to kidney membranes during cold ischemia: evidence of a role for calcium. *Transplantation*, 1989; **48:** 745–51.
44 Schrier RW, Conger JD, Burke TJ. Pathogenetic role of calcium in renal cell injury. In Hatamo M (ed) *Nephrology*, pp. 648–59. Tokyo: Springer-Verlag, 1991.
45 Burnier M, van Putten JJ, Schieppati A, Schrier RW. Effect of extracellular acidosis on Ca uptake in isolated hypoxic proximal tubules. *Am J Physiol* 1988; **254:** C839–C846.
46 Humes HD, Nguyen VD, Cieslinski DA *et al.* The role of free fatty acids in hypoxia-induced injury to renal proximal tubule cells. *Am J Physiol* 1989; **256:** F688–696.
47 Thornton MA, Zager RA. Brief intermittent reperfusion during renal ischemia: effects on adenine nucleotides, oxidant stress, and the severity of renal failure. *J Lab Clin Med* 1990; **115:** 564–571.
48 Zweier JL, Kuppusamy P, Lutty GA. Measurement of endothelial cell free radical generation: evidence for a central mechanism of free radical injury in post-ischemic tissues. *Proc Natl Acad Sci USA* 1988; **85:** 4046–50.
49 Molitoris BA. The potential role of ischemia in renal disease progression. *Kidney Int* 1992; **41:** S-21-S-25.
50 Gobe GC, Axelsen RA, Searle JW. Cellular events in experimental unilateral ischemic renal atrophy and in regeneration after contralateral nephrectomy. *Lab Invest* 1990; **63:** 770–999.
51 Reckelhoff JF, Samsell L, Day R *et al.* The effect of aging on glomerular hemodynamics in the rat. *Am J Kidney Dis* 1992; **20:** 70–5.
52 Tank JE, Vora JP, Houghton DC, Anderson S. Altered renal vascular responses in the aging rat kidney. *Am J Physiol* 1994; **266:** F942–F948.
53 Arendhorst WJ, Navar LG. Renal circulation and glomerular hemodynamics. In Schrier RW *et al.* (eds) *Diseases of the Kidney*, pp. 65–117. Boston: Little, Brown, 1993.
54 Arnold PE, van Putten VJ, Lumlertgul D *et al.* Adenine nucleotiide metabolism and mitochondrial Ca+2 transport following renal ischemia. *Am J Physiol* 1986; **250:** F357.
55 Biscoe TJ, Duchen MR. Monitoring pO2 by the carotid chemoreceptor. *News Physiol Sci* 1990; **5:** 229.

22

The epidemiology and clinical manifestations of atherosclerotic renal disease

JE SCOBLE

Introduction

Atherosclerotic renovascular disease unlike fibromuscular hyperplasia is a manifestation of a widespread vasculopathy.[1–3] The early study of Wollenweber *et al.*[1] found that of the 109 patients diagnosed as having atherosclerotic renovascular disease 33% had ischemic heart disease, 32% peripheral vascular disease and 11% cerebrovascular disease. Figure 22.1 illustrates a patient who had aortic aneurysmal and peripheral vascular disease (see p. 308). Although renal artery stenosis was present it was obviously only one of a number of serious medical problems for this patient. This is in contrast to fibromuscular hyperplasia where frequently the disease is confined to the renal arteries. Screening of angiograms performed for other reasons has shown a significant incidence of asymptomatic atherosclerotic renovascular disease (see Tables 22.5–22.7), but has not suggested the same for fibromuscular hyperplasia. It is likely that most fibromuscular disease is symptomatic but that much atherosclerotic disease may be occult. Because atherosclerotic renovascular disease may occur asymptomatically its precise epidemiology and natural history is unclear. Angiography is accepted as the gold standard in the diagnosis of this condition but it is an expensive and invasive procedure. Only when a sensitive and specific non-invasive test for atherosclerotic renovascular disease is available to screen a large asymptomatic population will a precise measure be possible. Without a large screening program interest will focus on the importance of atherosclerotic renovascular disease in specific clinical areas. For instance its importance in the older population has become more apparent recently.[4] New clinical presentations are being recognized for atherosclerotic renovascular disease as shown in Table 22.1. This chapter will review the epidemiology in relation to the clinical manifestations of atherosclerotic renovascular disease. Although these manifestations cannot provide a precise definition of the epidemiology, analysis of them can

Table 22.1. Various presentations of atherosclerotic renovascular disease

Presentation	Reference
Hypertension	Maxwell *et al.* 1972[9]; Ying *et al.* 1984[10]; Carmichael *et al.* 1986[11]
'Flash pulmonary edema'	Pickering *et al.* 1988[15]; Messina *et al.* 1992[16]; Connolly *et al.* 1994[17]
Acute renal failure +/– ACE inhibitors	Kalra *et al.* 1990[24]
Chronic renal failure	Scoble *et al.* 1989[3]; Meyrier *et al.* 1988[25]; Mailloux *et al.* 1988[26]
Atheroembolic disease	Vidt *et al.* 1989[29]
Asymptomatic at angiography	Harding *et al.* 1992[12]; Swartbol 1992[13]; Dustan *et al.* 1964[14]; Olin *et al.* 1990[30]; Valentine *et al.* 1993[31]; Wilms and Marchal 1990[34]; Choudhuri *et al.* 1990[35]; Ramirez *et al.* 1987[37]; Rackson *et al* 1990[57]

lead to a quantitative estimate when renovascular disease is compared with other forms of atherosclerotic disease.

Presentations

Postmortem

The most obvious method for the diagnosis of atherosclerotic renovascular disease is at autopsy (Table 22.2). The disadvantage with this method of assessment is that autopsies are carried out in only a small unrepresentative proportion of the deceased. The studies which have looked at this in detail have been on patients who have died in hospital.[5–7] These represent an incomplete analysis of autopsies for a particular population and only a small proportion of deaths within this population. These autopsies, however, were not requested on the basis of clinical suspicion of renovascular disease in any of the studies. Although imperfect due to the selection of patients for autopsy, these studies do give an important insight into the prevalence of asymptomatic atherosclerotic renovascular disease.

Table 22.2. Incidence of atherosclerotic renal artery stenosis at autopsy

Reference	Association	% (Total no)
Schwartz *et al.* 1964[6]	Postmortem	**24**(154)
Holley *et al.* 1964[5]	Postmortem,	
	All	**53**(295)
	Normotensive	**49**(256)
	Hypertensive	**77**(39)
Sawicki *et al.* 1991[7]	Postmortem	
	All	**4.3**(5194)
	Diabetes	**8.3**

Schwartz and White[6] in a prospective study gave an overall incidence of 24% for atherosclerotic renovascular disease in the 154 consecutive hospital autopsies studied. Table 22.3 shows the proportion of patients with disease in the different age groups in this study. Although only a small series it does illustrate the increased incidence of atherosclerotic renovascular disease with increasing age. This is both for the presence and the severity of the disease in that severe bilateral lesions were only found in patients over the age of 65 years. These authors reported a very high figure incidence of 86% for atherosclerotic renovascular disease in patients over the age of 75 years. The investigators however found no consistent relationship between the presence and severity of the renal artery stenosis at autopsy and the diastolic blood pressure recorded premortem. In the same year Holley *et al.*[5] in a prospective study using renal arteriography at necropsy found moderate to severe renal artery stenosis in 53% of 295 unselected patients with an incidence of 74% in those over the age of 70 years. Although the value is lower than found by Schwartz *et al.*[6] it is still considerable. Holley *et al.*[5] found that the incidence in those who were normotensive premortem was 49% and in those hypertensive premortem 77%. The larger retrospective study by Sawicki *et al.*[7] of 5194 consecutive autopsies found an overall incidence much lower than the earlier studies[5, 6] at 4.3%, although in 93% of these cases this was not diagnosed antemortem.

These studies illustrate the underdiagnosis of atherosclerotic renovascular disease by clinicians premortem and its lack of absolute linkage with hypertension. Both Holley *et al.*[5] and Schwartz and White[6] demonstrated that the inci-

Table 22.3. Incidence of postmortem atherosclerotic renovascular disease in various age groups

	Age (years)			
	<55	55–64	65–74	75+
	% total (*N*=26)	% total (*N*=29)	% total (*N*=48)	% total (*N*=45)
Renal artery stenosis	31	69	73	86
Moderate unilateral or bilateral	19	38	46	44
Severe unilateral stenosis	12	31	6	22
Severe bilateral stenosis	0	0	21	20

From Schwartz and White.[6]

dence of atherosclerotic renovascular disease markedly increases with age.

Hypertension

Since the early work of Goldblatt *et al.*[8] constriction of the renal artery had been widely recognized as a treatable cause of hypertension. Much effort has focused on the diagnosis of such cases because of the excellent clinical response to revascularization in some patients as discussed in later chapters. The epidemiology of renovascular hypertension is discussed in detail in Chapter 13. The presentation of fibromuscular dysplasia causing renal artery stenosis is invariably associated with hypertension. In our experience this is, however, a rare condition when compared with atherosclerotic renovascular disease. It is difficult to determine the incidence of atherosclerotic renovascular disease in patients with hypertension as no large study with angiography of all patients has been completed (Table 22.4). The Cooperative Study on Renovascular Hypertension which reported in 1972[9] attempted to answer this question. However, their conclusion of an incidence of 36% for renovascular disease as a cause of hypertension was an estimate without angiography in all patients. The patients studied were those who had been referred to the specialist hypertension clinics taking part in the study and not part of a population screening program.[9] The patients in the series from Ying *et al.*[10] and Carmichael *et al.*[11] all had angiograms because there was significant

Table 22.4. Incidence of renovascular disease in hypertensive patients

Reference	Association	% (Total no)
Maxwell *et al.* 1972[9]	Hypertension	36(2442)[a]
Munichoodappa *et al.* 1979[39]	Hypertension	48(104)
	Hypertension + diabetes mellitus	36(28)
Ying *et al.* 1984[10]	Hypertension	37(106)[b]
	Hypertension + renal impairment	48(21)
Carmichael *et al.* 1986[11]	Hypertension	36(235)

[a] Not all cases angiographically proven.
[b] Stenosis diagnosed if above 75% of lumen in addition to poststenotic dilatation or enhance collateral flow or both.

clinical suspicion of renal artery stenosis necessitating referral to those units (Table 22.4). In patients with hypertension and renal impairment reported by Ying *et al.*[10] the incidence was higher than in hypertension alone. In terms of the epidemiology of atherosclerotic renovascular disease as a whole there is a lack of absolute linkage of atherosclerotic renovascular disease and hypertension in either the postmortem or angiographic studies.[5–7, 12, 13] Dustan *et al*[14] found in an analysis of angiograms performed for occlusive arterial disease that diastolic hypertension was found in only 25% of those with renal artery stenosis and 16% of those with 'narrowing or roughening'. Swartbol *et al.*[13] observed that in patients who were found to have atherosclerotic renovascular disease at angiography for peripheral vascular disease, 20% were not hypertensive.

The incidence of atherosclerotic renovascular disease in the hypertensive community is unclear and atherosclerotic renovascular disease may occur in the absence of hypertension. The data from angiographic studies discussed later suggest that hypertension alone is not a good discriminant factor for atherosclerotic renovascular disease.

Pulmonary edema

Pulmonary edema can occur as a consequence of poor left ventricular function and consequent increase in pulmonary capillary pressure. Pickering *et al.*[15] though, described a fascinating group of patients in whom left ventricular function was not impaired but the patients went into unprovoked pulmonary edema. The patients in the Pickering *et al.*[15] series were completely cured of this problem by revascularization. This presentation has become known as 'flash pulmonary edema' and appears to be a specific presentation of renovascular disease. The original description was of either unilateral or bilateral disease. Since then Messina *et al.*[16] have reported that 94% of their patients with recurrent pulmonary edema with poorly controlled hypertension and renal insufficiency had bilateral occlusive disease and 54% an occluded renal artery. Once more these patients benefited from revascularization. Connolly *et al.*[17] found that 'flash pulmonary edema' related to occluded renal arteries rather than bilateral or unilateral disease. Missouris *et al.*[18] reported that relief of renal artery stenosis in two patients produced a dramatic diuresis and long-term relief of symptoms suggestive of congestive heart failure. These authors suggested that it may be a curable cause of chronic congestive cardiac failure.[18] Once more, as with hypertension, congestive cardiac failure is a common medical problem and without screening a whole population it will be impossible to ascertain the frequency of atherosclerotic renovascular disease in this group of patients. However, both of these modes of presentation are important as angiotensin converting enzyme (ACE) inhibitors are widely used and effective in prolongation of life in patients with left ventricular failure. Angiotensin converting enzyme inhibitors could, however, have a potentially catastrophic effect of patients with bilateral renovascular disease.[19, 20]

Acute renal failure

Atherosclerotic renovascular disease has been recognized as a cause of acute renal failure with renal artery occlusion since early reports of salvage of renal function with revascularization.[21–23] These early reports were mostly of individual cases often with excellent clinical outcomes. Kalra *et al.*[24] analyzed a large series of patients with acute renal failure and found that in 16% of cases atherosclerotic renovascular disease was, in their opinion, the cause (Table 22.5). The use of ACE inhibitors as a contributory factor in these cases was implicated in a third of these patients, that is 4% of the total cases. This series did not have angiograms in all cases and the incidence was an estimate. The increased use of ACE inhibitors has, however, become of significant clinical importance because there are now very powerful indications for ACE inhibition in patients with congestive cardiac failure and diabetic nephropathy as well as hypertension. The use of these agents can precipitate patients with mild impairment of renal function into acute renal failure[19, 20] by the mechanisms described in Chapter 15. Unfortunately these trials have always excluded patients with impaired renal function and it is unclear whether the same benefits would accrue given the risk of renovascular disease in patients with impaired renal function.

It is possible that the use of ACE inhibitors is making a greater proportion of patients with asymptomatic renovascular disease present with renal impairment. Atherosclerotic renovascular disease with or without the use of ACE inhibitors is now a relatively common cause of acute renal failure in the developed world, especially in the older population.

Chronic renal failure

Atherosclerotic renovascular disease has only recently been considered as a common cause of chronic renal failure (Table 22.5) and the incidence in the dialysis population will be discussed in detail in Chapter 23. In terms of the epidemiology of atherosclerotic renovascular disease patients are now being taken on to dialysis in many countries at an older age than previously and the incidence of atherosclerotic disease in general is common in the older age group.[4] A major problem has been that many patients do not have a specific renal diagnosis when taken on for renal replacement therapy. It

Table 22.5. Incidence of atherosclerotic renovascular disease in patients with renal failure

References	Association	% (total no.)
Mailloux *et al.* 1988[26]	Chronic renal failure	
	1970–3	7.9(63)[a]
	1974–7	7.9(152)[a]
	1978–81	6.7(135)[a]
	1982–5	16.5(182)[a]
Meyrier *et al.* 1988[25]	Chronic renal failure	
	Retrospective	0.3 (5891)
	Prospective	1.4 (1087)
Scoble *et al.* 1989[3]	Renal failure (>50 years of age)	14 (71)
Kalra *et al.* 1990[24]	Acute renal failure	16 (600)[a]
O'Neil *et al.* 1992[28]	Chronic renal failure, non-dialysis dependent	14(21)[b]

[a] not all cases angiographically proven.
[b] Stenosis diagnosed by renal duplex sonography.

is not a surprise then that as the index of suspicion for atherosclerotic renovascular disease has risen, more patients are diagnosed as having this condition. Meyrier *et al.*[25] found that within their unit the incidence of renovascular disease as a cause of chronic renal failure was low at 0.3%, but did increase to 1.4% when it was prospectively looked for rather than retrospectively assigned. This group of patients also included pediatric patients where there would be no atherosclerotic renovascular disease. Mailloux *et al.*[26] have also retrospectively calculated that the incidence on the basis of clinical suspicion or angiogram within their dialysis population has risen from 7.9% in 1970–3 to 16.5% in 1982–3. Scoble *et al.*[3] prospectively looked at patients being taken on to a dialysis programme in London and performed angiograms in patients without a histological renal diagnosis but with evidence of non-renal atherosclerotic disease. They found that atherosclerotic renovascular disease accounted for 14% of the patients over the age of 50 years being taken on for dialysis. This paper and a subsequent larger series[27] have documented the feature that half of these patients were on ACE inhibitors at the time of referral as the diagnosis of atherosclerotic renovascular disease had not been suspected. O'Neil *et al.*[28] looked at patients with chronic but not dialysis-dependent renal failure with renal duplex sonography and found 14% of their small series had atherosclerotic renovascular disease. In this series atherosclerotic renovascular disease was undiagnosed prior to ultrasound sonography.

Until all patients entering a renal replacement program are screened with a sensitive and specific test for atherosclerotic renovascular disease the precise proportion with this condition will remain unknown. What is clear, however, is that a significant proportion of the older population will be on dialysis as a consequence of atherosclerotic renovascular disease. The implications of this for the dialysis treatment in the future is discussed in Chapter 23. The apparent magnitude of the problem of atherosclerotic renovascular disease in renal failure will increase as the search for the condition intensifies.

Table 22.6. Incidence of atherosclerotic renovascular disease in patients with renal cholesterol embolic disease

Reference	Association	% (Total no)
Vidt *et al.* 1988[29]	Renal cholesterol emboli	79(24)

Atheroembolic disease

As discussed in Chapter 5 this probably is an underdiagnosed condition. In a retrospective analysis from the Cleveland Clinic, Vidt *et al.*[29] found that renal artery stenosis was present in 79% of patients in whom atheroembolic renal disease was diagnosed (Table 22.6). In patients whose renal function deteriorates after angiography most renal units do not routinely perform a renal biopsy. Thus the diagnosis of atheroembolic disease is usually entertained only if there is evidence of atheroembolic disease elsewhere. It is possible that there is considerable underrecognition of atheroembolic disease in patients with atherosclerotic renovascular disease. If, however, renal atheroembolic disease is diagnosed then the data from Vidt *et al.*[29] show that there is a high probability of atherosclerotic renovascular disease.

Incidental finding during investigation of other forms of atherosclerotic disease

Atherosclerosis, unlike fibromuscular dysplasia, is usually a widespread vasculopathy within an individual patient. Because renal angiography can be performed during angiography for symptomatic lesions in other vascular territories it is possible to get a precise estimate of the incidence of atherosclerotic renovascular disease in these patients. The importance of these angiographic studies is that the patients were not selected on the basis of possible renal disease but on the basis on the symptoms suggestive of atherosclerotic disease in another territory. Tables 22.7–22.9 show that different investigators have used different degrees of stenosis to indicate the presence of atherosclerotic renovascular disease. Often a significant stenosis is taken to be more than a 50% reduction in diameter on the basis of what is understood to cause

Table 22.7. Incidence of atherosclerotic renovascular disease in patients undergoing angiography for aortic disease

Reference	Association	% (Total no)
Rackson *et al.* 1990[57]	Aortic dissection	16(63)
Olin *et al.* 1990[30]	Abdominal aortic aneurysm	38(109)[a]
Olin *et al.* 1990[30]	Aorto-occlusive disease	33(21)[a]
Valentine *et al.* 1993[31]	Aneurysmal or occlusive vascular disease	28(346)[a]

[a] Stenosis diagnosed only if above 50%.

decreases in renal blood flow. The nature of atherosclerotic renovascular disease means the risk of progression and the association with atheroembolic disease, as discussed earlier in this chapter, could make any lesion significant for the patient.

In a number of retrospective studies of renal angiograms performed at the same time as those for aortic disease an incidence of between 16% (aortic dissection) and 38% (aortic aneurysm) was observed (Table 22.7). The incidence in the aneurysmal and occlusive disease seems consistent at between 28 and 38%.[30, 31] This suggests that atherosclerotic renovascular disease is not an uncommon association with these conditions as illustrated by the angiogram in Fig. 22.1.

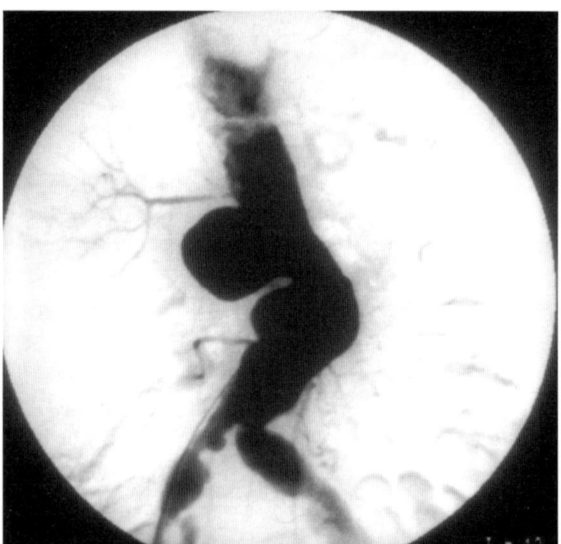

Figure 22.1. Patient with aortic aneurysmal and peripheral vascular disease.

Table 22.8. Incidence of atherosclerotic renovascular disease in patients undergoing angiography for peripheral vascular disease

Reference	Association	% (Total no)
Dustan *et al.* 1964[14]	Peripheral vascular disease	37(149)[a]
Olin *et al.* 1990[30]	Peripheral occlusive vascular disease	39(189)[a]
Wilms *et al.* 1990[34]	Peripheral vascular disease	22(100)[a]
Choudhri *et al.* 1990[35]	Peripheral vascular disease	59(100)[b]
Swartbol *et al.* 1992[13]	Peripheral vascular disease	49(450)
Missouris *et al.* 1994[36]	Peripheral vascular disease	45(127)

[a] Stenosis diagnosed only if above 50%.
[b] Including renal artery occlusion.

Another potential association with aortic occlusive disease is consequent renal occlusive disease. Streather *et al.*[32] have reported two cases of aortic occlusive disease with axillo-femoral bypass grafts where renal artery occlusion has been a late complication leading to renal failure. Reilly *et al.*[33] have, however, shown that surgical occlusion does not lead to this complication, suggesting that renal artery occlusion is related to the aortic disease rather than the occlusion *per se*. All these studies reinforce the clinical experience that atherosclerotic renovascular disease is a common accompaniment of aortic atherosclerotic disease.

The association of peripheral vascular disease with atherosclerotic renovascular disease has been observed since the early study of Dustan *et al.*[14] This has been followed by a number of further studies.[13, 30, 34–36] (Table 22.8). These all indicate a significant incidence in patients undergoing angiography for peripheral vascular disease. The proportion of patients with atherosclerotic renovascular disease appears overall to be the highest in this group of patients when compared with patients undergoing angiography for other indications (Tables 22.7–22.9). A number of authors have noted the correlation but not absolute linkage with hypertension.[13, 30, 34, 35] Missouris *et al.*[36] have demonstrated two other features. The first was that the presence of atherosclerotic renovascular disease correlated with the severity of the peripheral vascular disease.

The second was that patients with atherosclerotic renovascular disease had a increased mortality from operative intervention for peripheral vascular disease compared with patients without renal artery involvement. Thus peripheral vascular disease requiring angiography is a powerful predictor of the presence of atherosclerotic renovascular disease and the presence of atherosclerotic renovascular disease is a worse prognostic indicator for the operative outcome.

More recently investigators have looked at the incidence of atherosclerotic renovascular disease in patients undergoing coronary angiography (Table 22.9). Ramirez *et al.*[37] reported an incidence of 14% for atherosclerotic renovascular disease in these patients. This was a relatively small study compared with that reported by Harding *et al.*[12] of 1235 patients undergoing coronary angiography. These authors found an overall incidence of 30% for any form of atherosclerotic renovascular disease with 15% of patients having greater than 50% luminal stenosis and 15% less than 50% stenosis. Other studies have excluded atherosclerotic renovascular disease with a stenosis of less than 50% diameter as being insignificant, as discussed previously. The predictive factors for the presence of atherosclerotic renovascular disease which Harding *et al.*[12] found were age, severity of coronary artery disease, congestive heart failure, female gender and peripheral vascular disease. Hypertension was not an associated variable in keeping with the data from studies of postmortem examinations[5–7] and angiography for peripheral vascular disease.[13, 14, 30, 34, 35, 38]

The incidence of atherosclerotic renovascular disease is highest in patients undergoing angiography for peripheral vascular disease and peripheral vascular disease is a predictive factor for its occurence in patients undergoing coronary angiography. In terms of screening for atherosclerotic renovascular disease and avoiding inappropriate use of ACE inhibitors then peripheral vascular disease is the most important indication.

Table 22.9. Incidence of atherosclerotic renovascular disease undergoing angiography for coronary artery disease

Reference	Association	% (Total no)
Ramirez *et al.* 1987[37]	Coronary angiography	14(102)
Harding *et al.* 1992[12]	Coronary angiography	30(1235)

Diabetes

Sawicki *et al.*[7] in the postmortem series previously discussed found that the incidence of atherosclerotic renovascular disease was higher in diabetic patients at 8.3% and even higher in hypertensive diabetic patients at 10.1%. Overall, of those patients with atherosclerotic renovascular disease 73% were hypertensive and 53% diabetic antemortem.[7] Munichoodappa *et al.*[39] analyzing angiograms performed for the investigation of hypertension found an incidence of 36% atherosclerotic renovascular disease in the diabetic and 48% in the non-diabetic group. The number in the diabetic group was only 28 and in the non-diabetic group, 104.[39] Olin *et al.*[30] have reviewed the prevalence of diabetes mellitus in their patients and have concluded that it is similar for diabetic vs non-diabetic patients with aortic aneurysm or aorto-occlusive disease but was slightly higher in lower extremity occlusive disease. This would suggest that the association of atherosclerotic renovascular disease with other manifestations of atherosclerotic disease may be similar in diabetic patients but that atherosclerotic disease in other vascular territories may be more common in diabetics. This has implications for the use of ACE inhibitors in these patients, as discussed earlier.

What is the overall incidence?

Atherosclerotic renovascular disease may present in many different ways. Is it possible to estimate its incidence in the general population? The previous section illustrates that the strongest associations of atherosclerotic renovascular disease are with atheroembolic disease and angiography for peripheral vascular or coronary artery disease. The proportions of these patients with atherosclerotic renovascular disease in the latter groups were approximately 50% for peripheral vascular disease and 30% for coronary artery disease (Tables 22.8 and 22.9). In the United Kingdom general practitioners are responsible for the health care of specific groups of patients and are a reliable source of information on medical events occurring within this group. We collaborated with one rural practice with a stable patient population of 14 300. No patients were known within the practice to suffer from atherosclerotic renovascular disease but we posed the question of how many patients had angiography for either coronary artery or peripheral vascular disease in a 12-month period. In this practice three patients had angiography for peripheral vascular disease and none for coronary artery disease. Using the incidence data available this would suggest at least 1.5 new patients with atherosclerotic renovascular disease in this practice per year. If factored up this would represent a minimum of 105 new patients with atherosclerotic renovascular disease per 1 000 000 population per year. These calculations are speculative but are almost certainly an underestimate of the condition within the community.

Progression

There are many facets of progression of atherosclerotic renal disease to be considered. First, there is the progression of the degree of anatomical stenosis. Second, there is the progression of renal impairment in the stenosed kidney. Finally, there is the outcome for the patient which may be independent of the progression of the renal lesion alone. All of these play an important part in the natural history of patients with atherosclerotic renovascular disease.

Anatomical

Table 22.10 illustrates that angiographic studies on progression have not been systematic[1, 40–42] and angiograms have been performed at varying intervals after the initial diagnosis. The absence of a prospective angiographic study of the renal artery has meant that it is difficult to obtain a precise rate for progression of the stenosis. Lack of clinical symptoms or signs may not preclude progression of atherosclerotic renovascular disease. Weibull *et al.*,[43] as discussed below, have shown that progression of renal artery stenosis to occlusion was painless and without symptoms. Trials are under way of prospective angiographic examination of patients with atherosclerotic renovascular disease and these together with the duplex ultrasound studies may give a precise measure of the progression of renal artery stenosis in the future.

Anatomical progression of the lesion in atherosclerotic renovascular disease was established in the early studies including Meaney *et al.*[40] and Wollenweber *et al.*[1] Schreiber *et al.*[41] have shown that in a retrospective analysis atherosclerotic renovascular disease progressed in 44% of patients at reangiography which included progression to occlusion in 16% with a mean follow-up of 52 months. These authors also showed that the higher the degree of initial stenosis the higher the probability of progression to occlusion.[41] Weibull *et al.* have shown that in angiographically documented atherosclerotic renovascular disease progression to occlusion was only associated with a slight change in plasma creatinine without any symptoms or signs. Postma *et al.*,[44] in a small retrospective study, have shown that occlusion is more likely to occur in patients treated with an ACE inhibitor and diuretic. Although progression to bilateral occlusion may be associated with severe impairment in renal function the only conclusive way of diagnosing progression is repeat angiography.

Recently the use of duplex ultrasound has provided prospective data on the progression of atherosclerotic renovascular disease. Zierler *et al.*[45] showed that progression from less than 60% stenosis to greater than 60% stenosis or occlusion was 23% at 1 year and 42% at 2 years. Progression from greater than 60% stenosis to occlusion was 5% at 1 year and 11% at 2 years. The resolution of the ultrasound studies was only between less than 60% stenosis, greater than 60% stenosis and occlusion. This makes these studies difficult to compare with the angiographic studies where an attempt has been made for more precise grading of stenosis.[41] The strength of the study by Zierler *et al.*[45] was that it sequentially studied renal artery stenosis at set intervals which has not been performed with

Table 22.10. Rates of progression for atherosclerotic renovascular disease

Reference	Method of diagnosis	Number of patients/arteries	Criteria of progression	Rate % total	Follow-up (months)
Meaney *et al.* 1968[40]	Angiogram	39 patients	Angiogram progression Occlusion	26 10	Mean 33
Wollenweber *et al.* 1968[1]	Angiogram	30 patients	Angiogram progression New disease	33 10	Mean 28
Dean *et al.* 1981[46]	Angiogram	41 patients	Rise in creatinine Fall CrCl >10% ⇓ renal length Operation Occlusion	46 29.2 37 41 12	Variable
Schreiber *et al.* 1984[41]	Angiogram	169 patients	Angiogram progression (cumulative total)	4 10 12 14 16 21	12 24 26 48 60 >60
Postma *et al.* 1989[44]	Angiogram	78 patients	Occlusion	18	With occlusion 0–24 Without 0–118
Weibull *et al.* 1990[43]	Angiogram	485 patients	Occlusion	5	With occlusion 0–19
Dean *et al.* 1991[47]	Angiogram	58 patients	⇓ Estimated glomerular filtration rate	3.25% week	6
Tollefson *et al.* 1991[42]	Angiogram	48 patients 66 arteries	Angiogram progression Occlusion	53 11	15–180
Scoble *et al.* 1993[27]	Angiogram	28 patients	Death (no intervention)	45	60 (lifetable)
Guzman *et al.* 1994[48]	Duplex ultrasound	54 patients 101 arteries	1 cm ⇓ renal length: ≥=60% stenosis <60% stenosis ≥=60% stenosis	 26 0 19	 14.4 14.4 12 (lifetable)
Zierler *et al.* 1994[45]	Duplex ultrasound	84 patients 168 arteries	Ultrasound progression: <60% stenosis ⇒ >60% stenosis or occlusion >60% ⇒ occlusion	 23 42 5 11	 12 24 12 24

angiography. The anatomical progression rate is unclear from angiography studies, but the duplex ultrasound study of Zierler *et al.*[45] suggest that it is considerable.

Function

Progression in terms of worsening function in the individual kidney has been incompletely documented, as illustrated by the occurrence of asymptomatic renal artery occlusion.[43] Dean *et al.*[46] showed that in 46% of patients with atherosclerotic renovascular disease the serum creatinine increased by over 25%. Along with this the glomerular filtration rate fell by more than 25% in 29% of patients in a follow-up ranging from 6 to 78 months. Dean *et al.*[47] later demonstrated that the rate of decline of overall renal function was more rapid in patients with bilateral vs patients with unilateral disease. In terms of overall renal function Connolly *et al.*[17] have shown that the outcome is dependent on the initial angiographic findings. Actuarial survival of renal function sufficient to remain off dialysis at 2 years was 97% for patients with unilateral stenosis,

82% for patients with bilateral stenosis and 45% for those with unilateral occlusion and occlusion or stenosis on the contralateral side. Guzman *et al.*[48] have shown in kidneys with 60% or greater stenosis that there was a 19% chance that these would lose 1 cm or more of length in the succeeding 12 months. Although not a direct measure of individual kidney function, this loss of length is a marker for lessened function within these kidneys. They did not observe any decrease in length in kidneys with less than 60% stenosis.[48] These data have shown that progression in terms of renal function was related to the initial degree of stenosis.

Recent evidence suggests that the processes within the kidney with renal artery stenosis are complex, as discussed in Chapter 21. Features such as atheroembolic disease and the use of ACE inhibitors may play a role in progression of renal dysfunction which may be in addition to any progression of the anatomical lesion.[49–51]

Clinical outcome

The most important consideration is the morbidity and mortality of the individual patient with atherosclerotic renovascular disease. Patient survival has been shown to be diminished in patients with atherosclerotic renovascular disease. The original data from Wollenweber *et al.*[1] showed that a third of patients would be dead at 5 years. Connolly *et al.*[17] have shown that patient survival correlated with the initial angiographic finding.[17] Two-year actuarial patient survival was 96% for unilateral renal artery stenosis, 74% for bilateral renal artery stenosis and 47% for unilateral occlusion plus occlusion or stenosis on the contralateral side. This may be explained by the different angiographic findings at presentation in this study relating to different stages in the progression of atherosclerotic renovascular disease. As discussed in Chapter 23 Mailloux *et al.*[26] have shown that patient survival once on dialysis is worse than for any other cause of chronic renal failure with a 5-year survival on dialysis of only 12%.

The clinical outcome for patients with atherosclerotic renovascular disease is poor both in terms of mortality and progression to renal failure. The presence of atherosclerotic renovascular disease confers on to patients a worse prognosis when compared with patients with peripheral vascular disease alone[52] or with other dialysis patients.[26]

What of the future?

Is the natural history of atherosclerotic renovascular disease changing or is it becoming increasingly recognized? It is probable that with an increasingly aged population the diagnosis will become more common. The use of ACE inhibitors may have brought to medical attention patients[19, 20, 24, 44] who would not otherwise have been diagnosed and may accelerate the rate of decline of function in the affected kidney.[51] Later chapters suggest that atherosclerotic renovascular disease is a potentially reversible cause of renal failure and so it is a diagnosis that ought to be sought. At the present moment there are no randomized trials of drug therapy in atherosclerotic renovascular disrease which demonstrate a change in the rate of progression of renal impairment or of the lesion. Such studies do exist for atheromatous lesions in other vascular territories.[53–56] The challenge for the future is to identify patients with asymptomatic disease and arrest the natural history rather than intervene with end-stage atherosclerotic renovascular disease when some devastating complication such as renal failure has occurred.

Conclusion

Atherosclerotic renovascular disease is an underdiagnosed condition within the community at large and especially in those patients over 60 years of age. It may present in a number of ways (Table 22.1) and the strongest association is with peripheral vascular disease where the incidence approaches 50% in patients requiring angiography. The rate of progression is significant both in terms of the lesion itself and the clinical consequences. What is more difficult to determine is how many patients with asymptomatic disease will present with a clinical problem related to their renovascular disease. The likelihood of presentation with renal impairment is related to the initial angiographic findings. Our recognition of the importance of atherosclerotic renovascular disease within different presentations has increased but the exact prevalence within the community remains a mystery.

Acknowledgment

I am grateful to Dr C. Hunter for collaboration in the general practice survey.

References

1 Wollenweber J, Sheps SG, Davis GD. Clinical course of athersclerotic renovascular disease. *Am J Med* 1968; **21:** 60–70.
2 Hunt JC, String CG. Renovascular hypertension: mechanisms, natural history and treatment. *Am J Cardiol* 1973; **32:** 562–74.
3 Scoble JE, Maher ER, Hamilton G *et al.* Atherosclerotic renovascular disease causing renal impairment – a case for treatment. *Clin Nephrol* 1989; **31:** 119–22.
4 Scoble JE, Hamilton G. Atherosclerotic renovascular disease. *Br Med J* 1990; **300:** 1670–1.
5 Holley KE, Hunt JC, Brown AL *et al.* Renal artery stenosis: a clinical-pathological study in normotensive and hypertensive patients. *Am J Med* 1964; **37:** 14–22.
6 Schwartz CJ, White TA. Stenosis of renal artery: an unselected necropsy study. *Br Med J* 1964; **2:** 1415–21.
7 Sawicki PT, Kaiser S, Heinemann L *et al.* Prevalence of renal artery stenosis in diabetes mellitus – an autopsy study. *J Intern Med* 1991; **229:** 489–92.
8 Goldblatt H, Lynch J, Hanzal RF, Summerville WW. The production of persistent elevation of systolic blood pressure by means of renal ischemia. *J Exp Med* 1934; **59:** 347–78.
9 Maxwell MH, Bleifer KH, Franklin SS, Varady PD. Cooperative study of renovascular hypertension: demographic analysis of study. *JAMA* 1972; **220:** 1195–204.
10 Ying CY, Tifft CP, Garvas H, Chobanian AV. Renal revascularisation in the azotemic hypertensive patient resistant to therapy. *N Engl Med* 1984; **311:** 1070–5.
11 Carmichael DJS, Mathias CJ, Snell ME, Peart S. Detection and investigation of renal artery stenosis. *Lancet* 1986; **1:** 667–70.
12 Harding MB, Smith LR, Himmelstein SI *et al.* Renal artery stenosis: prevalence and associated risks factors in patients undergoing routine cardiac catheterization. *J Am Soc Nephrol* 1992; **2:** 1608–16.
13 Swartbol P. Renal artery stenosis in patients with peripheral vascular disease and its correlation to hypertension. A retropsective study. *Int Angiol* 1992; **11:** 195–9.
14 Dustan HP, Humphries AW, De Wolf VG, Page IH. Normal arterial pressure in patients with renal arterial stenosis. *JAMA* 1964; **187:** 1028–9.
15 Pickering TG, Herman L, Devereux RB *et al.* Recurrent pulmonary oedema in hypertension due to bilateral renal artery stenosis: treatment by angioplasty of surgical intervention. *Lancet* 1988; **2:** 551–2.
16 Messina LM, Zelenock GB, Yao KA, Stanley JC. Renal revscularization for recurrent pulmonary edema in patients with poorly controlled hypertension and renal insufficiency: a distinct subgroup of patients with arteriosclerotic renal artery occlusive disease. *J Vasc Surg* 1992; **15:** 73–8.
17 Connolly JO, Higgins RM, Walters HL *et al.* Presentation, clinical features and outcome in different patterns of atherosclerotic renovascular disease. *Quart J Med* 1994; **87:** 413–21.
18 Missouris CG, Buckenham T, Vallance PJT, MacGregor GA. Renal artery stenosis masquerading as congestive heart failure. *Lancet* 1993; **341:** 1521–2.
19 Hricik DE, Browning PJ, Kopelman R *et al.* Captopril-induced functional renal insufficiency in patients with bilateral renal-artery stenoses or renal-artery stenosis in a solitary kidney. *N Engl J Med* 1983; **308:** 373–6.
20 Hannedouche T, Godin M, Fries D, Fillastre JP. Acute renal thrombosis induced by angiotensin-converting enzyme inhibitors in patients with renovascular hypertension. *Nephron* 1991; **57:** 230–1.
21 Sheil AGR, May J, Stokes GS *et al.* Reversal of renal failure by revascularization of kidneys with thrombosed renal arteries. *Lancet* 1973; **2:** 865–6.
22 Baird RJ, Yndt ER, Firor WB. Anuria due to acute occlusion of the artery to a solitary kidney. *N Engl J Med* 1965; **272:** 1012–14.
23 Bengtsson U, Bergentz SE, Norback B. Surgical treatment of renal artery stenosis with impending uremia. *Clin Nephrol* 1974; **2:** 222–9.
24 Kalra PS, Mamtora H, Holmes AM, Waldek S. Renovascular disease and renal complications of angiotensin-converting enzyme inhibitor therapy. *Quart J Med* 1990; **282:** 1013.
25 Meyrier A, Buchet P, Simon P *et al.* Atheromatous renal disease. *Am J Med* 1988; **85:** 139–46.
26 Mailloux LU, Bellucci AG, Mossey RT *et al.* Predictors of survival in patients undergoing dialysis. *Am J Med* 1988; **84:** 855–62.
27 Scoble JE, Sweny P, Stansby G, Hamilton G. Patients with atherosclerotic renovascular disease

presenting to a renal unit: an audit of outcome. *Postgrad Med J* 1993; **69:** 461–5.

28 O'Neil EA, Hansen KJ, Canzanello VJ *et al.* Prevalence of ischemic nephropathy in patients with renal insufficiency. *Am Surg* 1992; **58:** 485–90.

29 Vidt DG, Eisele G, Gephardt GN *et al.* Atheroembolic renal disease: association with renal artery syenosis. *Cleve Clin J Med* 1989; **56:** 407–13.

30 Olin JW, Melia M, Young JR *et al.* Prevalence of atherosclerotic renal artery stenosis in patients with atherosclerosis elsewhere. *Am J Med* 1990; **88:** 1-46N–1-51N.

31 Valentine RJ, Clagett GP, Miller GL *et al.* The coronary risk of unsuspected renal artery stenosis. *J Vasc Surg* 1993; **18:** 433–9.

32 Streather C, Wlodarczyk ZC, Sneddon F *et al.* Progression of occlusive renal vascular disease and axillo-femoral bypass grafts. *Nephrol Dial Transplant* 1993; **8:** 1186–7.

33 Reilly LM, Sauer L, Weinstein ES *et al.* Stoney RJ. Infrarenal aortic occlussion: does it threaten renal perfusion or function? *J Vasc Surg* 1990; **11:** 216–25.

34 Wilms G, Marchal G. The angiographic incidence of renal artery stenosis in the arteriosclerotic population. *Eur J Radiol* 1990; **10:** 195–7.

35 Choudhri AH, Cleland JGF, Rowlands PC *et al.* Unsuspected renal artery stenosis in peripheral vascular disease. *Br Med J* 1990; **301:** 1197–8.

36 Missouris CG, Buckenham T, Cappucio FP, MacGregor GA. Renal artery stenosis: a common and important problem in patients with peripheral vascular disease. *Am J Med* 1994; **96:** 10–14.

37 Ramirez G, Bugni W, Farber SM, Curry AJ. Incidence of renal artery stenosis in a population having cardiac catheterization. *South Med J* 1987; **80:** 734–7.

38 Eyler WR, Clark MD, Gaeman JE *et al.* Angiography of the renal areas including a comparative study of renal arterial stenoses in patients with and without hypertension. *Radiology* 1962; **78:** 879–91.

39 Munichoodappa C, D'Elia JA, Libertino JA *et al.* Renal artery stenosis in hypertensive diabetics. *J Urol* 1979; **121:** 555–8.

40 Meaney TF, Dustan HP, McCormack LJ. Natural history of renal arterial disease. *Radiology* 1968; **91:** 881–7.

41 Schreiber MJ, Pohl MA, Novick AC. The natural history of atherosclerotic and fibrous renal artery disease. *Urol Clin North Am* 1984; **11:** 383–92.

42 Tollefson DFJ, Ernst CB. Natural history of atherosclerotic renal artery stenosis associated with aortic disease. *J Vasc Surg* 1991; **14:** 327–31.

43 Weibull H, Bergqvist D, Andersson I *et al.* Symptoms and signs of thrombotic occlusion of athersclerotic renal artery stenosis. *Eur J Vasc Surg* 1990; **4:** 161–5.

44 Postma CT, Hoefnagels WHL, Barentsz JO *et al.* Occlusion of unilateral stenosed renal arteries – relation to medical treatment. *J Human Hypertens* 1989; **3:** 185–90.

45 Zierler RE, Bergelin RO, Isaacson JA, Strandness DE. Natural history of atherosclerotic renal artery stenosis: a prospective study with duplex ultrasonography. *J Vasc Surg* 1994; **19:** 250–8.

46 Dean RH, Kieffer RW, Smith BM *et al.* Renovascular hypertension. *Arch Surg* 1981; **116:** 1408–15.

47 Dean RH, Tribble RW, Hansen KJ *et al.* Evolution of renal insufficiency in ischemic nephropathy. *Ann Surg* 1991; **213:** 446–56.

48 Guzman RP, Zierler RE, Isaacson JA *et al.* Renal atrophy and arterial stenosis: a prospective study with duplex ultrasound. *Hypertension* 1994; **23:** 346–50.

49 Truong LD, Farhood A, Tasby J, Gillum D. Experimental chronic renal ischemia: morphologic and immunologic studies. *Kidney Int* 1992; **41:** 1676–89.

50 Marcussen N. Atubular glomeruli in renal artery stenosis. *Lab Invest* 1991; **65:** 558–65.

51 Jackson B, Franze L, Sumithran E, Johnston CI. Pharmacological nephrectomy with chronic angiotensin converting enzyme inhibitor treatment in renovascular hypertension in the rat. *J Lab Clin Med* 1990; **115:** 21–7.

52 Criqui MH, Langer RD, Fronek A *et al.* Mortality over a period of 10 years in patients with peripheral arterial disease. *N Engl J Med* 1992; **326:** 381–6.

53 Brown G, Albers JJ, Fischer LD *et al.* Regression of coronary artery disease as a result of intensive lipd-lowering therapy in men with high levels of apolipoprotein B. *N Engl J Med* 1990; **323:** 1289–98.

54 Cashin-Hemphill L, Mack WJ, Pogoda JM *et al.* Beneficial effects of colestipol-niacin on coronary atherosclerosis. *JAMA* 1990; **264:** 3013–17.

55 Duffield RGM, Lewis B, Miller NE *et al.* Colchester ACF. Treatment of hyperlipidaemia retards progression of symptomatic femoral atherosclerosis. *Lancet* 1983; **2:** 639–42.

56 MAAS. Effect of simvastatin on coronary atheroma: the multicentre anti-atheroma study (MAAS). *Lancet* 1994; **344:** 633–8.

57 Rackson ME, Lossef SV, Sos TA. Renal artery stenosis in patients with aortic dissection: increased prevalence. *Radiology* 1990; **177:** 555–8.

23

Renal vascular end-stage renal disease

LIONEL U MAILLOUX, BARBARA NAPOLITANO, ALESSANDRO G BELLUCCI, RUBERT T MOSSEY, MELCHIORE A VERNACE, BARRY M WILKES

Introduction

The publication of the annual US Renal Data System (USRDS) report, based on Medicare and Health Care Financing Administration (HCFA) data, has dramatically increased our knowledge concerning the diagnoses of dialysis patients, their complications, outcomes and survival. Although the life expectancy of patients with end-stage renal disease (ESRD) has improved since the 1960s, it is still below 25% of the general population in the 49–59 age group (Table 23.1).[1–3] The most recent USRDS report showed a striking increase in ESRD from hypertension in white, elderly patients with poor 1-year and 5-year survivals respectively.[1,2] Our own program has observed an increase in ESRD patients with a diagnosis of renal vascular disease and a rise in the median age – from 47 to 61 years between 1970 and 1989. In the same period, 83 patients with a clinical diagnosis of renal vascular disease began dialysis. Hypertension should not be the diagnosis in ESRD elderly, white hypertensive patients if the clinical criteria suggest renal vascular disease. We hypothesize that many of the elderly, white patients in the USRDS report have major renal vascular disease rather than hypertension as the cause of their ESRD. There should be a concerted effort by nephrologists to make correct diagnoses in new ESRD patients.

This chapter reports the incidence, clinical correlations and outcome of dialysis patients meeting our clinical criteria for atherosclerotic renal vascular disease over a 20-year period of study.

Since 1970, a computerized database has been used to store basic information about all patients with ESRD at our center. (Data entry, patient characteristics and dialysis prescriptions have been described in recent publications[4–7].) The presence of associated medical conditions at the

Table 23.1. Expected remaining years of life for dialysis patients at various ages and compared with three cancers

	Age 40	Age 49	Age 59	Age ≥ 65
General population	37.4	29.8	21.6	12
Prostate cancer	NA	12.8	13.0	NA
Colon cancer	4.5	8.6	8.0	NA
ESRD	9.3	7.1	4.3	2.7
ESRD + DM	3.6	3.5	3.0	2.2
Lung cancer	1.3	2.7	2.5	1.1

Adapted from USRDS 1993 report and refs 1, 2, 17.
NA: not available.
ESRD: End-stage renal disease: ESRD + DM: End-stage renal disease due to diabetes mellitus.

initiation of dialysis we also entered into the database.

A total of 683 patients were admitted to our program between 1 January 1970 and 31 December 1989, with follow-up through to 31 December 1992, except for patients who underwent a dialysis modality switch which was noted as a time-dependent covariate.[6,8,9] All dialyses were performed to maintain normal blood pressures, dry weights and a clinical sense of well-being.

The starting dialysis years were grouped into five 4-year periods, 1970–3, 1974–7, 1978–81, 1982–5 and 1986–9. Diagnosis leading to ESRD was divided into seven categories for data analysis: chronic glomerulonephritis, polycystic kidney disease, diabetes mellitus, hypertension, renal vascular disease, interstitial diseases and 'other'. The same clinical criteria have been used since the first patient started dialysis in January 1970.

Clinical diagnosis of renal vascular disease

The clinical diagnosis of renal vascular disease was defined as: the clinical evidence of systemic atherosclerosis with either a positive renal angiogram or suggestive radionuclide studies in the absence of significant proteinuria and a benign urinary sediment, most often in a hypertensive setting. During our 20-year study, a diagnosis of renal vascular disease was made in 83 patients and has increased proportionately over time now accounting for approximately 14–16% of patients entering the program. There was also a significant relationship between the renal diagnoses and the dialysis starting periods ($p < 0.0001$, X^2 test).[6] Together with diabetes mellitus, these diagnoses have accounted for 40% of new dialysis patients since 1982.

There were 683 patients in our study: 383 males, 300 females, 600 whites, 63 blacks and 20 of other races. With a median age of 70 years, the 83 patients with renal vascular disease were significantly older than the other 600 patients ($p < 0.0001$, Mann-Whitney test) (Table 23.2). The median starting age increased significantly from 47 in the first start-year group (1970–3) to 61 years of age for patients entering during 1986–9 ($p < 0.0001$, Kruskal-Wallis test). In fact, 271 (40%) of the 683 patients were >61 years of age (Table 23.3).[6]

Estimates of survival

Estimates of survival revealed significant differences in terms of starting age, renal diagnoses, dialysis modality and race. The median survival for all 683 patients was 52 months with 44% 5-year and 23% 10-year survival periods.[6] There was a significant decrease in survival between the youngest and oldest patients, log-rank test, $p < 0.0001$, the median decreasing from 122 to 29 months respectively. Patients with renal vascular disease had the poorest survival estimates with a 25-month median survival and 18% 5-year and 5% 10-

Table 23.2. Median age at start by renal diagnoses[a]

Renal diagnosis	Median age (years)	Range (years)	nα
Diabetes mellitus	54	19–80	155
Chronic glomerulanephritis	49	18–81	212
Polycystic kidney disease	53	31–78	56
Renal vascular disease	70	37–86	83
Interstitial nephritis, chronic pyelonephritis, obstructive uropathy (congenital or aquired)	57	16–83	83
Other[b]	61	16–88	71
Malignant hypertension	55	27–69	23

[a] Renal vascular vs all other diagnoses, $p < 0.0001$, Mann-Whitney test.
[b] Other renal diagnoses include: amyloidosis, collagen vascular disease, myeloma, malignancies, toxic nephropathy, miscellaneous and unknown renal disorders.
From ref. 7 with permission.

Table 23.3. Renal diagnoses by age at start

Diagnoses	Ages at start of dialysis (%) 15–40 (*N* = 175)	41–60 (*N* = 237)	≥61 (*N* = 271)
Chronic glomerulonephritis	43	33	22
Diabetes mellitus	25	21	23
Polycystic kidney disease	3	17	3
Renal vascular disease	1	5	25
Interstitial nephritis, chronic pyelonephritis, obstructive uropathy (congenital or acquired)	17	10	12
Other[a]	11	14	15

[a] Other renal diagnoses include: amyloidosis, collagen vascular disease, malignant hypertension, myeloma, malignancies, toxic nephropathy, miscellaneous and unknown renal disorders.
From ref. 6 with permission.

Table 23.4. Survival estimates for selected renal diagnoses[a]

Diagnoses	Median (months)	Survival estimates 2 years %	5 years %	10 years %	15 years %
Polycystic kidney disease	133	91	77	59	32
Malignant hypertension	55	77	25	0	0
Renal vascular disease	25	56	18	5	0

[a] $p<0.0001$ log-rank test, hypertension vs polycystic kidney disease; $p<0.027$ log-rank test, hypertension vs renal vascular disease; $p<0.0001$, polycystic kidney disease vs renal vascular disease.
From ref. 6 with permission.

year survival periods. Table 23.4 compares these survival data with those of patients with three other ESRD diagnoses. The difference in survival is clearly observed when patients with polycystic kidney disease (the best survival rate of all diagnostic groups) are compared with those with renal vascular disease.

From 1970 to 1992, 59 of these 83 patients died. There were proportionally more others due to withdrawal or cardiac or vascular disease in this group than in the six other diagnostic groups (Table 23.6). Univariate analyses were performed to determine which factors were of significant prognostic importance to survival. Renal diagnosis, initial type of dialysis, starting age and race proved to be significant prognostic factors, ($p < 0.05$, log-rank test). Based on the Cox proportional hazards regression model, the risk of death for a dialysis patient with renal vascular disease is nearly 2.5 times greater than that for polycystic kidney disease, chronic glomerulonephritis or interstitial disease ($p < 0.0001$).[5, 6]

Associated conditions

At the initiation of dialysis, the most frequently occurring associated conditions were: documented pre-existing cardiac disease, peripheral vascular disease, hypertension, cerebrovascular disease/transient ischemic attack/stroke, abnormal electrocardiogram, low serum albumin and congestive heart failure. Patients with renal vascular disease had significantly increased frequency of these risk factors compared with those with other renal diagnoses (Table 23.5) ($p < 0.0001$, X^2 test). In fact, only hypertension in those patients with malignant hypertension leading to ESRD occurred more frequently. There was also an increase in these associated conditions in the later time periods of 1982–5 and

Table 23.5. Distribution of comorbid factors by renal diagnosis*

Diagnoses:	Diab	Glom	Other	Rvasc	HBP	PKD	Inter
N=	155	212	71	83	23	56	83
Factors	%	%	%	%	%	%	%
Pre-exist card	76	24	25	87	65	21	27
Periph vasc	79	17	20	83	48	18	23
Hypertension	86	59	46	93	100	45	43
Cong ht fail	50	17	23	54	39	7	14
Abnl ECG	90	32	48	93	87	25	42
Cerebrovascular	30	2	0	47	17	4	6

* p<0.0001 χ^2-test for pre-existing cardiac disease, peripheral vascular disease, hypertension, congestive heart failure, cerebrovascular disease and abnormal electrocardiogram vs renal diagnosis.

Diagnoses—Diab: diabetes mellitus: Glom: chronic glomerulonephritis; Rvasc: renal vascular disease: HBP: malignant hypertension; PKD: polycystic kidney disease; Inter: tubulointerstitial nephritides;
Other renal diagnoses include amyloidosis, collagen vascular disease, myeloma, toxic nephropathy, malignancies, miscellaneous and unknown renal disorders.

Factors—Pre-exist card: pre-existing cardiac disease, i.e. angina or previous myocardial infarction; Periph vasc: peripheral vascular disease, Cong ht fail: documented bouts of congestive heart failure; Abnl ECG: abnormal electrocardiogram; Cerebrovasc: presence of either major carotid or cerebral vascular disease with documented transient ischemic attacks or reversible ischemic neurological deficits or stroke.

From ref. 7 with permission.

Table 23.6. Causes of death by ESRD diagnosis Renal diagnosis

	Glom	Diab	Rvasc	Inter	Other	PKD	HBP
Deaths (N)	79	110	59	43	44	22	15
Total patient (*N*)	212	155	83	83	71	56	23
Cause of death	%	%	%	%	%	%	%
Infection	34	29	17	33	52	32	40
Withdraw	18	15	25	19	16	9	13
Cardiac	15	26	29	19		5	13
Sudden	11	18	5	9	2	18	7
Vascular	6	9	15	7	2	9	7
Other	16	3	9	13	19	27	20

Diagnosis—Diab: diabetes mellitus; Glom: chronic glomerulonephritis, Rvasc: renal vascular disease, HBP: malignant hypertension, PKD: polycystic kidney disease, Inter: tubulointerstitial nephritides.
Other renal diagnosis include: amyloidosis, collagen vascular disease, myeloma, toxic nephropathy, malignancies, miscellaneous and unknown renal disorders.

Causes of death—Infection: systemic infection with bacteremia not related to the access; Withdraw: withdrawal from dialysis with death due to uremia and not an underlying process; cardiac: death due to cardiac causes, e.g. myocardial infarction, congestive heart failure, arrhythmia: Sudden: sudden and unexpected death in a patient without known cardiac disease or hyperkalemia; Vascular: vascular accidents and/or ischemic episodes; Other: hyperkalemia, gastrointestinal bleeding, hemorrhagic episodes, trauma, cancer, respiratory failure and hepatic failure.

From ref. 7 with permission.

1986–8 compared with the first 12 years of the dialysis program.

Hypertensive neuropathy

Although it would appear that establishing the cause of a patient's ESRD should be simple, in reality this is extremely difficult except for polycystic kidney disease and clinically evident classic presentation of diabetic nephropathy. However, there has been substantial debate about making a diagnosis of diabetic nephropathy in older patients with Type II diabetes who may also have a substantial amount of systemic atherosclerosis and generalized vascular disease. The incidence of hypertension as a cause of ESRD is increasing more rapidly than all the other causes, except for diabetes mellitus, at an average annual rate of nearly 8%, especially in white adults over the age of 64 years.[1, 2] However, hypertensive nephropathy is a vague diagnosis because it is unclear whether non-malignant hypertension causes renal failure in non-blacks or if the hypertension is a consequence of an otherwise silent underlying primary renal disorder.

The diagnosis of hypertension or nephrosclerosis is popular because of the high incidence of elevated blood pressure in the pre-ESRD population, but this confounds morbidity and mortality statistics. Are these the same conditions or different entities? It is for all these reasons that some attention should be paid to making accurate renal diagnoses. Would it not seem logical that a substantial proportion of the elderly white patient population have ischemic nephropathy or major renal vascular disease leading to their ESRD.[1]

According to the 1992 USRDS report, there are similar 1 and 5-year survival periods for both black and white patients with hypertension up to the age of 39 years.[1]

Interestingly, compared with whites, the prevalence of hypertensive nephropathy decreases in black patients over 65 years of age. These data strongly suggest that hypertensive ESRD is different in the older, white patient population. Based on USRDS data, there are significantly poorer survival estimates for white patients than blacks over 65 years of age with 5-year survival periods of 20% for the 65–74 age group and 9% for patients >75 years of age. These survival estimate's are similar to those found in our study for renal vascular patients of a median age of 70 years (Table 23.4).

High-risk dialysis patients

Our clinical definition of atherosclerotic renal vascular disease appears to have identified a group of high risk dialysis patients. As mentioned earlier, these patients present to maintenance dialysis with more pre-existing cardiac, peripheral vascular and cerebrovascular disease (comorbid risk factors) than the other ESRD diagnostic groups (Table 23.5). Certainly, this is clinically logical, since renal vascular disease is only one manifestation of systemic atherosclerosis. This higher prevalence of vascular disease is also reflected in the greater proportion of cardiac and vascular deaths among these patients (Table 23.6).[7]

Over the last decade, there has been an increase in median patient age and the spectrum of renal diagnoses leading to dialysis has changed.[3, 10–13] Even though most nephrologists today recognize that patients put on dialysis are sicker, few reports have documented the increased number of concomitant risk factors for poor dialysis survival.[5, 10–13] In our experience, the proportion of patients with diabetes mellitus or renal vascular disease increased significantly between 1982 and 1989 and now accounts for 40% or more of the incoming patient population. Also, the patients with renal vascular disease are significantly older than the average dialysis patient. During the 1980s, Collins *et al.* demonstrated a near 12% increase in comorbid conditions in all age groups up to 99 years with the major single increase being in peripheral vascular disease.[11, 12] In their most recent study, they found that the number of ESRD patients over 60 years of age had risen by 15–20% annually since 1982.[12] Also, in non-diabetic, ESRD patients, the number diagnosed for vascular and hypertensive disease had doubled, with comorbidity now present in 66% of these patients.[12] As expected, the presence of these comorbid conditions has a direct negative effect on survival.

Renal artery stenosis is a well-recognized

cause of hypertension but is probably overlooked as a significant cause of renal failure.[14–19] In a study by Harding *et al.*, significant unilateral and/or bilateral renal artery stenosis (>50%) was demonstrated in 15% of 1302 patients undergoing cardiac catheterization for angina, but no data were reported about progression to renal failure.[20] Although the natural history of atherosclerotic renal vascular disease is not truly known, it is suspected that a significant number of patients with >50% renal artery stenosis will progress to total occlusion. Studies using serial angiography suggest that progressive stenosis will occur in 40–50% of renal arteries within several years.[17,18,21] Furthermore, the Cleveland Clinic Group has shown that total occlusion will develop in up to 40% of arteries with a 75% or greater initial stenosis.[18,21] The exact incidence of proven atherosclerotic occlusive renal vascular disease as a cause of ESRD is not known, but it seems likely that it is present in 12–15% of ESDR patients. These data highlight the need to establish a correct diagnosis earlier in the course of chronic renal insufficiency.

In a prospective angiographic study by Scoble *et al.* conducted over an 18-month period, atherosclerotic renal vascular disease was found to be the cause of ESRD in 14% of patients starting dialysis.[14] In another study in Scotland, of the 375 patients beginning dialysis between January 1985 and July 1991, 11% were diagnosed by angiography for renal vascular disease as the cause of their ESRD.[22] Not unexpectedly, the patient groups with poorer survival rates had significantly more peripheral vascular disease. These incidence rates of 11–15% are very close to our own study's rate of 14% for the years after 1982. Although our clinical diagnostic criteria appear well founded, they lack correlation with prospective renal angiography, in the case of most patients. In a recent study, Appel *et al.*[27] suggest an even higher prevalence of critical renovascular disease in older dialysis patients, accounting for as many as 22% of new ESRD patients.

Atherosclerotic vascular disorders causing renal failure are potentially correctable if diagnosed early while there is still viable renal tissue. Renal revascularization has frequently been shown to be successful in preventing further deterioration of renal function.[19,23–26] Hansen *et al.* have followed their patients prospectively and reported survival estimates based on the extent of atherosclerotic complications.[23] Although they did not have a group that had advanced to ESRD, the 'extreme' patients with significant peripheral vascular disease and advanced renal insufficiency had far better 4-year survival rates than our series of 83 patients. These data further emphasize the need for correct diagnoses. Unfortunately, there are no other data available for comparison of dialysis and surgical outcomes in patients with renal vascular disease.

Up to recent times (1989), the approved HCFA diagnoses made it difficult to properly ascribe ESRD to the so-called ischemic nephropathies, such as atherosclerotic occlusive disease, major renal vascular disease, atheroembolic issue, etc. Therefore, based on the USRDS data, it is difficult to identify the true extent of atherosclerotic renal vascular disease as a cause of ESRD since a large proportion of these patients may be identified as having hypertension. The marked increase in the incidence of ESRD due to 'hypertension', especially in whites over the age of 65 years, supports our initial hypothesis. In reality, a substantial number of these patients may be suffering from atherosclerotic renal vascular occlusive disease.

Summary

The true incidence rate of renal vascular disease leading to ESRD is not known. But it is more common than anticipated in elderly patients, probably being the correct diagnosis in 11–15% of ESRD patients. Early recognition of renal vascular disease could possibly lead to preventive and/or therapeutic measures. The fact that these patients have significantly more comorbid conditions than other ESRD patient groups most likely accounts for their poor dialysis survival rates.

The 1992 USRDS report showed decreasing survival periods for patients over 65 years of age, between 1978 and 1989 and that the median age of the general dialysis patient population was increasing and that the incidence of hypertension was rising rapidly. This, in view of their age and poor dialysis survival, all suggests that these elderly white patients, although having hypertension diagnosed as the cause of their ESRD, may actually have renal vascular disease.[1] More clinical studies are required to enable correct ESRD diagnosis and assist nephrologists with proper therapeutic regimens.

References

1 US Renal Data System. *USRDS 1992 Annual Data Report*. Bethesda, MD: The National Institutes of Health, National Institute of Diabetes and Digestive and Kidney Disease, 1992.

2 US Renal Data System. *USRDS 1993 Annual Data Report*. Bethesda, MD: The National Institutes of Health, National Institute of Diabetes and Digestive and Kidney Disease, 1993.

3 Eggers PW, Connerton R, McMullan M. The Medicare experience with end-stage renal disease: trends in incidence, prevalence, and survival. *Health Care Finan Rev* 1984, **5:** 69–88

4 Mailloux LU, Bellucci AG, Mossey RT *et al.* Predictors of survival in patients undergoing dialysis. *Am J Med* 1988 **84:** 855–62.

5 Mailloux LU, Bellucci AG, Wilkes BM *et al.* Mortality in dialysis patients: analysis of the causes of death. *Am J Kidney Dis* 1991, **18:** 326–35.

6 Mailloux LU, Bellucci AG, Napolitano B *et al.* Survival estimates for 683 patients starting dialysis from 1970 through 1989: identification of risk factors for survival. *Clin Nephrol* 1994; **42:** 127–35.

7 Mailloux LU, Napolitano B, Bellucci Ag *et al.* Renal vascular disease causing end-stage renal disease, incidence, clinical correlates and outcomes: a 20-year clinical experience. *Am J Kidney Dis* 1994 **24:** 662–9.

8 Lee ET. *Statistical Methods for Survival Data Analysis*; pp. 12–14 Belmont, CA: Lifetime Learning Publications 1980.

9 Kaplan EL, Meier P. Non-parametric estimation from incomplete observations. *J Am Statist Ass* 1958 **53:** 457–81.

10 Hylander B, Lundblad H, Kjellstrand CM. Changing patient characteristics in chronic hemodialysis. *Scand J Urol Nephrol* 1991 **25:** 59–63.

11 Collins AJ, Hanson G, Umen A *et al.* Changing risk factor demographics in end-stage renal disease patients entering hemodialysis and the impact on long-term mortality. *Am J Kidney Dis* 1990, **15:** 422–32.

12 Collins AJ, Ma JZ, Umen A, Keshaviah P. Urea index and other predictors of hemodialysis patient survival: Hemodialysis and the impact on long-term mortality. *Am J Kidney Dis* 1994, **23:** 272–82.

13 Shapiro FL, Umen A. Risk factors in a hemodialysis patient survival. *Am Soc Artif Intern Organs* 1983; **6:** 176–84.

14 Scoble JE, Maher ER, Hamilton *et al.* Atherosclerotic renovascular disease causing renal impairment — a case for treatment. *Clin Nephrol* 1989; **31:** 119–22.

15 Jacobson HR. Ischemic renal disease: an overlooked clinical entity? *Kidney Int* 1989; **34:** 729–37.

16 Meaney TF, Dustan HP, McCormack LJ. The natural history of renal arterial disease. *Radiology* 1968; **21:** 881–96.

17 Rimmer JM, Gennari FJ. Atherosclerotic renovascular disease and progressive renal failure. *Ann Int Med* 1993; **118:** 712–19.

18 Schreiber MJ, Pohl MA, Novick AC. The natural history of atherosclerotic and fibrous renal artery disease. *Urol Clin North Am* 1984; **11:** 383–90.

19 Messina LM, Zelenock GB, Yao KA, Stanley JC. Renal revascularization for recurrent pulmonary edema in patients with poorly controlled hypertension and renal insufficiency: a distinct subgroup of patients with arteriosclerotic renal artery occlusive disease. *J Vasc Sur* 1992; **15:** 73–82.

20 Harding MB, Smith LR, Himmelstein *et al.* Renal artery stenosis: prevalence and associated risk factors in patients undergoing routine cardiac catheterization. *J Am Soc Nephrol* 1992; **2:** 1608–14.

21 Pohl MA, Novick AC. Natural history of atherosclerotic and fibrous renal artery disease: clinical implications. *Am J Kidney Dis* 1985; **5:** 120–8.

22 Khan IH, Catto GRD, Edward N *et al.* Influence of coexisting disease on survival on renal-replacement therapy. *Lancet* 1993; **341:** 415–18.

23 Hansen KJ, Starr SM, Sands E *et al.* Contemporary surgical management of renovascular disease. *J Vasc Surg* 1992; **16:** 319–31.

24 Libertino JA, Bosco PJ, Ying CY *et al.* Renal revascularization to preserve and restore renal function. *J Urol* 1992; **147:** 1485–90.

25 Novick AC, Ziegelbaum M, Vidt DG. Trends in surgical revascularization for renal artery disease. *JAMA* 1987; **257:** 498–505.

26 Novick AC. Current concepts in the management of renovascular hypertension and ischemic renal failure. *Am J Kidney Dis* 1989; **13** (Suppl. 1): 33–41.

27 Appel RG, Bleyer AJ, Reavis S, Hansen KJ. Renovascular disease in older patients beginning renal replacement therapy. *Kidney Int* 1995; **48:** 171–6.

24

Patient selection for intervention to preserve renal function in ischemic renal disease

ANDREW C NOVICK

Introduction

Atherosclerosis is the most common cause of renal artery disease and accounts for 70% of all renal artery lesions. This disease predominantly affects men over 50 years of age but is not uncommon in women of a similar age or in younger adults. The disease may be limited to the renal artery (15–20% of cases) but is more often a manifestation of diffuse atherosclerosis involving the abdominal aorta, coronary, cerebral or lower extremity vessels (80–85% of cases). The development of chronic renal failure from atherosclerotic renal artery disease, termed ischemic nephropathy, has become an important clinical issue that is separate and distinct from the problem of renovascular hypertension.

Recent epidemiologic studies indicate that atherosclerotic renal artery disease is quite common in patients with generalized atherosclerosis obliterans, regardless of whether or not renovascular hypertension is present. These studies have involved obtaining renal angiography in patients with a documented abdominal aortic aneurysm, aorto-occlusive disease or lower extremity occlusive disease.[1–7] In such patients, the overall incidence of atherosclerotic renal artery stenosis (ARAS) has ranged from 31 to 61%, with significant (>50%) ARAS present in 14–42% of patients (Table 24.1). In the most detailed of these studies by Olin *et al.*, significant ARAS was present in 41 of 108 patients (38%) with an abdominal aortic aneurysm, 7 of 21 patients (33%) with aorto-occlusive disease, and 74 of 189 patients (39%) with lower extremity occlusive disease.[3]

Other studies have evaluated the prevalence of atherosclerotic renal artery disease in patients with coronary artery disease by obtaining abdominal aortography at the time of coronary angiography (Table 24.2). Vetrovec noted significant (>50%) ARAS in 22 of 76 patients (29%) with coronary artery disease.[8] In a much larger study, Harding found significant (>50%)

Table 24.1. Prevalence of ARAS in patients with peripheral vascular disease

Study	No. of patients	No. with <50% ARAS	No. with >50% ARAS
Choudri *et al.* 1990[1]	100	17 (17%)	42 (42%)
Wilms *et al.* 1990[2]	100	NA	22 (22%)
Olin *et al.* 1990[3]	318	71 (22%)	122 (38%)
Salmon *et al.* 1990[4]	374	64 (17%)	52 (14%)
Swartbol *et al.* 1992[5]	450	117 (26%)	104 (23%)
Valentine *et al.* 1993[6]	98	36 (37%)	24 (24%)
Missouris *et al.* 1994[7]	127	22 (17%)	35 (28%)

NA = Not available.

Table 24.2. Prevalence of ARAS in patients with coronary artery disease (CAD)

Study	No. of patients with CAD	No. of patients with >50% ARAS
Vetrovec *et al.* 1989[8]	76	22 (29%)
Harding *et al.* 1992[9]	817	164 (20%)

ARAS in 164 of 817 patients (20%) with coronary artery disease.[9] In the latter study, the prevalence of significant ARAS was greater in patients with more severe coronary artery disease; significant ARAS was present in 29% of patients with three-vessel disease and in 39% of patients with left-main disease.

Another recent study has shown an increased prevalence of ARAS in patients with diabetes mellitus. Sawicki *et al.* evaluated 5194 consecutive autopsy protocols from patients who died between 1980 and 1988.[10] Significant (>50%) ARAS was present in 4.3% of all patients but in 8.3% of all diabetic patients; all but one of the latter had non-insulin-dependent diabetes mellitus. Bilateral ARAS was found in 30% of non-diabetic patients with ARAS but in 43% of diabetic patients with ARAS. These data suggest that the presence of non-insulin-dependent diabetes mellitus increases the risk of ARAS and that the latter is more likely to involve both kidneys.

The above studies show that ARAS is commonly present in patients with generalized atherosclerosis, particularly those with peripheral vascular disease or coronary artery disease. Although hypertension is also commonly present in such older patients with ARAS, it is far more likely to be idiopathic (essential) than renovascular in origin. Therefore, the prevalence of anatomical ARAS is much greater than that of atherosclerotic renovascular hypertension.

Natural history of atherosclerotic ischemic renal disease

The natural history of atherosclerotic renal artery disease has been studied by obtaining sequential abdominal aortography or duplex ultrasound scanning in patients with documented renal artery lesions who have been treated medically (Table 24.3).[11–16] The largest and most recent of these studies have shown that progressive arterial obstruction occurs in 42–53% of patients with atherosclerotic renal artery disease, often within the first 2 years of radiographic follow-up. The incidence of progression to complete renal artery occlusion in these studies has ranged from 9 to 16%, and this has occurred more often in arteries that initially showed high degrees of stenosis.

In a study at the Cleveland Clinic, we reviewed the natural history of ARAS in 85 patients who were followed with sequential renal angiograms obtained 3–172 months after an initial diagnostic angiogram.[13] Progressive obstruction of the renal artery due to atherosclerosis occurred in 37 patients (44%), including 14 (16%) in whom such progression eventuated in complete occlusion of the involved renal artery. In patients in whom progressive disease developed, it occurred primarily within the first 2 years of angiographic follow-up (Fig. 24.1). The rate of progression of ARAS correlated directly with the degree of stenosis on the initial angiogram. The majority of renal arteries with mild (<50%) or moderate (50–75%) stenosis on the initial angiogram were unchanged on follow-up angiograms. In contrast, 39% of renal arteries with >75% stenosis on the initial angiogram progressed to complete occlusion. Other studies have since validated this observation that progression to 100% occlusion

Table 24.3. Natural history of ARAS

	No of patients	% Progression obstruction	% Complete occlusion
Wollenweber *et al.* 1968[11]	30	63	NA
Stewart *et al.* 1970[12]	39	36	8
Schreiber *et al.* 1984[13]	85	44	16
Zucchelli *et al.* 1987[14]	36	40	NA
Tollefson and Ernst 1991[15]	48	53	9
Zierler *et al.* 1993[16]	80	42	11

NA = Not available.

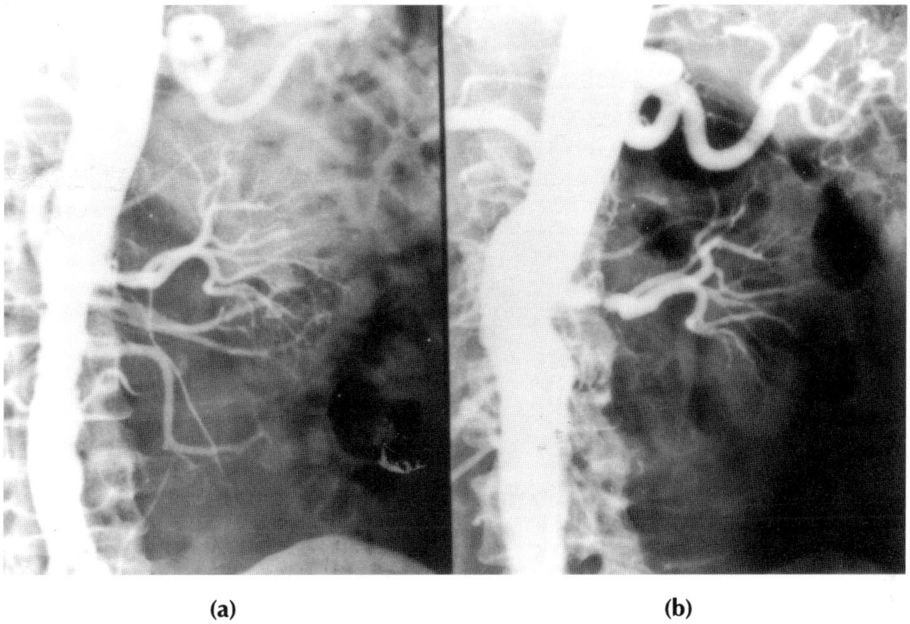

Figure 24.1. Initial aortography (a) shows mild stenosis of the artery to a solitary left kidney. Follow-up aortography 2 years later (b) shows high grade stenosis of the left renal artery.

occurs more often and more rapidly in renal arteries that are initially involved with a high degree of stenosis.[15,16]

Clinical follow-up of patients in our study also revealed that significantly more patients with progressive disease developed deterioration of overall renal function compared with patients with stable disease. Interestingly, serial blood pressure control was equivalent in these two groups indicating that the latter is not a useful clinical marker for progressive ARAS.

The above natural history data clearly show that atherosclerotic renal artery disease progresses in many patients and that loss of functioning renal parenchyma is a common sequela of such progression. It is now further appreciated that progressive atherosclerotic renal artery obstruction can eventuate in end-stage renal failure (ESRD). The typical occurrence is in older patients with generalized atherosclerosis who are not candidates for transplantation and whose prognosis on chronic dialysis is poor in terms of both quality of life and longevity. In an early study, we identified 25 patients in whom ESRD was clearly a consequence of advanced atherosclerotic renal artery disease.[17] Seventeen of these patients were maintained on chronic dialysis and, of these, 13 died within 1 year (mean survival 8.7 months). The causes of death on dialysis were myocardial infarction (6), infection (2), gastrointestinal bleeding (1), ruptured aortic aneurysm (1), mesenteric infarct (1), cardiogenic shock (1), and cerebrovascular accident (1). In a subsequent study, Mailloux analyzed survival of patients started on dialysis from 1970 to 1985 according to the primary renal diagnosis.[18] Patients with renal vascular disease as the cause of ESRD had the poorest survival with a 27-month median survival rate and 12% five-year survival rate. These data further highlight that ESRD from atherosclerotic renal artery disease does not respond well to renal replacement therapy.

The exact incidence of ESRD caused by atherosclerotic renal artery disease in the United States is not known. In a report from England, Scoble *et al.* prospectively performed renal arteriography in all new patients with ESRD during an 18-month period.[19] Atherosclerotic renal artery disease was the cause of ESRD in 6% of all patients, and in 14% of patients over 50 years of age. Approximately 150 000 patients in the United States are currently being maintained on chronic dialysis. Their median age is over 60 years and a majority have evidence of generalized atherosclerosis obliterans. Although the exact number of patients with ESRD caused by atherosclerotic renal artery disease is not known, based on the above data, there appear to be several thousand patients in this category.

Identification of patients with atherosclerotic ischemic renal disease

The screening of patients for atherosclerotic renal artery disease is based in part on an early study by Gifford *et al.*[20] These investigators found that in 53 of 75 older patients (71%) with unilateral renal atrophy, the renal atrophy was caused by stenosing atherosclerotic renal artery disease. Of equal importance was the finding that 22 of these 53 patients (42%) also had unsuspected atherosclerotic renal artery disease involving the opposite normal-sized kidney. Subsequently, Lawrie *et al.* reviewed 40 patients with renal atrophy caused by total arterial occlusion and noted contralateral ARAS in 31 patients (78%).[21] These observations underscore the high incidence of renal artery disease, often bilateral, in patients with generalized atherosclerosis and diminished renal size. The additional finding of even mild azotemia in this setting further enhances the likelihood that underlying large vessel occlusive disease is present.

Harding *et al.* recently evaluated clinical variables associated with ARAS in a study of 1235 patients undergoing simultaneous cardiac catheterization and abdominal aortography.[9] A multivariate logistic-regression analysis identified the following five risk factors as strongly predictive of significant ARAS: higher age, coronary artery disease, a history of congestive heart failure, female gender and peripheral vascular disease. An elevated serum creatinine level was also predictive of ARAS by univariate logistic-regression analysis. Hypertension was not helpful in identifying patients with ARAS.

Another important clinical clue to the presence of significant ARAS is the development of progressive azotemia following medical control of the blood pressure in patients with significant hypertension. This problem strongly suggests the presence of perfusion-dependent renal function due to significant underlying renal artery obstruction.[22] In addition to reducing flow across a stenotic renal artery by lowering the systemic blood pressure, antihypertensive medications can impair renal function in such patients through other mechanisms as well. β-Adrenergic blockers produce a fall in cardiac output, which may occasionally diminish effective renal plasma flow and glomerular filtration rate (GFR). Angiotensin converting enzyme inhibitor agents can lead to deterioration of renal function through loss of efferent arteriolar vasoconstrictor tone in the kidney.[23]

Finally, atherosclerotic renal artery disease should also be suspected in older patients with renal insufficiency and no obvious cause for the latter. Corradi *et al.* recently obtained renal angiography in 51 consecutive patients with the following criteria: age > 60 years, creatinine clearance <50 ml/min, no analgesic abuse, proteinuria < 1 g/day, clinical signs of generalized atherosclerosis, and no biochemical or radiographic findings indicative of glomerulopathy, diabetic nephropathy, polycystic disease, obstructive nephropathy or pyelonephritis.[24] Angiographic studies revealed significant (<70%) renal artery stenosis in 29 patients (56.8%); renal artery stenosis was present bilaterally in 10 patients (19.6%) and unilaterally in 19 patients (37.2%).

The above studies indicate that clinical screening for atherosclerotic renal artery disease is appropriate in older patients with most or all of the following features: (1) evidence of generalized atherosclerosis, (2) a decrease in the size of one or both kidneys, (3) renal insufficiency, even of a mild extent, particularly in patients with no obvious underlying cause, (4) the development of progressive azotemia following restoration of normotension with medical antihypertensive therapy, (5) coronary artery disease, (6) a history of congestive heart failure and (7) peripheral vascular disease. It should be emphasized that patients with atherosclerotic renal artery disease may or may not have significant hypertension, and this should not influence the decision to investigate the patient for this disease.

Patient selection for intervention to preserve renal function

Anatomical severity and extent of renal artery disease

Following angiographic diagnosis of atherosclerotic renal artery disease, and with knowledge of the natural history of this disease, one can identify those patients in whom such disease poses a significant threat to overall renal function. This designation applies to patients with high grade (>75%) arterial stenosis affecting their entire renal mass, namely where such stenosis is present bilaterally or involves a solitary kidney (Fig. 24.2). In these patients, the risk of complete renal arterial occlusion is significant, and if this occurs, the clinical outcome is a critical decrease in functioning renal mass with resulting renal failure. Intervention to restore normal renal arterial blood flow is indicated in such patients for the purpose of preserving renal function. In a study from the Cleveland Clinic, surgical revascularization for preservation of renal function was performed in 161 patients with ARAS bilaterally or in a solitary kidney.[25] Postoperatively, renal function was improved in 93 patients (58%), stable in 50 patients (31%) and deteriorated in only 18 patients (11%).

The benefit of undertaking revascularization for preservation of renal function in patients with unilateral ARAS and an unobstructed contralateral renal artery is not established. If the contralateral kidney is anatomically and functionally normal, revascularization for this purpose is clearly not warranted. If the opposite kidney is functioning but involved with some type of parenchymal disorder, revascularization of the ischemic kidney may benefit some patients but specific indications for this approach are not well defined. Dean and associates reviewed the renal functional outcome following surgical revascularization in 53 patients with ischemic nephropathy.[26] The postoperative

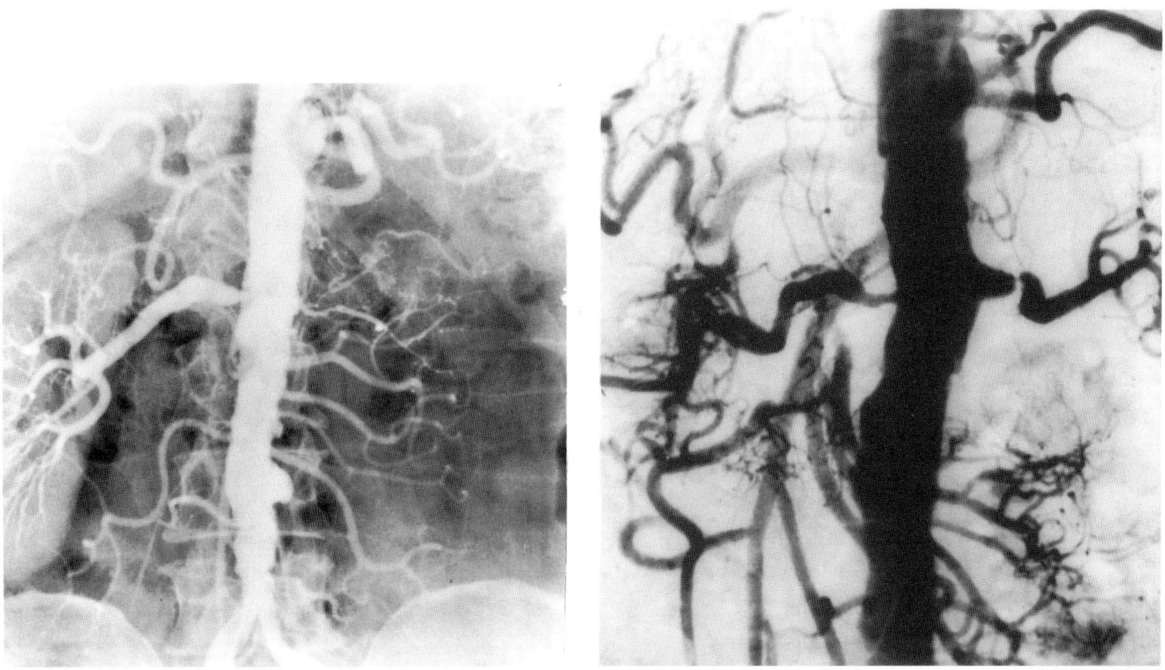

(a) (b)

Figure 24.2. Atherosclerotic renal artery disease poses the greatest threat to overall renal function in patients with: (a) high grade arterial stenosis to a solitary (right) kidney, and (b) bilateral high grade renal artery stenosis, as demonstrated on these abdominal aortograms.

estimated GRF was improved significantly in 41 patients treated for bilateral ARAS but was unaltered in 12 patients with unilateral ARAS.

Complete occlusion of the renal artery most often eventuates in irreversible ischemic damage of the involved kidney. However, in some patients with gradual arterial occlusion, the viability of the kidney can be maintained through the development of collateral arterial supply.[27–29] Helpful clinical clues suggesting renal salvability in such cases include the following: (1) angiographic demonstration of retrograde filling of the distal renal arterial tree, by collateral vessels on the side of total arterial occlusion (Fig. 24.3); (2) a renal biopsy showing well-preserved glomeruli, (3) kidney size >9 cm; and (4) function of the involved kidney on isotope renography or intravenous pyelography. When such criteria are present, restoration of normal renal arterial flow can lead to recovery of renal function.

Level of renal function

In general, revascularization to preserve renal function in patients with ARAS is most likely to be beneficial in those who have not yet sustained severe, permanent impairment of overall renal function. In a study from the Cleveland Clinic, we evaluated the effect of baseline renal function on the outcome of surgical revascularization in elderly patients with ARAS.[30] The majority of these patients had preoperative serum creatinine levels of <3.0 mg/dl; postoperative renal function was stable or improved in 89% of patients in this category.

Revascularization to preserve renal function is generally not worthwhile in patients with severe azotemia (serum creatinine >4.0 mg/dl), because advanced underlying renal parenchymal disease is inevitably present and obviates improvement in renal function with restored perfusion. This observation has been recorded by several groups including our own.[31, 32] Severe nephrosclerosis is the most common form of renal parenchymal disease in such patients; however, renal cholesterol embolization may be an additional complicating feature[33] (Fig. 24.4). In patients with atherosclerotic ischemic renal disease and a serum creatinine level >4.0 mg/dl, our policy is to perform a renal biopsy to evaluate the severity of renal parenchymal involvement from one or both of these disorders (see section below).

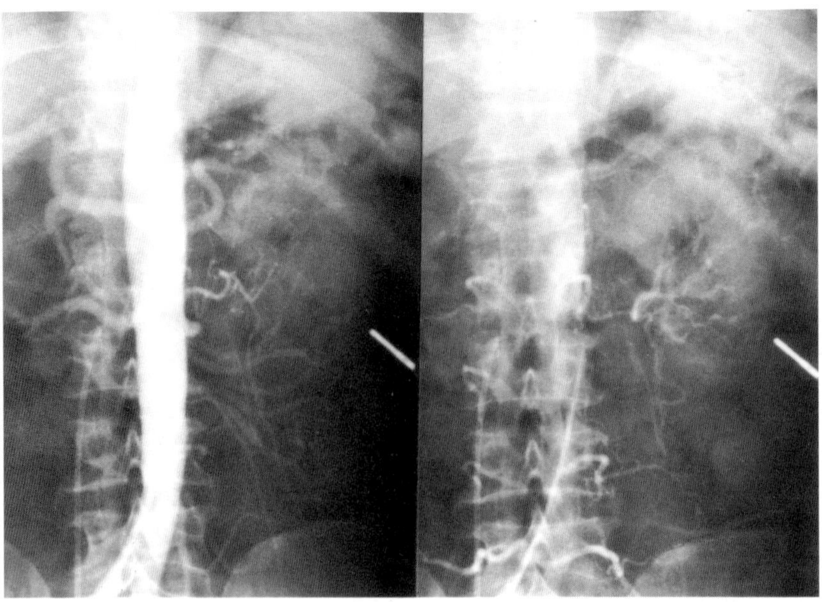

(a) (b)

Figure 24.3. Abdominal aortogram reveals complete occlusion of the left renal artery (a) with filling of the distal renal artery branches from an extensive collateral supply on delayed films (b).

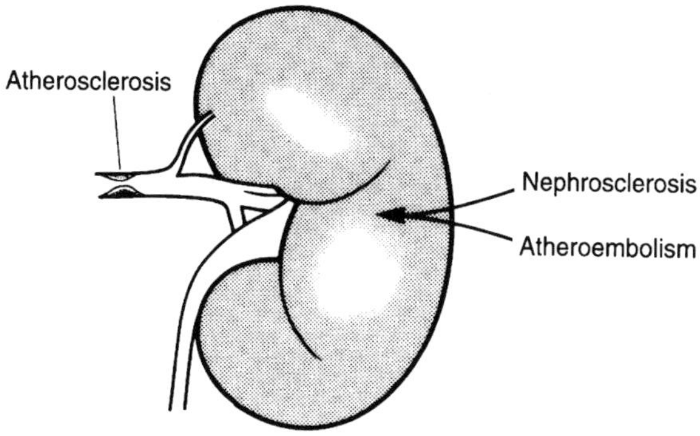

Figure 24.4. Patients with atherosclerotic renal artery disease often have renal parenchymal involvement with varying degrees of nephrosclerosis or atheroembolic disease.

Some patients will present with severe impairment of overall renal function which has developed acutely following initiation of medical antihypertensive therapy.[22, 23] As discussed previously, such rapidly progressive renal insufficiency may be a manifestation of perfusion-dependent renal function due to underlying ARAS. If this problem is detected promptly, renal function will often improve following discontinuation of the offending antihypertensive medications. Intervention to relieve renal arterial obstruction can prevent permanent renal damage in patients with this type of severe acute renal insufficiency.

In addition to the absolute level of renal function, the rate of decline in overall renal function is an important determinant of the outcome following intervention in atherosclerotic ischemic renal disease. In a study by Dean and associates, patients with a rapid rate of deterioration in estimated GFR during the 6 months preceding surgical revascularization achieved the greatest benefit in terms of postoperative improvement of estimated GFR.[26] Unfortunately, their data precluded definition of a critical rate of decline in estimated GFR that would predict retrieval of renal function by revascularization. Nevertheless, rapid deterioration of overall renal function in association with ARAS suggests a strong possibility of retrieval of function by intervention to restore normal renal arterial flow.

Occasional patients with ESRD from ischemic nephropathy have been encountered in whom renal function has been salvable with revascularization.[34, 35] The basis for this has been the presence of chronic bilateral total renal arterial occlusion where, fortuitously, the viability of one or both kidneys has been maintained through collateral vascular supply. In such cases, revascularization can yield dramatic recovery of renal function (Fig. 24.5). Unfortunately, this clinical presentation is rare and a less favorable outcome of bilateral arterial occlusion on renal viability is far more common.

We recently reported nine patients with ESRD caused by atherosclerotic renal artery occlusion who underwent surgical revascularization with subsequent recovery of renal function.[35] The duration of dialysis preoperatively ranged from 1 to 13 months. In all cases, renal viability was being maintained by collateral vascular supply. Postoperatively, renal function improved immediately and no patient required subsequent dialysis. Excellent overall rehabilitation was achieved in all patients. Six patients are alive at a mean interval of 4.0 years postoperatively and with satisfactory renal function (mean serum creatinine 2.7 mg/dl). Three patients died at a mean interval of 6.8 years postoperatively, and they all maintained satisfactory renal function (mean serum creatinine 3.0 mg/dl) until death. While some patients with ESRD caused by atherosclerotic arterial occlusion can be salvaged in this manner, in most such cases irreversible loss of renal function will have occurred. Therefore, the most effective approach is to relieve arterial obstruction before the development of ESRD.

Finally, it is important to emphasize that patients with ESRD and atherosclerotic renal artery stenosis without complete occlusion are not appropriate candidates for revascularization to restore function. In such cases, main renal arterial blood flow is preserved, albeit at a reduced level, and yet the supplied renal parenchyma is without function. The basis for this is the presence of severe unalterable parenchymal damage that precludes recovery of renal function with improved perfusion.

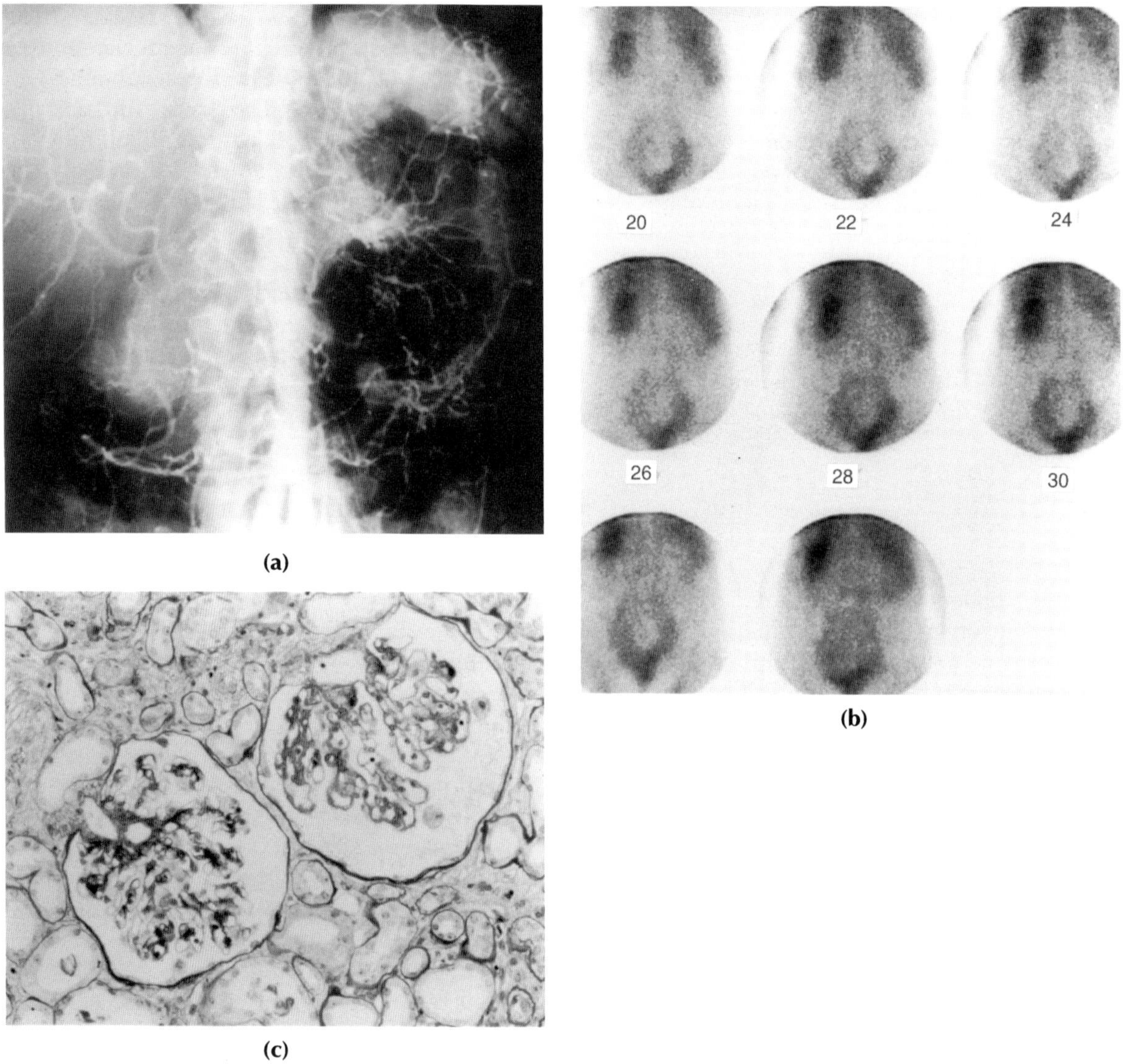

Figure 24.5. (a) This abdominal aortogram was obtained in a 60-year-old woman who had been undergoing chronic dialysis for 9 months with no urine output. The aortogram shows complete bilateral renal artery occlusion with evidence of collateral vascular supply to the left kidney. (b) A technetium renal scan confirms blood flow to the left kidney (left) from collateral supply. (c) A left renal biopsy shows hypoperfused but viable glomeruli indicating a salvageable kidney. Left renal revascularization led to recovery of renal function and discontinuation of dialysis in this patient.

Renal histopathology

Evaluation of renal histopathology can help to determine the presence of salvable renal function in selected patients with atherosclerotic renal ischemic disease. In patients with ARAS and severe existing impairment of overall renal function (serum creatinine >4.0 mg/dl) renal biopsy findings can help to predict whether revascularization is likely to forestall further progressive renal insufficiency. In patients with atherosclerotic renal artery occlusion, renal biopsy findings can indicate whether the involved kidney is viable and functionally salvable on the basis of collateral vascular supply. The two predominant morphologic lesions in such patients are arteriolar nephrosclerosis and atheroembolic renal disease, with the former being more often encountered.

Both of these diagnoses can be established upon a frozen section histopathologic examination and, therefore, the renal biopsy can be done at the same time as surgical revascularization, if the biopsy findings are favorable. In patients with arteriolar nephrosclerosis, the most important favorable criterion is histologic evidence that a majority of examined glomeruli are intact and viable.[28, 29] The presence of tubular atrophy, interstitial fibrosis and arteriolar sclerosis are of lesser importance and do not necessarily preclude recovery of renal function; these findings may merely reflect the histologic changes of chronic reversible renal ischemia. However, the finding of widespread

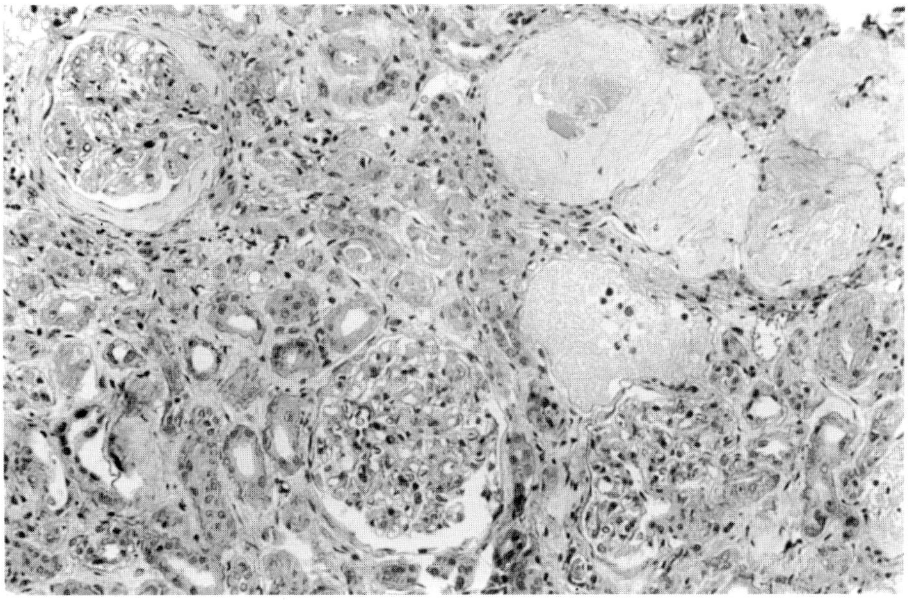

(a)

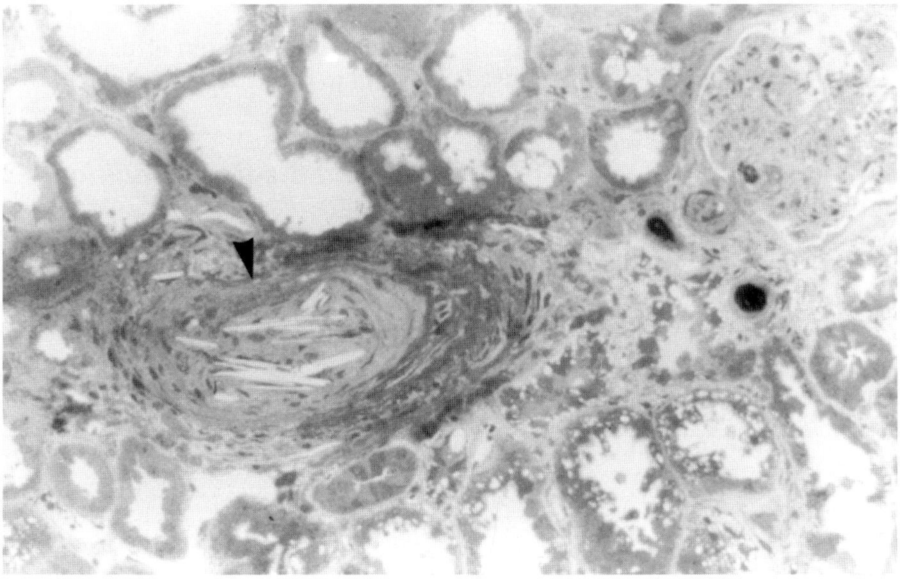

(b)

Figure 24.6. (a) Light microscopic findings upon biopsy of a kidney with total arterial occlusion demonstrates extensive glomerular hyalinization which precludes any benefit from revascularization. (b) Biopsy of a kidney in another patient demonstrates atheroembolic disease (arrow).

glomerular hyalinization indicates irreversible ischemic renal injury which obviates any benefit from relief of renal arterial obstruction (Fig. 24.6a). The finding of extensive atheroembolic disease would also preclude renal revascularization (Fig. 24.6b). With respect to the technique for renal biopsy in such patients, a more representative specimen of renal tissue is obtained with an open surgical wedge biopsy than with a closed needle biopsy.

Hemodynamic evaluation

Renal hemodynamic evaluation may be helpful in confirming the functional significance of atherosclerotic renal arterial occlusive disease. Several years ago, Textor and associates developed a test involving an intravenous infusion of sodium nitroprusside to define the hemodynamic limits posed by vascular disease on overall renal function in such patients.[36] The premise was that such limits might be seen as loss of renal function when perfusion is reduced in a controlled fashion. This test involves measuring effective renal plasma flow (ERPF) and GFR in the basal (hypertensive) state, following a stable graded reduction in blood pressure to normal with an intravenous infusion of sodium nitroprusside, and again following blood pressure recovery to the basal level. Sodium nitroprusside was used for this test because it is a pure vasodilating agent with minimal direct effects on renal hemodynamics.

The nitroprusside infusion study was employed to evaluate 16 patients with bilateral (N=7) or unilateral (N=9) atherosclerotic renal artery stenosis. All of these patients were tested upon their initial evaluation, and patients with bilateral disease were retested following renal revascularization. The results of such testing are outlined in Table 24.4. Initial studies in patients with bilateral disease showed a marked drop in ERPF and GFR when blood pressure was reduced, which was no longer present following revascularization (Fig. 24.7). By contrast, reduction in blood pressure produced no changes in ERRF or GFR in patients with unilateral disease. The latter finding is most likely attributable to the functional reserve offered by a normal contralateral kidney in these patients, which allows autoregulation of renal function over a range of systemic blood pressures.

These data indicate that renal hemodynamic and functional evaluation during graded blood pressure reduction with sodium nitroprusside provides a means of identifying a pathophysiologic limit on perfusion pressure required for renal function in patients with severe atherosclerotic renal artery stenosis bilaterally or in a solitary kidney. These data further demonstrate that this level of critical perfusion pressure is altered after renal revascularization and that subjects with unilateral vascular disease demonstrate no such limits. This approach allows more detailed evaluation of the functional significance of atherosclerotic ischemic renal disease and can assist in the selection of patients for revascularization to preserve renal function.

General medical condition

In therapeutic decision-making for atherosclerotic ischemic renal disease, it is important to consider the general medical condition of the

Table 24.4. Results of sodium nitroprusside infusion study in patients with atherosclerotic renovascular disease[36]

	Bilateral disease (N=7)			Unilateral disease (N=9)		
	Basal	BP Reduction	BP Recovery	Basal	BP Reduction	BP Recovery
Initial evaluation						
ERPF (ml/min)	148 ± 32	57 ± 12*	145 ± 27	266 ± 27	264 ± 35	248 ± 25
GFR (ml/min)	38 ± 9	15 ± 3*	39 ± 8	82 ± 76	76 ± 11	73 ± 8
Postoperative evaluation						
ERPF (ml/min)	196 ± 81	202 ± 84	204 ± 75			
GFR (ml/min)	44 ± 7	44 ± 7	43 ± 8			

* p<0.1.

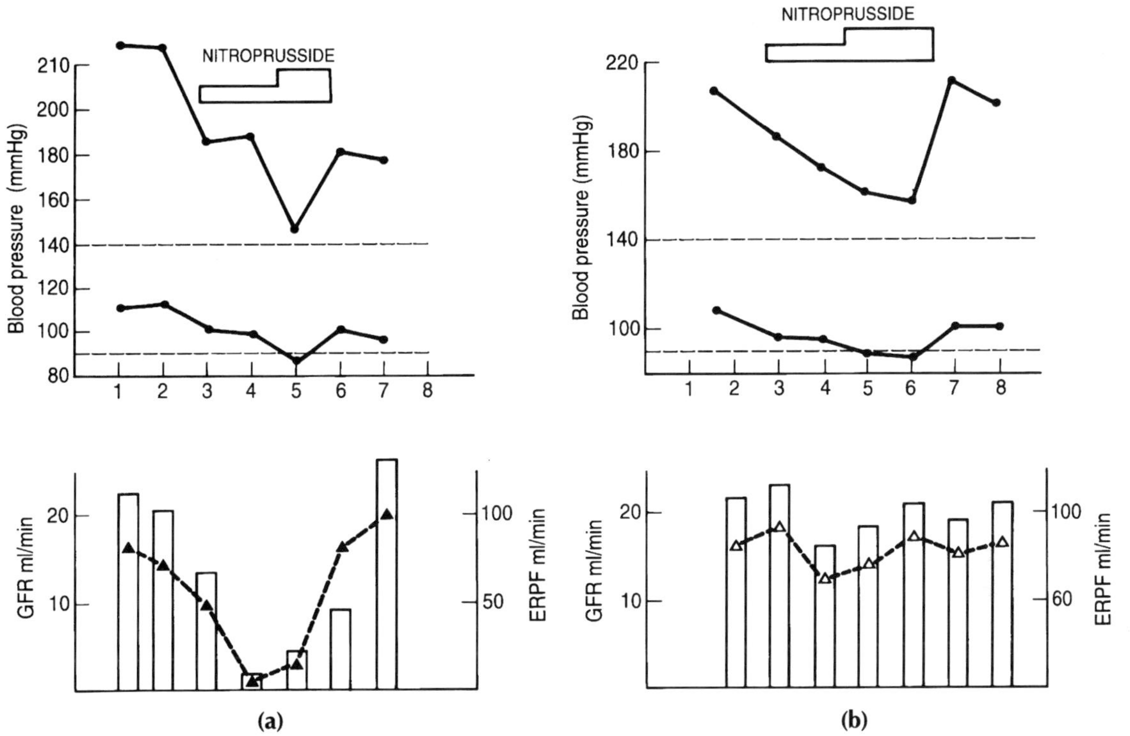

Figure 24.7. Results of sodium nitroprusside infusion testing in a patient with high grade arterial stenosis involving a solitary kidney. (a) The preoperative blood pressure, ERPF and GFR before, during and after infusion of sodium nitroprusside. Pressure reduction to normotensive levels produced a significant reduction in renal function. (b) The results of repeat sodium nitroprusside infusion testing following renal revascularization. Note that blood pressure reduction now no longer reduces the ERPF and GFR, demonstrating restored normal autoregulation.

patient as an assessment of both anticipated longevity and the risk of possible surgical intervention. The medical evaluation must include a diligent search for evidence of generalized atherosclerosis. Particularly important are a history of angina pectoris, congestive heart failure, myocardial infarction, transient ischemic attacks, cerebrovascular accidents or intermittent claudication. On physical examination, careful attention should be paid to the presence of carotid bruits, focal neurologic deficits suggesting a prior cerebral infarct, third and fourth heart sounds, precordial left ventricular heave, arterial pulsations in the extremities and the presence of an aortic aneurysm on examination of the abdomen.

The patient's evaluation should include a careful search for coronary artery disease because this has been the leading cause of late mortality in patients with atherosclerotic renal artery stenosis; this is also the main cause of operative death following surgical treatment in such patients.[37] In addition to a careful history, physical examination and electrocardiogram, all patients at our center undergo a thallium cardiac stress test. If any of the latter assessments suggest the presence of coronary artery disease, coronary cine angiography and left ventriculography are done. Myocardial revascularization should be strongly considered in patients with significant correctable coronary artery disease, along with treatment of atherosclerotic ischemic renal disease. In such patients who require treatment with surgical renal revascularization, the risk of the latter can be reduced by performing preliminary myocardial revascularization. Coronary artery bypass grafting has been a safe operation with only a 1% incidence of postoperative myocardial infarction or death at our institution.[38] Patients with either mild to moderate or advanced but compensated coronary artery disease do not require myocardial revascularization. For patients with severe non-correctable coronary artery disease or irreversible myocardial impairment, aggressive treatment of atherosclerotic ischemic renal disease is best deferred except for the most dire of circumstances.

Cerebrovascular accident is another important cause of late mortality in patients with atherosclerotic renal artery disease, albeit less common than myocardial infarction. The approach in patients whose history or examination suggests the presence of extracranial cerebrovascular disease is similar to that used in patients with suspected coronary artery disease. In such patients, duplex ultrasound of the carotid arteries is performed, and if significant occlusive disease is found, more detailed angiographic imaging is undertaken. Carotid endarterectomy is then considered in patients with significant symptomatic occlusive disease.

Summary

The development of chronic renal failure from progressive atherosclerotic renal arterial occlusive disease, termed ischemic nephropathy, is an important clinical problem in older patients with generalized atherosclerosis obliterans. Studies on the natural history of atherosclerotic renal artery disease have made it possible to identify those patients in whom this disease poses a significant threat to overall renal function. Several factors must be considered in evaluating the renal functional benefit of intervention to relieve arterial obstruction. These include the severity and extent of renal artery obstruction, the level of renal function, renal histopathologic information and the general medical condition of the patient. Renal hemodynamic testing may also occasionally be useful. Intervention to restore normal renal arterial blood flow is indicated in selected patients to prevent deterioration of renal function that may culminate in the need for dialytic replacement therapy.

References

1 Choudhri AH, Cleland JGF, Rowlands PC *et al.* Unsuspected renal artery stenosis in peripheral vascular disease. *Br Med J* 1990; **301:** 1197–8.

2 Wilms G, Marchal G, Penne P, *et al.* The angiographic incidence of renal artery stenosis in the atherosclerotic population. *Eur J Radiol* 1990; **10:** 195–7.

3 Olin JW, Melia M, Young JR *et al.* Prevalence of atherosclerotic renal artery stenosis in patients with atherosclerosis elsewhere. *Am J Med* 1990; **188:** 46–51.

4 Salmon P, Brown MA. Renal artery stenosis and periphral vascular disease: implications for ACE inhibitor therapy. *Lancet* 1990; **336:** 321.

5 Swartbol P, Thorvinger BOT, Parsson H *et al.* Renal artery stenosis in patients with peripheral vascular disease and its correlation to hypertension: a retrospective study. *Int Angio* 1992; **11:** 195–9.

6 Valentine RJ, Myers SI, Miller GL *et al.* Detection of unsuspected renal artery stenosis in patients with abdominal aortic aneurysms: refined indications for preoperative aortography. *Ann Vasc Surg* 1993; **7:** 220–4.

7 Missouris CG, Buchenham T, Cappuccio FP, MacGregor GA. Renal artery stenosis: a common and important problem in patients with peripheral vascular disease. *Am J Med* 1994; **96:** 10–14.

8 Vetrovec GW, Landwehr DM, Edwards VL. Incidence of renal artery stenosis in hypertensive patients undergoing coronary angiography. *J Interv Cardiol* 1989; **2:** 69–76.

9 Harding MB, Smith LR, Himmestein SI *et al.* Renal artery stenosis: prevalence and associated risk factors in patients undergoing routine cardiac catheterization. *J Am Soc Nephrol* 1992; **2:** 1608–16.

10 Sawicki PT, Kaiser S, Heinenmann L *et al.* Prevalence of renal artery stenosis in diabetes mellitus: an autopsy study. *J Intern Med* 1991; **229:** 489–92.

11 Wollenweber J, Sheps SG, Davis DG. Clinical course of atherosclerotic renovascular disease. *Am J Cardiol* 1968; **21:** 60–71.

12 Stewart BH, Dustan HP, Kiser WS *et al.* Correlation of angiography and natural history in evaluation of patients with renovascular hypertension. *J Urol* 1970; **104:** 231–8.

13 Schreiber MJ, Pohl MA, Novick AC. The natural history of atherosclerotic and fibrous renal artery disease. *Urol Clin North Am* 1984; **11:** 383–92.

14 Zucchelli P, Chiarini C, Zuccala A, Delgi Espositi E. Renal ischemic is the real problem in renovascular hypertension in Glorioso N (ed.). *Renovascular Hypertension.* pp. 273–8. New York: Raven Press, 1987.

15 Tollefson DE, Ernst CB. Natural history of atherosclerotic renal artery stenosis associated with aortic disease. *J Vasc Surg* 1991; **14:** 327–31.

16 Zierler RE, Bergelin RO, Isaacson JA *et al.* Natural history of renal artery stenosis: a prospective study with duplex ultrasound. *J Vasc Surg* 1994; **19:** 250–8.

17 Novick AC, Textor SC, Bodie B *et al.* Revascularization to preserve renal function in patients with atherosclerotic renovascular disease. *Urol Clin North Am* 1984; **11:** 477–90.
18 Maillous LU, Bellucci AG, Mosey RT *et al.* Predictors of survival in patients undergoing dialysis. *Am J Med* 1988; **84:** 855–62.
19 Scoble JE, Maher ER, Hamilton G *et al.* Atherosclerotic renovascular disease causing impairment: a case for treatment. *Clin Nephrol* 1989; **31:** 119–22.
20 Gifford RW, McCormack LJ, Poutasse EF. The atrophic kidney: its role in hypertension. *Mayo Clin Proc* 1965; **40:** 834–52.
21 Lawrie GM, Morris CGJR, DeBakey ME. Long-term results of treatment of the totally occluded renal artery in 40 patients with renovascular hypertension. *Surgery* 1980; **88:** 753–9.
22 Textor SC, Novick AC, Steinmuller D, Streem S. Renal function limiting antihypertensive therapy as an indication for renal revascularization. *Arch Int Med* 1983; **143:** 2208–11.
23 Hricik DE, Browning PJ, Kopelman R *et al.* Captopril-induced functional renal insufficiency in patients with bilateral renal artery stenosis or renal artery stenosing in a solitary kidney. *N Engl J Med* 1983; **308:** 373–6.
24 Corradi B, Malberti F, Farini M *et al.* Chronic renal failure due to atheromatous renovascular disease in the elderly. *Contrib Nephrol* 1993; **105:** 167–71.
25 Novick AC, Ziegelbaum, Vidt DG *et al.* Trends in surgical revascularization for renal artery disease: ten years' experience. *JAMA* 1987; **257:** 498–501.
26 Dean RH, Tribble RW, Hansen KJ *et al.* Evolution of renal insufficiency in ischemic nephropathy. *Ann Surg* 1991; **213:** 446–56.
27 Morris GC, Heider CF, Moyer JH. The protective effect of subfiltration arterial pressure on the kidney. *Surg Forum* 1956; **6:** 623–7.
28 Zinman L, Libertino JA. Revascularization of the chronic totally occluded renal artery with restoration of renal function. *J Urol* 1977; **118:** 517–21.
29 Schefft P, Novick AC, Stewart BH *et al.* Renal revascularization in patients with total occlusion of the renal artery. *J Urol* **124:** 1980; **124:** 184–86.
30 Bedoya L, Ziegelbaum M, Vidt DG *et al.* The effect of baseline renal function on the outcome following renal revascularization. *Cleve Clin J Med* 1989; **56:** 415–21.
31 Mercier C, Piquet P, Alimi Y *et al.* Occlusive disease of the renal arteries and chronic renal failure: the limits of reconstructive surgery. *Ann Vasc Surg* 1990; **4:** 166–70.
32 Chaikof EL, Smith RB, Salam AA *et al.* Ischemic nephropathy and concomitant aortic disease. A ten-year experience. *J Vasc Surg* 1994; **19:** 135–48.
33 Vidt DG, Eisle G, Gephart GN *et al.* Atheroembolic renal disease: an association with renal artery stenosis. *Cleve Clin J Med* 1988; **56:** 407–13.
34 Wasser WG, Krakoff LR, Haimov *et al.* Restoration of renal function after bilateral renal artery occlusion. *Arch Int Med* 1981; **141:** 1647–51.
35 Kaylor W, Novick AC, Ziegelbaum M *et al.* Reversal of end-stage renal failure with surgical revascularization in patients with atherosclerotic renal artery occlusion. *J Urol* 1989; **141:** 486–8.
36 Textor SC, Novick AC, Tarazi RC *et al.* Critical perfusion pressure for renal function in patients with bilateral atherosclerotic renal vascular disease. *Ann Int Med* 1985; **102:** 308–14.
37 Novick AC, Straffon RA, Stewart BH *et al.* Diminished operative morbidity and mortality following revascularization for atherosclerotic renovascular disease. *JAMA* 1981; **246:** 749–53.
38 Loop FD, Cosgrove DM, Lytle BW *et al.* An eleven-year evolution of coronary arterial surgery (1968–1978). *Ann Surg* 1979; **190:** 444–55.

PART V

Treatment

25

Medical management of renovascular hypertension

MARC A. POHL

Introduction and general principles

High blood pressure in patients with renal artery stenosis (RAS) has historically evoked the assumption that the RAS causes the hypertension. However, it has long been known that not all patients with angiographically demonstrated stenotic lesions of the renal artery are cured of their hypertension by either surgical revascularization or percutaneous transluminal renal angioplasty. Further, some patients with RAS, particularly those with atherosclerotic renal artery disease, are not hypertensive,[1–3] and the great majority of hypertensive patients with atherosclerotic renal artery disease have essential or primary hypertension. Thus, it is critical to distinguish between RAS in which a stenotic lesion is present but is not necessarily causing hypertension, and 'renovascular hypertension' (RVH), wherein sufficient arterial stenosis is present to produce renal tissue ischemia and initiate the sequence of pathophysiologic events leading to hypertension. In the final analysis, proof that a patient has RVH rests with the demonstration that the hypertension, presumed to be 'renovascular', is eliminated or substantially ameliorated by removing the stenosis by surgical revascularization or angioplasty, or by removing the kidney distal to the stenosis.

The pathologic and clinical features of atherosclerotic and fibrous renal artery disease are frequently associated with hypertension. The more severe the hypertension, the greater the likelihood that it is 'renovascular' in origin. In general, younger patients with fibrous renal artery disease respond well to intervention with either surgery or angioplasty, but results in patients with atherosclerotic renal artery disease are less favorable, as many of them are older and almost certainly have coexisting primary or essential hypertension.[4–8] Thus, there are several scenarios: (1) true RVH, in which atherosclerotic or fibrous renal artery disease is the sole cause of the hypertension; (2) pure essential hypertension, in which atherosclerotic or fibrous renal artery disease is present but does not contribute to the hypertension at all; and (3) essential hypertension with superimposed RAS producing a renovascular contribution to the underlying essential hypertension. Therefore, the medical management of patients with *presumed* RVH is really an effort to control the blood pressure in patients with renovascular disease.

Despite the uncertainty in knowing whether a patient with hypertension and coexisting RAS has 'RVH', the goals of medical therapy in such patients are to control the blood pressure, minimize target-organ damage, avoid adverse drug side-effects, and maintain renal function.[6, 9] Although hypertension in patients with true RVH is more severe than in most patients with primary or essential hypertension,[5, 10, 11–13] RVH does, indeed, respond to standard antihypertensive drug therapy. The degree of hypertension and the response to drug therapy are highly variable in patients with presumed RVH, and one should not assume that every patient with RAS and coexisting hypertension will need surgical revascularization, angioplasty or nephrectomy to control their blood pressure. This is particularly true now that a number of potent antihypertensive agents with a variety of pharmacologic properties are available which, when used appropriately and in proper combinations, can successfully control the blood pressure. In addition, medical antihypertensive therapy is necessary to optimize blood pressure control before planned surgery or angioplasty and for patients whose blood pressure is not normalized by surgery or angioplasty.

The main indications for antihypertensive drug therapy (medical management) of presumed RVH include advanced age, poor surgical risk, atherosclerotic lesions, situations wherein renal revascularization or angioplasty are not feasible owing to technical difficulties of these treatment modalities or irreversible atrophy of the kidney distal to the stenosis, doubtful significance of the RAS lesion by angiographic criteria, long duration of hypertension (which suggests concomitant, essential hypertension or arteriolar nephrosclerosis or both), and patients who simply choose medical management.[5, 7, 8, 10, 11, 13]

Before the early 1970s, pharmacologic therapy for presumed RVH was empirical and quite similar to that of essential hypertension. The degree of hypertension and response to drug therapy are, not unexpectedly, highly variable for patients with RAS, and one should not assume that every patient with RAS will respond readily to antihypertensive drug treatment or to treatment with only one or two drugs. The physician also cannot assume that patients with hypertension and RAS will necessarily need surgery, angioplasty or nephrectomy to control the blood pressure, even when clinical clues predicting that such interventions will cure or markedly improve the hypertension are present. Patients undergoing medical treatment of presumed RVH must be closely monitored for continuing hypertension, intolerable drug side-effects and progressive atrophy of the kidney distal to the stenosis. Surgical therapy or angioplasty for presumed RVH should be strongly considered for patients whose hypertension is refractory to medical management, for younger patients, for patients who are good surgical risks and when progressive arterial stenosis poses a threat to renal function.

Responses to medical treatment

Considerable controversy surrounds the issue of how best to treat presumed RVH: medical management, surgery or percutaneous transluminal renal angioplasty. Unfortunately, no prospective randomized trials have addressed the long-term benefits, risks and successes of these three treatment modalities. Nonetheless, there is sizable successful experience in the medical therapy of hypertension associated with renovascular disease.[14] The first substantial series of patients with presumed RVH, treated medically, was described by Dustan *et al.* in 1963.[15] A thiazide diuretic and either hydralazine or guanethidine or both were used in 32 patients, who were followed up for 1–6 years. Treatment successfully controlled the hypertension in 41% and failed in 28%; 31% of the patients died during follow-up. Results of antihypertensive drug therapy during the late 1960s and the 1970s yielded somewhat better results, i.e. controlled or much improved blood pressures.[16–22] Dramatic improvements in the medical treatment of presumed RVH evolved with the development of β-adrenergic blocking agents (β-blockers) and subsequently with the use of angiotensin converting enzyme (ACE) inhibitors.[20, 22–39] These two classes of antihypertensive agents are particularly effective because they interfere with specific steps in the renin–angiotensin–aldosterone system, which plays a pivotal role in the pathogenesis of RVH.[30]

As depicted in Figs 25.1 and 25.2, the pathophysiology of classic two-kidney, one-clip Goldblatt hypertension produces ischemia of the 'stenotic kidney', activating the renin–angiotensin–aldosterone system and producing a vasoconstrictor type of hypertension.[30] β-Adrenergic blockade, by suppressing renin release,[31–34] blunts the generation of angiotensin I and, subsequently, angiotensin II, the primary vasoconstrictor substance operative in the early stages of classic two-kidney, one-clip Goldblatt hypertension.[35, 36] In addition, β-blockers also lower blood pressure by reducing cardiac output, suppressing the central nervous system, reducing peripheral vascular resistance, resetting the baroreceptor levels and preventing the pressor response to catecholamines with exercise and stress.[35, 36] As depicted in Fig. 25.2, ACE inhibitors interfere with the conversion of angiotensin I to angiotensin II, again reducing the concentration of this potent endogenous vasoconstrictor. Improved responses to medical management with β-blockers and ACE inhibitors are

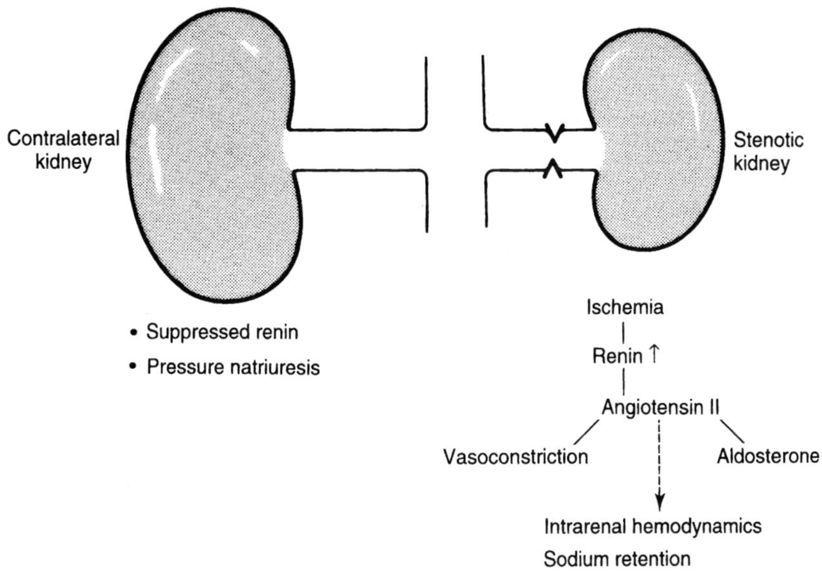

Figure 25.1. Schematic representation of two-kidney renovascular hypertension. The presence of a hemodynamically significant renal arterial narrowing initiates a sequence of events within the affected kidney based fundamentally upon the stimulation of the renin–angiotensin system. Vasoconstriction and sodium retention result, leading to the systemic elevation of blood pressure and suppression of renin and enhanced excretion of sodium by the contralateral kidney. From ref. 30, with permission.

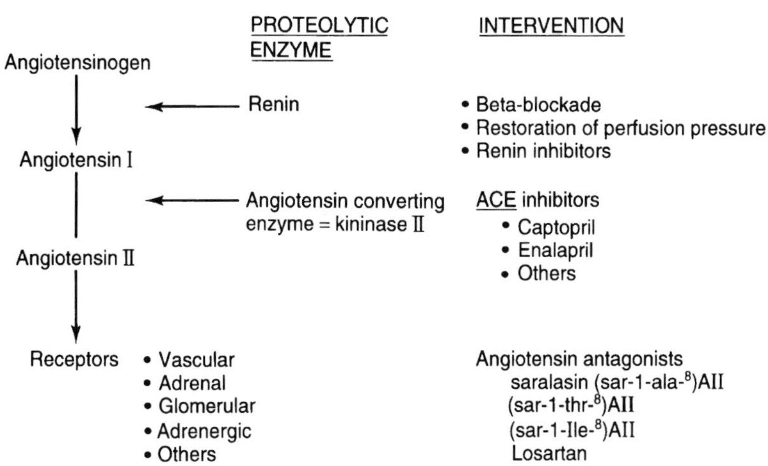

Figure 25.2. Progressive activation of the renin–angiotensin system by proteolysis of circulating angiotensinogen. This mechanism transmits changes in kidney perfusion into widespread vasoconstriction and sodium retention, which tend to restore perfusion pressure at the expense of systemic hypertension. From ref. 30, with permission.

therefore not surprising, at least in the early stages of RVH, since these two classes of antihypertensive agents directly affect the renin–angiotensin system. Interference with the generation of angiotensin II is not, however, the entire explanation for the blood pressure lowering effects of ACE inhibitors: they also potentiate bradykinin, and some ACE inhibitors are associated with increased levels of vasodilatory prostaglandins.[37]

Medical antihypertensive therapy in a patient with RAS becomes more difficult if hypertension has lasted longer than 3–5 years (particularly for patients with atherosclerotic renal artery disease), if a patient has coexisting chronic renal insufficiency with concomitant extracellular fluid volume expansion, or if there is a major element of essential hypertension or arteriolar nephrosclerosis or both. Treatment with a β-blocker or an ACE inhibitor alone (or in combination) is often ineffective in controlling the blood pressure in these circumstances. The same observations are true for patients with bilateral atherosclerotic renal artery stenosis. In patients with unilateral RAS of long duration, and in particular with poor blood pressure control, the high pressure initially generated by the 'stenotic kidney' (Fig. 25.1), is transmitted to the 'contralateral' kidney via the contralateral patent renal artery, producing substantial small-vessel disease, i.e. arteriolar nephrosclerosis in the kidney supplied by the patent renal artery. Therefore, over time, and especially in the presence of uncontrolled blood pressures, the two-kidney, one-clip hypertension escalates to an analog of two-kidney, two-clip hypertension with pathophysiologic features similar to chronic renal failure, associated with extracellular fluid volume expansion.[30] Volume control is necessary for such patients, usually with dietary salt restriction and diuretics, and it has been well documented that the effectiveness of β-blockers and ACE inhibitors is markedly augmented when they are used in conjunction with diuretics.[6, 7, 38] Thus, in contrast to the choice of antihypertensive drugs in initiating therapy for patients with essential hypertension (wherein the pathogenesis and pathophysiology are multifactorial and poorly understood), the pathophysiology of RVH allows for a more mechanism-oriented approach to drug selection and focused treatment interfering with elements of the renin–angiotensin system.

Reports of the effectiveness of captopril in patients with RVH are especially encouraging, particularly since some of these patients were resistant to alternative medical regimens, including the use of β-blockers.[26, 27, 14] In a series of 269 patients, the efficacy of captopril was unequivocal, even though 40% of the patients were azotemic and 136 of 269 had either a solitary kidney or advanced bilateral renal artery disease (Table 25.1).[27] Captopril was ineffective

Table 25.1. Reported responses to medical therapy in RVH

Investigator	*N*	Follow-up	Agents[a]	Results (%) Controlled or much improved	Intermediate	Failure	Deaths
Dustan *et al.* 1963[15]	32	1–6 years	Hydralazine, guanethidine	41	31	28	31
Peart 1967[16]	42	0–8 years	–	45	36	19	–
Shapiro *et al.* 1969[17]	72	34 months	–	–	–	–	40
Kjelbo *et al.* 1970[18]	165	0.5–10 years	–	46	30	24	30
Owen, 1973[19]	83	5 years	–	35	34	31	34
Buhler *et al.* 1973[20]	11	1–180 days	Propranolol	45	27	18	–
Hunt and Strong 1976[21]	114	1–8 years	Methyldopa	81	19	3	–
	59	7–14 years		46		39	
Streeten and Anderson 1979[22]	44	<6 months	Propranolol	59	23	18	–
	16		No propranolol	29	18	63	
Studer *et al.* 1981[23]	12	6 months	Captopril	92	8	0	–
Atkinson *et al.* 1982[24]	15	6 weeks	Captopril	62	23	15	–
Hollifield *et al.* 1982[25]	53	2–3 years	Captopril	68	20	17	–
Case *et al.* 1982[26]	21	28 ± 3 months	Captopril	90	10	0	–
Hollenberg 1983[27]	269	0.3–2 years	Captopril	77	18	0.37	–

a In most patients, a thiazide diuretic was also used.
Adapted from ref. 14, with permission.

in only 5% of patients, and more than 80% of the patients achieved marked improvement or goal blood pressure. The pharmacologic features of β-blockers and ACE inhibitors are detailed in Tables 25.2[35, 36] and 25.3.

Calcium antagonists have been found to be quite effective in patients with presumed RVH.[39, 40] Their antihypertensive effect is primarily due to direct arteriolar vasodilation. The calcium antagonists are a chemically, pharmacologically and therapeutically heterogeneous group of agents. Their clinical effects are related to blocking the L-class of voltage-gated calcium channels in a variety of tissues. In general, the calcium antagonists act by selective inhibition of calcium influx through the cell membrane. This interference appears to interact with selective blockade of the slow channel for transmembrane calcium influx. Since calcium ions play an important role in the contractile process of smooth muscle, calcium antagonists, by preventing this influx, produce arteriolar relaxation.[41, 42]

The precise mechanisms of action of the calcium antagonists are under active investigation, but the effects of calcium antagonists on the elements of the renin–angiotensin system are complex. In general, an increase in intracellular calcium produces an increase in hormone release and synthesis, and blockage of calcium entry might be expected to blunt this response. However, calcium antagonists stimulate the synthesis and release of renin in juxtaglomerular cells.[43, 44] Therefore, the antihypertensive effect of calcium antagonists in RVH is probably not due to decreasing renin release, but is more likely secondary to direct peripheral arteriolar vasodilation. One potential benefit of calcium antagonists in the treatment of hypertensive patients with renovascular disease is their favorable effect on renal function in comparison with ACE inhibitors.[45–47]

Table 25.2. Pharmacodynamic properties of β-blockers used in hypertension

Drug	β_1-Blockade potency ratio (propranolol = 1.0)	Relative β_1-selectivity	Intrinsic sympathomimetic activity	Membrane-stabilizing activity
Acebutolol	0.3	+	+	+
Atenolol	1.0	++	0	0
Betaxolol	1.0	++	0	+
Bisoprolol[a]	10.3	++	0	0
Carteolol	10.0	0	+	0
Labetalol[b]	0.3	0	+	0
Metoprolol	1.0	++	0	0
Nadolol	1.0	0	0	0
Penbutolol	1.0	0	+	0
Pindolol	6.0	0	++	+
Propranolol	1.0	0	0	++

[a]Bisoprolol is also approved as a first-line antihypertensive therapy in combination with a very low dose diuretic.
[b]Labetalol has additional α_1-adrenergic blocking activity and direct vasodilatory activity (β_2-agonism); it is available for use in intravenous form for hypertensive emergencies.
From refs 35, 36, with permission.

Table 25.3. Currently available ACE Inhibitors[a]

Drug	Daily dose (mg)	Frequency of administration
Captopril	25–100	Twice or three times daily
Enalapril	2.5–20	Daily or twice daily
Lisinopril	5–40	Daily
Benazepril	5–40	Daily or twice daily
Ramipril	2.5–10	Daily
Quinapril	5–20	Daily or twice daily
Fosinopril	10–40	Daily or twice daily

[a] Several of the above also exist in fixed combinations with thiazide diuretics.

Calcium antagonists have had a major impact on the treatment of hypertension of all types and ischemic heart disease. Their well-documented effectiveness in lowering blood pressure has resulted in widespread use of these agents.[45–48] It is beyond the scope of this chapter to discuss all of the cardiac and hemodynamic effects of calcium antagonists, but the dosage and cardiac and hemodynamic effects of clinically available calcium antagonists are listed in Tables 25.4 and 25.5. The dihydropyridine calcium antagonist nifedipine, when it was first introduced in clinical medicine, was characterized by a short half-life and extensive first-pass metabolism in the liver. Frequent dosing was required (three times a day) to maintain an adequate hypotensive clinical response. Subsequently, a number of slow-release formulations have been developed that can be taken once or twice daily (Table 25.4). Nifedipine has little suppressive effect on myocardial tissue, having its major effects in blocking vasoconstriction in large to medium-sized arteries. Increased sympathetic nervous system activity is noted with the use of this class of calcium antagonists, and side-effects include reflex tachycardia, headache, palpitations and a burning sensation in the face and legs. Verapamil, a phenylalkylamine-type calcium antagonist, is less directly vasodilatory than the dihydropyridines (e.g. nifedipine). Further, verapamil depresses sinoatrial and atrioventricular nodal activity, and should be used with caution in patients with heart block. Diltiazem, a benzothiazepine-type calcium antagonist, has properties closely related to those of verapamil, but its effect on the heart rate is more variable and appears to be dose dependent (Tables 25.4 and 25.5).

Because of the potential of interfering more specifically with the actions of angiotensin II at the receptor level,[49] angiotensin II receptor blockers (A II-receptor blockers) are under active investigation and development. The first A II-receptor blocker, saralasin, was used in the early 1970s, mainly to explore the effects of inhibition of the renin–angiotensin–aldosterone system.[50] Although widely used in clinical investigation, its complex peptide structure and quick hydrolysis after oral administration made it impractical

Table 25.4. Dosage and administration of currently available calcium antagonists

Drug	Daily dose (mg)	Frequency of administration
Amlodipine	2.5–10	Once daily
Diltiazem CD	120–360	Once daily
Diltiazem XR	120–480	Once daily
Felodipine	5–20	Once daily
Isradipine	5–20	Twice daily
Nicardipine SR	60–120	Twice daily
Nifedipine XL	30–120	Once daily
Verapamil SR	120–480	Once daily (twice daily when daily dose exceeds 240 mg once daily)
Verapamil CR	120–480	Once daily

Adapted from ref. 48, with permission.

Table 25.5. Cardiac and hemodynamic effects of calcium antagonists in patients with normal ejection fractions

Effect	Amlodipine	Diltiazem	Felodipine	Isradipine	Nicardipine	Nifedipine	Verapamil
Arteriolar dilation	++++	++	++++	++++	++++	++++	++
Coronary vasodilation	++++	++	++++	++++	++++	++++	++
Cardiac after load	↓↓	↓	↓↓	↓↓	↓↓	↓↓	↓
Cardiac contractility[a]	0	↓	0	0	0	0/↓[b]	↓
Heart rate	→ or ↑ (acute), then →	↓ or →	→ or ↑ (acute), then →	→ or ↑ (acute), then →	↑ (acute), then →	↑	↓ or →
AV conduction	0	↓	0	0	0	0	↓↓
SA automaticity	0	↓↓	0	↓ (slight)	0	0	↓

[a] Net effect (direct cardiac effect plus influence of activation of sympathetic nervous system, etc.).
[b] Depends on type of patient and extent of sympathetic stimulation; nifedipine may decrease contractility in susceptible patients.
Adapted from ref. 48, with permission.

as an antihypertensive drug.[51] Recently, a number of non-peptide molecules that interfere with A II-receptors and lower blood pressure have been synthesized.[52] The prototype blocker of this type of agent is losartan (which should be available by the time this book is published). Other A II-receptor blockers are being investigated as well. The hope is that these agents, which interfere farther down the renin–angiotensin system cascade than do the ACE inhibitors (see Fig. 25.2), may not cause some of the troublesome side-effects associated with ACE inhibition, e.g. cough and angioedema. Whether these agents will be as effective as currently available ACE inhibitors in patients with presumed RVH remains to be determined. At present, there is no clear information as to whether losartan differs significantly from the available ACE inhibitors in causing hyperkalemia, mild reductions in glomerular filtration rate[53] or frank acute renal failure, but at least one report suggests less adverse effects on renal function with A II-receptor blockade.[54]

A detailed discussion of the many additional types of antihypertensive agents, e.g. diuretics, α-1 agonists, α-blockers, peripheral neurogenic inhibitors and the vasodilators hydralazine and minoxidil, is beyond the scope of this chapter. In general, use of these agents in the medical management of patients with renovascular disease and presumed RVH follows the usual guidelines when these agents are used in essential hypertension. However, when RVH is suspected, the first step should be to use either an ACE inhibitor, a β-blocker or a calcium antagonist. The combination of an ACE inhibitor and a calcium antagonist is extremely effective. The conjoint use of an ACE inhibitor and a β-blocker is also effective. Caution must be exercised in using a β-blocker in combination with verapamil or diltiazem, especially in patients with a tendency to bradycardia or any electrocardiographic evidence of heart block, since the conjoint use of these two drug classes might dangerously slow the heart rate or precipitate congestive heart failure. The next drug to be added would ideally be a diuretic agent, particularly in conjunction with an ACE inhibitor and a β-blocker. Clonidine is also effective, often as a third drug in patients with severe hypertension in association with renovascular disease; clonidine is especially effective in lowering the systolic blood pressure in elderly hypertensives.

Complications and liabilities of medical management of RVH

The side-effects of the many antihypertensive drugs used in treating RVH are well known and beyond the scope of this chapter. However, several untoward metabolic or physiologic effects of medical antihypertensive therapy are of particular interest in managing patients with renovascular disease, including, but not limited to, hypokalemia, hyperkalemia, acute renal failure, reduced renal perfusion pressure, 'flash' pulmonary edema, and ischemic shrinkage of the kidney distal to the stenosis. In the classic model of two-kidney, one-clip Goldblatt hypertension, aldosterone levels increase as a consequence of activation of the renin–angiotensin–aldosterone system (Fig. 25.1). Accordingly, secondary aldosteronism ensues, and hypokalemia is a cardinal feature of true RVH. Given the propensity to hypokalemia in patients with *bona fide* RVH, the use of diuretic agents, either alone on in conjunction with other drugs, has the potential to produce severe hypokalemia. The clinical syndrome of hyporeninemic hypoaldosteronism is not uncommon in patients with renovascular disease and essential hypertension (not true RVH), particularly in the presence of mild to moderate azotemia, diabetes, and old age. This condition produces hyperkalemia, which may be aggravated to dangerous levels with the use of ACE inhibitors and β-blockers, both of which increase the serum potassium level.

Acute renal failure in conjunction with ACE inhibition in patients with bilateral RAS or high grade stenosis of an artery to a solitary kidney is well described;[55–63] this is often the limiting factor in drug treatment of patients with presumed RVH. Indeed, acute deterioration in renal function in patients undergoing medical treatment for presumed RVH is frequently the clinical observation that prompts the physician to discontinue medical therapy and consider angioplasty or renal revascularization in suitable candidates. This phenomenon has been observed in up to 23% of patients with high grade RAS who take ACE inhibitors.[64] Fortunately, renal function usually recovers when the ACE inhibitor is discontinued.[58–60, 63] Although clear evidence of permanent structural damage in the kidney distal to the stenosis in such situations is lacking in humans, renal artery thrombosis in such situations has been described.[64–67] Whether shrinkage of the kidney distal to the stenosis in patients treated long-term with ACE inhibitors is due to ACE inhibition *per se* or to progressive arterial stenosis (or both) is unclear, but progressive renal atrophy is an indication to abandon medical management and proceed with angioplasty or surgery if technically feasible.

Calcium antagonists appear to induce less impairment of renal function in patients with RVH than do ACE inhibitors.[45, 46] In two studies comparing the effects of captopril and nifedipine, both agents demonstrated excellent antihypertensive effects. Nifedipine, however, produced a smaller decrement in glomerular filtration rates than did captopril in patients with unilateral, bilateral or solitary-kidney RAS. Calcium antagonists may maintain renal blood flow and function better because of their preferential afferent arteriolar vasodilatory effect. Finally, any type of antihypertensive therapy that effectively lowers the blood pressure may decrease renal blood flow and glomerular filtration rate if the blood pressure is lowered below a 'critical' renal perfusion pressure.[68–70] Diuretic-induced extracellular fluid volume contraction would obviously potentiate this untoward effect of reduced perfusion pressure on renal function.

Flash pulmonary edema has been described in association with unilateral or bilateral RAS.[70] Episodes of acute pulmonary edema in the absence of overt cardiac disease in patients with a reasonable left ventricular ejection fraction are being observed more frequently in the aging population with disseminated vascular disease involving the renal arteries. If the blood pressure in such patients is not rigorously controlled, interventional procedures on the renal artery are required, not only to help control the blood pressure, but to avoid recurrent bouts of flash pulmonary edema.

Additional therapeutic maneuvers

The discussion above has focused on a pathophysiologic approach to the drug treatment of presumed RVH. But regardless of the pharmacologic regimen employed to control blood pressure in such patients, long-term adherence to therapy remains a major problem, as it does in patients with essential hypertension. Failure to control blood pressure adequately leaves such patients at risk for the cardiovascular complications of stroke and congestive heart failure. Which drugs to use, and the choice of medical, surgical, or angioplasty treatment must be individualized carefully. In general, medical management is preferred for older patients, especially those with serious cardiovascular risk factors for surgery. On the other hand, surgical therapy is preferable for patients with fibrous renal artery disease and for younger patients with atherosclerosis, particularly if they have acceptable surgical risk factors. For all patients managed medically, meticulous follow-up is required to ensure that the systolic blood pressure remains less than 140–150 mmHg and the diastolic pressure less than 90 mmHg. Cardiac function, renal excretory function and possible atherosclerotic complications such as transient ischemic attacks and peripheral vascular disease should be monitored closely. Optimal medical care of such patients, particularly those with atherosclerotic renal artery disease, demands modification of cardiovascular risk factors such as smoking cessation, lipid control and regular exercise. Whether current or future antihyperlipidemic drugs, e.g. HMG CoA reductase inhibitors, will have a meaningful impact on atherosclerotic renal artery stenosis remains to be determined, but their benefits in promoting regression of atherosclerosis in other vascular beds is promising.

References

1 Eyler WR, Clark MD, Garman JE *et al.* Angiography of the renal areas including a comparative study of renal arterial stenosis in patients with and without hypertension. *Radiology* 1962; **78:** 879.

2 Dustan HP, Humphries AW, deWolfe VG *et al.* *JAMA* 1964; **187:** 138.

3 Holley KE, Hunt JC, Brown HL Jr *et al. Am J Med* 1964; **37:** 14.
4 Shapiro AP, Perez-Stable E, Scheib ET *et al.* Renal artery stenosis and hypertension. Observations on current status of therapy from a study of 115 patients. *Am J Med* 1969; **47:** 175–93.
5 Hughes JS, Dove HG, Gifford RW Jr, Feinstein AR. Duration of blood pressure elevation in accurately predicting surgical cure of renovascular hypertension. *Am Heart J* 1981; **101:** 408–13.
6 Working Group on Renovascular Hypertension. Detection, evaluation and treatment of renovascular hypertension. *Arch Int Med* 1987; **147:** 820–9.
7 Ram CVS. Renovascular hypertension. *Cardiol Clin* 1988; **6:** 483–508.
8 Pohl MA. Renovascular hypertension: an internist's point of view. In Punzi HA, Flamenbaum W (eds) *Hypertension*. Mt Kisco, NY: Futura, 1989.
9 Vidt DG. Advances in the medical management of renovascular hypertension. *Urol Clin North Am* 1984; **11:** (3) 417–24.
10 Pickering TG. Medical management of renovascular hypertension. In Kaplan NM, Brenner BM, Laragh JH (eds) *The Kidney in Hypertension*. New York: Raven Press, 1987.
11 Kaplan NM. *Clinical Hypertension*, 5th edn. Baltimore: Williams and Wilkins, 1990.
12 Smith MC, Dunn MJ. Renovascular and renal parenchymal hypertension. In Brenner BM, Rector RL Jr (eds) *The Kidney*. Philadelphia: WB Saunders, 1986.
13 Sheps SG, Osmundson PJ, Hunt JC *et al.* Hypertension and renal artery stenosis. Serial observations on 54 patients treated medically (Commentary). *Clin Pharmacol Ther* 1965; **6:** 700–9.
14 Hollenberg NK. The treatment of renovascular hypertension: surgery, angioplasty, and medical therapy with converting-enzyme inhibitors. *Am J Kidney Dis* 1987; **10:** (Suppl. 1): 52–60.
15 Dustan HP, Page IH, Poutasse EF *et al.* An evaluation of treatment of hypertension associated with occlusive renal arterial disease. *Circulation* 1963; **27:** 1018–33.
16 Peart WS. Treatment of hypertension associated with renal artery stenosis. In Engel A, Larsson T (eds) *Stroke: Thule International Symposium*. Stockholm: Nordiska Bokhandeins Forlag, 1967.
17 Shapiro AP, Perez-Stable E, Scheib ET *et al.* Renal artery stenosis and hypertension. *Am J Med* 1969; **47:** 175–93.
18 Kjelbo H, Lund N, Bergentz SE. Renal artery stenosis and hypertension. *Scand J Nephrol* 1970; **4:** 43–7.
19 Owen K. Results of surgical treatment in comparison with medical treatment of renovascular hypertension. *Clin Sci Mol Med* 1973; **45:** (Suppl. 1) 95.
20 Buhler FR, Laragh JH, Vaughan ED Jr *et al.* The antihypertensive action of propranolol. Specific antirenin responses in high and normal renin forms of essential, renal renovascular and malignant hypertension. In Laragh HD (ed.) *Hypertension Manual*, pp. 873–98. New York: York, 1976.
21 Hunt JC, Strong CG. Renovascular hypertension: mechanisms, natural history and treatment. In Laragh HD (ed.) *Hypertension Manual*, pp. 509–36. New York: York, 1976.
22 Streeten DHP, Anderson GH Jr. Outpatient experience with saralasin. *Kidney Int* 1979, **15:** 44–52.
23 Studer A, Luscher T, Griminger P *et al.* Captopril in therapy-resistant essential and renovascular hypertension. In Brunner HT, Gross F (eds) *Recent Advances in Hypertensive Therapy*, pp. 31–40. Amsterdam: Excerpta Medica, 1981.
24 Atkinson AB, Brown JJ, Cumming ANM *et al.* Captopril in the management of hypertension with renal artery stenosis: its long-term effect as a predictor of surgical outcome. *Am J Cardiol* 1982; **49:** 1460–6.
25 Hollifield JW, Moore LC, Winn SD *et al.* Angiotensin converting enzyme inhibition in renovascular hypertension. *Cardiovasc Rev Rep* 1982; **3:** 673–6.
26 Case DB, Atlas SA, Marion RM *et al.* Long term efficacy of captopril in renovascular and essential hypertension. *Am J Cardiol* 1982; **49:** 1440–6.
27 Hollenberg NK. Medical therapy of renovascular hypertension: efficacy and safety of captopril in 269 patients. *Cardiovasc Rev Rep* 1983; **4:** 852–79.
28 Prichard BNL. Propranolol as an antihypertensive agent. *Am Heart J* 1970; **79:** 128–33.
29 Buhler FR, Laragh JH, Vaughan ED Jr *et al.* The antihypertensive action of propranolol. Specific antirenin responses in high and normal renin forms of essential, renal renovascular and malignant hypertension. *Am J Cardiol* 1973; **32:** 511–22.
30 Textor SC. Pathophysiology of renovascular hypertension. *Urol Clin North Am* 1984; **11:** (3) 373–81.
31 Vander AJ, Luciano JR. Neural and humoral control of renin release in salt depletion. *Circ Res* 1967; **21:** (Suppl. 2) 69–77.
32 Nomura G, Kurosaki M, Takabatake T *et al.* Reinnervation and renin release after unilateral renal denervation in the dog. *J Appl Physiol* 1972; **33:** 649–55.
33 Davis JO. The control of renin release. *Am J Med* 1973; **55:** 333–50.
34 Bravo EL, Tarazi RC, Dustan HP. On the mechanism of suppressed plasma renin activity during beta-adrenergic blockade with propranolol. *J Lab Clin Med* 1974; **83:** 119–28.
35 Frishman WH. β-Adrenergic blockers. *Med Clin North Am* 1988; **72:** 37–81.
36 Frishman WH. *Clinical Pharmacology of the β-Adrenoreceptor blocking drugs*, 2nd edn. Norwalk, CT: Appleton-Century-Crofts, 1984.

37 Erdos EG. Angiotensin converting enzyme and the changes in our concepts through the years. *Hypertension* 1990, **16:** 363–70.
38 Franklin SS, Smith RD. A comparison of enalapril plus hydrochlorothiazide with standard triple therapy in renovascular hypertension. *Nephron* 1986; **44:** (Suppl. 1) 73–82.
39 Epstein M. Calcium antagonists in the management of hypertension. In Epstein M (ed.) *Calcium Antagonists in Clinical Medicine*, pp. 49–67. Philadelphia: Hanley and Belfus, 1992.
40 Bursztyn M, Grossman R, Rosenthal T. Nifedipine as a substitute for converting enzyme inhibitors in the treatment of renovascular hypertension. *Clin Exp Hypertension* 1985; **A7:** 1187–97.
41 Triggle DJ. Calcium antagonists. In Antonaccio MJ (ed.) *Cardiovascular Pharmacology*, 3rd edn, pp. 107–60. New York: Raven Press, 1990.
42 Morris AD, Meredith PA, Reid JL. Pharmacokinetics of calcium antagonists: implications for therapy. In Epstein M (ed.) *Calcium Antagonists in Clinical Medicine*, pp. 49–67. Philadelphia: Hanley and Belfus, 1992.
43 Churchill PG. Second messengers in renin secretion. *Am J Physiol* 1985; **249:** F175–F184.
44 Hackenthal E, Paul M, Ganten D, Taugner R. Morphology, physiology, and molecular biology of renin secretion. *Physiolog Rev* 1990; **70:** 1067–116.
45 Ribstein J, Mourad G, Mimron A. Contrasting acute effects of captopril and nifedipine on renal function in renovascular hypertension. *Am J Hypertension* 1988; **1:** 239–44.
46 Miyamoti R, Yasubara S, Matsubara T *et al.* Comparative effects of captopril and nifedipine on split renal function in renovascular hypertension. *Am J Hypertension* 1988; **1:** 359–63.
47 Fiorentini C, Galli C, Tamborine G *et al.* Hemodynamic and renin responses to nifedipine in renovascular hypertension. *Am Heart J* 1990; **119:** 353–6.
48 Weir MR. Calcium entry blockers. In Izzo JL, Black HR (eds) *Hypertension Primer*, pp. 311–14, Dallas: American Heart Association, 1993.
49 Timmermans PB, Chiu AT, Herblin WR *et al.* Angiotensin II receptor subtypes. *Am J Hypertension* 1992; **5:** 406–10.
50 Brunner HR, Gavvas H, Laragh JH, Keenon R. Angiotensin II blockade in man by SAR1-A1a8-angiotensin II for understanding and treatment of high blood pressure. *Lancet* 1973; **3:** 1045–8.
51 Case DB, Laragh JH. Reactive hyperreninemia in renovascular hypertension after angiotensin blockade with saralasin or converting enzyme inhibitor. *Ann Int Med* 1979; **91:** 153–60.
52 Smith RD, Chin AT, Wong PC *et al.* Pharmacology of non peptide angiotensin II receptor antagonists. *Ann Rev Pharmacol Toxicol* 1992; **32:** 135–65.
53 Kon V, Fogo A, Ichikawa I. Bradykinin causes selective efferent arteriolar dilation during angiotensin I converting enzyme inhibition. *Kidney Int* 1993; **44:** 545–50.
54 Mimron A, Jover B, Saladini D. Effect of losartan and enalapril in 1-kidney 1-clip sodium restricted rats. *J Am Soc Nephrol* 1994; **5:** 546.
55 Hricik DE, Browning PJ, Kopelman R *et al.* Captopril-induced functional renal insufficiency in patients with bilateral renal artery stenosis or renal artery stenosis in solitary kidney. *N Engl J Med* 1993; **308:** 373–6.
56 De Zeevu D *et al.* The angiotensin converting enzyme inhibitor enalapril and its effect on renal function. *J Hypertension* 1983; **1:** (Suppl. 1) 93.
57 Tillman DM, Malatino LS, Cumming AM. Enalapril in hypertension with renal artery stenosis: long term follow-up and effects on renal function. *J Hypertension* 1984; **2:** (Suppl. 2) S93–S100.
58 Chrysant SG, Dunn M, Marples D, DeMasters K. Severe reversible azotemia from captopril therapy. *Arch Int Med* 1983; **143:** 437–41.
59 Murphy BF, Whitworth JA, Kincaid-Smith P. Renal insufficiency with combinations of angiotensin-converting enzyme inhibitors and diuretics. *Br Med J* 1984; **288:** 844–5.
60 Hodsmon GP, Brown JJ, Cumming AM *et al.* Enalapril in the treatment of hypertension with renal artery stenosis: changes in blood pressure, renin, angiotensin I and II, renal function, and body composition. *Am J Med* 1984; **77:** (2A) 52–60.
61 Jackson B, Murphy BR, Johnston CI *et al.* Renovascular hypertension: treatment with the oral angiotensin-converting enzyme inhibitor enalapril. *Am J Nephrol* 1986; **6:** 182–6.
62 Kalra PA, Mamtora H, Holmes AM, Waldek S. Renovascular disease and renal complication of angiotensin-converting enzyme inhibitor therapy. *Quar J Med* 1990; **77:** 1013–18.
63 Toto R, Mitchell H, Lee H *et al.* Reversible renal insufficiency due to angiotensin-converting enzyme inhibitors in hypertension nephrosclerosis. *Ann Int Med* 1991; **115:** 513–19.
64 Postma CT, Hoefnagels W, Barentz JO *et al.* Occlusion of unilateral stenosed renal arteries: relation to medical treatment. *J Human Hypertens* 1989; **3:** 185–90.
65 Williams PS, Herdy MS, Ackrill P. Captopril-induced acute renal artery thrombosis and persistent anuria in a patient with documented pre-existing renal artery stenosis and renal failure. *Postgrad Med J* 1984; **60:** 561–3.
66 Hoefnagels W, Thien R. Renal artery occlusion in patients with renovascular hypertension treated with captopril. *Br Med J* 1986; **292:** 24–5.
67 Hannedouche T, Godin M, Fries D, Fillastue JP. Acute renal thrombosis induced by angiotensin-converting enzyme inhibitors in patients with renovascular hypertension. *Nephron* 1991; **57:** 230–1.
68 Textor SC, Novick AC, Tarazi RC *et al.* Critical perfusion pressure for renal function in patients

with bilateral atherosclerotic renal vascular disease. *Ann Int Med* 1985; **102:** 308–14.
69 Ying CY, Tifft CP, Gavvas H, Chobanian AV. Renal revascularization in the azotemic hypertensive patient resistant to therapy. *N Engl J Med* 1984; **311:** 1070–5.
70 Pickering TG, Herman L, Devereauz RB *et al.* Recurrent pulmonary oedema in hypertension due to bilateral renal artery stenosis: treatment by angioplasty or surgical revascularization. *Lancet* 1988; **2:** 551–2.

26

Medical management of atherosclerotic renovascular disease

P SWENY

Introduction

Atherosclerosis in general and atherosclerotic renal artery stenosis (ARAS) in particular is a progressive disease.[1] Restenosis after vascular surgery or angioplasty is common.[2] Aggressive medical therapy can reverse atherosclerosis.[3] For these three reasons the medical management of ARAS should be receiving increasing attention. A multidisciplinary approach is essential: vascular surgeon, physician and dietitian. In one sense treatment has only just begun after successful bypass surgery or angioplasty.

Etiological factors in atherosclerosis

The pathogenesis of atherosclerosis has recently been reviewed.[4] The principal cells involved in the process (platelets, macrophages, endothelial cells and smooth muscle cells) produce a wide range of cytokines and growth factors. The initiating event appears to be endothelial injury with subsequent recruitment and interaction of these cell types with coagulation factors and dyslipidemia. As indicated in Table 26.1, even a partial understanding of these factors opens up possible avenues of treatment.

Table 26.1. Etiological factors in atherosclerosis: avenues for intervention

Pathogenesis	Intervention
Smoking	Abstain
Diet	Healthy eating
Hypertension	Drugs
Hyperlipidemia	Diet and drugs
Oxidized LDL	Antioxidants (probucol, vitamin E)
Endothelial injury: expression of adhesion molecules	
Cytokines, chemoattractants and growth factors	ACE inhibitors, α_2-macroglobulin
Smooth muscle migration and proliferation	Heparin
Production of extracellular matrix	
Platelets-fibrinogen-coagulation	Aspirin, EPA
Mural thrombosis	
Arachidonic acid metabolites	Aspirin, EPA
Macrophages	
T-Lymphocytes	
Fibroblasts—fibrosis (TGF-β)	
Glucose intolerance	Diet, drugs
Excessive alcohol	Moderation
Genetic factors	Liver transplantation

Assessment

There are many precedents for a multidisciplinary approach to medical problems. A full assessment of etiological factors and end organ damage is essential. Vascular surgeons need to assemble a team that can produce the specialized dietary, metabolic, hypertension and renal advice to limit progression and prevent recurrence. This is as important as the dramatic repair of the vascular disease.

Fasting lipids need to be checked and rechecked after adherence to an appropriate diet. In patients with borderline elevations of total cholesterol, high/low density lipoprotein (HDL/LDL) ratios can indicate those who would benefit from treatment. Drug therapy can then be chosen appropriately. Lipid studies need to be extended to include measurements of lipoprotein (a) (Lp (a)) as drugs are appearing that can reduce Lp (a) levels. Fibrinogen measurement is required as elevated levels can be treated. Fasting plasma glucose and glucose tolerance test may be required to define patients with diabetes mellitus or insulin resistance. The importance of hypothyroidism as a risk factor for atherosclerosis, particularly in older females needs emphasizing. Apolipoprotein phenotyping is important in identifying high risk patients.

Angiograms provide a measurement of the severity of the stenosis, but often are a poor indicator of vessel wall thickness and can therefore underestimate the severity of atherosclerosis. The etiological factors underlying atherosclerosis predominantly affect wall thickness rather then stenosis *per se*. Non-invasive B-mode ultrasound techniques have been developed to assess wall thickness in extracranial carotid arteries and are being used to assess regression under pravastatin therapy.[5]

Progression of renal failure

There are several aspects of progressive renal failure that need discussion. Atherosclerotic renal artery stenosis is known to be progressive,[1] but progressive renal impairment may be due to the downstream effects of cholesterol emboli.[6] Acute or chronic renal failure in macrovascular renal artery disease due to angiotensin converting enzyme (ACE) inhibitor drugs is well recognized.[7] A similar effect on renal function can be produced by non-steroidal anti-inflammatory drugs (NSAID) which not only reduce renin production, but also reduce the production of vasodilating renal prostaglandins.

Following Brenner's hypothesis of hyperperfusion—hyperfiltration and progressive renal disease[8] the general area of insidious deterioration of kidney function to end-stage chronic renal failure has been widened to encompass a view that progression is also mediated by a glomerular process very similar to atherosclerosis.[9]

Table 26.2. Relationship between serum creatinine and GFR

GFR (ml/min)	Serum creatinine (μmol/l)
120	60
60	120
30	240
15	480
7.5	1000
<5	>1500

Both the onset and progression of renal disease is often recognized late by non-nephrologists. This is because the published normal range for serum creatinine is often too wide. Serum creatinine is affected by glomerular filtration rate (GFR) and muscle mass. The average 60–70 kg adult has a serum creatinine of 60–70 μmol/l. As GFR halves, serum creatinine will double, giving the well-known exponential relationship between GFR and serum creatinine (Table 26.2). Thus a serum creatinine just outside the normal upper limit of 120 μmol/l usually means the loss of half total renal function. Medical or surgical intervention that is only triggered by a creatinine of 200–300 μmol/l means that the disease process is already very advanced.

Blood pressure

Hypertension is one of the most important treatable etiological factors for atherosclerosis and its progression. The question that immediately arises is what is a normal blood pressure for the population with renal artery stenosis, usually older males. The best definition of an abnormally elevated blood pressure is that pressure at which there is an increased risk of end organ damage or, put another way, it is that pressure at which treatment confers benefit. This approach has taught us that hypertension in the elderly is worth treating.[10, 11] Targets are difficult to set in this older patient group with rigid blood vessels as side-effects of drugs are common, particularly postural hypotension. New United States criteria have recently been published[12] and suggest that a blood pressure in excess of 140 systolic or 90 diastolic is to be considered elevated in all adults whether or not they are elderly. Even isolated systolic hypertension in a patient under the age of 85 has been shown to be worth treating. Indeed, increased systolic blood pressure is a more potent risk factor than increased diastolic blood pressure.[13]

Blood pressure evaluation is an essential part of the management of ARAS. Many of these patients are elderly and it needs to be remembered that blood pressure is more variable in the elderly, so frequent measurements should be made. Postural hypotension is common so that postural measurements should be recorded at each visit. Standing blood pressure should be used as the guide for treatment. Non-pharmacological methods of blood pressure lowering (reduction of weight, reduction of salt intake, moderation of alcohol consumption and increase in exercise) should be tried before and as well as drug therapy.[14]

The choice of the antihypertensive agent used will be affected by the presence of renal artery stenosis, associated risk factors and age. There is an increasing body of evidence that suggests that the renin–angiotensin–aldosterone system plays an important part in vascular remodeling and pathology. The use of ACE inhibitors has improved the prognosis of scleroderma renal crisis[15] and radiation nephritis.[16] In both conditions there is an obliterative endarteritis. Similar evidence of efficacy is available for ACE inhibition in chronic rejection in renal transplants.[17] Angiotensin converting enzyme inhibitors are also lipid neutral and do not adversely affect glucose tolerance. Once renal artery stenosis has been corrected, patients with renovascular disease can be considered for therapy with an ACE inhibitor. There seems little to choose between the rival agents although captopril is also a free radical scavenger and the increased renal tissue binding of quinalopril may be relevant.

There is evidence that suggests that with unilateral renal artery stenosis treatment with an ACE inhibitor preserves renal function better in the unaffected kidney, but hastens ischemic atrophy of the affected kidney. Whether this implies a requirement of angiotensin II as a trophic hormone or represents tubular atrophy secondary to a reduced glomerular filtration and loss of tubular growth factors is unknown.[18, 19] Angiotensin converting enzyme inhibitors should therefore not be used until renal revascularization has been successful, unless it is desired to hasten autonephrectomy, e.g. in an inoperable dialysis-dependent patient with severe hypertension or in patients with severe unilateral disease not amenable to surgical nephrectomy. As mentioned earlier, atherosclerotic renal disease can be broadened to include atherosclerotic-like processes affecting small intrarenal vessels, particularly the glomeruli. Some have considered the glomeruli to be hemiarterioles. One side is a leaky capillary through which filtration occurs, while the other side is contractile smooth muscle-like mesangial cell. The glomerulus is therefore heir to disease processes that affect small arterioles, such as hypertension, as well as diseases which damage capillaries, such as diabetes and the thrombotic microangiopathies. Again there is increasing evidence of beneficial effects of ACE inhibitors in a variety of renal conditions including a reduction of proteinuria,[20] preservation of GFR[21] and a reduction of glomerular scarring,[22] particularly in animal models. In a rat model of atherosclerosis ACE inhibitors have been shown to reduce smooth muscle proliferation.[23] Whether this beneficial effect is due to a reduction in glomerular blood pressure or related to beneficial effects on cytokines and mitogens in the local glomerular capillary is unknown.

Calcium channel blockers have been shown in some studies to reduce atherosclerosis.[24] As a class they are also lipid and carbohydrate metabolism neutral. Some agents such as nifedipine and nicardipine may dilate the afferent glomerular arteriole and increase glomerular blood pressure and proteinuria while others are less likely to do so (verapamil and diltiazem). The antianginal properties of this class of blood pressure lowering drugs makes them particularly suitable for use in patients with widespread atherosclerosis. α-Blockers such as prazosin and doxazosin are also of value in patients with atherosclerosis and also improve the dyslipidemia. An incidental advantage may be improved bladder emptying in elderly males. Postural hypotension and nasal stuffiness can be difficult.

Once GFR is much below 50%, thiazide diuretics do not work and potassium sparing agents become ineffective and have the attendant risk of hyperkalemia. Loop diuretics have a good dose—response curve extending into severe renal failure. Bumetanide is less diabetigenic than others in this class. Although thiazides are diabetogenic, patients with normal renal function, particularly the elderly, respond well to very low doses of thiazide diuretics with minimal side-effects.

β-Blockers are valuable in the control of angina, but vasculopaths may find that their claudication worsens. β-Blockers can also precipitate congestive cardiac failure in patients with poor myocardial function and they worsen dyslipidemia.

Table 26.3. Dietary intervention

Increase
Fruit
Vegetables
(complex carbohydrates and soluble fibre)
(unsaturated fats: linoleic, oleic, EPA, olive oil)
Decrease
Refined carbohydrate
Animal fats
Eggs, butter (saturated fats)
Total calorie intake
Alcohol
Substitute
Olive oil for cooking with animal fats
Olive oil-based spreads for butter
Fish and chicken for fatty red meat
Grill, don't fry or bake
Skimmed milk for full cream milk

Dietary management

All patients (and their medical advisors) should follow healthy eating guidelines.[25] It has to be acknowledged that it is difficult to persuade patients to change the habits of a lifetime, at least until after a major medical event has overtaken them. Nevertheless we should try. The general principles to be followed include a diet to reduce weight appropriate to the age, sex and height of the patient. All agree that a reduction in animal fats (saturated fats) and an increase in polyunsaturated fats is appropriate. The recent concerns about the risk of *trans*-isomers of the naturally occurring *cis*-isomers of unsaturated fats particularly in butter substitutes has not been confirmed.[26] Cooking with reused vegetable oils, particularly coconut oil,[27] increases the intake of potentially toxic oxidized fatty acids and may increase the risk of atherosclerosis. Currently an increase in olive oil-based spreads and olive oil for frying and cooking is recommended.[28] The merits of a high fibre diet have been well aired and patients should be encouraged to increase their intake of fruit and vegetable fiber. Such advice makes a reduction in the intake of refined carbohydrates easier. The assistance of an enthusiastic dietitian is essential if patients are to change ingrown patterns of eating.

Hypertriglyceridemic patients usually respond well to a reduction in the intake of total unsaturated fats with an increase in the intake of complex carbohydrates. This results in a reduced conversion of VLDL to LDL and to a decrease in insulin resistance.

Central obesity, fat intake (especially of saturated fats), cholesterol intake and boiled unfiltered coffee have been shown to increase plasma cholesterol. A high fiber diet and certain types of plant proteins, for example soya, can reduce plasma cholesterol. Dietary efforts can reduce total cholesterol levels by only about 10%. An increase in intake of soluble dietary fiber may act by increasing the rate of excretion of cholesterol in bile, e.g. an increase in the intake of oats, beans and fruit. Table 26.3 summarizes the major dietary interventions. Dietary therapy should be considered for some 3–6 months before recourse to lipid lowering drugs.

Exercise

Regular exercise plays an important part in the management of both coronary and peripheral vascular disease. It is an important addition to weight reducing diets. In particular, exercise through claudication pain may encourage collateral circulation. Patients should not exercise to the point of angina, fatigue or breathlessness. In the elderly and in those with arthritis,

Table 26.7. Medical management of ARAS

Stop smoking
Lose weight
Take more exercise
Adopt healthy eating habits
Obsessional control of blood pressure; choose agents carefully
Control dyslipidemia
Consider other measures to retard atherosclerosis; platelet inhibitors antioxidants

reduce associated risk factors. Treatment should be based on a multidisciplinary approach and continue indefinitely. Many of the patients are elderly and special care and thought needs to be given to blood pressure and lipid control. Preventing progression and restenosis are as important as the initial surgical correction (Table 26.7).

References

1 Wollenweber J, Sheps SG, Davis GD. Clinical course of atherosclerotic renovascular disease. *Am J Cardiol* 1968; **21:** 60–71.
2 Califf RM, Ohman M, Frid DJ. Restenosis: the clinical issues. In Topol EJ (ed.) *Textbook of Interventional Cardiology*, pp. 363–94. Philadelphia: WD Saunders, 1990.
3 Loscalzo J. Regression of coronary atherosclerosis. *N Engl J Med* 1990; **323:** 1337–9.
4 Ross R. The pathogenesis of atherosclerosis: a perspective for the 1990s. *Nature* 1993; **362:** 801–9.
5 Crouse JR, Thompson CJ. Evaluation of methods for quantifying lumen stenosis and atherosclerosis. *Circulation* 1993; **87:** (Suppl. 11) 17–33.
6 Meyrier A, Buchet P, Simon P *et al.* Atheromatous renal disease. *Am J Med* 1988; **85:** 139–46.
7 Hrick DE, Browning PJ, Kopelman R *et al.* Captopril induced functional renal insufficiency in patients with bilateral renal artery stenoses or renal artery stenosis in a solitary kidney. *N Engl J Med* 1983; **308:** 373–6.
8 Brenner BM, Meyer TW, Hostetter TH. Dietary protein intake and the progressive nature of kidney disease. *N Engl J Med* 1982; **307:** 652–9.
9 Diamond J-R. Analagous pathobiologic mechanisms in glomerulosclerosis and atherosclerosis. *Kidney Int* 1991; **39:** S29–S34.
10 MRC Working Party. Medical Research Council trial of treatment of hypertension in older adults: principal results. *Br Med J* 1992; **304:** 405–12.
11 The systolic hypertension in the elderly program (SHEP) cooperative research group prevention of stroke by antihypertensive drug treatment: final results of SHEP. *JAMA* 1991; **265:** 3255–64.
12 Joint National Committee on detection, evaluation and treatment of high blood pressure. The fifth report of the Joint National Committee on detection, evaluation and treatment of high blood pressure. *Arch Int Med* 1993; **153:** 154–83.
13 Bennet NE. Hypertension in the elderly. *Lancet* 1994; **344:** 447–52.
14 Alderman MH. Non-pharmacological treatment of hypertension. *Lancet* 1994; **344:** 307–11.
15 Steen VD, Constantino JP, Shapiro AP, Medsger TA Jr. Outcome of renal crisis in systemic sclerosis: relation to availability of angiotensin converting enzyme inhibitor. *Ann Int Med* 1990; **113:** 352–7.
16 Cohen EP, Fish BL, Moulder JE. Treatment of radiation nephropathy with captopril. *Radiat Res* 1992; **132:** 346–50.
17 Morales JM, Andres A, Montoyo C *et al.* Effect of captopril, an angiotensin converting enzyme inhibitor on the massive proteinuria due to chronic rejection after renal transplantation—a prospective study. *Transplant Proc* 1992; **24:** 92–3.
18 Michael J-B, Menard J, Dussaule J-C *et al.* Effects of antihypertensive treatment in one-clip two kidney hypertension in rats. *Kidney Int* 1986; **29:** 1011–20.
19 Jackson B, Franze L, Sumithran E, Johnston CI. Pharmocological nephrectomy with chronic angiotensin converting enzyme inhibitor treatment in renovascular hypertension in the rat. *J Lab Clin Med* 1990; **115:** 21–7.
20 Praga M, Hernandez E, Montoyo C *et al.* Long term beneficial effects of angiotensin converting enzyme inhibition in patients with nephrotic syndrome. *Am J Kidney Dis* 1992; **20:** 240–8.
21 Lewis EJ, Hunsicker LG, Bain RP, Rhohde RD. The effect of angiotensin converting enzyme inhibition on diabetic nephropathy. *N Engl J Med* 1993; **329:** 1456–62.
22 Anderson S, Rennke HG, Brenner BM. Therapeutic advantage of converting enzyme inhibitors in arresting progressive renal disease associated with systemic hypertension. *J Clin Invest* 1986; **77:** 1993–2000.
23 Daemen MJ, Lombardi DM, Bosman FT, Scwartz SM. Angiotensin II induces smooth muscle cell proliferation in the normal and injured rat arterial wall. *Circ Res* 1991; **68:** 450–6.
24 Armstrong ML, Heistad DD, Lopez JAG. Regression of atherosclerosis: a role for calcium antagonists. *Am J Hypertension* 1991; **4:** 503S–511S.
25 Department of Health. *Report on Health and Social Subjects 46. Nutritional Aspect of Cardiovascular Disease*. London: HMSO, 1994.
26 McKeigue P. Trans fatty acids and coronary heart

disease: weighing the evidence against hardened fat. *Lancet* 1995; **345:** 269–70.
27 Grundy SC, Denke MA. Dietary influences of serum lipids and lipoproteins. *J Lipid Res* 1990; **31:** 1149–72.
28 Keys A, Menotti A, Karvonen MJ *et al.* The diet and 15 year death rate in the seven countries study. *Am J Epidemiol* 1986; **124:** 903–15.
29 Rossouw JE, Lewis B, Rifkind BM. The value of lowering cholesterol after myocardial infarction. *N Engl J Med* 1990; **323:** 1112–19.
30 Rossouw JE. Canner PL, Hulley SB. Deaths from injury, violence and suicide in secondary prevention trials of cholesterol lowering. *N Engl J Med* 1991; **325:** 1813.
31 Davies MJ, Thomas A. Thrombosis and acute coronary-artery lesions in sudden cardiac ischemic death. *N Engl J Med* 1984; **310:** 1137–40.
32 Brown BG, Zhao X-Q, Sacco DE, Albers JJ. Lipid lowering and plaque regression. New insights into prevention of plaque disruption and clinical events in coronary disease. *Circulation* 1993; **87:** 1781–91.
33 Laker M, Neil A, Wood C (eds) *British Hyperlipidaemia Association Symposium. Cholesterol Lowering Trials: Advice for the British Physician.* London: Royal College of Physicians, 1993.
34 Durrington P. Lipid lowering studies and management protocols: what should we be doing today? *Br J Cardiol* 1994; **1:** (Suppl. 1): 28–9.
35 Davey Smith G, Song F, Sheldon TA. Cholesterol lowering and mortality: the importance of considering initial level of risk. *Br Med J* 1993; **306:** 1367.
36 La Rosa JC, Applegate W, Crouse JR III *et al.* Cholesterol lowering in the elderly: results of the cholesterol reduction in seniors program (CRISP) pilot study. *Arch Int Med* 1994; **154:** 529–39.
37 Betteridge DJ, Dodson PM, Durrington PN *et al.* Management of hyperlipidaemia: guidelines of the British Hyperlipidaemia Association. *Postgrad Med J* 1993; **69:** 359–69.
38 Leaf A, Weber PC. Cardiovascular effects of n-3 fatty acids. *N Engl J Med* 1988; **318:** 549–57.
39 Antiplatelet Trialists' Collaboration. Secondary prevention of vascular disease by prolonged antiplatelet treatment. *Br Med J* 1988; **296:** 320–31.
40 Mortensen JZ, Schmidt EB, Nielsen AH, Dyerberg J. The effect of N6 and N3 polyunsaturated fatty acids on hemostasis, blood lipids and blood pressure. *Thromb Haemostas* 1983; **50**(2): 543–6.
41 Sweny P, Wheeler DC, Lui SF *et al.* Dietary fish oil supplements preserve renal function in renal transplant recipients with chronic vascular rejection. *Nephrol Dial Transplant* 1989; **4:** 1070–75.
42 Steinberg D, Pathasarathy S, Carew TE *et al.* Beyond cholesterol: modification of low density lipoprotein that increase its atherogenicity. *N Engl J Med* 1989; **320:** 915–24.
43 Rimm EB, Stampfer MJ, Ascherio A *et al.* Vitamin E consumption and the risk of coronary heart disease in men. *N Engl J Med* 1993; **328:** 1450–6.
44 Stampfer MJ, Hennekens CH, Manson JE *et al.* Vitamin E consumption and the risk of coronary disease in women. *N Engl J Med* 1993; **328:** 1444–9.
45 Mackness MI, Abbott CA, Arrol S, Durrington PN. The role of high density lipoprotein and lipid soluble anti-oxidant vitamins inhibiting low denisty lipoprotein oxidation. *Biochem J* 1993; **294:** 829–4.
46 Kannel WB, Wolf PA, Castelli WP, D'Agostino RB. Fibrinogen and risk of cardiovascular disease. The Framingham Study. *JAMA* 1987; **258:** 1183–6.
47 Sullivan JM, Van der Zwagg R, Hughes JP *et al.* Estrogen replacement and coronary artery disease—effect on survival in post menopausal women. *Arch Int Med* 1990; **150:** 2557–62.
48 Ost C-R, Stenson S. Regression of peripheral atherosclerosis during therapy with high dose of nicotinic acid. *Scand J Clin Lab Invest* 1967; **99:** (Suppl.) 241–5.
49 Brown G, Albers JJ, Fisher LD *et al.* Regression of coronary artery disease as a result of intensive lipid lowering therapy in men with high levels of apolipoprotein B. *N Engl J Med* 1990; **323:** 1289–98.
50 Pearson TA, Marx HJ. The rapid reduction in cardiac events with lipid lowering therapy. Mechanisms and implications. *Am J Cardiol* 1993; **72:** 1072–3.
51 Fanelli C, Aronoff R. Restenosis following coronary angioplasty. *Am Heart J* 1990; **119:** 357–68.
52 Simons M, Leclerc G, Safian RD *et al.* Relation between activated smooth muscle cells in coronary artery lesions and restenosis after atherectomy. *N Engl J Med* 1993; **328:** 608–13.
53 Herrman JPR, Hermans WRM, Vos J, Serruys PW. Pharmacological approaches to the prevention of restenosis following angioplasty. *Drugs* 1993; **46**(1): 18–52.
54 Nikol S, Isner JM, Pickering JG *et al.* Expression of transforming growth factor-β1 is increased in human vascular restenosis lesions. *J Clin Invest* 1992; **90:** 1582–92.
55 Blankenhorn DN, Nessim SA, Johnson RL *et al.* Beneficial effects of combined colestipol-niacin therapy on coronary atherosclerosis and coronary venous by-pass grafts. *JAMA* 1987; **257:** 3233–40.
56 Pauletto P, Sartore S, Pessina AC. Smooth muscle cell proliferation and differentiation in neointima formation and vascular restenosis. *Clin Sci* 1994; **87:** 467–79.
57 Chan P, Patel M, Betteridge L *et al.* Abnormal growth regulation of vascular smooth muscle by heparin in patients with restenosis. *Lancet* 1993; **341:** 341–2.
58 Clowes AW. Prevention and management of recurrent disease after arterial reconstruction:

new prospects for pharmacological control. *Thromb Haemostas* 1991; **66:** 62–6.

59 O'Connor GT, Malenka DJ, Olmstead EM *et al.* A meta-analysis of randomised trials of fish oil in the prevention of restenosis following coronary angioplasty. *Am J Prev Med* 1992; **8:** 186–92.

60 Sirtori CR. Hypoalphalipoproteinaemia: from a mutation to drug development. In Schonfeld G, Seidel D, Shepherd J, Kritchevsky D (eds) *Atherosclerosis* IO, Oct 1994 Montreal, Canada. Amsterdam: Elsevier, 1995.

61 Topol EJ, Califf RM, Weisman HF *et al.* Randomised trial of coronary intervention with antibody against platelet IIb/IIIa integrin for reduction of clinical restenosis: results at 6 months. *Lancet* 1994; **343:** 881–6.

62 Agishi T, Wood W, Gordon B. LDL apheresis using the liposorber LA-15 system in coronary and peripheral vascular disease associated with severe hypercholesterolaemia. *Curr Ther Res* 1994; **55**(8)**:** 879–904.

27

Percutaneous transluminal angioplasty in fibrous dysplasia and children

CHARLES J TEGTMEYER, ALAN H MATSUMOTO, JOHN F ANGLE

Introduction

Renovascular hypertension, seen in approximately 4% of the hypertensive population in the United States, poses the double threat of severe high blood pressure (with its complications) and progressive renal insufficiency. If the renal artery is severely narrowed, lowering the blood pressure by medical therapy causes further reduction in renal blood flow and may result in ischemic atrophy or even renal infarction. It is therefore desirable to correct the lesion wherever clinically possible. Both surgery and percutaneous transluminal renal angioplasty (PTRA) have been utilized to correct renal artery lesions.

Fibromuscular dysplasia in adults

The best results for both surgery and PTRA in correcting renovascular hypertension have been achieved in patients with fibromuscular dysplasia (FMD). Fibromuscular dysplasia was first described in the renal arteries in 1938.[1] Subsequently, it was recognized that the disease affects other arteries.[2] The condition has been demonstrated in the carotid, celiac, iliac, vertebral, subclavian brachial, splenic, mesenteric, axillary, coronary and hepatic arteries as well. It occurs with greatest frequency in the renal and carotid arteries. There is also an apparent association with cerebral aneurysms. The Cooperative Study on Renovascular Hypertension examined 884 patients with renal artery lesions. Atherosclerosis was the etiology in 577 (63%), and FMD in 286 (32.4%) and miscellaneous disease entities in 41 (4.6%).[3] In the University of Virginia Series,[4] FMD was the cause of the renal artery lesion in 24% of the hypertensive patients. Therefore, FMD is the second most prevalent cause of renal artery lesions in adults.

The cause of FMD remains unknown. The disease seems to be that of a generalized arterial dysplasia. Because the disease is seen predominantly in the renal and carotid arteries, some authors have suggested a relationship between increased blood flow and the development of these lesions. Other theories include a hormonal influence, trauma, hypermobility of the kidney, embryonic alteration of the vessel and immunologic injury to the vessel wall. The disease is a chronic progressive disease with variable rates of progression. Although the disease may be seen at any age in either sex, it affects young adult and middle-age women more often than men and is often bilateral. Fibromuscular dysplasia appears to affect the right renal artery more often than the left. When contrasted to atherosclerotic disease, the patients with hypertension secondary to FMD are usually younger (mean age 39 years) predominantly female, and more likely to have no family history of hypertension. The patients often have an upper quadrant abdominal or a flank bruit. The bruit is of a systolic-diastolic or continuous nature.

McCormack *et al.*[5, 6] classified the lesions of FMD according to primary sites of involvement in the arterial wall, and they correlated the histological findings with angiographic appearances. Their classification includes intimal fibroplasia, medial fibroplasia, fibromuscular hyperplasia and subadventitial fibroplasia. The classification in the present analysis is based solely on the angiographic appearance of the lesion because histological material was not available. In this report, intimal fibroplasia consists of symmetrical narrowing of the artery with poststenotic dilatation or an irregularly dilated segment. Because there has been considerable difficulty separating intimal fibroplasia from fibromuscular hyperplasia angiographically, these lesions have been grouped together as intimal fibroplasia[7] (Fig. 27.1). These are the so-called 'focal' lesions (Fig. 27.2). Medial fibroplasia consists of the classic 'string of beads' appearance, with the diameter of the 'beads'

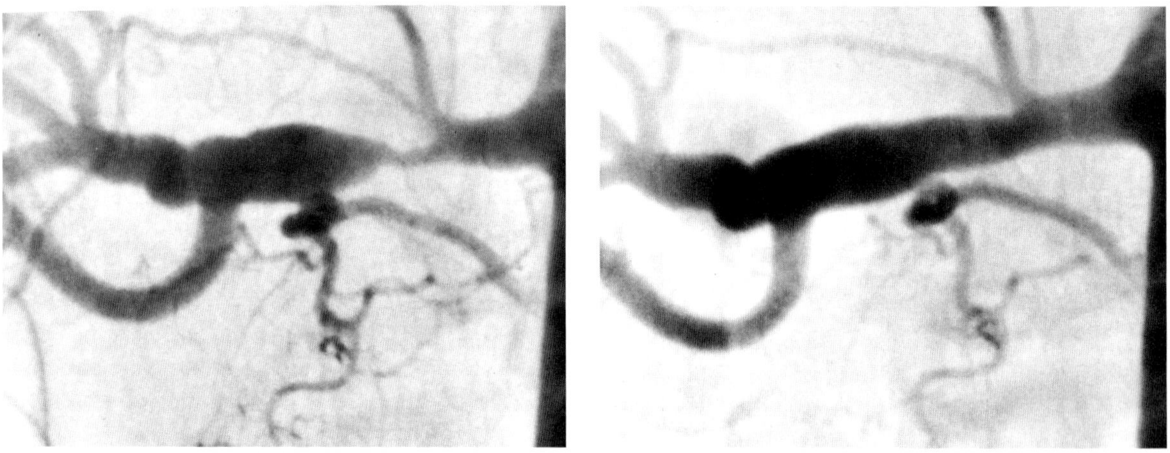

(a) (b)

Figure 27.1. Intimal fibroplasia is illustrated in a hypertensive middle aged man. (a) The arteriogram demonstrates a tight smooth stenosis in the right renal artery. (b) Immediately after PTRA the vessel is wide open.

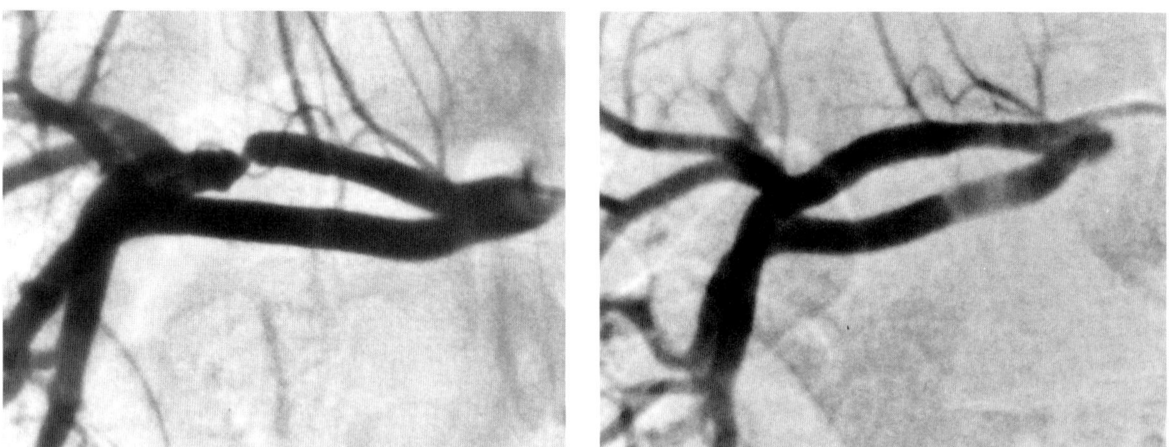

(a) (b)

Figure 27.2. A focal lesion is demonstrated in a 27-year-old woman with a 4.5 year history of hypertension. (a) The arteriogram shows a tight isolated stenosis in the dorsal branch of the right renal artery. (b) The lesion cannot be detected on a follow-up arteriogram obtained 27 months after PTRA. From ref. 82, with permission.

exceeding the expected diameter of the renal artery in the affected region (Fig. 27.3). Lesions were classified as subadventitial fibroplasia when they appeared as areas of severe, uneven stenosis. 'Beading' may be present in the artery; however, the width of the 'beads' does not exceed the original diameter of the vessel (Fig. 27.4).

The most common type of FMD is medial

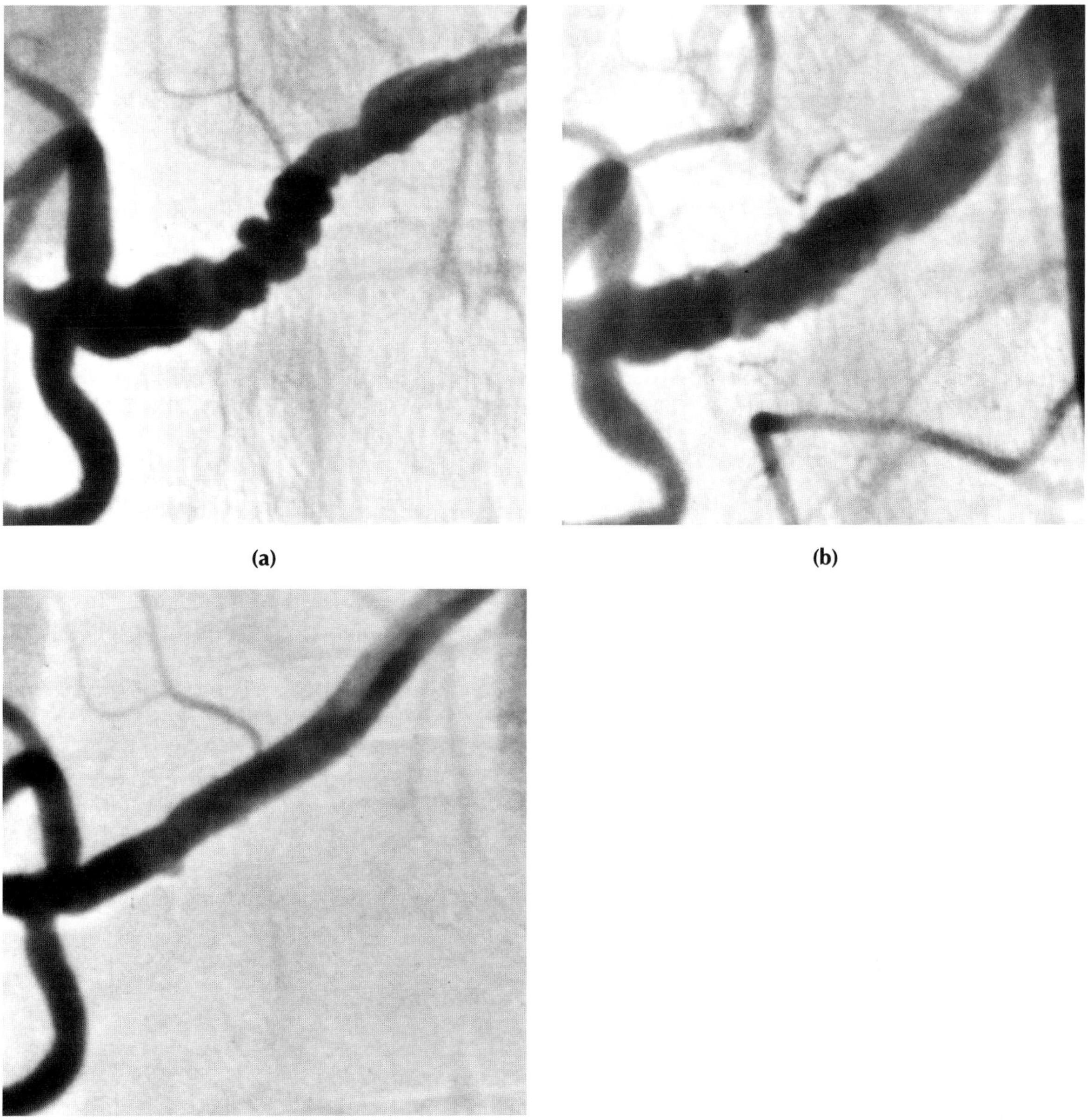

(a) **(b)** **(c)**

Figure 27.3. The long-term results of PTRA are shown in a 51-year-old woman with medial fibroplasia. (a) The renal arteriogram reveals the beaded appearance of extensive medial fibroplasia in the right renal artery. (b) Immediately following PTRA with a 5 mm balloon, the vessel appears irregular but there is good flow through the vessel. This appearance is typical immediately after PTRA in FMD lesions. (c) The arteriogram obtained 12.5 months later shows no evidence of the former lesion. This is the usual long-term appearance after PTRA of medial lesions. From ref. 4, with permission.

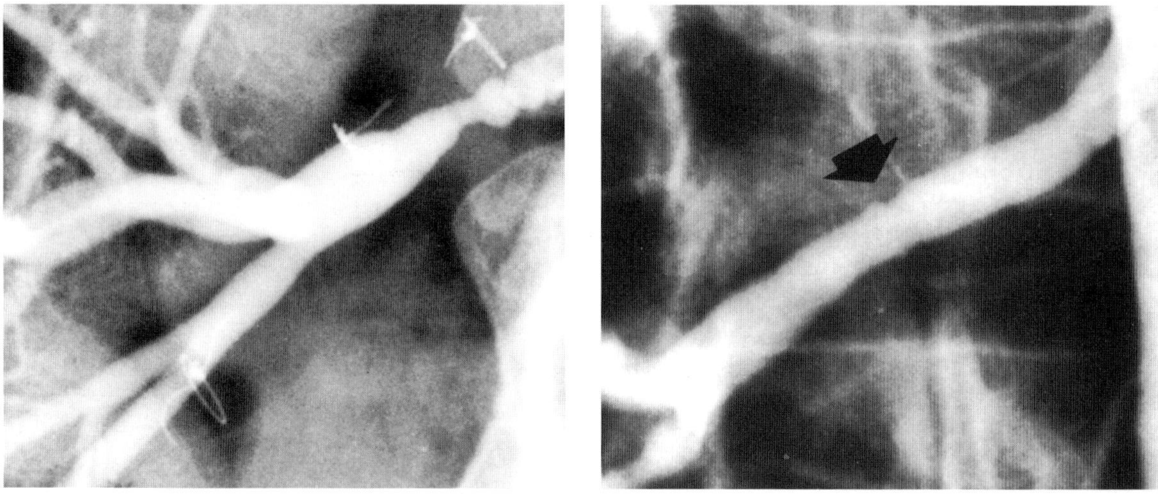

(a) (b)

Figure 27.4. Subadvential fibroplasia is demonstrated in a 24-year-old hypertensive woman. (a) Selective renal arteriogram shows a tight subadvential stenosis in the right renal artery. (b) Immediately following the dilatation, the lesion has opened up (arrow). From ref. 16, with permission.

fibroplasia.[8] In the University of Virginia series,[9] 46 (70%) of the 66 patients had medial fibroplasia. Intimal disease was present in 13 (20%) patients and 5 (8%) had subadventitial fibroplasia. One patient had a combination of medial and intimal fibroplasia and one patient had a combination of medial and subadventitial fibroplasia.

It is interesting to review the evolution of the treatment of FMD. The first patient known to have the disease, a 5-year-old boy, was successfully treated with a nephrectomy in 1938.[1] Surgical treatment subsequently evolved to the use of autologous vein grafting, autogenous tissue grafts or autotransplantation. In 1968 Morris *et al.*[10] reported on the intraoperative dilatation of stenoses in the carotid arteries caused by FMD. They had no recurrences up to 4 years later. Then in 1970, Fry *et al.*[11] described the use of small graduated surgical dilators, following surgical exposure of the renal artery, to treat three patients with FMD involving the renal arteries. In 1979, Houck[12] exposed a renal artery and used a Fogarty balloon to treat a 49-year-old woman with FMD. Simultaneously, percutaneous transluminal angioplasty was evolving. In 1964, Dotter and Judkins[13] described the use of coaxial vessel dilators, inserted percutaneously, to treat patients with atherosclerotic peripheral vascular disease. A decade later, Grüntzig and Hopff[14] developed the flexible double-lumen balloon catheter for the percutaneous treatment of arterial lesions. The versatility of the balloon catheter revolutionized the procedure and facilitated the treatment of stenosis and occlusions throughout the vascular tree. Grüntzig *et al.*[15] utilized PTRA to treat the first renal artery lesion, an atherosclerotic stenosis in a left renal artery in 1978. Considering the evolution of the treatment of FMD it was natural that PTRA would be used to treat renal artery stenosis due to FMD.[9, 16] Today it is apparent that PTRA is the treatment of choice in patients with FMD.

Technique

The techniques of renal angioplasty have been refined and simplified[17] since Grüntzig[15] first described the procedure. Renal angioplasty, however, remains more complex than peripheral angioplasty. It is far from innocuous and should be performed only by angiographers who have gained considerable experience dilating peripheral vessels.

A high quality preliminary midstream arteriogram is necessary to determine the best approach.

If an arteriogram has not been obtained within the previous month, a midstream abdominal arteriogram should be performed before selectively catheterizing a stenotic renal artery. The midstream arteriogram will reveal any recent change in the artery and its very helpful in determining the size of the angioplasty balloon. Characteristically the lesions of FMD involve the middle and distal portions of the main renal artery. Involvement of the proximal renal artery is uncommon. Kincaid *et al.*[8] found that the lesions extended into the renal artery branches in 39% of their 125 cases and isolated branch involvement was present in 6% of patients. Aberrant arteries, when present, were involved 44.4% of the time. Therefore the vascular architecture of the kidneys has to be evaluated in detail. This often necessitates selective oblique angiograms to evaluate fully the intrarenal branches.

It is very important to complete the diagnostic portion of the study before proceeding to PTRA. The characteristics and locations of all the lesions should be known before attempting to cross and dilate the lesions. This approach avoids undetected lesions and turns in the arteries that can lead to poor results.

The renal artery is approached either from the femoral or the left axillary artery. Most patients, however, can be treated from the femoral approach. Either the standard over-the-wire balloon or the coaxial TEGwire ST system may be employed. The stenoses in FMD tend to occur in the distal two-thirds of the main renal artery and may involve the branches of the renal artery. This makes it more difficult to cross the lesions with the over-the-wire technique. Therefore we prefer the TEGwire ST system for most cases (Fig. 27.5).

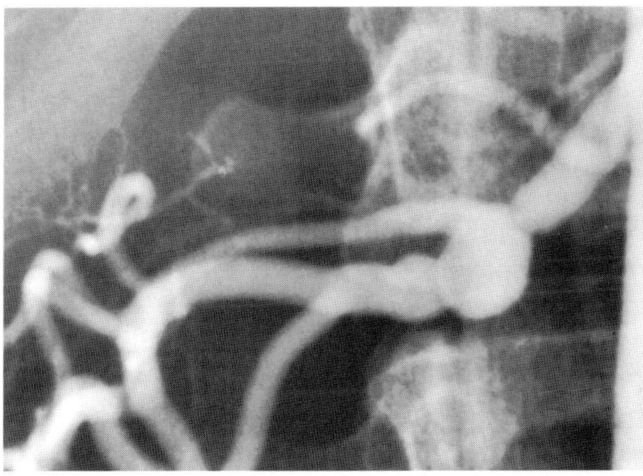

(a)

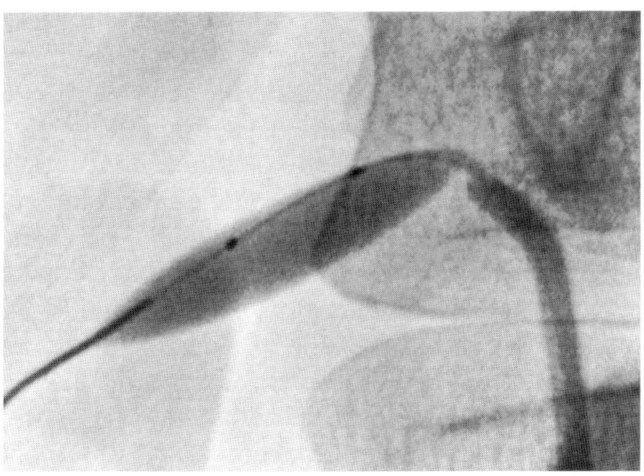

(b)

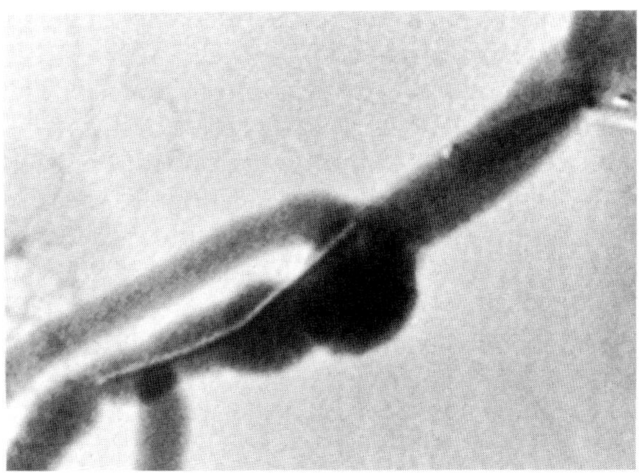

(c)

Figure 27.5. The technique of PTRA with the TEGwire ST system employed in a 38-year-old woman with a 15-year history of hypertension. (a) The midstream arteriogram reveals bilateral FMD. Several tight pleats are seen in the midportion of the right renal artery. The disease extends into the main branches. (b) The orifice of the renal artery is selected with the guiding catheter and a 6 mm TEGwire is used to dilate the lesion. (c) The follow-up angiogram obtained through the guiding catheter shows a good result. The balloon is still across the lesion.

The TEGwire ST system has simplified the conventional coaxial technique.[18] It consists of a low profile polyethylene teraphthalate balloon mounted on a highly torqueable 0.035 inch guidewire shaft. The TEGwire ST has a flexible, 2 cm long, 0.014 inch shapeable tip. The balloon is available in 3, 4, 5, and 6 mm diameters. The 3 and 4 mm balloons fit through a 6 F guide. A 7 F guiding catheter is necessary for the 5 and 6 mm balloons. The balloons are available in 1.3 cm and 2 cm lengths for renal angioplasty.

The appropriately shaped guiding catheter is inserted through a 7 F sheath over a 0.035 inch guidewire. The guidewire is removed, and the renal artery is gently selected. The TEGwire 1.3 cm length balloon is inserted in the guiding catheter. The position of the guiding catheter is checked with a gentle injection of contrast material. The TEGwire balloon catheter is directed across the stenosis. Contrast material is injected through the guiding catheter to confirm the position of the balloon. Heparin 2000–5000 iu, and verapamil 2.5 mg, are then injected through the guiding catheter. The balloon is positioned across the stenosis and inflated. The result is checked by performing dignital subtraction angiography (DSA) through the guiding catheter while the deflated balloon remains across the lesion.

The TEGwire ST system has several advantages. It simplifies renal angioplasty by eliminating the need for guidewire and catheter exchanges. The low profile balloon on a 0.035 inch shaft is ideal for crossing tight renal artery stenosis. The balloon has great torque control, so it can be directed across the long tortuous lesions often seen in FMD. The follow-up renal angiogram is easily obtained through the coaxial guiding catheter, while the deflated balloon is still in place across the lesion. A disadvantage of the system is that balloons above 6 mm are not currently available; however, they will be in the near future.

Treatment and prevention of vascular spasm

Spasm of the main renal artery or of a major arterial branch is a frequent occurrence during renal angioplasty[19] (Fig. 27.6). It is especially pronounced in children and young adult patients with FMD. This is usually caused by mechanical stimulation of the vessel wall by the guidewire or catheter and may occur locally or at a distance. If possible, the guidewire should not be placed within the segmental branches of the renal artery. Focal spasm may also be produced in the area adjacent to the angioplasty site or even in distal small branches. Calcium channel blockers are highly effective in preventing and reversing spasm in the renal arteries. At the University of Virginia, adult patients are prophylactically given 2.5 mg of verapamil hydrochloride intra-arterially through the diagnostic or guiding catheter as soon as the lesion is crossed. If spasm is encountered, another 2.5 mg of verapamil is given intra-arterially. There has been a marked decrease in the number of patients experiencing spasm during PTRA since we instituted this protocol. Alternatively adult patients scheduled for renal angioplasty can be pretreated with nifedipine in a dose of 10–20 mg orally or sublingually, 30 min before the procedure. If spasm occurs in spite of the calcium channel blockers, nitroglycerine in a dose of 100–200 μg is given intra-arterially. Nitroglycerine is very effective in relieving spasm, but its mechanism of action is different from that of the calcium channel antagonists. It has an additive effect when given with calcium channel blockers, so it is very effective when spasm is encountered after the blocker has been administered. We prefer to use the calcium channel blockers initially because the duration of action is longer than that of nitroglycerine. Verapamil has the advantage of being available in a liquid parenteral form. Nifedipine, on the other hand, is the most potent vasodilator of the calcium channel blockers available. Calcium channel blockers may induce hypotension, so they should be used with caution in patients who have known cardiac conduction defects. Verapamil has a greater effect on cardiac conduction than the other calcium channel blockers. It is also important to remember that the guidewire is the major cause of spasm and that continued stimulation of the vessel wall will cause spasm to recur. All catheter and guidewire manipulations should be kept to a minimum, and the most effective treatment of spasm is to remove the catheter and guidewire.

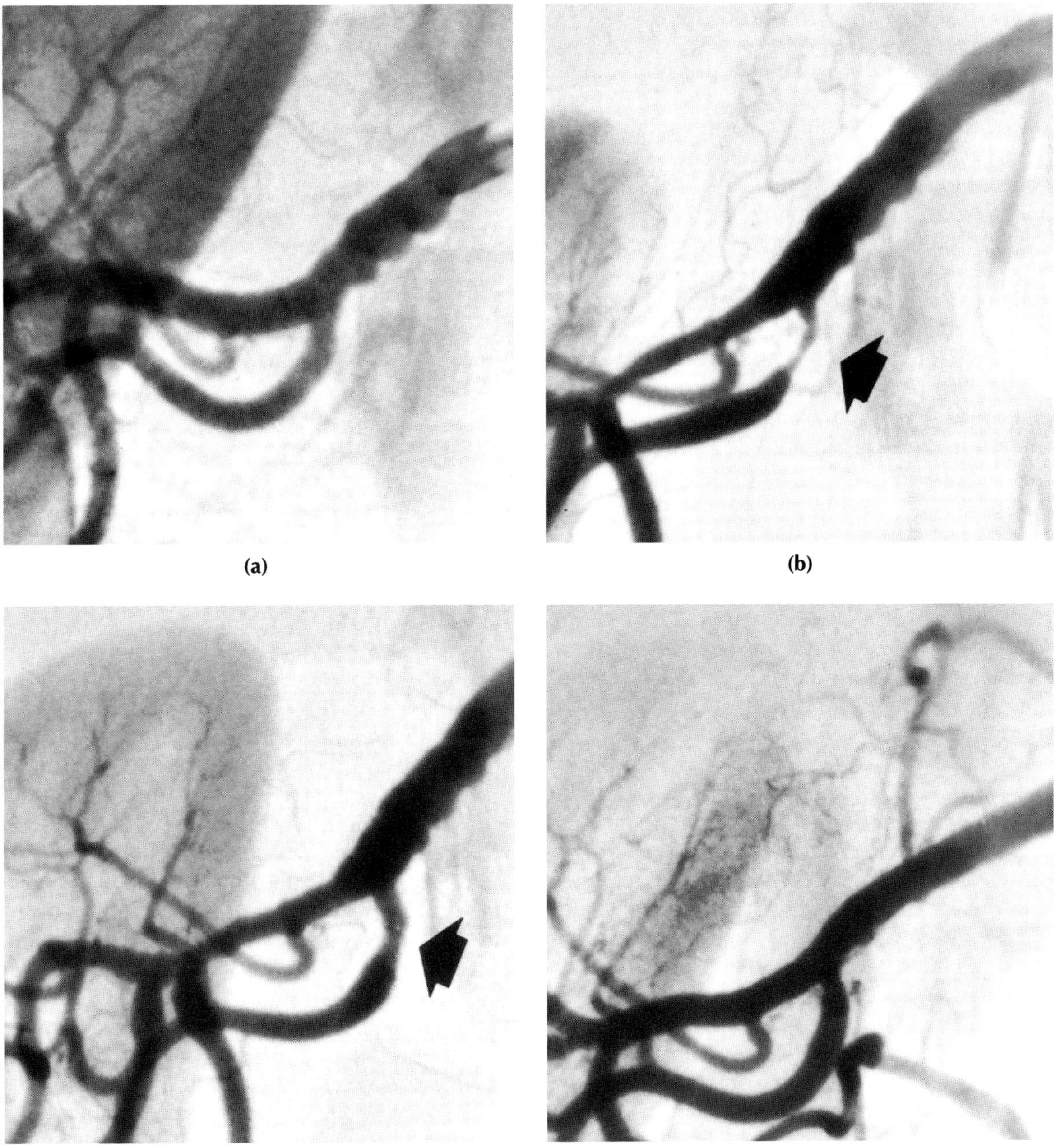

Figure 27.6. Spasm caused by inflating the angioplasty balloon is illustrated in a 38-year-old hypertensive woman. (a) The selective renal arteriogram shows medial fibroplasia. (b) Immediately following PTRA, the lesion is widely patent, however severe narrowing is noted in a major branch of the renal artery (arrow). (c) Following administration of an antispasmodic drug, the vessel has opened up (arrow). (d) A follow-up arteriogram obtained 4.5 months later shows that the previously dilated lesion has smoothed up considerably and that the spastic branch is wide open. From ref. 16, with permission.

Patient periprocedure management

Proper treatment of candidates for renal angioplasty requires a team approach. The proper selection of patients and the periprocedural management of the blood pressure require the close cooperation of a hypertension specialist. Inadvertent occlusion or rupture of the renal artery may create a surgical emergency. Therefore, the procedure should be performed only when a skilled vascular surgeon is available, because the complexity of renal reconstruction may be increased after PTRA.[20] Before renal angioplasty, the patient's blood pressure should be controlled by angiotensin converting enzyme inhibitors, such as captopril or enalopril, whenever possible. These agents pharmacologically inhibit the production of angiotensin II, the active hypertensive substance in renin-mediated renovascular hypertension. The pharmacological action of these agents is physiologically the same as that of a successful renal angioplasty. For this reason, sudden drastic drops of blood pressure due to removal of the renin–angiotensin–aldosterone effect following successful angioplasty are not as pronounced when patients are treated with these drugs.

Because of the complexity of the procedure and the potential for volatile changes in blood pressure following the procedure, renal angioplasty should not be considered an outpatient procedure. The blood pressure must be monitored very carefully during the first 24–48 h following PTRA because profound changes may, nevertheless, occur. If the diastolic pressure rises above 110 mmHg, the blood pressure should be controlled by a repeat dose of captopril or nifedipine, or with a rapid and short-acting, parenteral antihypertensive drugs such as labetolol. A drop in blood pressure can usually be controlled by rapid intravenous infusion of normal saline. Therefore, all patients undergoing renal angioplasty should have an intravenous line in place prior to the procedure.

At the University of Virginia, the adult patient receives 2000 iu of heparin subcutaneously every 6 h following PTRA unless it contraindicated. Heparin administration is begun 8 h after the procedure and continued for 2 days. Patients also receive 75 mg dipyridamole (Persantin®; Boehringer Ingelheim, Ridgefield, CO) orally twice a day and 325 mg of aspirin once a day beginning the day of angioplasty and continuing for at least 6 months. Patients are encouraged to stop smoking. After angioplasty, the patient should be checked by a physician who specializes in the control of high blood pressure. The patient's blood pressure medication will need to be adjusted following the procedure. Therefore, the patient's blood pressure must be monitored closely. If the blood pressure rises in the ensuing months, repeat arteriography should be performed.

Complications

The complication rate following renal angioplasty varies from 5 to 10%. A meta-analysis of the literature reveals that in 1118 patients undergoing PTRA the complications rate is 9.3%.[21] Renal failure was excluded in the analysis. In the University of Virginia series[9] 12 complications were seen in 93 procedures performed on patients with FMD (Table 27.1). Spasm was the most prevalent complication. In all cases the spasm was relieved by antispasmodic medication (Fig. 27.6). Perforation of the renal artery is more prevalent in fibromuscular lesions than in atherosclerotic lesions. This is because of the corrugated tortuous nature of the medial and subadventitial lesions. The lesions are also easier to perforate than atherosclerotic lesions. In our series, two patients experienced perforation of their renal arteries. Both patients were successfully handled percutaneously. In one, the perforation was successfully sealed by recrossing the lesion and dilating the lesion. In the other, a renal branch artery was perforated and

Table 27.1. Twelve complications in 93 renal procedures (10 patients)

Complications	Patients (*N*)
Spasm of renal artery	5
Upper pole branch occluded	1
Perforation of renal artery	2
Brachial plexus injury	1
Blood loss (transfused 2 units packed cells)	2
Exacerbation of chronic renal insufficiency	1
Total	12

From ref. 9, with permission.

the branch was successfully occluded with a Gianturcco coil. The renal artery was successfully dilated. Subsequent to the analysis of this series another patient had the artery perforated during PTRA. The lesions were successfully dilated but the perforation did not seal. The balloon was inflated and intermittently deflated controlling the leak. The patient was taken to the operating room and the perforation was sutured. Fibromuscular lesions are more difficult to cross than atherosclerotic lesions so care must be taken when crossing the lesions to avoid perforation or subintimal dissection. It is often helpful to have the patients take a deep breath to straighten the artery before attempting to cross the lesion.

Results of PTRA in FMD

Renal angioplasty is a highly effective method for treating renal artery lesions in experienced hands. The best results are achieved in patients with FMD.[9, 16] When compared with atherosclerotic disease, the patients are usually younger and have less associated risk factors. In the University of Virginia series[9] the mean age of the patients was 45 years, the median age was 47 years. The average duration of hypertension was 8.2 years and the hypertension was refractory to medical management in 46 of the 66 patients. The disease is frequently bilateral and in our series 34 of the 66 patients had bilateral lesions of 50% or greater.

A meta-analysis of 370 FMD patients treated with PTRA for angiotensinogenic hypertension reveals that 94% of the 345 patients in whom the data was available were considered technically successful, (Table 27.2). Following successful PTRA the long-term follow-up reveals that 49% of the patients were classified as cured and 43% of the patients were considered improved. Therefore of the 324 reported long-term results 92% of the patients benefited from the procedure.

In the University of Virginia series,[9] all 66 patients with 85 FMD lesions received an initial benefit. In our series, life-table analysis revealed a 10-year predicted long-term patency rate of 87.07% (Fig. 27.7 and Table 27.3). This analysis excluded secondary patency. Klinge *et al.*[25] achieved similar results with a cumulative 5-year patency rate of 89%.

The primary patency rate in the literature analysis was 85% and the secondary patency, which includes those patients requiring a second PTRA procedure, was 93%. In our series[9] the primary patency rate was 91% and the secondary patency rate was 98%. The restenosis rate in our series was 8% of lesions and 10% of patients.[9] Martin *et al.*[21] reported a similar 11.5% rate of restenosis in FMD lesions in a meta-analysis of the literature. Analysis of the six recurrences in

Table 27.2. Results of PTRA–hypertension in FMD

Series	No. of patients	Technical success *N*	Technical success %	Cure *N*	Cure %	Clinical results[a] improve *N*	Clinical results[a] improve %	Benefits *N*	Benefits %	Follow-up (months) range
Rodríguez-Pérez *et al.* 1994[22]	27	25/27	92	6/12	50	3/12	25	9/12	75	96
Tegtmeyer *et al.* 1991[9]	66	66/66	100	26/66	39	39/66	59	65/66	98	1–121
Baert *et al.* 1990[23]	22	19/22	86	11/19	58	4/19	21	15/19	79	6–72
Greminger *et al.* 1989[24]	34	30/34	88	14/30	47	16/30	53	30/30	100	6–48
Klinge *et al.* 1989[25]	52	47/52	90	18/47	38	26/47	55	44/47	94	
Beebe *et al.* 1988[26]	9	9/9	100	3/9	33	5/9	55	8/9	88	6–60
Simonetti *et al.* 1987[27]	25			15/25	60	6/25	24	21/25	84	
Bell *et al.* 1987[28]	8	7/8	88	5/7	71	2/7	29	7/7	100	12
Kremer Hovinga *et al.* 1986[29]	10	10/10	100							4
Grim *et al.* 1986[30]	26	26/26	100	15/26	58	9/26	35	24/26	92	1
Martin LG *et al.* 1985[31]	20	20/20	100	5/20	25	12/20	60	17/20	85	3–36
Miller *et al.* 1985[32]	15	15/15	100	11/13	85	2/13	15	13/13	100	6–36
Sos *et al.* 1983[33]	31	27/31	87	16/27	59	9/27	33	25/27	93	4–40
Mahler *et al.* 1982[34]	6	6/6	100	5/6	83	1/6	17	6/6	100	12–47
Colapinto *et al.* 1982[35]	11	9/11	82	4/9	44	5/9	55	9/9	100	1–36
Martin EC *et al.* 1981[36]	8	8/8	100	5/8	63	1/8	13	6/8	75	4–25
	370	324/345	94	159/324	49	140/324	43	299/324	92	

[a]Initial technical failures are excluded.

Table 27.3. Long-term response: life-table analysis of 66 FMD patients

Follow-up period (months)	Patient arteries (*N*) Beginning of interval	End follow-up	Recurrences (*N*)	Failure rate (%)	Patency rate (%)	Cumulative patency rate (%)	SEM of cumulative patency rate (%)
0–12	66	13	2	3.36	96.64	100.0	0.0
12–24	51	12	2	4.44	95.56	96.64	2.34
24–36	37	4	2	5.71	94.29	92.34	3.71
36–48	31	8	0	0.0	100.0	87.07	5.04
48–60	23	7	0	0.0	100.0	87.07	5.04
60–72	16	5	0	0.01	100.0	87.07	5.04
72–84	11	3	0	0.01	100.0	87.07	5.04
84–96	8	2	0	0.0	100.0	87.07	5.04
96–108	6	5	0	0.0	100.0	87.07	5.04
108–120	1	1	0	0.0	100.0	87.07	5.04

From ref. 9 with permission.

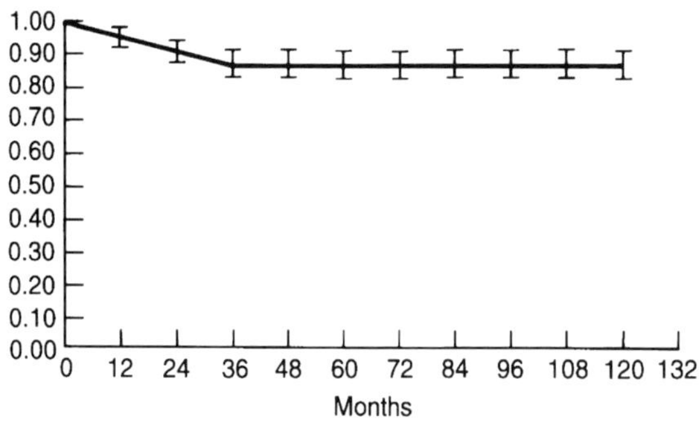

Figure 27.7. Plot of long-term response for 66 patients with fibromuscular disease. Patients were followed for as long as 121 months after PTRA. Life-table method of analysis was used to calculate predicted long-term patency rate. From ref. 9, with permission.

our series shows that four lesions were initially underdilated (Table 27.4). The underdilated lesions were due to medial fibroplasia. It is often difficult to select the correct balloon size in medial fibroplasia because the 'beads' are larger than the original size of the artery. It is prudent to be conservative rather than overdilating and rupturing the artery. Five of the six recurrent lesions were successfully redilated. The one long-term failure was a patient with a smooth tubular stenosis, intimal fibroplasia. We have experienced other examples of failure to dilate focal smooth lesions since reporting the series. This unusual manifestation of FMD may be difficult to dilate. Higher balloon pressures are often necessary to dilate the lesions. Archibald *et al.*[37] successfully dilated focal lesions in four out of five patients and reviewed the literature finding that 81% of these focal lesions responded satisfactorily to PTRA. Medial and subadventitial lesions are more difficult to cross with the balloon but respond better to PTRA than intimal (focal) stenoses.

Recurrent FMD lesions are generally easier to dilate than the initial lesions.[38, 39] This is because the plicae have been disrupted and follow-up studies indicate that most fibromuscular lesions smooth up with time. Therefore it is much easier to cross the lesion during repeat dilatation. It is also clear that it is important to obtain a good initial result. If a 30% or greater residual stenosis remains, the lesion is likely to recur.[39]

Segmental renal arteries are involved in 39% of the cases with FMD. Controversy exists with regards to the optimal treatment of FMD lesions when the segmental branches are involved. Some surgeons feel that branch stenoses increase the technical difficulty of PTRA and that this type of lesion should be treated surgically.[40] However, surgical revascularization is much more complicated when the disease extends into the branches. Cluzel *et al.*[41] have recently reported on the results of PTRA involving the renal branch arteries. They treated 20 consecutive patients with 25 branch artery stenoses caused by FMD. They were technically successful in 21 of the 25 stenoses (84%). The stenoses recurred in 9% of the lesions, however, these lesions were easily redilated. The results of Cluzel *et al.* confirm our experience (Fig. 27.8). Renal artery branch stenoses due to FMD are amenable to PTRA. Improvement in equipment and techniques now allow these lesions to be success-

Table 27.4. Analysis of patients with recurrent FMD stenoses

Age (years)/sex	Classification of FMD side	Initial stenosis	Side dilated	Time of recurrence (months)	Redilated (*N*)	Long-term response (months)
40/F	Medial R	80	R	3	1	I (112)
	Medial L	25				
50/F	Medial R	Cannot grade	R	0	1	I (36)
	Medial L	Cannot grade	L	27[a]		
66/F	Medial R	Cannot grade	R	27	1	I (36)
	Medial L	10			(dilated L)	
20/F	Intimal R	80	R	6	2	NI (21)
		Small aneurysms	L			
40/F	Medial R[b]	99	R	16[a]	1	I (25)
	Medial L	90	L	16[a]	1	
43/F	Medial L	80	L	15[a]	1	C (18)
	R nephrectomy					

C: cure; I: improved; NI: not improved.
[a] Underdilated initially.
[b] Atherosclerotic lesion also dilated.
In one additional patient, one atherosclerotic recurrence was redilated twice.
From ref. 9 with permission.

fully dilated. The procedure is more complex than dilating the main renal artery and only angioplasters experienced in treating renal lesions should attempt these lesions. However, it is clear that in experienced hands the first-line treatment for hypertension due to renal branch stenosis in FMD should be PTRA. Surgery should be reserved for the lesions in which PTRA is unsuccessful.

Conclusion

Clearly PTRA is the initial treatment of choice in hypertension caused by fibromuscular dysplasia. The initial success rate is high and the restenosis rate is low. The fibromuscular lesions continue to improve dramatically with time after PTRA. In many patients, minimal or no disease is seen on long-term angiographic follow-up. It is easy to redilate the recurrences because the lesions are easier to cross the second time.

Pediatric renal angioplasty

Hypertension is being increasingly recognized in children, because of a heightened awareness. Approximately 2% of all children have hypertension and 10% of these children have severe hypertension.[42] A child younger than 12 years of age who has a diastolic blood pressure over 90 mmHg or one 13–18 years of age who has a diastolic pressure over 100 mmHg should be considered to have severe hypertension.[43] Although essential hypertension occurs in this age group, the incidence of secondary hypertension is much higher than in the adult population. In the etiology of severe persistent hypertension in the pediatric age group, renovascular lesions rank second in importance after renal parenchymal disease. In children with renal arterial disease the clinical findings are often non-specific and the customary adult screening procedures are often negative.[44] The child with hypertension is often asymptomatic but may present with headaches, epistaxis, anorexia or a failure to thrive. Because it is a potentially correctable condition that can permanently damage renal function it is important not to overlook the diagnosis of renovascular hypertension. The child with a high index of suspicion for having angiotensingenic hypertension based on the presence of unexplained severe hypertension should undergo angiography.[45] The yield is high, renovascular lesions account for up to 25% of the secondary hypertension in children who undergo renal arteriography for hypertension.[46, 47]

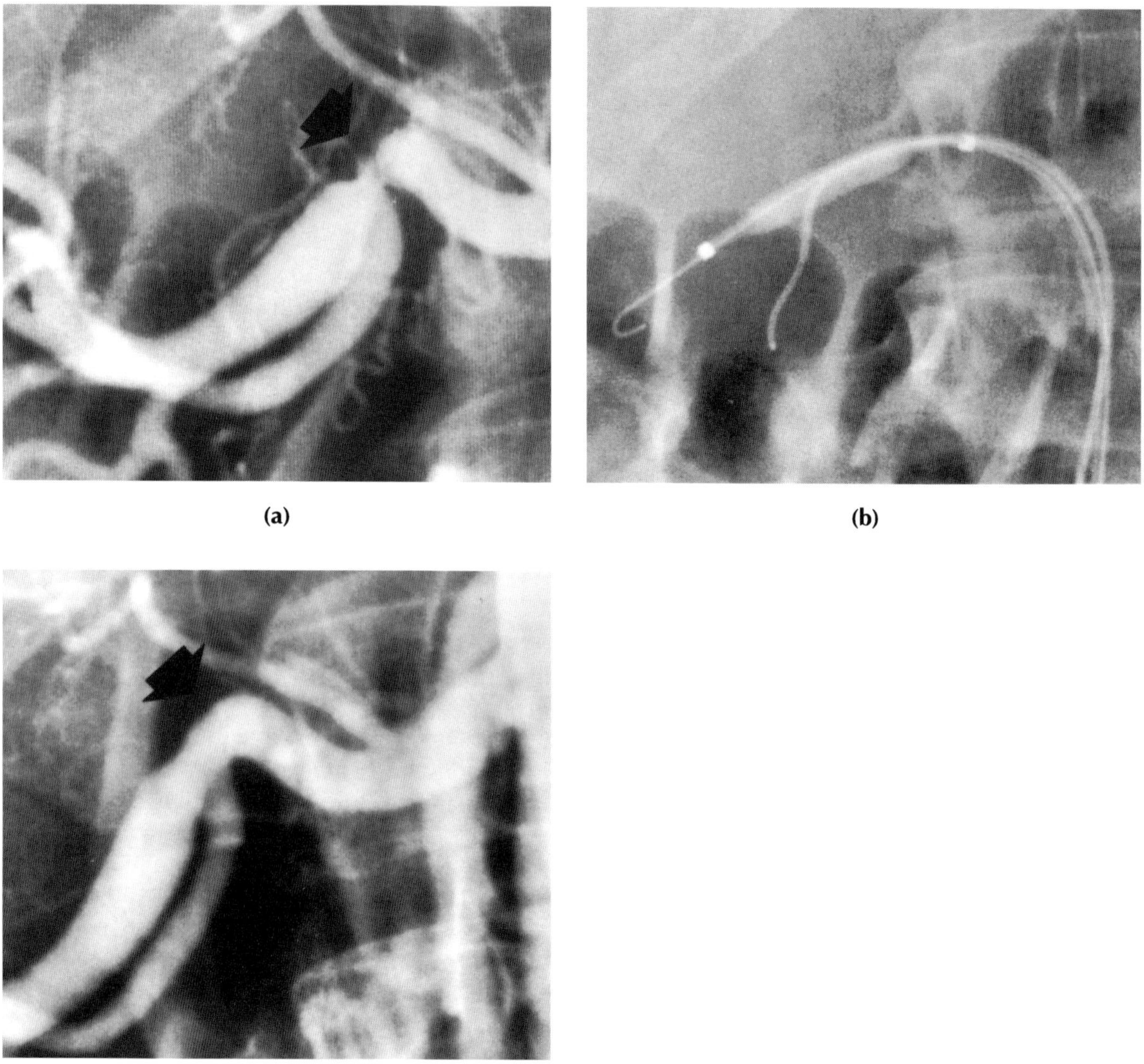

(a) (b) (c)

Figure 27.8. PTRA in a branch stenosis is demonstrated. (a) A selective arteriogram shows a tight stenosis at the junction of the dorsal and ventral branches of the renal artery. (b) The spot film shows the balloon inflated across the upper branch, dilating the lesion, a catheter is in the lower branch protecting the orifice of the artery. (c) Immediately after PTRA, the renal artery and both branches are widely patent. From ref. 17, with permission.

Techniques

A high quality midstream arteriogram should always be performed prior to selecting the renal artery, unless an arteriogram has already been performed within the previous month. The diagnostic arteriogram is usually performed through the femoral approach in children. In young children a 4 F pigtail catheter is employed; in older children a 4 or 5 F catheter is utilized. Following the midstream arteriogram, detailed selective renal arteriograms in the oblique projections should be performed. Selective angiograms are necessary because branch stenoses are more prevalent in the pediatric population (Fig. 27.9). If stenoses are seen in the main renal arteries, a lateral view of the aorta should also be obtained to show the origins of the mesenteric vessels.

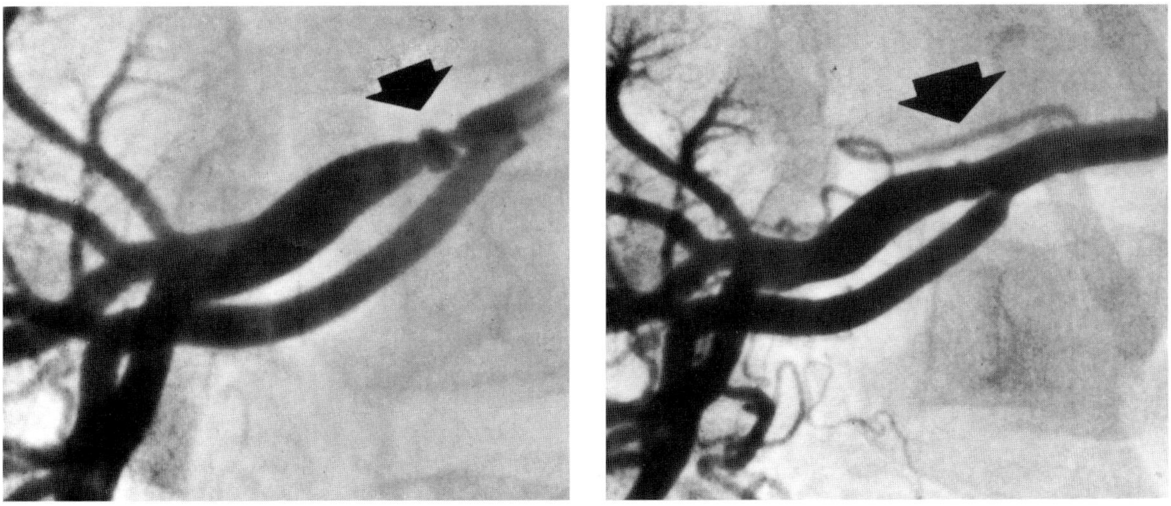

(a) (b)

Figure 27.9. PTRA is illustrated in a 9-year-old girl with hypertension (160/120 mmHg). (a) The selective renal arteriogram reveals a short tight lesion due to FMD in her dorsal branch (arrow). (b) Immediately following PTRA the vessel is widely patent (arrow). She is normotensive 63 months following PTRA (117/78). From ref. 16, with permission.

Robinson *et al.*[48] found the mesenteric vessels were involved in 62.5% of their cases of middle aortic syndrome and in 33% of their cases with neurofibromatosis. FMD may also involve the mesenteric vessels. Digital subtraction angiography is very helpful to reduce the contrast levels in pediatric patients.

Once the diagnosis is established, the involved renal artery is carefully selected with a 4 or 5 F diagnostic catheter, usually a 'shepherds crook' catheter is utilized. A soft-tipped wire, such as a Bentson wire or a 0.014 guidewire with a 0.035 open-ended guidewire over it is advanced across the stenosis under fluoroscopic control. The diagnostic catheter is then advanced across the stenosis over the guidewire. Once the catheter is in position, the wire is removed and diluted contrast material is injected to ascertain the intraluminal position of the catheter. Next, to reduce problems with thrombi and vasospasm, heparin (50 iu/kg) and verapamil (1.0–2.5 mg) are injected through the catheter. A tight J-movable core guidewire or a Rosen wire is inserted and in younger children with small arteries a 4 F catheter is employed. The diagnostic catheter is exchanged for the appropriate balloon catheter. In older children, we now prefer to use the TEGwire ST system for renal angioplasty whenever possible.

An alternative technique is utilized in some cases. If the stenosis is located in the distal branches of the renal artery, and there is not enough room distally to park the tip of the TEGwire balloon, the Grüntzig-guided coaxial system is used (Fig. 27.10). This system is the same as that used for coronary dilatation. The system employs an 8 F guiding catheter, which is used to select the orifice of the renal artery and a 4 F coaxial balloon catheter. The balloon catheter is passed through the guiding catheter and into the main renal artery. A 0.014 inch steerable guidewire is threaded through the balloon catheter and directed across the stenosis under fluoroscopic control. The balloon catheter is then passed over the guidewire and across the lesion and the stenosis is dilated. Contrast can be injected through the guiding catheter to monitor the progress of the dilatation.

Etiology

The causes of renal artery stenosis in children are different from those of adults.[44, 49] In adults

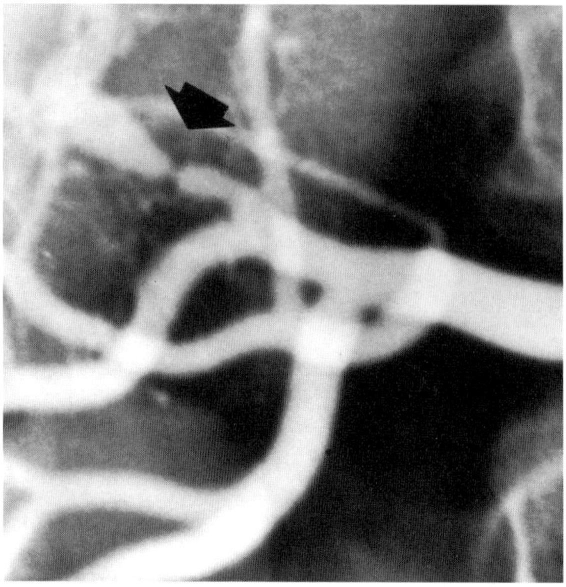

(a)

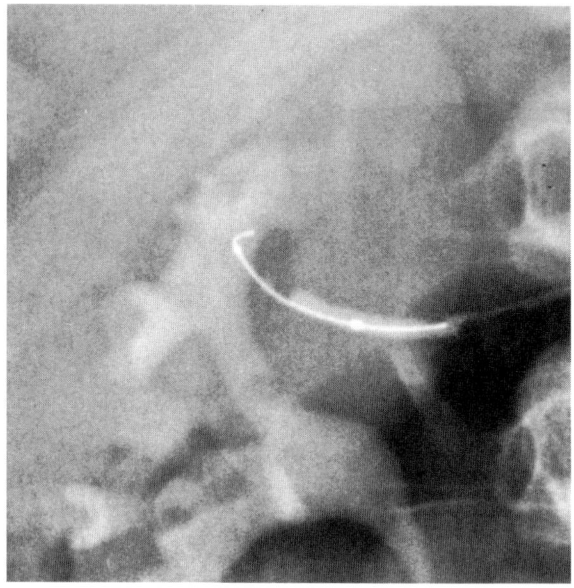

(b)

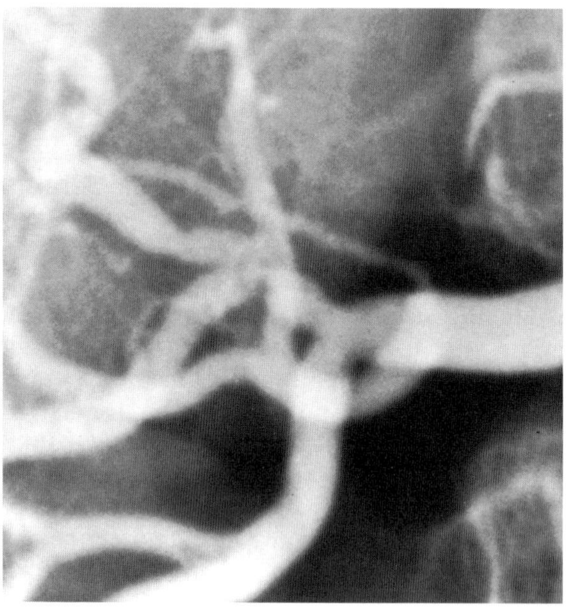

(c)

Figure 27.10. Coronary system is used to dilate an intrarenal branch stenosis in an 11-year-old boy with hypertension. (a) The selective renal arteriogram demonstrates a tight stenosis (arrow) in an interlobar branch to the upper pole. Note the poststenotic dilatation. (b) The balloon is shown dilating the lesion. (c) Immediately following PTRA the branch is widely patent. The blood pressure was 106/56 mmHg, 6 months post-PTRA. From ref. 52, with permission.

atherosclerosis is the most common cause of renal artery disease and FMD accounts for most of the remaining cases. In children there is a greater range of etiologies. The causes of renal artery disease include: fibromuscular dysplasia, neurofibromatosis, Williams' syndrome, arteritis, middle aortic syndrome and trauma.

Fibromuscular dysplasia

Renal artery stenoses in the majority of children are caused by FMD.[43, 44, 50] Moreover, stenoses in the renal artery branches are seen as often as major renal artery disease in children.[43] In adults main artery disease is more common. The classic 'string of beads' appearance of medial fibroplasia is not as common in children as it is in adults. In children focal or tubular stenoses, due to intimal fibroplasia or fibromuscular hyperplasia, are seen most frequently.

In children, PTRA for correction of FMD is more difficult than in adults because the vessels are smaller and access is more difficult. The lesions often involve the branches and very tight stenoses are usually seen (Fig. 27.10). The lesions are more resistant to balloon angioplasty in contrast to adult FMD lesions, and frequently require high balloon pressures to open the arteries. However, with the development of miniballoon catheters many of these lesions can be reached and crossed with balloon catheters.

Analysis of the results of PTRA in children is complicated by the fact that segmental stenoses often seen in children can have different etiologies. Therefore some authors[47, 51] have chosen to categorize their results according to the location and length of the stenosis, rather than by etiology. Some of the patients in these reports are undoubtedly due to FMD, but because no etiology is ascribed to these patients, they are excluded from this analysis. A review of the literature and the experience at the University of Virginia[52] reveals that at least 25 pediatric patients with lesions described as due to FMD have undergone PTRA (Table 27.5). There were 12 males and 12 females, in one patient no sex was designated. The initial technical success rate was high. Twenty-three (92%) patients were described as having undergone a completely successful PTRA procedure. One patient, a 19-year-old female, was described as a partial success, because one side was corrected initially. The other side was subsequently corrected by PTRA at another institution.[59] The only short-term failure was in our series. In our case the smooth tight lesions in the proximal portions of both renal arteries, required high pressure but appeared to respond initially to PTRA. However, the blood pressure did not respond and a follow-up angiogram 22 days later showed no change in the arteries. The failure was due to

Table 27.5. Results of pediatric PTRA–hypertension in FMD

Series	Age (years)	Sex	Technical success	Clinical results Cure	Improve	Benefits	Months	Follow-up	Result
McCook *et al.* 1980[53]	3,6/12	F	Good	✓		✓	5	(90/60)	Normotensive
Mathias *et al.* 1981[54]	5	M	Good	✓		✓	10	(126/80)	Normotensive
Paolini *et al.* 1981[55]	16	M	Good	✓		✓	8	(110/80)	Normotensive
	17	M	Good	✓		✓	5	(110/70)	Normotensive
Ghisla *et al.* 1983[56]	4, 6/12	M	Good	✓		✓	18	(102/70)	Normotensive
Lund *et al.* 1984[57]	13	M	Good			❍		(160/104)	Residual hypertension Contralateral disease
	15	M	Good	✓		✓		(120/70)	Normotensive
Stanley *et al.* 1984[58]	11	M	Good			❍	10	(126/92)	Rx recurrence surgery
	1,10/12	F	Good	✓		✓	24	(100/60)	Normotensive
	7	F	Good	✓		✓	12	(100/60)	Normotensive
	12	M	Good	✓		✓	18	(126/74)	Normotensive
Millan *et al.* 1985[59]	19	F	Partial one side	✓		✓	62	(130/90)	PTRA otherside later Normotensive
	10	M	Good	✓		✓	44	(118/68)	Normotensive
	12	F	Good	✓		✓	25	(100/70)	Normotensive
Fallo *et al.* 1986[60]	11, 6/12	F	Good	✓		✓	15	(105/70)	Normotensive
	9, 2/12	F	Good	✓		✓	14	(110/70)	Normotensive
	22	F	Good		✓	✓	19	(150/100)	BP easier to control
	4, 2/12	F	Good	✓		✓	8	(100/60)	Normotensive
Robinson *et al.* 1991[48]	3		Good		✓	✓			
	6	F	Good		✓	✓	10		
Tegtmeyer (present series)	9	F	Good	✓		✓	63	(117/78)	Normotensive
	11	M	Good	✓		✓	6	(106/56)	Normotensive
	17	M	Good	✓		✓	95		Normotensive
	12	M	Fair			❍	1	(140/95)	Rx surgery
	1,2/12	M	Good	✓		✓			

Rx: treated with

elastic recoil of the lesions. The lesions were subsequently corrected with surgery. The pathology reports showed medial fibroplasia with severe secondary intimal fibroplasia.

Although follow-up is short, 22 patients (88%) received a long-term benefit from the procedure. There have been only three failures. The cure rate is surprisingly high. Nineteen patients (76%) have been described as cured by PTRA. They are all normotensive and off all antihypertensive medications. The results of PTRA in children suggest that in experienced hands PTRA should be the initial treatment of choice for FMD lesions in the pediatric age groups.

Neurofibromatosis

Neurofibromatosis was first described by Von Recklinghausen in 1882 as a hamartomatous disorder derived from the neural crest involving ectodermal, neuroectodermal and mesodermal tissue. It is an inherited disorder, transmitted as a simple dominant trait with variable penetrance.

Hypertension in patients with neurofibromatoses may result from either coarctation of the aorta, pheochromocytoma or renal artery stenosis. In elderly patients the hypertension is usually secondary to pheochromocytoma, however, in younger patients the hypertension is usually due to renal artery stenoses. Vascular lesions are more common in patients with neurofibromatoses than is generally recognized.[61] Angiographic abnormalities that have been described include: aortic coarctation (usually abdominal), aortic branch lesions and arterial aneurysms. Involvement of the renal arteries is the most frequently reported site.[62] Associated narrowing of the abdominal aorta is seen in approximately 25% of patients. Analysis of the 12 patients who underwent PTRA for correction of renal arterial lesions (Table 27.6) shows that three of these patients had angiographically detectable involvement of the abdominal aorta. The disease may be unilateral or bilateral. It was reported as bilateral in 6 of the 12 patients undergoing PTRA.

Itzchak *et al.*[63] described the distinctive angiographic features of aortic branch lesions seen in many cases of neurofibromatosis. The involved arteries have a smooth stenotic segment continuing into an enlarged funnel-shaped channel. These changes, however, are also seen in other entities such as Takayasu's disease. Reubi[61] and Feyrter[64] were the first to define the histopathology of the vascular lesions in the kidney seen in neurofibromatosis. Their descriptions were extended by the Salyers.[62] There are four types: pure intimal, advanced intimal, intimal aneurysmal and nodular. There is frequently an overlap of features, including intimal proliferation, thinning of the media, fragmentation of the elastic tissue and fibrosis giving the lesions a variable appearance. The Salyers suggested a common pathogenesis that of proliferation of Schwann cells within the arterial walls and secondary degenerative changes.

Table 27.6. Results of PTRA—neurofibromatosis

Series	Age (years)	Sex	Technical success	Clinical results Cure	Improve	Benefits	Months	Follow-up	Result
Martin, EC *et al.* 1980[66]	10	F	Poor initially	✓		✓	6		Normotensive
Baxi *et al.* 1981[67]	19	F	Good	✓		✓	3	(120/60)	Normotensive
Guzzetta *et al.* 1983[68]	3	M	Failure						Rx surgery
Lund *et al.* 1984[57]	10	M	Poor					(140/90)	Rx surgery
Millan *et al.* 1985[59]	13	M	Poor						Rx surgery
	20	M	Partial one side						Rx surgery
	15	M	Poor						Rx surgery
Mallman and Roth 1986[69]	12	F	Good		✓	✓	81		Mild controlled hypertension
Mali *et al.* 1987[51]	13	F	Poor initially		✓	✓	14	(145/55)	Rx medically
Gardiner *et al.* 1988[70]	29	M	Poor initially	✓		✓	5		Normotensive
Robinson *et al.* 1991[48]	5	M	Poor × 2						Rx surgery One side failed
Tegtmeyer (present series)	9	M	Fair × 2	✓		✓	50		Normotensive

Rx: treated with

There are two basic categories of vascular lesions associated with the disease.[65] The first involves larger vessels such as the aorta and proximal renal arteries. The vessels are surrounded with neurofibromatous or ganglioneuromatous tissue. The vessel wall itself may be involved with changes as well. The second type is seen in the vessel walls and may involve all the layers of the wall. These changes are felt to reflect a mesodermal dysplasia.[65] The changes occur in multiple arteries and involve the small intrarenal branches. The changes, when present in the small branches, make both surgical repair and PTRA difficult.

Neurofibromatosis is a relatively uncommon condition so experience with PTRA in these patients is infrequent. It is clear that these lesions are difficult to dilate. However, PTRA appears to be successful in selected cases (Table 27.6). An analysis of 11 reported cases and one patient from this institution reveals that 6 cases benefited long-term and 6 cases were failures. Four patients were described as cures and two patients had improved blood pressure control. It is interesting to note that in the six patients that underwent clinically successful PTRA, good initial results were only seen in three lesions. However, several authors[51, 66, 70] all reported poor initial results with long-term good results. Gardiner *et al.*[70] reangiogramed their patient 5 months after PTRA with a poor initial result and discovered the artery was wide open. Most of these cases involved the proximal third of the renal artery. An exception was the 19-year-old woman reported by Baxi *et al.*[67] This patient had an isolated midrenal artery lesion that was successfully dilated. We have experience with only one case, a 9-year-old boy with a long, smooth, proximal stenosis of the right renal artery. This lesion has been dilated twice and initially the results appeared fair with residual stenoses greater than 33%. No delayed improvement was seen on the follow-up angiogram. The patient, however, has remained normotensive for 50 months since the initial PTRA procedure.

Therefore the results of PTRA in neurofibromatosis show that 50% of the reported cases have benefited from the procedure. The initial results may not look good angiographically but a delayed response is seen in some cases.

Takayasu's arteritis

Takayasu's arteritis is an uncommon chronic inflammatory arterial disease which characteristically involves the aorta, its main branches and the pulmonary arteries. The etiology remains unknown. The disease can produce stenosis, occlusion, dilatation and aneurysm formation. Although the disease is more common in the East, the disease has a worldwide distribution. It is most common in woman in their second and third decades of life.

The histology of Takayasu's disease is characterized by a non-specific chronic arteritis. There is marked thickening of the intima, media and adventitia. Thickening and fibrotic changes are more pronounced in the intima than in the media and adventitia. Premature atheroscleroses may be seen.

Stenoses or obstructions are the most common manifestations and frequently involve the abdominal aorta and the renal arteries. Renal artery stenosis is common and often bilateral. The adjacent aorta is involved in up to 70% of cases. Clinically there are two phases. The early phase is characterized by mild systemic symptoms: arthralgia, fever, night sweats, chest and abdominal pain, skin rashes, and accompanied by an elevated sedimentation rate. A late occlusive or pulseless phase occurs when the systemic symptoms subside and are replaced by symptoms due to occlusions or stenosis of the arteries. Hypertension secondary to renal artery stenosis is common. The disease tends to be chronic, progressive and the prognoses is poor. Wiggelinkhuizen and Cremin[71] examined eight children with Takayasu's disease and hypertension and found that all the children had clinical evidence of left ventricular hypertrophy.

Total aortography is felt to be mandatory for the diagnoses and treatment of the disease. Reports in the literature[72–75] describe the technical difficulties with performing diagnostic aortography and PTRA in Takayasu's disease. The accompanying severe stenosis in the aorta makes the lesions hard to cross and the lesions are resistant to dilatation necessitating high inflation pressures and prolonged dilatation times. The initial results are encouraging. Doug *et al.*[74] had an initial success in 86.4% of 32 patients including adults (average age 17.3 years) with renal artery lesions treated by PTRA. Sharma *et al.*[75] had an initial success in 85% of 20 patients, including adults (average age 16 years). Sharma's failures were in patients with coexistent abdominal aortic disease. The lesions were described as tough and non-compliant. Sharma *et al.*[76] in a separate communication, reported on PTRA in eight children with Takayasu's arteritis. The initial success rate was 80%. Restenoses occurred in one patient after 5.5 months. The lesion was successfully redilated. The follow-up period in these studies was short. Fava *et al.*[77] recently reported their long-term experience. Twelve patients underwent PTRA. The initial success was high (83%); however, the 5-year patency rate was only 33.3%. Their conclusion is that, as with other modes of therapy, including surgery and steroid therapy, PTRA is only palliative. The initial and short-term results of PTRA in Takayasu's arteritis are encouraging, however, more long-term studies are necessary to determine the true long-term response.

The middle aortic syndrome

The middle aortic syndrome[48, 78, 79] is characterized by severe diffuse narrowing of the distal thoracic and abdominal aorta. Involvement of the visceral and renal branches is common. This rare syndrome is usually seen in children usually in the second decade of life and appears to arrest at puberty. While intimal and medial fibroses is found histologically, the etiology of this condition remains unknown.

Isolated stenoses of the abdominal aorta are known to be caused by several entities: Takayasu's Type 3 Post-rubella syndrome, neurofibromatosis, Williams' syndrome[80] and middle aortic syndrome. In many cases the etiology of the stenoses in the abdominal aorta can be defined. However, in some cases, it cannot, these cases have been called the middle aortic syndrome.

Arteriography shows a smooth high grade stenosis of the abdominal aorta. The stenosis is variable in length usually extending from just above the celiac artery to just below the renal arteries. The renal arteries are frequently involved. The lesions are usually confined to the orifice. The visceral arteries are also frequently involved necessitating lateral aortograms for complete analysis. The experience with angioplasty is limited. Nanni *et al.*[81] treated a 12-year-old hypertensive boy with successful dilatation of the abdominal aorta. At 1-year follow-up he was asymptomatic and his blood pressure was much easier to control. Lewis *et al.*[79] attempted preoperative PTRA in two patients. Both patients failed at long-term follow-up.

Conclusion

In the pediatric age group; PTRA is complex because the vessels are smaller, access is more difficult and management of the patients is complicated. In order to obtain optimum results, a team approach involving a pediatric nephrologist, an interventional radiologist and a vascular surgeon maximizes the chances of safe, successful and long-term correction and management of hypertension due to renal artery stenoses. The procedure should be performed only by experienced interventional radiologists and only after careful preparation of the patient by a pediatrician experienced in the management of hypertension. An experienced surgeon should be available to deal with possible complications or to electively repair the vessel if PTRA should be unsuccessful.

As expected from the adult experience, short, isolated, non-ostial stenoses respond best to PTRA. Isolated lesions in branch arteries respond as favorably as lesions in the main renal artery. Long tubular lesions or those lesions involving the ostium are less likely to have a good long-term response. Etiology is important and lesions due to FMD have the most favorable response. In the meta-analyses reported here, 88% of the pediatric patients with FMD had a beneficial long-term response.

References

1 Leadbetter WF, Burkland CE. Hypertension in unilateral renal disease. *J Urol* 1938; **39:** 611.
2 Palubinskas AJ, Ripley HR. Fibromuscular hyperplasia in extrarenal arteries. *Radiology* 1964; **82:** 451–4.
3 Veterans Administration Cooperative Study Group

on Anti-hypertensive Agents. Effects of treatment of morbidity in hypertension: results in patients with diastolic blood pressures averaging 115 through 129 mm Hg. *JAMA* 1967; **202:** 1028–34.

4 Tegtmeyer CJ, Kellum CD, Ayers C. Percutaneous transluminal angioplasty of the renal arteries: results and long-term follow-up. *Radiology* 1984; **153:** 77–84.

5 McCormack LJ, Poutasse EF, Meaney TF *et al.* A pathologicarteriographic correlation of renal artery disease. *Am Heart J* 1966; **72:** 188–98.

6 McCormack LJ, Dustan HP, Meaney TF. Selected pathology of the renal artery. *Semin Roentgenol* 1967; **2:** 126–38.

7 Meaney TF, Dustan HP, McCormack LJ. Natural history of renal arterial disease. *Radiology* 1968; **91:** 881–7.

8 Kincaid OW. Fibromuscular dysplasia of the renal arteries. *Am J Roentgenol* 1968; **104:** 271–82.

9 Tegtmeyer CJ, Selby JB, Hartwell GD *et al.* Results and complications of angioplasty in fibromuscular disease. *Circulation* 1991; **83:** I–155–I–161.

10 Morris GC, Lechter A, DeBakey ME. Surgical treatment of fibromuscular disease of the carotid arteries. *Arch Surg* 1968; **96:** 636–43.

11 Fry WJ, Brink BE, Thompson NW. New techniques in the treatment of extensive fibromuscular disease involving the renal arteries. *Surgery* 1970; **68:** 959–67.

12 Houck WS. Renovascular hypertension secondary to arterial fibrodysplasia: treatment by dilation using a fogarty balloon. *JAMA* 1979; **242:** 1396–7.

13 Dotter CJ, Judkins MP. Transluminal treatment of arteriosclerotic obstruction: description of a new technique and preliminary report of its application. *Circulation* 1964; **30:** 654–70.

14 Grüntzig A, Hopff H. Perkutane Rekanalisation chronischer arterieller Verschlüsse mit einem neuen Dilatationskatheter: Modifikatin der Dotter-Technik. *Deutsch Med Wochenschr* 1974; **99:** 2502–11.

15 Grüntzig A, Kuhlmann U, Vetter W *et al.* Treatment of renovascular hypertension with percutaneous transluminal dilation of a renal artery stenosis. *Lancet* 1978; **1:** 801–2.

16 Tegtmeyer CJ, Elson J, Glass TA *et al.* Percutaneous transluminal angioplasty: the treatment of choice for renovascular hypertension due to fibromuscular dysplasia. *Radiology* 1982; **143:** 631–7.

17 Tegtmeyer CJ, Sos TA. Techniques of renal angioplasty. *Radiology* 1986; **161:** 577–86.

18 Tegtmeyer CJ. Guide wire angioplasty balloon catheter: preliminary report. *Radiology* 1988; **169:** 253–4.

19 Beinart C, Sos TA, Saddekni S *et al.* Arterial spasm during renal angioplasty. *Radiology* 1983; **149:** 97–100.

20 Dean RH, Callis JT, Smith BM *et al.* Failed percutaneous transluminal renal angioplasty: experience with lesions requiring operative interven- tion. *J Vasc Surg* 1987; **6:** 301–7.

21 Martin LG, Rees CR, O'Bryant T. Percutaneous angioplasty of the renal arteries. In Strandness DE, van Breda A (eds) *Vascular Diseases: Surgical and Interventional Therapy*, pp. 721–41. New York, Churchill Livingstone, 1994.

22 Rodríguez—Pérez JC, Plaza C, Reyes R *et al.* Treatment of renovascular hypertension with percutaneous transluminal angioplasty: experience in Spain. *J Vase Intervent Radiol* 1994; **5:** 101–9.

23 Baert AL, Wilms G, Amery A *et al.* Percutaneous transluminal renal angioplasty: initial results and long-term follow-up in 202 patients. *Cardiovasc Intervent Radiol* 1990; **13:** 22–8.

24 Greminger P, Steiner A, Schneider E, *et al.* Cure and improvement of renovascular hypertension after percutaneous transluminal angioplasty of renal artery stenosis. *Nephron* 1989; **51:** 362–6.

25 Klinge J, Mali WPTM, Puijlaert CBAJ *et al.* Percutaneous transluminal renal angioplasty: initial and long-term results. *Radiology* 1989; **171:** 501–6.

26 Beebe HG, Chesebro K, Merchant F *et al.* Results of renal artery balloon angioplasty limit its indications. *J Vasc Surg* 1988; **8:** 300–6.

27 Simonetti G, Urigo F, Sergiacomi GL *et al.* Percutaneous transluminal renal angioplasty: follow-up at 48 months. In Glorioso N *et al.* (eds) *Renovascular Hypertension*, pp. 499–509. New York: Raven Press, 1987.

28 Bell GM, Reid J, Buist TAS. Percutaneous transluminal angioplasty improves blood pressure and renal function in renovascular hypertension. *Quart J Med* 1987; **241:** 393–403.

29 Kremer Hovinga TK, de Jong PE, de Zeeuw D *et al.* Restenosis prevalence and long-term effects on renal function after percutaneous transluminal renal angioplasty. *Nephron* 1986; **44** (Suppl. 1): 64–7.

30 Grim CE, Yune HY, Donohue JP *et al.* Renal vascular hypertension: surgery vs. dilation. *Nephron* 1986; **44** (Suppl. 1): 96–100.

31 Martin LG, Price RB, Casarella WJ *et al.* Percutaneous angioplasty in clinical management of renovascular hypertension: Initial and long-term results. *Radiology* 1985; **155:** 629–33.

32 Miller GA, Ford KK, Braun SD *et al.* Percutaneous transluminal angioplasty vs. surgery for renovascular hypertension. *Am J Roentgenol* 1985; **144:** 447–50.

33 Sos TA, Pickering TG, Sniderman K *et al.* Percutaneous transluminal renal angioplasty in renovascular hypertension due to atheroma or fibromuscular dysplasia. *N Engl J Med* 1983; **309:** 274–9.

34 Mahler F, Probst P, Haertel M *et al.* Lasting improvement of renovascular hypertension by transluminal dilatation of atherosclerotic and nonatherosclerotic renal artery stenoses: a follow-up study. *Circulation* 1982; **65:** 611–17.

35 Colapinto RF, Stronell RD, Harries—Jones EP *et al.* Percutaneous transluminal dilatation of the renal artery: follow-up studies of renovascular hypertension. *Am J Roentgenol* 1982; **139:** 727–32.
36 Martin EC, Mattern RF, Baer L *et al.* Renal angioplasty for hypertension: predictive factors for long-term success. *Am J Roentgenol* **137:** 921–4.
37 Archibald GR, Beckmann CF, Libertino JA. Focal renal artery stenosis caused by fibromuscular dysplasia: treatment by percutaneous transluminal angioplasty. *Am J Roentgenol* 1988; **151:** 593–6.
38 Tegtmeyer CJ, Dyer R, Teates CD *et al.* Percutaneous transluminal dilatation of the renal arteries. *Radiology* 1980; **135:** 589–99.
39 Tegtmeyer CJ, Teates CD, Crigler N *et al.* Percutaneous transluminal angioplasty in patients with renal artery stenosis. *Radiology* 1981; **140:** 323–30.
40 Novick AC. Management of renovascular disease. A surgical perspective. *Circulation* 1991; **83:** I–167–I–171.
41 Cluzel P, Raynaud A, Beyssen B *et al.* Stenoses of renal branch arteries in fibromuscular dysplasia: results of percutaneous transluminal angioplasty. *Radiology* 1994; **193:** 227–32.
42 Dillion MJ. Investigation and management of hypertension in children: a personal perspective. *Pediatr Nephrol* 1987; **1:** 59–69.
43 Guzzetta PC, Potter BM, Ruley EJ *et al.* Renovascular hypertension in children: current concepts in evaluation and treatment. *J Pediatr Surg* 1989; **24:** 1236–40.
44 Stanley P, Gyepes MT, Olson DL *et al.* Renovascular hypertension in children and adolescents. *Radiology* 1978; **129:** 123–31.
45 Norling LL, Chevalier RL, Gomez RA, Tegtmeyer CJ. Use of interventional radiology for hypertension due to renal artery stenosis in children. *Child Nephrol Urol* 1992; **12:** 162–6.
46 Korobkin M, Perloff DL, Palubinskas AJ. Renal arteriography in the evaluation of unexplained hypertension in children and adolescents. *J Pediatr* 1976; **88:** 388–93.
47 Watson AR, Balfe JW, Hardy BE. Renovascular hypertension in childhood: a changing perspective in management. *J Pediatr* 1985; **106:** 366–72.
48 Robinson L, Gedroyc W, Reidy J *et al.* Renal artery stenosis in children. *Clin Radiol* 1991; **44:** 376–82.
49 Stanley JC, Fry WJ. Pediatric renal artery occlusive disease and renovascular hypertension. *Arch Surg* 1981; **116:** 669–76.
50 Clayman, AS, Bookstein JJ. The role of renal arteriography in pediatric hypertension. *Radiology* 1973; **108:** 107–10.
51 Mali WP, Puijlaert CB, Kouwenbert HJ *et al.* Percutaneous transluminal renal angioplasty in children and adolescents. *Radiology* 1987; **165:** 391–4.
52 Chevalier RL, Tegtmeyer CJ, Gomez RA. Percutaneous transluminal angioplasty for renovascular hypertension in children. *Pediatr Nephrol* 1987; **1:** 89–98.
53 McCook TA, Mills SR, Kirks DR *et al.* Percutaneous transluminal renal artery angioplasty in a 31/2-year-old hypertensive girl. *J Pediatr* 1980; **97:** 958–60.
54 Mathias K, Struck E, Schindera F *et al.* Percutaneous treatment of renovascular hypertension. *Pediatr Radiol* 1981; **11:** 154–6.
55 Paolini RM, Marcondes M, Widman A *et al.* Percutaneous transluminal angioplasty of renal artery stenosis. *Acta Radiol Diag* 1981; **22:** 571–5.
56 Ghisla R, Mahler F, Haertel M *et al.* Lasting antihypertensive effect of percutaneous transluminal angioplasty of renal artery stenoses in a child. *Am J Dis Child* 1983; **137:** 600–1.
57 Lund G, Sinaiko A, Castaneda-Zuniga W *et al.* Percutaneous transluminal angioplasty for treatment of renal artery stenosis in children. *Eur J Radiol* 1984; **4:** 254–57.
58 Stanley P, Hieshima G, Mehringer M. Percutaneous transluminal angioplasty for pediatric renovascular hypertension. *Radiology* 1984; **153:** 101–4.
59 Millan VG, McCauley J, Kopelman RI *et al.* Percutaneous transluminal renal angioplasty in nonatherosclerotic renovascular hypertension. *Hypertension* 1985; **7:** 668–74.
60 Fallo F, Oberfield SE, Levine LS *et al.* Perctuaneous transluminal renal angioplasty in the treatment of renovascular hypertension in children. *Clin Exp Theory Prac* 1986; **A8:** 887–91.
61 Reubi F. Neurofibromatose et lesions vasculaires. *Schweiz Med Wochenschr* 1945; **75:** 463–5.
62 Salyer WR, Salyer DC. The vascular lesions of neurofibromatosis. *Angiology* 1974; **25:** 510–19.
63 Itzchak Y, Katznelson D, Boichis H *et al.* Angiographic features of arterial lesions in neurofibromatosis. *Am J Roentgenol* 1974; **122:** 643–7.
64 Feyrter F. Ober die Vasculare Neurofibromatose Nach Untersuchungen am Menschlichen Magen-Darmschlauch. *Virchows Arch Pathol Ana Physiol* 1949; **317:** 221–65.
65 Greene JF, Fitzwater JE, Burgess J. Arterial lesions associated with neurofibromatosis. *Am J Clin Pathol* 1974; **62:** 481–7.
66 Martin EC, Diamond NG, Casarella WJ. Percutanous transluminal angioplasty in non-atherosclerotic disease. *Radiology* 1980; **135:** 27–33.
67 Baxi R, Epstein HY, Abitbol C. Percutaneous transluminal renal artery angioplasty in hypertension associated with neurofibromatosis. *Radiology* 1981; **139:** 583–4.
68 Guzzetta PC, Potter BM, Kapur S *et al.* Reconstruction of the renal artery after unsuccessful percutaneous transluminal angioplasty in children. *Am J Surg* 1983; **145:** 647–51.
69 Mallman R, Roth FJ. Treatment of neurofibromatosis associated renal artery stenosis with hypertension by percutaneous transluminal angioplasty. *Clin Exp Theory Prac* 1986; **A8**; 893–9.
70 Gardiner GA, Freedman AM, Shlansky-Goldberg R. Percutaneous transluminal angioplasty: delayed

response in neurofibromatosis. *Radiology* 1988; **169:** 79–80.

71 Wiggelinkhuizen J, Cremin BJ. Takayasu arteritis and renovascular hypertension in childhood. *Pediatric* 1978; **62:** 209–17.

72 Hiramatsu K, Iwata Y, Kohda E *et al.* Percutaneous transluminal renal angioplasty in Takayasu's arteritis. *Int Angio* 1983; **2:** 69–73.

73 Cook PG, Wells IP, Marshall AJ. Case report: renovascular hypertension in Takayasu's disease treated by percutaneous transluminal angioplasty. *Clin Radiol* 1986; **37:** 583–4.

74 Doug Z, Li S, Lu X. Percutaneous transluminal angioplasty for renovascular hypertension in arteritis: experience in china. *Radiology* 1987; **162:** 477–9.

75 Sharma S, Saxena A, Talwar KK. Renal artery stenosis caused by nonspecific arteritis (Takayasu disease): results of treatment with percutaneous transluminal angioplasty. *Am J Roentgenol* 1992; **158:** 417–22.

76 Sharma S, Rajani M, Shrivastava S *et al.* Non-specific aorto-arteritis (Takayasu's disease) in children. *Br J Radiol* 1991; **64:** 690–8.

77 Fava MP, Foradori GB, Garcia CB *et al.* Percutaneous transluminal angioplasty in patients with Takayasu arteritis: five-year experience. *J Vasc Intervent Radiol* 1993; **4:** 649–52.

78 Messina LM, Goldstone J, Ferrell LD *et al.* Middle aortic syndrome. *Ann Surg* 1986; **204:** 331–9.

79 Lewis VD, Meranze SG, McLean GK *et al.* The midaortic syndrome: diagnosis and treatment. *Radiology* 1988; **167:** 111–13.

80 Daniels SR, Loggie JM, Schwartz DC *et al.* Systemic hypertension secondary to peripheral vascular anomalies in patients with Williams syndrome. *J Pediatr* 1985; **106:** 250–1.

81 Nanni GS, Hawkins IF, Alexander JA. Percutaneous transluminal angioplasty of an abdominal aortic coarctation. *Am J Roentgenol* 1983; **140:** 1239–41.

82 Tegtmeyer CJ *et al.* Renal angioplasty: current status. *Am J Roentgenol* 1984; **142:** 17–21.

28

Percutaneous transluminal angioplasty in atherosclerosis

GG GEYSKES

Introduction

Intra-arterial dilatation was practised as early as 1964 when the pioneer Dotter[1] dilated iliac and femoral atheromatous stenoses with coaxial catheters of increasing diameter. Thanks to his contribution his name is connected with intra-arterial dilatation. The verb 'to Dotter' is now frequently used to replace the more elaborate expression percutaneous transluminal angioplasty (PTA) or, in case of renal arteries, PTRA.

Because with Dotter's technique the puncture site limited catheter diameter, a major breakthrough was the development of an inflatable balloon catheter by Grüntzig. In 1978 and 1979 the first reports of successful dilatation of coronary and renal artery stenosis (RAS) with the balloon catheter were published by Grüntzig's group.[2] Their first case report of a patient with unilateral atheromatous RAS was followed by an equally successful dilatation in a patient with fibromuscular dysplasia (FMD).[3]

After some years of experience with the balloon technique in femoral and iliac arteries our own experience with renal artery dilatation started when a patient with severe renovascular hypertension, who refused surgery, read about the new balloon dilatation in the newspaper. This dilatation, performed at his own request, was uneventful and a success mainly because after withdrawal of his antihypertensive medication he regained his sexual abilities, an improvement of his quality of life. In the following years reports on first small and later larger series of patients were published, detailing frequent technical success of balloon dilatation of RAS of atheromatous as well as other renal artery diseases. These were mainly different forms of FMD but also stenosis in the surgical anastomosis of transplantation or bypass surgery and in RAS is caused by Takayasu's arteritis.

Over the years it became clear that the technical and antihypertensive results of PTRA differed between patients with FMD and atheromatous disease. This warrants special chapters about these two diseases in this book. This chapter will be confined to the problems of treatment with PTRA of RAS caused by atheromatous disease.

Angiographic and clinical subgroups of atheromatous renal artery stenosis

At angiography different lesions and combinations of lesions can be distinguished. Some of these lesions have a different hypertensive renal pathophysiology and prognosis. They need different approaches for treatment as well as for diagnostic procedures.

In *unilateral* RAS, with a normal contralateral kidney and renal artery, different lesions can be seen in the artery of the affected kidney (see Fig. 28.1). Some kidneys show multiple renal

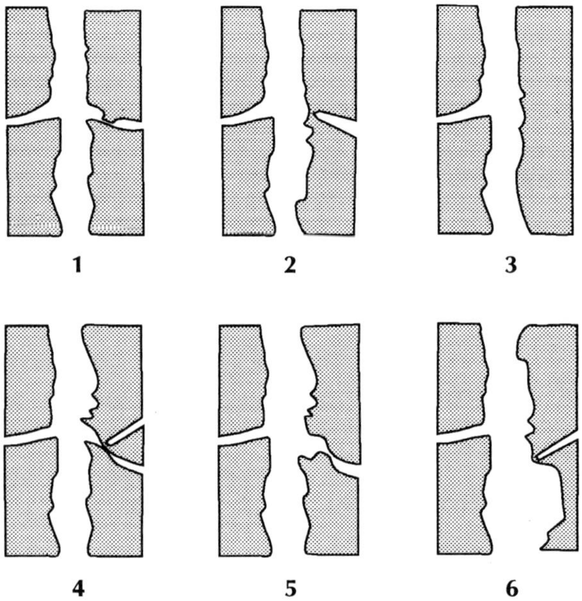

Figure 28.1. Different presentations of atheromatous renal artery disease (from the upper left to the bottom right): 1. truncal; 2. ostial; 3. complete obstruction; 4. long and segmental; 5. in ulcer, ostial; 6. in aneurysm, second artery occluded? All combinations may occur in bilateral lesions. Ostial lesions can be missed when the contrast column in the aorta projects over the ostium: oblique views are necessary. Margins of the contrast represent the blood column, not the wall of the aorta: Ostial stenosis may have a 'pseudo' wide entrance within a thick atheromatous layer.

arteries of a smaller diameter which can also be stenosed. These multiple renal arteries are rather frequent and do not supply specifically either the upper or lower poles of the kidney. The nephrographic phase of the angiogram can show a normal kidney but frequently the kidney is shrunken, in some cases severely. This is especially the case when the main renal artery is completely occluded. This shrinkage is caused mainly by tubular atrophy and interstitial fibrosis but in atheromatous disease it is frequently caused by cholesterol microemboli (see Fig. 28.2). In this instance the nephrogram may show irregular contours and circulation, caused by infarcts (segmental occlusions). The kidney parenchyma may also be affected by other, non-related pathology: reflux, stones, cysts, even carcinoma. This can happen because angiography in many patients was indicated because screening revealed renal, anatomic or functional abnormalities. *Unilateral* renal artery stenosis with an intact contralateral renal artery and kidney is from a pathophysiological standpoint the classic Goldblatt high renin hypertension. In the affected kidney there is a low arterial pressure, a diminished renal blood flow and glomerular filtrate rate (GFR) and a high renin production. In the unaffected contralateral kidney there is in contrast a high blood pressure and a suppressed renin. This causes the typical differences between the two kidneys in the diagnostic workup: the renal vein renin ratio, the rapid sequence intravenous pyelogram and renography with or without converting enzyme inhibition. When the RAS is repaired, complete recovery of renovascular hypertension can be expected. Problems arise when long-standing hypertension causes the contralateral kidney to develop nephrosclerotic lesions. This may inhibit a return to a normal blood pressure after repair of the stenosis. This occurrence had been noted in the years before PTRA when antihypertensive results of renovascular surgery were analyzed.

In atherosclerotic RAS, lesions are frequently *bilateral* and all combinations of lesions as described with unilateral disease are possible. A frequent combination is total occlusion with a shrunken kidney on one side and stenosis on the other side in the artery of the contralateral kidney. The pathophysiology of the hypertensive mechanisms in bilateral lesions is more complicated because there is no normal contralateral kidney with a high arterial pressure and a high sodium and water output. This causes more volume overload and less elevated renin concentrations when compared with unilateral artery stenosis. Pathophysiologically there is one more and one less affected kidney, whereby the less affected kidney behaves to some extent as the contralateral kidney in unilateral artery stenosis, although limited in its excretory function by its own RAS. Clinically, the overall renal function is frequently diminished and, because of the volume overload, recurrent pulmonary edema may occur. Converting enzyme inhibition causes overall renal failure by diminishing GFR in both kidneys. Differences between the two kidneys, a hallmark of most diagnostic tests, are less obvious.

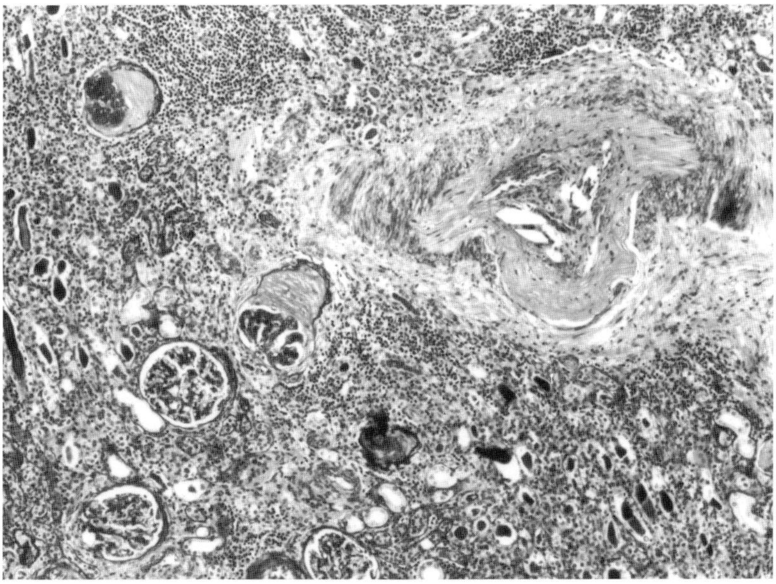

(a)

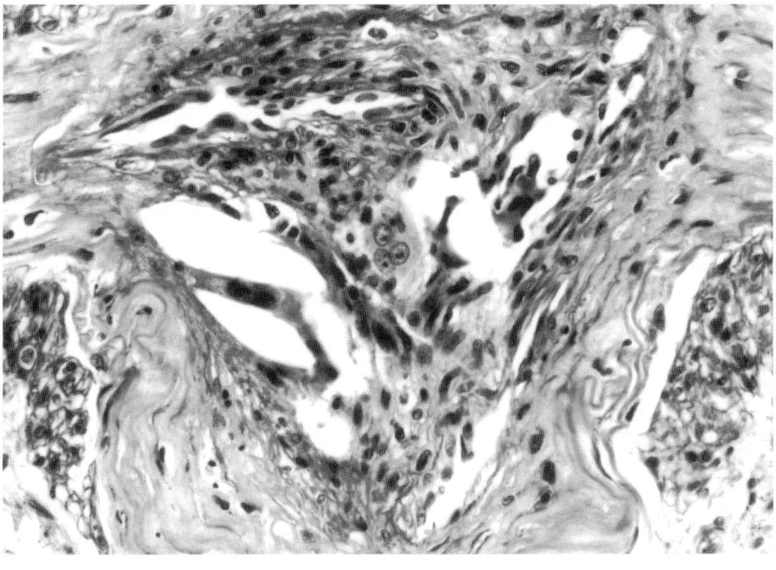

(b)

Figure 28.2. (a) Renal tissue of a small kidney behind an occluded renal artery. Spontaneous cholesterol emboli in arteriole. Note giant cell eating cholesterol. PTRA, not done in this patient, would have solved only part of the hypertensive renal mechanisms. After nephrectomy, however, this patient became normotensive. (b) Enlargement of part 2(a). Courtesy of Professor Th.M. Vroom, Department of Pathology, University Hospital, Utrecht.

When the RAS is bilaterally dilated and the renal parenchyma is undamaged, cure of the renovascular hypertension can be expected, but this is a relatively rare occurrence. When only one renal artery is sufficiently dilated, and the other is completely occluded or otherwise not satisfactory repairable, renovascular hypertension has been changed from bilateral to unilateral, then no result on the blood pressure can be expected. Moreover, in bilateral RAS there is more chance of unilateral or bilateral renal parenchymal damage. This prevents return of the blood pressure to normal even if the renovascular component has been taken care of. These factors may explain why the blood pressure response after PTRA in patients with bilateral RAS is lower than in patients with unilateral RAS.

Unilateral or bilateral RAS occurs frequently in combination with other atherosclerotic lesions of the abdominal aorta. In patients with complicating iliac stenosis this can be dilated in the same session as the renal artery dilatation. In cases of aortic aneurysm our policy is to dilate the renal artery(ies) first and replace the aneurysm by a vascular prothesis thereafter. Only patients with an acute abdominal aorta aneurysm are treated first by the vascular surgeon, who replaces the aorta and connects the prothesis with the renal artery(ies) in one session. This policy is based on reports of an increasing number of complications when surgery of the abdominal aorta is combined with renal bypass surgery.

Indications for PTRA

The two main indications for PTRA are:

1 *Relief of renovascular hypertension.* When atherosclerotic RAS shows up at angiography there also should be evidence that renal perfusion is low, causing renovascular hypertensive mechanisms.
2 *Conservation of renal function.* Loss of overall kidney function is very probable when renal function is dependent on only one kidney with a severe RAS, the other kidney being absent or shrunken with minimal function. However, the danger of loss of kidney function sufficient to require renal replacement therapy is a reality in all patients with atherosclerotic RAS because the disease is progressive and frequently bilateral.

Demonstration of a renovascular component of hypertension

In the workup of a patient with renovascular hypertension there are several investigations that to some extent can predict a fall of blood pressure after correction of the stenosis, showing that a renovascular cause of hypertension was operative.

The angiographic appearance

An estimation can be made of the severity of stenosis. This is expressed as a percentage by measuring the diameters of the smallest part and a normal part of the artery distal to the stenosis. Although frequently used, it has several pitfalls. At angiography the stenosis is not always projected at its maximum in the posterior anterior projection. Furthermore, the poststenotic area may be dilated by the jet stream of the stenosis. Renovascular mechanisms start at about 50% stenosis but more than 70% stenosis is a more likely indication of renovascular mechanisms. Other indications of a significant stenosis are a small kidney, a slow washout of contrast in the smaller arterioles and a collateral circulation.

The demonstration of an activated, asymmetric renin system

Although of important theoretical interest, the value in decision-making of such tests in the therapy of renovascular hypertension is much debated. It is not the demonstration of an RAS at angiography but a decline of blood pressure after successful correction of the stenosis that is the gold standard for renovascular hypertension. All tests should be weighed against this and not against the angiographic appearances.

The practical importance of the diagnostic tests has become less important since surgery has been replaced by PTRA. The test or the group of tests should be less cumbersome for the patient, less costly and at the same time close to the reliability of a diagnostic angiography, eventually extended by PTRA.

Peripheral plasma renin activity (see Chapter 14) may be a good screening test because it is cheap, but only when standard conditions are in place such as discontinuation of all medications—which is not always attractive.

Testing of the renin dependency of the blood pressure by converting enzyme inhibition is an unreliable test to differentiate between renovascular hypertension and essential hypertension.

Collection of split renal vein renin is close to angiography in many aspects but has frequent false negative results.

In recent years renography with converting enzyme inhibition has been developed as a rather reliable test for renovascular hypertension, probably because it combines the demonstration of an elevated renin and a low GFR in the kidney involved. Both are functional changes in a kidney demonstrating a stenosis. When compared with the blood pressure fall after PTRA, the test's sensitivity is even higher than the finding of a 50% stenosis at angiography (see Table 28.1). It can replace angiography for screening and is useful for follow-up after PTRA when the blood pressure does not return to normal, as is the case in most patients after PTRA of an atheromatous lesion. It can demonstrate that the pathophysiology of the residual hypertension has changed from renovascular to some other cause and the patient can be treated accordingly.

As with the other tests, the captopril renogram is most productive in unilateral RAS with an intact contralateral kidney. Difficulties arise when the contralateral kidney is also involved and there is a diminished GFR. This can be caused by parenchymal diseases (nephrosclerosis, cholesterol emboli), concomitant bilateral RAS, occlusion of the artery or any other reason (reflux nephropathy, dysplasia, cysts). This will modify the pathophysiologic changes at renography, and specific renovascular changes in the less involved or a single kidney can be difficult to demonstrate or exclude.

A study from our department[4] together with other studies[5,6,7], have shown that the antihypertensive results of PTRA in patients with a negative captopril renogram are minimal. For this reason, in our department, further evaluation by angiography is done only in exceptional cases when captopril renography is negative, i.e. shows two symmetric curves.

Table 28.1. Number of patients receiving PTRA and showing cure improvement or no change of their blood pressure after PTRA

	Blood pressure PTRA	Cured/ improved	No change
Captopril renogram[a]	59	53	6
Angiography[b]	77	58	19
Difference[c]	18	5	13

The golden standard of angiography challenged.
The predictive value for cure or improvement of the blood pressure after successful PTRA is for captopril renography 90% and for angiography 73%, demonstrating the difference between renovascular hypertension and RAS.
The table shows differences in results between two policies: in patients with hypertension and suspicion for renovascular hypertension on clinical grounds:
[a] Captopril renogram used as a selection criterion for PTRA. Angiography and PTRA are performed only when the captopril renogram is positive.
[b] Angiography and PTRA are performed when a stenosis of 50% or more is shown, independent of captopril renography.
[c] The differences between the two policies are the results of PTRA in patients with a stenosis of 50% more at angiography, but with a negative captopril renogram.
From ref. 4, with permission.

Renal failure after angiotensin converting enzyme inhibition

Patients with bilateral RAS, a single kidney with RAS or other reasons why most of their renal function is dependent on kidney tissue behind an RAS, may demonstrate a rise in serum creatinine and oliguria after angiotensin converting enzyme (ACE) inhibition. Although not worked out as a diagnostic test, the incidental occurrence of this side-effect of ACE inhibition in hypertensive patients has brought many patients with renovascular hypertension to the attention of physicians. In some patients ACE inhibition alone does not produce this effect but only when combined with diuretics. This should be borne in mind before excluding bilateral involvement in the absence of renal failure during ACE inhibition. Any patient who has deterioration of renal function after ACE inhibition should be investigated for renovascular involvement especially as these are the patients in whom renal function is at risk.

Protection of kidney function

The second indication for PTRA is protection of kidney function. Generally, the loss of one kidney in a patient with a normal contralateral kidney is of no importance for that patient's overall kidney function. However, in atheromatous renal artery disease patients frequently have bilateral involvement. Atheromatous lesions are progressive in nature. In patients with bilateral involvement or with a single functioning kidney with a stenosed artery, protection of loss of kidney function is of the utmost importance. There are currently no convincing data from comparative trials to demonstrate that PTRA protects kidney function. However, many incidental data in the literature showing improvement of sometimes severe renal failure support following an aggressive diagnostic and therapeutic procedure. This is in the hope that an important number of patients can be saved from renal replacement therapy. Studies have shown that patients who have lost their kidney because of renovascular disease constitute about 10–15% of the population of dialysis units.

Contraindications of PTRA

Cholesterol emboli are an important complication of intra-arterial catheter manipulation. As a consequence, spontaneous cholesterol emboli or cholesterol emboli during previous intra-arterial catheterization are considered a contraindication for PTRA (see Colour plate 3). In our department cholesterol emboli in the lower part of the body after PTRA are seen less frequently since we initiated a relatively long introduction sheath through which other catheters are changed. Other contraindications are relative and should be weighed against the benefits. Contrast allergy can be prevented by antihistamines and prednisone. To minimize acute tubular necrosis especially in patients with only one functioning kidney, we use low osmolar non-ionic contrast media. Patients with atheromatous renal artery disease frequently have atheromatous lesions in other organs, with or without symptoms. In contrast to vascular surgery these are not contraindications but support the procedure because relief of renovascular high renin hypertension may prevent further arterial disease. The same holds true for renal insufficiency. If this is caused by vascular disease the advantages of better renal perfusion outweigh the disadvantages of contrast-induced temporary tubular change.

Technique

Before PTRA the patients should be informed about the procedure itself and more importantly, about both the positive and negative possible outcomes. It is explained to a patient with atheromatous RAS that the expectation is of better blood pressure control with less medication. It is also explained that there may be a chance of a cure of the hypertension dependent on the individual pathology. The patient is also informed about an albeit relatively small chance of losing the kidney, especially if there is a single kidney. The patient should agree on renal replacement therapy in case their kidney function is lost and is also informed about the risk of emergency vascular surgery in case of hemorrhage. At least 1 day before the PTRA we start aspirin 300 mg/day.

The patient can have a light breakfast. All the antihypertensive medication is withheld to prevent periods of hypotension after the procedure. One hour before the intervention the patient receives a long-acting calcium antagonist and a sedative. After local anesthesia an introduction sheath is placed. Anticoagulation is promoted with 2500–5000 units heparin. A midstream angiogram is performed with a pigtail catheter just above the expected origin of the renal arteries, if necessary at different angles. A guidewire with a soft platina tip is introduced into the renal artery using the most appropriate catheter: cobra or sidewinder. A balloon catheter of the same diameter as the intact part of the renal artery is positioned in the stenosis and inflated three times for 30 s. The balloon catheter is deflated and withdrawn, the pigtail catheter repositioned and a control angiogram performed. When no satisfactory dilatation is achieved the procedure is repeated. If it is still unsatisfactory the procedure can be terminated and the clinical result can be awaited because intimal tears may mimic insufficient dilatation. Alternatively, an intravascular stent can be placed. In the case of bilateral RAS we start with the less affected kidney because this is the most important kidney for the patient, and it takes less time to dilate this kidney than the more severely affected kidney. The second kidney can be treated in the same session, dependent on patient tolerance. After withdrawal of all catheters the puncture site is compressed first by hand and later by bandages. Observation of vital signs, leg circulation and urinary output is carried out every 2 hours until the next morning. In a patient with a single kidney, urinary output is checked by bladder catheterization.

Patients frequently suffer backache and nausea. Severe lumbar pain, a palpable mass, signs of shock and a drop of hemoglobin concentration are signs of arterial leakage. Oliguria, hypertension and an increase in serum creatinine indicate a possible arterial thrombosis. If necessary, depending on the blood pressure, previous antihypertensive medication is reintroduced successively. As fluctuations of the blood pressure may occur in the days after PTRA, the results of PTRA on blood pressure are determined after about 6 weeks when the blood pressure is stabilized with or without medication. To ensure unbiased observation of the changes in blood pressure induced by PTRA it is important to reintroduce only those antihypertensive drugs that were used during the initial blood pressure observations before PTRA.

For this reason, antihypertensive medication is simplified, not just withdrawn, as much as possible prior to PTRA, preferably allowing some hypertension and, as a consequence, showing some antihypertensive effect of PTRA. An exception to this rule is the patient in whom no antihypertensive result of PTRA is expected because of contralateral or ipsilateral distal renal artery stenosis kidney tissue produces renin thus maintaining renovascular hypertension. A typical example is bilateral RAS, unilaterally treated. The same pathophysiology may be seen in one kidney with several stenosed arteries, only one of which is successfully dilated. Such patients are treated by PTRA to preserve kidney function during treatment of their hypertension with an ACE inhibitor.

After PTRA the dose of aspirin is lowered to 80 mg/day. At 6 weeks a control captopril renogram is performed and compared with the captopril renogram prior to PTRA, because a successful PTRA will induce improvement of the renogram (see Fig. 28.6).

Technical results

There will always be patients who are very difficult to treat with PTRA. This is, of course, to a large part dependent on the skills of the group in the angiography room. A typical example is the patient without palpable femoral arteries. The axillary route can be used but our first choice is aortic replacement. Another example is the patient with a total occlusion of the renal artery. Occasionally a catheter can be passed through the occlusion and the artery reopened. Frequently the catheter cannot be pushed or pulled (with the sidewinder) through the obstruction and the PTRA is classified as a technical failure. Some renal arteries have curves which cannot be passed by the guidewire or by the somewhat stiffer balloon catheter, for instance a sharp downward angle of the origin or segmental arteries in the first part of the renal artery (see Fig. 28.3). Catheters may perforate parts of the arterial wall and cause bleeding or arterial thrombosis with total occlusion (see Fig. 28.3 and 28.4). In the case of a tight stenosis even an experienced angiographer cannot pass a guidewire into an artery.

Another category of technical failures is in patients who show immediate reoccurence of the stenosis after successful dilatation. This may be caused by a flap that functions as a valve or, more frequently, by an atheromatous mass in the aortic wall around the origin of the renal artery. This is pushed away during balloon inflation but returns to the original position immediately after deflation. This category of ostium stenosis is frequently non-responsive to PTRA and is a candidate for bypass surgery or for arterial stenting. These and many other examples are technical failures. They are treated by medication, by bypass surgery, by stenting, by nephrectomy, or in case of a relative small kidney with an intact contralateral kidney (eventually after PTRA of its artery) by embolization (see Fig. 28.5).

The percentage of technical failures varies between groups from 0 to 44% with an average of 12%. A successful technical result can be obtained when the initial constriction of the balloon after inflation is smoothed, and when, the stenosis has decreased to less than 50% at control angiography after the retraction of the

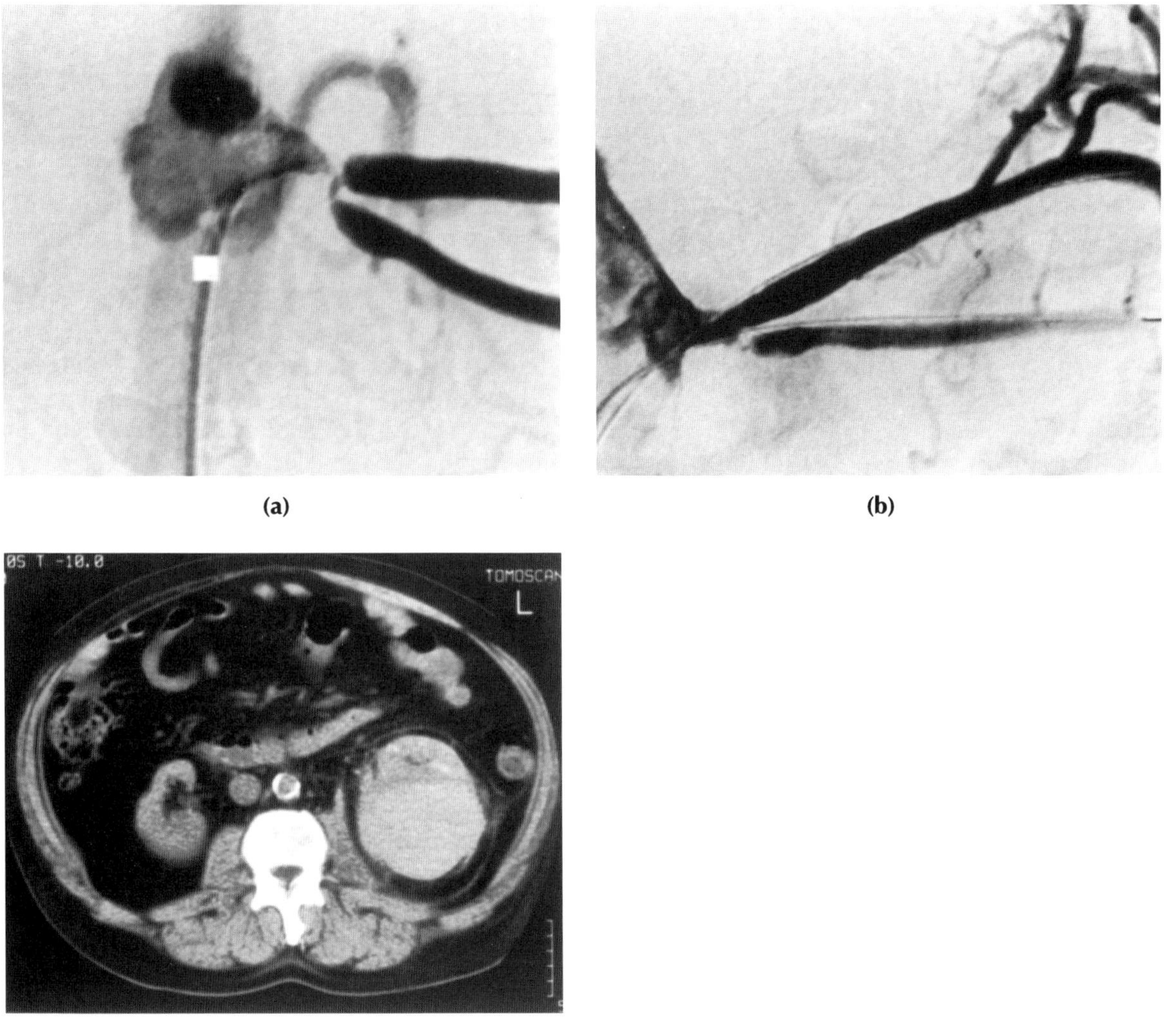

(a) (b) (c)

Figure 28.3. Complication of bleeding in 57-year-old man. (a) Atheromatous stenosis in an early branch of the left renal artery. (b) Dilatation of the upper branch, but the balloon could not be moved over the guiding wire in the lower branch. The patient experienced left lumbar pain. (c) Next day a CT scan showed massive hematoma in the left kidney. The exact site of the bleeding remains obscure.

balloon. This is not always easily shown because of arterial tears that mimic residual stenosis. If there is any doubt, a second series of dilations can be performed. If again there is no improvement of the arteriogram, the effects on blood pressure or renal function must be awaited. It can happen that the residual stenoses have disappeared and the inner arterial wall has become smooth at repeat angiography months later.[8]

We do not perform pressure gradients because they are dependent on flow. Other groups report pressure gradients to be diminished to 10% in patients after technical success of PTRA.

Technical or angiographic results after longer time have been studied in patients with reoccurrence of the original high blood pressure. Recently, a systematic study of reoccurrence of stenosis after the first PTRA, independent of the blood pressure obtained, showed that after an average of 8.8 months restenosis at angiography was more frequent in atheromatous disease: more than 50% stenosis was seen in 5 of 59 patients

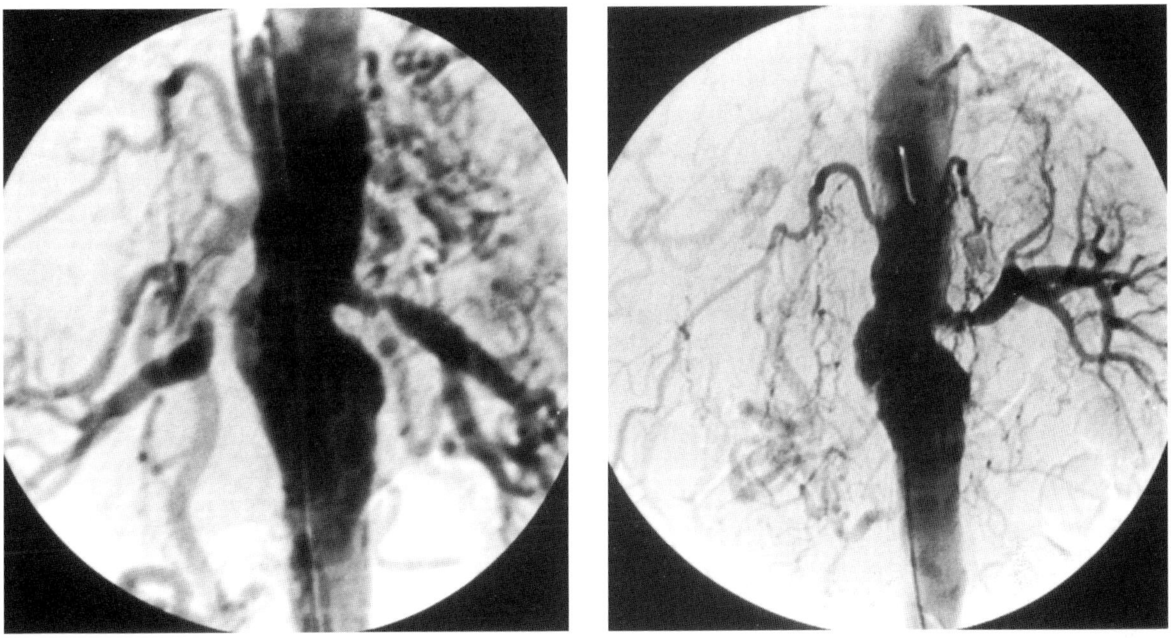

(a) (b)

Figure 28.4. Complication of thrombosis in 60-year-old woman. (a) Bilateral RAS (right more severe) of the ostium, probably covered by a thrombus. (b) After bilateral PTRA, improvement on the left side, but disappearance of the right renal artery. Because the right kidney represented only 20% of the total renal perfusion as shown by MAG_3 renography before PTRA, no action was taken to save the right kidney. Patient's blood pressure did not change initially, became normal after converting enzyme inhibition, with unchanged mild renal insufficiency.

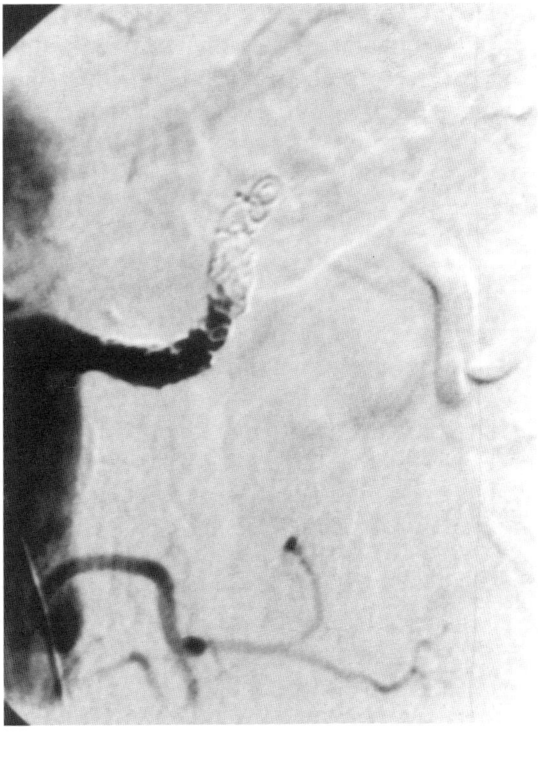

Figure 28.5. Artificial thrombosis after bleeding in a 81-year-old woman. Bleeding from the left artery after PTRA (not shown here) stopped by several coils in the artery. Right renal artery intact. Normal blood pressure and unchanged mild renal insufficiency after ACE inhibition.

with atheromatous disease, but in none of those with fibromuscular disease. In the atheromatous groups, restenosis, defined as one of five grades of stenosis more than directly after PTRA, was seen significantly more frequently in ostial (3/9 patients) than in non-ostial (8/50 patients) lesions. Restenosis was also more frequently seen when the stenosis was long (≥ two diameters) or more severe (> 75%), or when atheromatous disease was present in the aorta or elsewhere. Restenosis was also seen more frequently in patients who were older or who smoked.

Effect on blood pressure

The results of PTRA in patients with atheromatous renal artery disease are colored by generalized and progressive atheromatous arterial disease. Compared with FMD, the results of PTRA on blood pressure of patients with atheromatous disease are less favorable. This difference in antihypertensive effect is not exclusive to PTRA and has also been reported for surgical treatment. Several reasons may explain this difference. In patients with atheromatous disease cholesterol emboli may have occurred in the affected or in the contralateral kidney. Patients with atheromatous disease have more frequent reoccurrences of stenosis. Patient with atheromatous RAS frequently have underlying essential hypertension with secondary atheromatous arterial disease (see Fig. 28.6 and Table 28.2). Because the patients are older and may have a longer duration of hypertension, the function of the contralateral kidney and thereby the overall renal function can be diminished and contribute to residual hypertension. In the atheromatous patients the artery of the more affected kidney may have a complete obstruction which cannot be dilated, with a small contracted kidney which loses its exocrine function but is still actively producing renin: the 'endocrine kidney'. In these patients PTRA of the less affected kidney only corrects to a limited extent the pathophysiologic hypertensive mechanisms. The patient shifts from bilateral to unilateral RAS. Complete antihypertensive therapy is achieved only after additional nephrectomy of the kidney with the occluded artery or after ACE inhibition. The latter now can be given without fear of renal insufficiency.[9] Without these additional therapies PTRA will have only a minimal effect on blood pressure.

It is difficult to compare the results of PTRA with the results of the previously most used therapy, vascular surgery. When the antihypertensive results of series in the literature are compared they seem slightly to favor surgical repair, although this may be due to differences in patient selection. Does this imply that surgery is the first choice? Certainly not! The somatic and psychological morbidities of the two procedures are very different and favor PTRA. Even if the average blood pressure response were better after surgery then the first choice should still be PTRA. The discussion should not concentrate on blood pressure response but on the question as to how RAS can be treated and the flow or pressure gradient normalized most permanently with the least harm to the kidney and patient. For many patients the answer to this question will be PTRA. Surgery can be reserved for those patients in whom PTRA is not a technical success or in patients with a frequent reoccurrence of the stenosis. However, a recent innovation, placement of an intravascular stent, may extend the role of PTRA.

Vascular surgery in our hospital is reserved for patients with specific lesions which cannot be treated by less invasive techniques such as PTRA or stenting. This includes complete occlusion of the renal artery with a relatively intact kidney that maintains more than 25% of overall renal function. Patients with an acute arterial thrombosis, with dissection of the renal artery, with renal artery aneurysms and with bleeding after a PTRA procedure are also candidates for surgery. It should be mentioned that both procedures, PTRA and renal vascular surgery, should be concentrated in larger medical centers with sufficient experience in invasive radiology and vascular surgery. In such a centre the renovascular group will use PTRA, stenting and surgery in combination. In a review of the effect of PTRA on blood pressure in eight published series up until 1988, we summarized the results after a follow-up period of 0–60 months.[10] After PTRA, blood pressure was brought down to normal without antihypertensive medication in only a

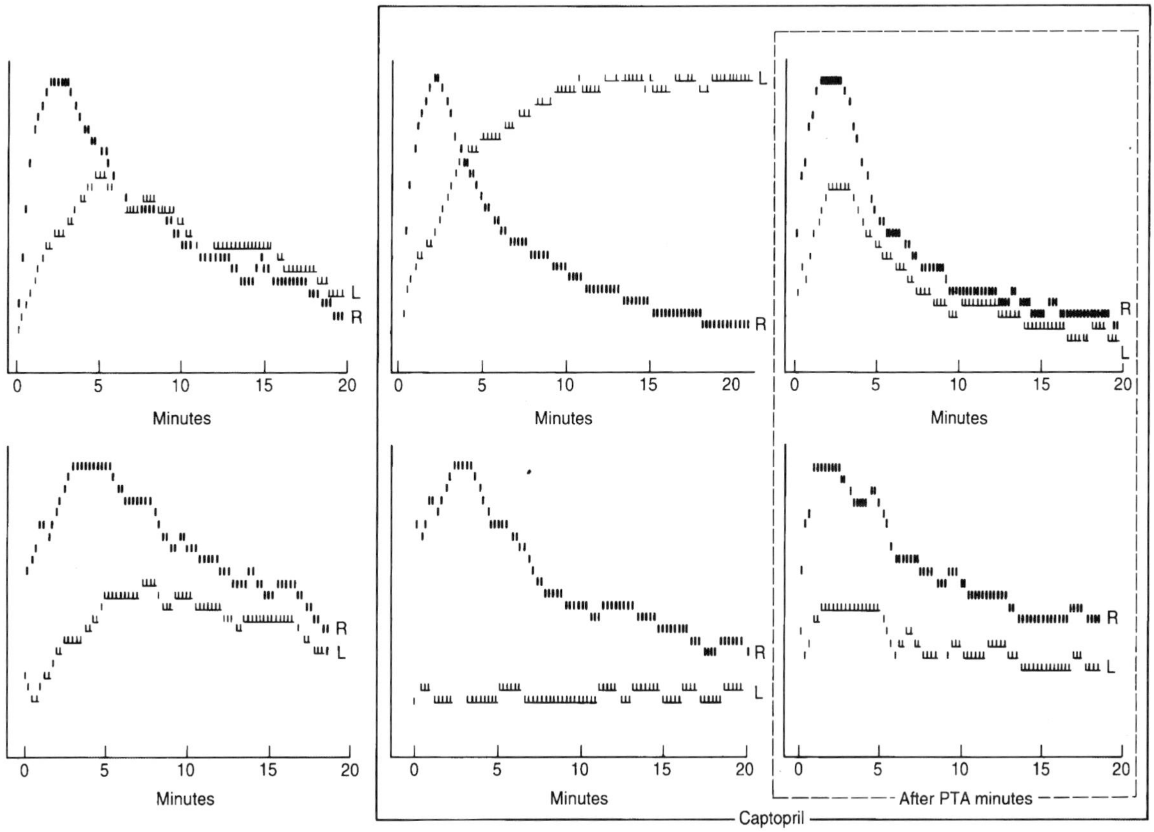

(a)

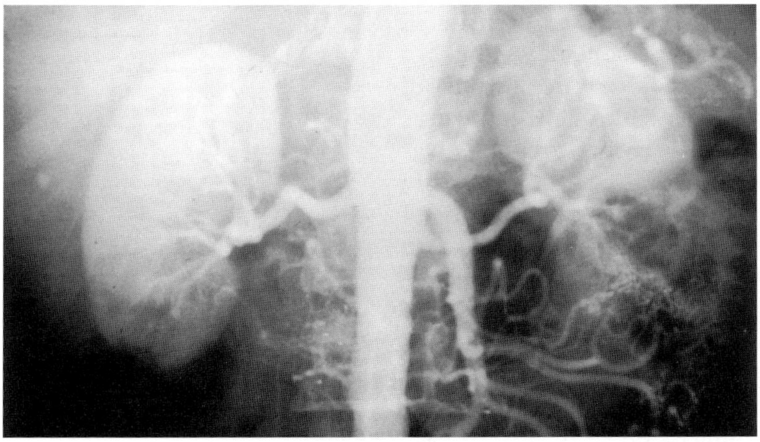

(b)

Figure 28.6. Captopril renography and control angiography in a patient with residual hypertension after PTRA, the blood pressure being improved, not cured. (a) From left to right, ^{131}I orthoiodohippurate sodium renography curves before PTRA, with and without captopril premedication, and after PTRA with captopril premedication. Bottom, technetium-99m diethylenetriaminepentaacetic acid (DPTA) curves made at identical times and conditions. R indicates right; L, left. Before PTRA, captopril induced the specific changes in the hippurate and DTPA time—activity curves, which disappeared after PTRA. (b) Resolution of the renovascular component of this patient hypertension is confirmed by a normal arteriography after PTRA. The residual hypertension of this patient is non-renovascular.

Table 28.2. Better results of nephrectomy compared with PTRA on blood pressure in patients with one small kidney, demonstrating residual hypertensive mechanisms in a shrunken kidney after PTRA.

57 patients with a small kidney (radiohippurate uptake < 25 per cent of total) because of renal artery stenosis (28 patients) or occlusion (29 patients)

	Intervention in the small kidney			Total
	None	Percutaneous transluminal arterioplasty	Nephrectomy	
Number of patients	11	18	28	57
Normotensive				
without medication		5	16	21
with medication	10	8	9	27
Hypertensive				
with medication	1	5	3	9

Intervention in the artery of the small kidney and the blood pressure achieved at termination of the study period (average: 31.5, range: 2–79 months). In 24 patients a stenosis in the artery of the contralateral kidney was successfully dilated by PTRA.
From ref. 20, with permission from Oxford University Press.

minority of patients (4–37%). This was lower than in the FMD group of whom 37–85% were cured. Improvement of the blood pressure was achieved in 26–59%, with no improvement in 6–69%. In an analysis published in 1990,[11] which comprised two more studies, hypertension in atheromatous disease was cured in 19%, improved in 52% and showed no improvement in 30%.

The classification of cure, no result or improvement of blood pressure as used in all studies is derived from the Cooperative Study of Renovascular Hypertension on the results of surgery on blood pressure.[12] In the Cooperative Study, improvement of blood pressure was defined as a decrease of diastolic blood pressure of 15% or more, and a diastolic blood pressure of 91–109 mmHg, measured without medication after as well as before the procedure. None of the PTRA studies has fulfilled these stringent criteria. As a consequence the percentage of patients showing improvement varies in the different studies. However, the antihypertensive effect of PTRA shows a sliding scale from no result to cure and it seems likely from the published reports that 50% or more of patients with atheromatous RAS do benefit to some extent. In a study of 39 patients with atheromatous RAS the blood pressure response after PTRA changed from an average of 191/107 to 167/90 mmHg. This was a significant difference for systolic and diastolic blood pressure, and concomitantly the number of antihypertensive drugs used fell significantly from 1.4 to 1.9.[13] These results can be improved when patients are carefully selected—i.e. excluding patients unlikely to benefit, e.g. those with ostial stenosis or bilateral disease. In a review of

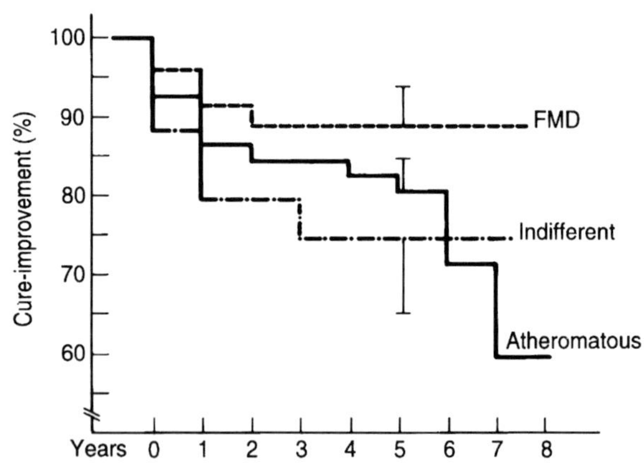

Atheromatous	115	94	66	51	41	35	13	4	1
FMD	47	40	37	30	21	20	6	2	–
Indifferent	25	16	15	11	11	10	4	1	–

Figure 28.7. Life-table of cure or improvement ± SEM of the blood pressure after technical successful PTRA in 187 patients, divided in three subgroups according to the etiology of their renal arterial disease. The decline during the years is caused only by recurrence of the hypertension (change from cured or improved to no result). Patients with no result from the beginning cause the curves to start below 100%. In the atheromatous group recurrence continues after 5 years' follow-up 13.2 ± 4%. From ref. 10, with permission.

six published series of patients with non-ostial unilateral stenosis Pickering[14] reported 89.5% successful dilatations; 28.5% of these were cured and 41% improved. In the long term recurrence of stenosis will occur, causing recurrence of hypertension. Recurrence of hypertension is shown in the life-table in Fig. 28.7. Starting with 115 patients with atheromatous RAS and 47 patients with FMD. Recurrence of hypertension were seen throughout follow-up in the atheromatous group, whereas the FMD group showed recurrence only in the first 2 years. At 5 years' follow-up the percentage cure and improvement in the atheromatous group declined from an initial 93% to 80% due to recurrence of the initial hypertension in 13%. After 5 years, recurrence of hypertension continued in the atheromatous group, but a quantitative calculation became less valuable because of the small number of observations. In contrast, the recurrence rate of hypertension in the FMD group remained at 7% after the second year. The highest recurrence rate (20%) was seen in a subgroup of 25 patients with atheromatous stenosis at the origin of the renal artery. Another factor that increased the recurrence rate retrospectively was an undersized balloon diameter. Oversized balloons did not influence recurrence.

Effect on renal function

In a recent review, Rimmer[15] compiled papers presenting the effect of PTRA on renal function in patients with atheromatous RAS. Improvement of renal function occurred in 43% (25/57) of patients, data comparable with results from surgical treatment. Martin[16] described a significant decrease of 20% in serum creatinine after PTRA in 61% of patients with bilateral stenosis, but also in 38% of patients with unilateral stenosis and a normal contralateral blood flow. In patients with severe RAS already on hemodialysis, the effect of PTRA was successful only in one of nine patients. As shown by Meyrier[17] in 32 patients with atheromatous renal disease, severe renal insufficiency is not only due to main RAS, but also to complex intrarenal lesions with multiple stenosis of intrarenal vascularity and cholesterol embolism. The same criterion, a 20% reduction in serum creatinine after PTRA, was observed in 40% of 60 patients with a baseline serum creatinine greater than 150 mmol/l, 10% showed deterioration.[18] In 26% of kidneys with a >60% artery stenosis, an average decrease in length of 1.90 cm was observed during an average follow-up of 14.4 months.[19]

In a study of 57 patients[20] with one shrunken kidney (less than 25% perfusion) caused by RAS or occlusion, cholesterol emboli and/or renal infarcts could be demonstrated in 15 of 28 (53%) of the kidneys after nephrectomy (see Fig. 28.8). These irreversible intrarenal parenchymatous lesions may explain why renal function (and blood pressure) recover only partly after correction of the stenosis in the main renal artery. That study did indeed show improvement of renal function (and blood pressure) after nephrectomy of the small kidney if combined with PTRA of a stenosis in the contralateral kidney. In ten such patients serum creatinine improved from 163 to 127 mmol/l on average. This improvement was of course due to PTRA in the contralateral kidney, in combination with relief of a highly stimulated renin–angiotensin–aldosterone system by removal of the shrunken kidney. Notwithstanding the limitations of intrarenal parenchymal disease, reports have been published describing patients with dramatic improvement of renal function (as in the patient presented in Fig. 28.8),[21] some patients even come off regular hemodialysis after PTRA.[22]

Atheromatous disease is progressive in nature and artery stenosis may progress to occlusion and a shrunken kidney with minimal exocrine function. This has been shown in several studies. Some of these studies show a high variability in the speed of progression between patients. Progression has been shown in 36–63% of patients and total vessel obstruction is observed relatively often (10–16%) during a follow-up period from 6 months to 7 years. Occlusion can also occur during ACE inhibition. As a consequence loss of renal function can be expected, especially when all renal function is dependent on one kidney with a severely stenosed artery, as in patients with severe stenosis on one side and complete obstruction with a shrunken kidney on the other side, or in patients with a single

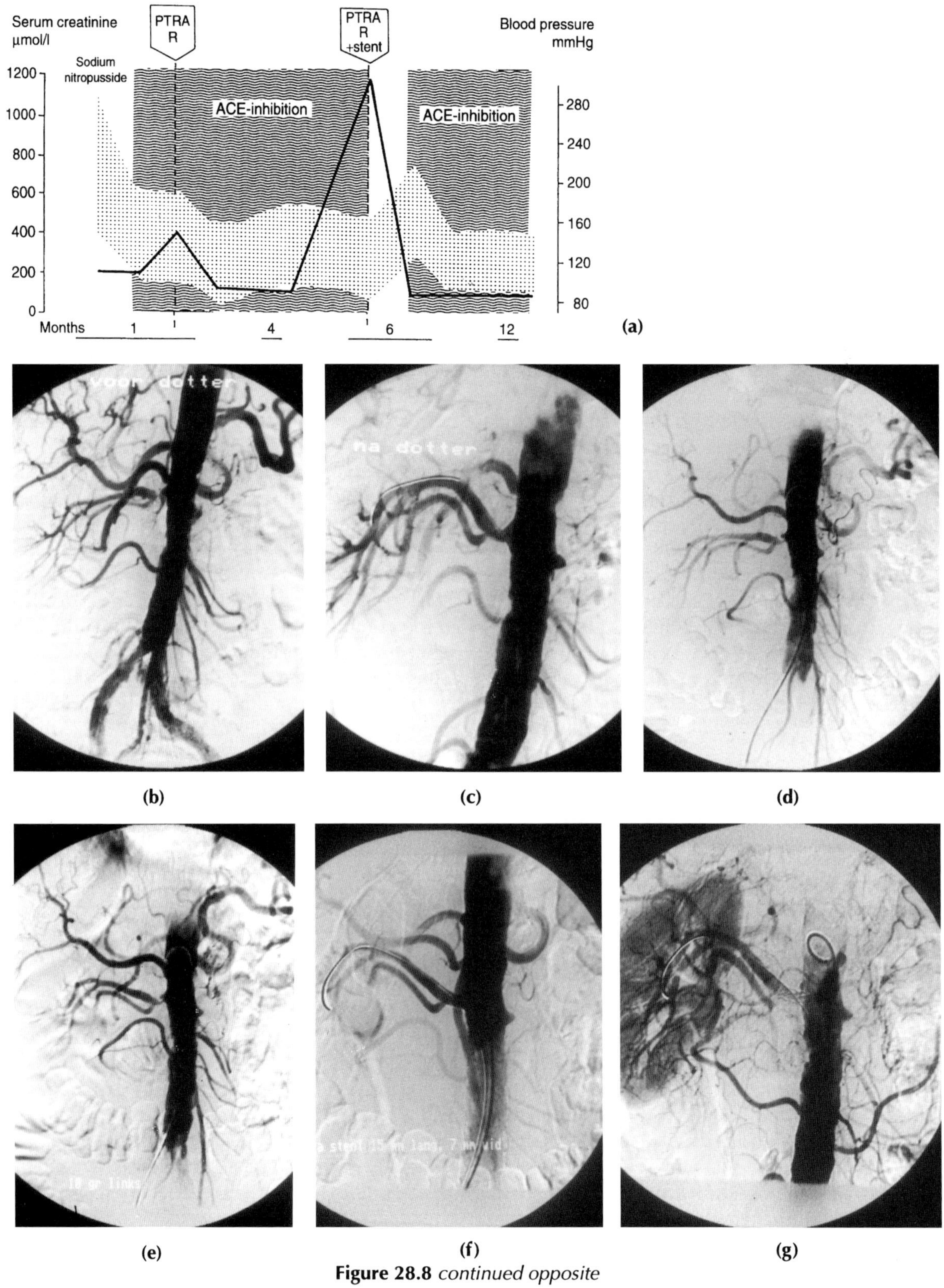

(a)

(b) (c) (d)

(e) (f) (g)

Figure 28.8 *continued opposite*

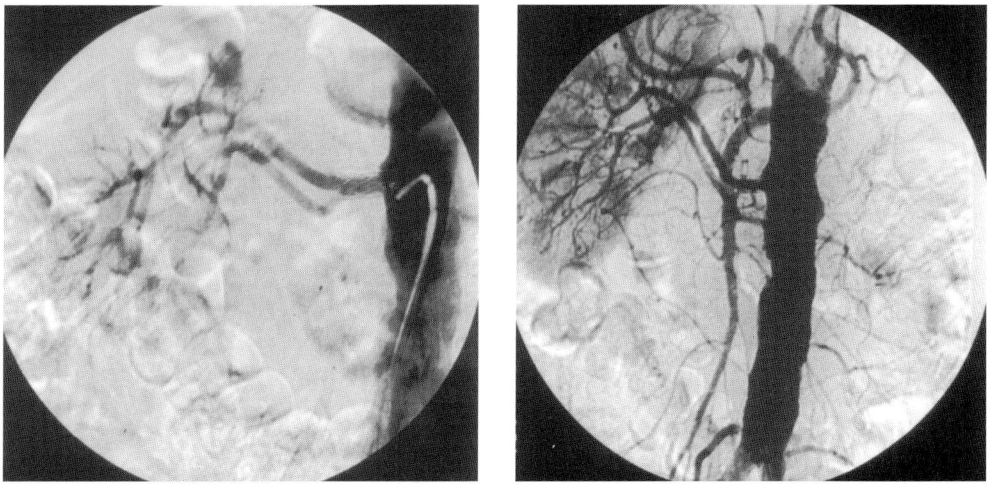

(h) (i)

Figure 28.8. Bilateral renal artery obstruction. Renal failure during ACE inhibition (ACEI) relieved by unilateral PTRA. Restenosis during ACEI, shown mainly as renal failure, treated by PTRA and stent. A 74-year-old woman was admitted because of pulmonary edema and hypertension. Eight years previously she suffered a myocardial infarction and thereafter was frequently admitted with recurrent pulmonary edema. After initial intravenous sodium nitroprusside she was treated with ACE inhibition. This resulted in renal failure. Arteriography showed an occluded left renal artery and 80% stenosis at the origin of her right renal artery. After PTRA of the right renal artery she continued treatment by ACE inhibition. This was tolerated well with good blood pressure control and near normal serum creatinine values for 5 months. She was then admitted because of anuria following a day of vomiting. At admission she was not dehydrated, had a normal blood pressure but a very high serum creatinine of 1200 μmol/1 (a). Immediate angiography showed restenosis of her right renal artery. PTRA was not very successful, after deflating the balloon catheter the control angiography showed restenosis by an intimal flap which was the reason for placing a vascular Palmaz stent. Her renal function recovered and remained stable when the blood pressure was again treated with ACE inhibition. A year later her blood pressure and serum creatine were constant and a repeat angiogram showed patency of the vascular stent. Angiograms were as follows: (b) before the first PTRA; (c) after the first PTRA; (d) before the second PTRA; (e) after the second PTRA; (f) immediately after placement of the stent; (g) the same, later phase of angiogram; (h) 6 months later, early phase of angiogram; (i) the same, later phase of angiogram.
This patient shows several aspects of atheromatous renal artery stenosis: 1. recurrent pulmonary edema in a patient with renovascular hypertension due to bilateral RAS; 2. renal failure during ACE inhibition but not during nitroprusside as a symptom of bilateral RAS; 3. recurrence of an atheromatous stenosis at the origin of the renal artery; 4. an intimal flap after PTRA, resolved by placement of a Palmaz stent; 5. continuation of renovascular hypertension after successful reopening of the artery of the larger kidney, caused by the shrunken contralateral kidney still behind an occluded renal artery: 6. effective medical treatment with ACE inhibition in a patient with unilateral, renovascular hypertension; 7. prevention of the need for renal replacement therapy as the main indication for PTRA.

kidney and severe artery stenosis. With conservative management in such patients there seems to be a severe risk of a sudden total loss of kidney function, death or dependence on renal replacement therapy in a relatively short period. However, PTRA itself is not without risk in the short term of loss of kidney function. Complete loss of kidney function directly after PTRA is not, however, a frequent occurrence. When it does occur, the patient is under close observation and can be treated accordingly by dialysis, repeated PTRA or vascular surgery.[23, 24]

Currently, data of results of PTRA on renal function cannot be compared with data of the natural course in this particular group of patients. It is possible that such data will never be produced because of the possibility of success with PTRA. In our hospital about 100 patients with a single functioning kidney have been treated by PTRA and complete loss of renal function necessitating dialysis has occurred in only two of them. Pickering[25] attempted PTRA in 55 patients with atheromatous renovascular hypertension and progressively worsening azotemia. In 26 (47%) of the patients the serum creatinine declined and remained stable during the 2 years' follow-up. The procedure induced renal failure requiring hemodialysis in three patients (5%). However, dialysis was necessary during follow-up in 14 of 23 (47%) patients with unsuccessful PTRA, making the risk/benefit ratio for haemodialysis 5:47%, justifying PTRA in this high risk group.

In conclusion, prevention of loss of renal function seems more important than recovery from renal insufficiency that has already developed. An aggressive attitude in the diagnosis and treatment of atheromatous renal disease in the protection of renal insufficiency is warranted.

PTRA with arterial stent

The placement of intra-arterial stents has been attempted to prevent recurrence of stenosis after dilatation of arteries (see Chapter 29). In a renal artery restenosis is most frequent in atheromatous ostial lesions. Sometimes this restenosis occurs directly after deflating the balloon, causing early recurrence or technical failure of the PTRA. After successful PTRA, we have found a recurrence of hypertension in 20% of patients with atheromatous stenosis at the origin of the renal artery. The percentage of restenosis is higher because our study did not include technical failures (early restenosis) and no control angiography was done in patients without recurrence of hypertension. About the same percentage of restenosis of ostitial lesions has been shown by Sos[26] and by the working group on renovascular hypertension.[27] In a recent study of reangiography performed 8.8 months after a first successful angioplasty, independently of the blood pressure response, restenosis was observed in 35% of ostial stenosis.[28]

Canzanello reported no improvement in the blood pressure in 20 of 30 patients with ostial lesions, in 14 because of a restenosis. This has raised doubt about the indication for PTRA in patients with atheromatous ostial stenosis. However, patients with ostial lesions are frequently not the best candidates for surgery because they suffer from other complications of atheromatous arterial disease which are contraindications for surgery. Besides, extensive atheromatous disease of the aorta and other large arteries may complicate bypass surgery. Medical treatment has the disadvantage of progression of stenosis to occlusion and loss of kidney function. Placement of arterial stents may have a lower risk for the patient than surgery and a better immediate and long-term arterial dilatation when compared with PTRA. We use the Palmaz stent (non-articulated),[29] a balloon-mounted stent which is expanded during inflation and remains expanded in the stenotic area when the balloon is deflated and withdrawn. Placing this stent exactly in the stenosis is less difficult than other stents. The first reports of the use of a stent in RAS are promising. Joffre[30] obtained preserved patency in 19 of 21 patients with persistent stenosis after several PTRA attempts or with recurrent stenosis. Kuhn[31] obtained successful stent placement in eight of ten patients after failed PTRA or end arteriectomy. Rees,[32] however, observed seven recurrences of stenosis after an average follow-up period of 8 months in 28 patients. We used a stent in four patients with recurrent atheromatous ostial stenosis of a single functioning kidney. After at least 1 year these stents have remained open (see patients in Fig. 28.8 and Colour plate 4. Currently we are conducting a trial to investigate the additional value of primary stents in patients treated by PTRA for origin stenosis; the results are awaited.

Acknowledgements

We thank Professor Willem P.Th.M. Mali and his staff in the Department of Radiology, University Hospital Utrecht, for their cooperation within our renovascular working group. We also thank Laurien de Boer for excellent secretarial assistance.

References

1 Dotter CT, Judkins MP. 1964; *Circulation*, **30:** 654.
2 Grüntzig A, Vetter W, Meier B, *et al.* Treatment of renovascular hypertension with percutaneous

transluminal dilatation of a renal-artery stenosis. *Lancet* 1978: **i:** 801–2.

3 Millan VG, Madias NE. Percutaneous transluminal angioplasty for severe renovascular hypertension due to renal-artery medical fibroplasia. *Lancet* 1979; **i:** 993–5.

4 Geyskes GG, AJ de Bruyn. Captopril renography and the effect of percutaneous transluminal angioplasty on blood pressure in 94 patients with renal artery stenosis. *Am J Hypertension* 1991; **4:** 685S–689S.

5 Fommei E, Ghione S, Hilson AJ *et al.* Captopril radionuclide test in renovascular hypertension: a European multicentre study. European Multicentre Study Group. *Eur J Nucl Med* 1993; **20:** 617–23.

6 Setaro JF, Saddler MC, Chen CC *et al.* Simplified captopril renography in diagnosis and treatment of renal artery stenosis. *Hypertension* 1991; **18:** 289–98.

7 Gruenewald SM, Collins LT, Antico VF *et al.* Can quantitative renography predict the outcome of treatment of sclerotic renal artery stenosis? *J Nucl Med* 1984; **30:** 1946–54.

8 Wilms GE, Baert AL, Amery AK *et al.* Short-term morphologic results of percutaneous transluminal renal angioplasty as determined with angiography. *Radiology* 1984; **170:** 1019–21.

9 Kumagai H, Suzuki H, Matsukawa S *et al.* Captopril therapy following percutaneous transluminal angioplasty for bilateral renal artery stenosis. *Arch Int Med* 1990; **149:** 1973–6.

10 Geyskes GG. Treatment of renovascular hypertension with percutaneous transluminal renal angioplasty. *Am J Kidney Dis* 1988; **12**(4): 253–65.

11 Ramsay LE, Waller PC. Blood pressure response to percutaneous transluminal angioplasty for renovascular hypertension: an overview of published series. *Br Med J* 1990; **300:** 569–72.

12 Maxwell MH, Bleifer KH, Franklin SS, Varady PD. Cooperative Study of Renovascular Hypertension: demographic analysis of the study. *JAMA* 1972; **22:** 1195–204.

13 Marshall FI, Hagen S, Mahaffy RG *et al.* Percutaneous transluminal angioplasty for atheromatous renal artery stenosis—blood pressure response and discriminant analysis of outcome predictors. *Quart J Med* 1990; **75:** 483–9.

14 Pickering TG, Sos TA, Laragh JH. (1988) Percutaneous angioplasty in renovascular hypertension. *Lancet* 1988; **i:** 4–5.

15 Rimmer JM, Gennari FI. (1988) Atherosclerotic renovascular disease and progressive renal failure. *Ann Int Med* 1993; **118:** 712–119.

16 Martin LG, Casarella WJ, Gaylord GM. Azotemia caused by renal artery stenosis: treatment by percutaneous angioplasty. *Am J Radiol* 1988; **150:** 839–44.

17 Meyrier A, Buchet P, Simon P *et al.* Atheromatous renal disease. *Am J Med* 1988; **85:** 139–46.

18 Pattison JM, Reidy JF, Rafferty MJ *et al.* Percutaneous transluminal renal angioplasty in patients with renal failure. *Quart J Med* **85:** 883–8.

19 Guzman RP, Zierler RE, Isaacson JA *et al.* Renal atrophy and arterial stenosis: a prospective study with duplex ultrasound. *Hypertension* **23:** 346–50.

20 Geyskes GG, Oei HY, Klinge J *et al.* Renovascular hypertension: the small kidney updated. *Quart J Med* 1988; **251:** 203–17.

21 O'Donovan RM, Guttierrez OH, Izzo JL Jr. Preservation of renal function by percutaneous renal angioplasty in high-risk elderly patients: short-term outcome. *Nephron* 1992; **60:** 187–92.

22 Beraud JJ, Calvet B, Durand A, Mimran A. Recanalization of an atherosclerotic renal artery occlusion. *J Hypertension* 1989; **7:** 909–11.

23 Martinez AG, Novick AC, Hayes JM. Surgical treatment of renal artery stenosis after failed percutaneous transluminal angioplasty. *J Urol* 1990; **144:** 1094–6.

24 Kazmers A, Moneta GL, Harley JD *et al.* Treatment of acute renal artery occlusion after percutaneous transluminal angioplasty. *J Vasc Surg* **9:** 487–92.

25 Pickering TG, Sos TA, Saddek S *et al.* Renal angioplasty in patients with azotemia and renovascular hypertension. *J Hypertension* 1986; **4:** (Suppl.6) S667–S669.

26 Sos TA, Saddekni S, Pickering TG, Laragh JH. Technical aspects of percutaneous transluminal angioplasty in renovascular hypertension. *Nephron* 1986; **44:** (suppl. 1) 45–50.

27 Working Group on Renovascular Hypertension. Final report: detection, evaluation, and treatment of renovascular hypertension. *Arch Int Med* 1987; **147:** 820–9.

28 Plouin PF, Darne B, Chatellier G *et al.* Restenosis after a first percutaneous transluminal renal angioplasty. *Hypertension* **21:** 89–96.

29 Palmaz JC. Intravascular stenting: from basic research to clinical application. *Cardiovasc Intervent Radiol* 1992; **15:** 279–84.

30 Joffre F, Rousseau H, Bernadet P *et al.* Midterm results of renal artery stenting. *Cardiovasc Intervent Radiol* 1992; **15:** 313–18.

31 Kuhn FP, Kutkuhn B, Torsello G, Modder U. Renal artery stenosis: preliminary results of treatment with the Strecker stent. *Radiology* 1991; **180:** 367–72.

32 Rees CR, Palmaz JC, Becker GJ *et al.* Palmaz stent in atherosclerotic renal arteries: preliminary report of a multicenter study. *Radiology* 1991; **181:** 507–14.

29

Endovascular stents

DAVID TROST, THOMAS A SOS

Introduction

It is now well accepted that fibromuscular dysplasia of the main and branch renal arteries is best treated by percutaneous transluminal renal angioplasty (PTRA). Technical success rates exceed 90% with approximately 50% of the patients being cured and an additional 40% being improved.[1] This is true for adults as well as children.[2]

Angioplasty of atheromatous stenoses more than 1 cm away from the aortic wall has a 90% technical success rate in several series.[1] Hypertension is cured in 20% of these patients, and 50% are improved. The remainder are technical failures or are partially or completely due to concurrent essential hypertension and therefore fail to respond.

The major reason for failure of renal angioplasty has been the presence of an ostial renal artery lesion[3] (Fig. 29.1). Only one series by Martin *et al.*[4] demonstrated satisfactory results of angioplasty in ostial renal artery lesions; however others have failed to duplicate these authors' success. Because of the frustratingly high (over 80%) immediate or short-term recurrence of ostial stenoses following dilation, other technologies have been tried.[3, 5–7] These have included lasers and atherectomy devices.[8] Unfortunately, most of these have not proven to have any lasting benefit. Recent experience by several investigators with metallic intravascular stents has shown improved initial success and lasting benefit at least in the immediate and intermediate terms.

Metallic stents for intravascular use were first proposed by Charles Dotter in 1969. He employed simple stainless steel coils.[9] These crude devices were effective in normal canine arteries but were not used in humans. Stent development was stagnant until the early 1980s when Maass *et al.* started to experiment with self-expanding spring coils.[10] This prosthesis, constructed of stainless steel, consisted of two bands in the form of a double helix spiral. These stents were

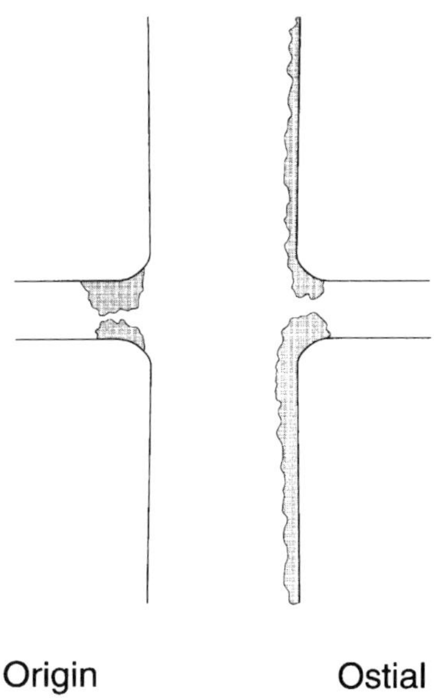

Figure 29.1. 'True' ostial vs origin disease.

designed for large vessels such as the vena cava and the aorta and were produced in various sizes up to 35 mm in diameter. The stent had a somewhat large, 7 mm diameter, but flexible delivery system and had to be placed through an arterial or venous cutdown. Smaller versions up to 10–15 mm diameter were designed for percutaneous insertion. Once released the stent was held in place by its self-expanding force. Double helix spiral stents were placed into two patients with dissecting aortic aneurysms, and for post-operative stenoses in large veins,[11] making it the first stent used clinically. Maass also experimented with an endoprosthesis made from polyester/polyurethane with an implanted metal mesh for the treatment of aortic aneurysms and to occlude arteriovenous fistulas non-surgically.[12]

Since Maass' efforts there have been many other stents created which have been successful to a greater or lesser degree.

There are three basic categories of stent designs; shape memory alloy stents, balloon-expanded stents and self-expanding stents.

Shape memory alloy designs rely on a property of certain metal alloys specifically nitinol (nickel-titanium). This metal exhibits unique thermal recovery properties. If nitinol wire is formed into a shape such as a coil and heated to a high temperature ~500° C it will memorize that shape. The coil can then be placed in ice water and straightened out. This wire can be inserted into a vessel through a catheter. When the wire is warmed by the blood it reforms the memorized shape. Dotter[13] and Cragg[14] both developed nitinol coil stents but these early designs were difficult to place and produced significant intimal proliferation in animal testing. Research continues using nitinol as a stent material. Rabkin *et al.*,[15–16] Zollikofer *et al.*[12] and McNamara *et al.*[17] have each designed stents which do not appear to incite significant intimal proliferation. However, the stents are still difficult to place mainly due to the long wire needed to form a useful stent.

The second type of stent is the balloon-expanded stent. These stents are mounted on balloon angioplasty catheters and are expanded by balloon inflation. Two of these types of stents are commercially available, the Palmaz stent (Johnson and Johnson Interventional Systems, Warren, NJ, USA) and the Strecker stent (Boston Scientific, Natick, MA, USA).

The Palmaz stent (Fig. 29.2) was developed in

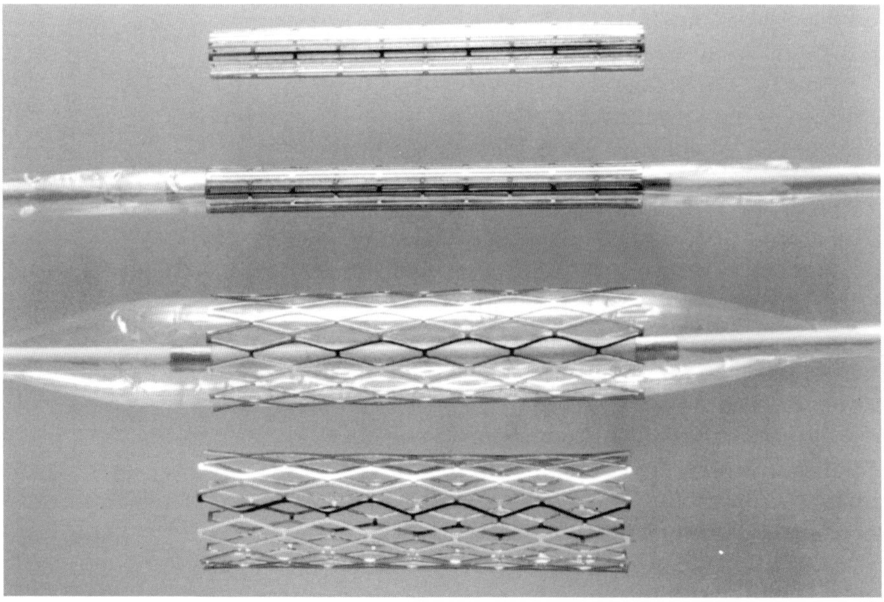

Figure 29.2. Palmaz stent unexpanded and expanded. Courtesy of Johnson and Johnson Interventional Systems, Warren NJ, USA.

the 1980s by Julio Palmaz.[18] This stent is the only stent approved for use by the United States Food and Drug Administration (FDA) and is specifically approved for use only in the iliac and the coronary arteries. The stent is a tube of stainless steel with staggered parallel slots etched through the wall. The stent is crimped on a balloon and delivered through a sheath. After the sheath is withdrawn the stent is expanded and the slots form diamond shapes. The stent is fairly rigid making it difficult to place through or in very tortuous vessels, however it has a very predictable expansion and can be accurately placed. The stent has mainly been placed in iliac and coronary arteries but trials of renal stenting with the Palmaz stent are underway.[19]

The Strecker stent (Fig. 29.3) is also a balloon-expandable stent.[20] It is made of a single fine tantalum filament. The wire is woven into a series of loops which makes the stent more flexible in both the longitudinal and radial directions. The collapsed stent is held in place on the balloon by silicone sleeves. As the balloon is expanded the sleeves retract and the stent is released. As with the Palmaz stent the Strecker stent is mainly used in the iliac arteries, however renal applications are being explored.

The last type of stent is the self-expanding stent. These stents expand by their inherent radial expansion to a predetermined diameter. There are two commercially available self-expanding stent designs, Gianturcco stent (Cook Inc, Bloomington, IN, USA) and the Wallstent (Schneider, Minneapolis, MN, USA).

The Gianturcco stent consists of stainless steel wire bent in a zigzag pattern. The stent is compressed and placed through an 8–12 French sheath. These stents are fairly rigid and have been mainly used in the vascular system for stenting large vessels such as the vena cava.[21] These stents have not been used in the renal arteries.

The Wallstent (Fig. 29.4) consists of multiple fibers of stainless steel woven in a criss-cross tubular pattern. The fibers are not fixed together thus making the stent very flexible and allowing a very small delivery system for the size of the stent being placed. Unfortunately the stent is difficult to place accurately because it shortens greatly as it is being deployed and

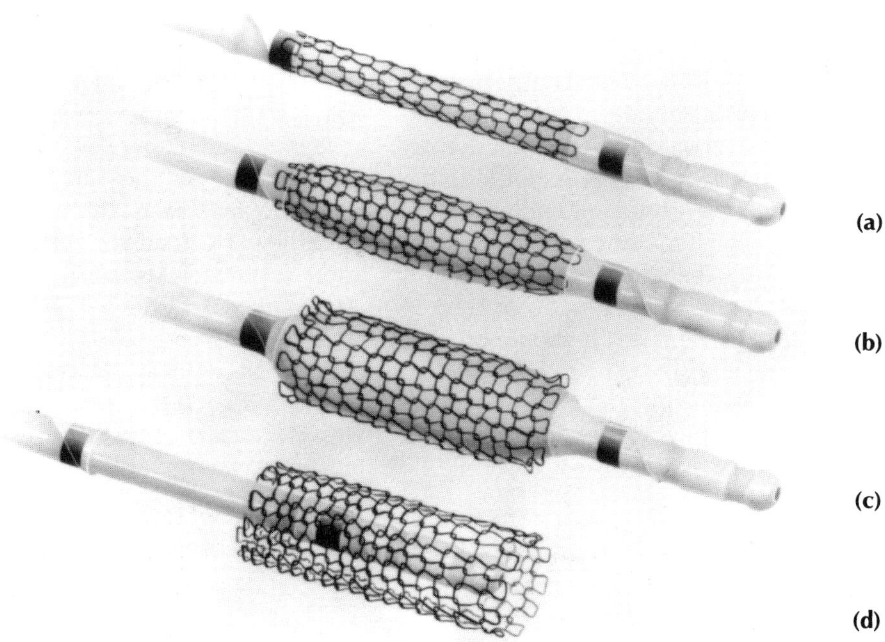

Figure 29.3. Strecker stent. (a) Preloaded stent; (b) inflation begins; (c) sleeves release stent; (d) catheter is withdrawn. Courtesy of Medi-Tech/Boston Scientific Corporation, Natick, MA, USA.

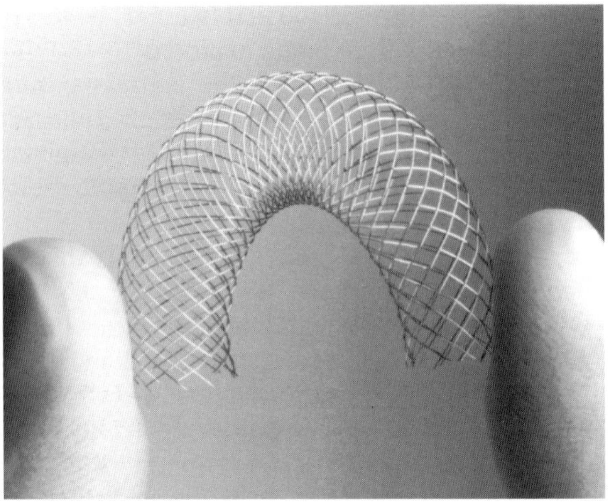

Figure 29.4. Demonstration of the flexibility of the Wallstent. Courtesy of Schneider Inc., Minneapolis, MN, USA.

it can be difficult to see on fluoroscopy. These stents have been used in the coronary and peripheral arteries since 1986.[22] They have also been used in the renal arteries.[23]

Each of these designs has its own unique strengths and weaknesses but as of yet no one has designed the perfect stent for any or all applications.

The ideal stent should have several important characteristics. It has to be biologically inert. It has to be flexible to negotiate tortuous vessels. The delivery system should have a small diameter to minimize the puncture hole required in the access artery and a low profile to facilitate crossing of the lesion, thus increasing technical success and decreasing the chance of cholesterol embolization. It should be very radio-opaque to facilitate proper placement and it should be easy to position, deploy and size. The expanded stent should be able to conform to curved and tortuous vessels, it should have a high hoop strength (radial force to keep lesions open). It should be radially elastic and spring back if it is compressed allowing it to be placed across joints or in locations where the vessel might be externally compressed. It should have a minimum surface area and possibly a negative charge which may help decrease its thrombogenicity.[14, 24] It should be made of a material which causes no magnetic imaging resonance artifacts allowing future noninvasive imaging. The characteristics of stents commonly used in the renal arteries are summarized in Table 29.1.

Patient selection for renal stenting

The evaluation of patients with suspected renovascular hypertension (RVH) is described in Part III of this book. Due to our referral pattern at the New York Hospital our patients have a high prevalence of renovascular disease. We usually perform intra-arterial digital subtraction angiography (DSA) concurrently with renal vein renin (RVR) sampling early in the patient's evaluation especially if a previous screening test such as peripheral plasma renin activity (PRA) with or without captopril or a nuclear scan with or without captopril has been positive. If an angiographically significant stenosis is demonstrated, it is treated at the same sitting, with angioplasty or with angioplasty and stent placement. Lesions which are not clearly significant by angiographic appearance are either selectively catheterized for pressure gradient measurement or the procedure is terminated. Standard balloon angioplasty is initially performed on main and branch renal artery lesions; unless there is a poor result, stents are not placed. Ostial lesions are now treated differently. Until recently, we performed standard balloon angioplasty on ostial lesions and only placed a stent for a suboptimal result. Patients with restenosis of an initially successful angioplasty of an ostial lesion were also stented.

Table 29.1. Characteristics of clinically used renal stents

		Stent				Delivery system		
Type	Alloy	Radiopacity	Conformability	Elasticity	MRI effect	Size	Flexibility	Ease of postioning
Palmaz	Stainless	++	–	–	+	7.5–8Fr	+	++
Wallstent	Stainless	+	+++	+++	++	7Fr	++	+
Strecker	Tantalum	+++	+++	+	–	8Fr	++	++

Currently, we place stents primarily for all ostial lesions due to atheroma.

Mechanism of angioplasty at the renal ostium

In order to understand the reason why angioplasty of the renal ostium does not work well, the ostial lesion must be defined.

Ostial renal artery stenoses consist of two entities: (1) aortic plaque encroaching on the renal artery orifice and (2) disease of the renal artery origin (Fig. 29.1). These two can be difficult or impossible to discriminate on arteriography. Frequently the disease is a combination of the two types.[25]

Angioplasty works by 'controlled trauma'. The atheroma is fractured longitudinally and circumfrentially. The cracks extend into the intima and the media. The muscle fibers of the media are injured and paralyzed, the adventitia is overdilated, and the atheromatous material is redistributed radially and laterally into the overdilated adventitia, thus leaving a large central lumen which is kept open by the increased flow; this is true for lesions within the renal artery. In ostial stenoses the sheet of atheroma surrounding the renal artery ostium is acted upon in a longitudinal rather than a radial fashion by the dilating balloon. Soon after deflation of the balloon the atheroma recoils and the stenosis recurs. Stents are useful in preventing this recoil.

Renal artery stenting

While stents are approved for several locations in the vascular system by the FDA, there are none approved for use in the renal arteries. Stents placed in this location are currently under evaluation and several large multicenter trials have been completed or are underway in the United States, Europe and Australia. Renal artery stents are probably best used for ostial stenoses, restenoses following PTRA, complications of PTRA and for other lesions which responded poorly to conventional angioplasty. As more data are collected it appears clear that stenting of ostial stenoses has a higher initial success rate[26] and a greatly improved intermediate term patency rate over balloon angioplasty alone. This information justifies primary placement of stents for ostial disease regardless of the appearance of the angioplasty.

Technical considerations

Placing renal stents is associated with a set of considerations not normally encountered by the interventionist who only performs conventional balloon angioplasty. While angioplasty does not usually affect subsequent surgical renal artery revascularization, stenting can. Stents in the ostial location prevent the performance of aortorenal endarterectomy, a procedure which waxes and wanes in popularity but is recently becoming popular again. A proximally placed stent will not usually have an effect on most bypass procedures, unless the stent extends near the branching of the artery. Placement of stents further out in the renal artery will severely limit the options for subsequent surgical reconstruction.

Positioning the stent in the stenosis is of utmost importance and is much more critical than in angioplasty alone. It is essential that the renal artery is imaged in the proper oblique so that the lesion is exactly in profile, especially if the lesion is ostial. Only in that oblique can the stent be accurately positioned (Fig. 29.5). The major technical failure in stent placement is malpositioning of the stent. Positioning is especially difficult with the Wallstent.[27, 28] The goal is to place the stent so that it covers the lesion and extends 1–2 mm past it on both sides. For ostial lesions the proximal end should extend 1–2 mm into the aorta to ensure that it covers the ostium adequately. It is much better to err having too much stent in the aorta rather than risk not adequately covering the renal ostium.

Most ostial disease can be treated with a 10–15 mm long stent. Most US angiographers use the Palmaz 10 or 15 mm long non-articulated stent which can be dilated from 4–9 mm in diameter. Other stent designs such as the Wallstent and the Strecker stent[29] are being used in the renal arteries in Europe.

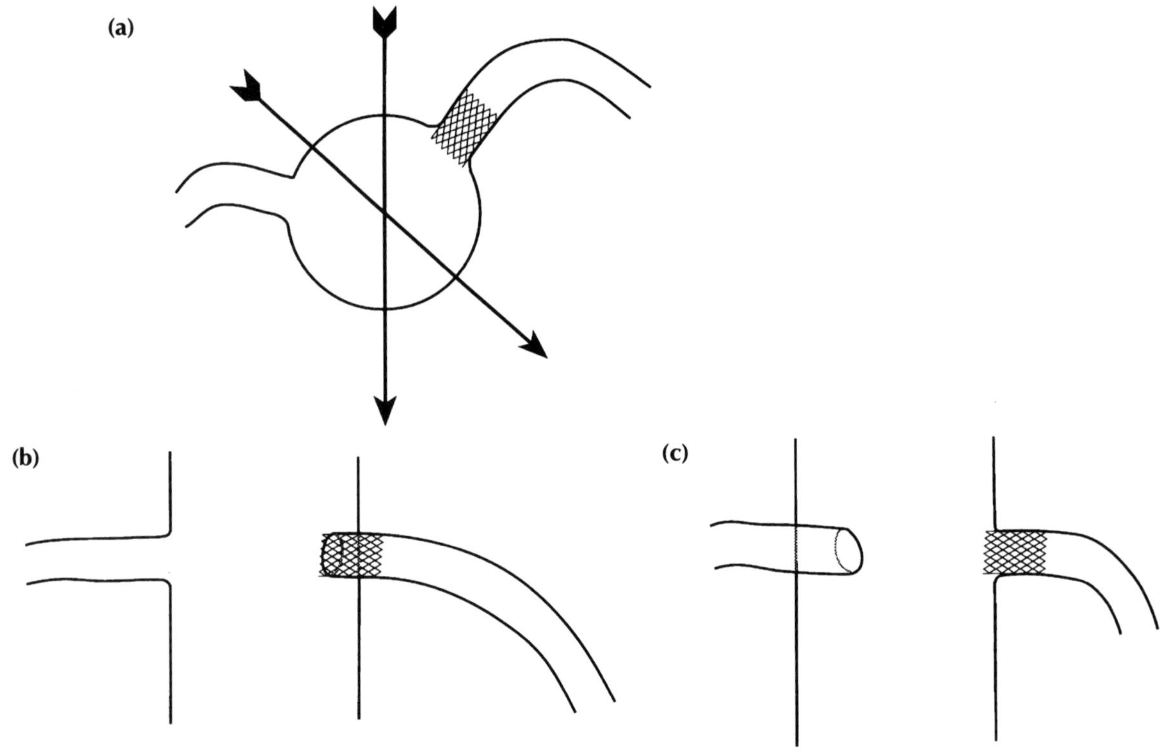

Figure 29.5. Diagram illustrating the importance of imaging the renal artery in the proper oblique (a). Note the projected overlap of the stent on the anterioposterior view (b). The true overlap is seen on the right anterior oblique view (c).

Stenting technique

Prior to the placement of a stent an angiogram is performed using the standard technique described by Tegtmeyer and Sos.[30]

Performing the completion angiogram following PTRA (or stenting) with a technique which preserves wire position across the stenosis facilitates repeated interventions including stent placement and decreases complications by obviating the need to recross the lesion.[31]

The following description applies to the placement of a Palmaz stent (Figs 29.6 and 29.7). The stent/balloon is placed into a 7 French sheath or an angled 8 French guiding catheter positioned so that the tapered tip of the balloon catheter is just protruding out of the guide but the stent is kept covered. Proper positioning of the stent is the most critical step of the procedure especially for an ostial lesion. In standard PTRA the balloon is usually 2 cm long and it is easily placed so that the entire stenosis is covered and dilated, thus, the positioning is relatively noncritical. The balloon should not extend far into the renal artery past the lesion but it can extend back into the aorta. The positioning of a stent is much more critical. The balloon/stent/guide combination is advanced to the renal artery ostium and an angiogram in the previously determined optimal oblique is performed through the guide. The balloon/stent/guide is advanced into the renal artery over a previously placed rigid guidewire (we prefer the TAD II [Peripherial Systems Group]), using the arteriogram as a reference. The shortening of the stent when expanded must be taken into account as it is positioned. When satisfied with the position, the guide catheter is withdrawn to just out of the renal artery while the balloon/stent catheter is kept in the anticipated optimal position. An angiogram is performed through the guiding catheter to confirm positioning. The position

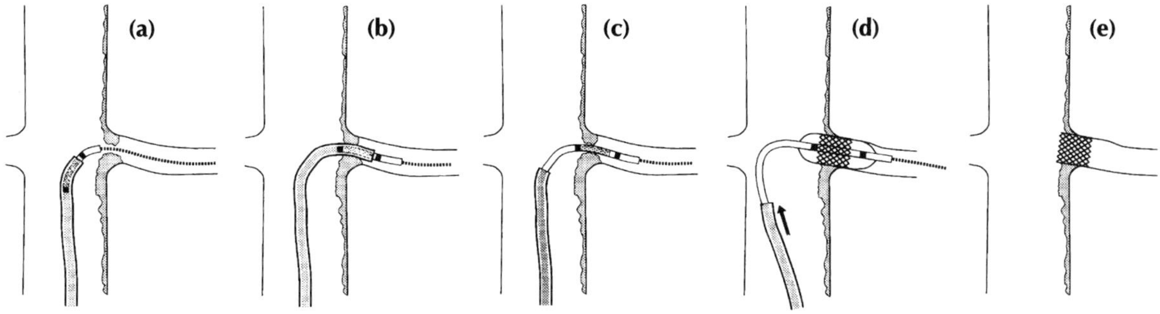

Figure 29.6. Renal stent placement. (a) Stent system in position for placement angiogram through the guiding catheter. (b) Stent system positioned in renal artery. (c) Guiding catheter pulled back for final positioning angiogram. (d) Stent expanded while balloon is played out to help align the stent to the artery (arrow). (e) The expanded stent in the renal ostium.

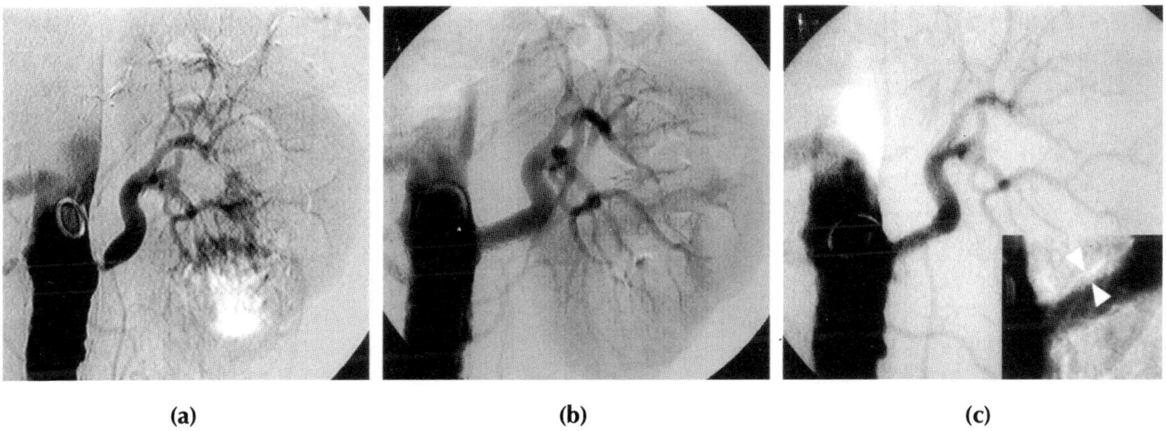

Figure 29.7. Uninephric 57-year-old female with hypertension. (a) Initial angiogram demonstrating a severe ostial stenosis of the left renal artery. (b) Immediately post-stent placement. (c) 7 Months post-stent placement. Inset: the white arrows delineate the neointima growth.

should be close to if not exactly correct, however if needed it can usually be moved relatively easily by gently pushing or pulling on the balloon catheter. The stent is then expanded, the guidewire left in position and the balloon catheter withdrawn being careful to avoid moving the stent and a completion angiogram performed through the guiding catheter. If the stent does not cover the entire lesion, a second stent can be placed to overlap the first.

The complications of stent placement are the same as those of renal angioplasty, although there are some additional complications specific to stents.[32] Potential problems with stent placement include malpositioning, migration, embolization of the stent and difficulty removing the balloon from the stent. Malpositioning can be minimized by performing the procedure in the proper oblique and taking the time to position the stent carefully as described above.

Post procedure care

Immediately postprocedure patients are hydrated as vigorously as they can tolerate. The heparin given during the procedure is not reversed, but additional doses of heparin are not used following stent placement. Blood pressure, intake and output as well as the serum creatinine are monitored closely. Deterioration of the patient's renal status may warrant reangiography, further intervention or surgical bypass. We recommend that our angioplasty and stent patients take an antiplatelet agent usually aspirin p.o. 80–300 mg four times daily postprocedure indefinitely. We do not routinely give systemic anticoagulation except to patients with known hypercoagulable states.

Results

Early reports of stenting of the renal arteries are now being published. Rees presented the results of a multicenter trial of the Palmaz-Schatz stent, at the 1994 meeting of the Cardiovascular and Interventional Radiological Society of Europe.[19] In Rees' study 304 stents were placed in 296 arteries in 263 patients. Technical success was 95%; 80% of the lesions were ostial; 98% of lesions were atherosclerotic. At 6-month follow-up 64% had improvement or cure of hypertension. In 123 patients with renal insufficiency (creatinine >1.5 mg/dl), there was improvement in 34%, stability in 39% and deterioration in 27%. Angiographic follow-up at 6 months was performed in 150 patients. Angiographic restenosis (diameter <50%) occurred in 32.7%. Restenosis was lower in males 23% ($p<0.05$), for stents dilated to <6 mm (26%, $p<0.05$), and lowest for males >6 mm (10.5%).

At the New York Hospital we have placed 25 Palmaz stents in 23 arteries of 21 patients.[33] Twenty-two of these were used for atheromatous ostial stenoses. All patients were hypertensive, 11 had serum creatinine ≥1.5 mg/dl and 8 ≥2.0 mg/dl; 30% of the patients were functionally or anatomically uninephric. Technical success was achieved in 95% of procedures. Repeat angiography was performed in half of the patients at a mean of 7.5 months. Restenosis of 50% or greater luminal diameter occurred in 36% of patients; however, in only one patient was this accompanied by deterioration of renal function and worsening of hypertension. Mean clinical follow-up was 11.2 months with a range of 1–21 months; however, ten patients were followed for a minimum of 15 months. Cure or improvement of hypertension was achieved in 71% of patients. All patients with serum creatinine ≤1.5 mg/dl were stable at last clinical follow-up. Of eight patients with serum creatinine ≥ 2.0 mg/dl three were improved, three were stable and two deteriorated (one of whom had microcholesterol embolization).

In 1994, Henequin, Joffre and Rousseau *et al.* reported the longterm follow-up of 25 Wallstents placed in 21 patients.[23] The stents were placed for restenosis after previous balloon angioplasty (N=13) or inadequate immediate postangioplasty response (N=8). Indications for angioplasty were: hypertension in all patients and renal preservation in seven. The stenoses were atheromatous in 15 patients and involved the ostium in seven. Initial stent placement was successful in 91% (19/21) patients. In two patients the initial stent did not cover the lesion and an additional stent was placed at 2 and 3 months. At follow-up angiography (range: 12–60 months) mean 29 ± 14.22 months, four patients (20%) had stent restenosis. Of these, three had undergone treatment for restenosis after angioplasty and three had ostial lesions. Cumulative primary patency rate was 95%, 85% and 77% at 7, 9 and 15 months, respectively. The cumulative secondary patency was 92% at 15 months. Hypertension was improved in all cases and felt to be cured in three. Renal function was improved in one patient, worse in one patient and unchanged in the remainder. There were three complications: thrombosis of a small branch vessel (N=1), renal hilar hemorrhage (N=1) and progressive renal dysfunction thought to be secondary to cholesterol embolization (N=1).

Also in 1994, Raynaud *et al.* reported their experience with the Wallstent.[34] These investigators eployed 25 stents in 18 renal arteries in 18 patients: 15 were atheromatous lesions, four of which were ostial; 13 were placed for PTRA failures, and the others were placed for post PTRA dissections. Five patients required a second stent because the initial stent was malpositioned. There were two stent-related complications: one acute thrombosis 15 days postplacement and an early restenosis or thrombosis. Hypertension at 6 months was cured in one patient, improved in eight and unchanged in eight. Follow-up angiograms were performed in 16 of the 18 patients at a mean of 11 months. One patient had a restenosis greater than 50% and one was occluded.

In 1992 Kuhn *et al* reported their use of the Strecker flexible balloon-expandable tantalum stent for treatment of renal artery stenosis.[35] Indications were inadequate immediate postangioplasty response ($N = 16$) and obstructing intimal flaps following transaortic endarterectomy ($N = 2$). Seventeen were hypertensive, one was normotensive. In two of the patients renal artery stenosis had developed after kidney transplantation. Stent placement was technically successful and patency was preserved in 14 patients. Midterm results (mean: 12–13 months) of 11 patients showed restenoses (greater than 50%) in two patients, and improvement of hypertension in eight patients.

The current literature is encouraging with regard to the immediate and intermediate results of the use of stents in the renal arteries, however longer follow-up is needed to really prove the durability of stents in comparison with surgical reconstruction. The available stent designs are working well but there is still room for improvement in the stents themselves and the delivery systems. Many researchers are currently working on improvements to the current designs and exploring radically new concepts such as covered, biodegradable and chemically impregnated stents.

Based on the literature and our own experience we recommend that renal artery disease including ostial lesions be treated by percutaneous methods either by balloon angioplasty alone or in combination with stents. However, good long-term results and patient benefit are best served by cooperation and communication between the radiologist, nephrologist and surgeon.

References

1 Pickering TG, Laragh JH, Sos TA. Renovascular hypertension. In Schrier RW, Gottschalk CW (eds) *Diseases of the Kidney*, 5th edn, Vol. II, 88: pp. 1451–74. Boston, Toronto and London: Little, Brown, 1993.

2 Sos TA, Saddekni S. Pediatric renovascular hypertension: the role of renal angioplasty. *Dialog Ped Urol* 1985; **8**(12)**:** 7–9.

3 Cicuto KP, McLean GK, Oleaga JA *et al.* Renal artery stenosis: anatomic classification for percutaneous transluminal angioplasty. *Am J Roentgenol* 1981; **137:** 599–601.

4 Martin LG, Cork RD, Kaufman SL. Long term results of angioplasty in 110 patients with renal artery stenosis. *J Vasc Intervent Radiol* 1992; **3:** 619–26.

5 Sos TA, Pickering TG, Sniderman KW, Saddekni S *et al.* Percutaneous transluminal renal angioplasty in renovascular hypertension due to atheroma or fibromuscular dysplasia. *New Engl J Med* 1983; **309:** 274–9.

6 Baert AL, Wilms G, Amery A *et al.* Percutaneous transluminal renal angioplasty: initial results and long term follow-up of 202 patients. *Cardiovasc Intervent Radiol* 1990; **13:** 22–8.

7 Klinge J, Mali WP, Puylaert C *et al.* Percutaneous transluminal angioplasty: initial and long term results. *Radiology* 1989; **171:** 501–6.

8 Tegtmeyer CJ. Atherectomy and renal artery stenosis. Abstract presented at the IV course on Vascular and Interventional Radiology as a Therapeutic Alternative, Las Palmas, Canary Islands, Spain, 1994.

9 Dotter CT. Transluminally-placed coilspring endarterial tube grafts: long-term patency in canine popliteal artery. *Invest Radiol* 1969; **4:** 329–32.

10 Maass D, Kropf L, Egloff L *et al.* Transluminal implantation of intravascular 'double helix' spiral prostheses: technical and biological considerations. *ESAO Proc* 1982; **9:** 252–6.

11 Maass D, Zollikofer, Largiader F, Senning A. Radiological follow-up of transluminal inserted vascular endoprostheses: an experimental study using expanding spirals. *Radiology* 1984; **152:** 659–63.

12 Zollikofer C, Antonucci F, Stuckman G *et al.* Historical overview on the development and characteristics of stents and future outlooks. *Cardiovasc Intervent Radiol* 1992; **15:** 272–8.

13 Dotter CT, Buschmann RW, McKinney MK, Rosch J. Transluminally expandable nitinol coil stent grafting: preliminary report. *Radiology* 1983; **147:** 259–60.

14 Cragg A, Lund G, Rysavy J *et al.* Nonsurgical placement of arterial endoprostheses: a new technique using nitinol wire. *Radiology* 1983; **147:** 261–3.

15 Rabkin JK, Natzvlishvili ZG, Kavteladze ZA. *Seven years experience with Rabkin technology nitinol prostheses for vessels after balloon, lasers, and rotor recanalization.* Moscow: National Research Center of Surgery, 1991.

16 Rabkin IH, Natzvlishvili ZG, Rabkin DI, Bajzhigitov BB. Nitinol endoprostetic reconstruction of renal arteries. *J Intervent Radiol* 1991; **6:** 87–91.

17 McNamara TO, Mednik G. Nitinol spiral stent: Results in porcine arteries. Abstract presented at 18th Annual Scientific Meeting of SCVIR, New Orleans, LA, USA, 1993.

18 Palmaz JC, Sibbitt RR, Reuter SR *et al.* Expandable intraluminal graft: a preliminary study. *Radiology* 1985; **156:** 73–7.
19 Rees CR, Niblett R, Snead D. United States multicenter study of Palmaz–Schatz stents in the renal arteries. CIRSE Annual Meeting and Postgraduate Course of the Cardiovascular and Interventional Radiological Society of Europe, Crete, June 1994.
20 Strecker EP, Liermann D, Barth K *et al.* Expandable tubular stents for treatment of arterial occlusive diseases: experimental and clinical results work in progress. *Radiology* 1990; **175:** 97–102.
21 Rosch J, Bedell JE, Putnam J *et al.* Gianturcco expandable wire stents in the treatment of superior vena cava syndrome recurring after maximum-tolerance radiation. *Cancer* 1987; **60:** 1243–6.
22 Joffre F, Puel J, Imbert C *et al.* Use of a new type of self expanding vascular stent prosthesis: early clinical results. Presented at the 72nd Scientific Assembly and Annual Meeting of the Radiological Society of North America, Chicago, IL, USA, 1986.
23 Hennequin LM, Joffre FG, Rousseau HP *et al.* Renal artery stent placement: long-term results with the Wallstent endoprosthesis: *Radiology* 1994 **191**(3): 713–9.
24 Sawyer PN, Stanczewski B, Srinivasan S *et al.* Electron microscopy and physical chemistry of healing in prosthetic heart valves, skirts and struts. *J Thoracic Cardiovasc Surg* 1974; **67:** 25–43.
25 Cicuto KP, McLean GK, Oleaga JA *et al.* Renal artery stenosis: anatomic classification for percutaneous transluminal angioplasty. *Am J Reentgenol* 1981; **137:** 599–601.
26 Dorros G, Prince C, Mathiak L. Stenting of a renal artery stenosis achieves better relief of the obstructive lesion than balloon angioplasty. *Cath Cardiovas Diagn* 1993; **29:** 191–8.
27 Joffree F, Rousseau H, Bernadet AL *et al.* Midterm results of renal artery stenting. *Cardiovasc Intervent Radiol* 1992; **15:** 31–18.
28 Wilms GE, Peene P, Baert AL *et al.* Renal artery stent placement with the use of the Wallstent endoprosthesis. *Radiology* 1991; **179:** 457–62.
29 Kuhn FP, Kuthkuhn B, Torsello G, Moedder U. Renal artery stenosis: preliminary results of treatment with the Strecker stent. *Radiology* 1991; **180:** 367–72.
30 Tegtmeyer CJ, Sos TA. Techniques of renal angioplasty. *Radiology* 1986; **161:** 577–86.
31 Khilnani NM, Trost D *et al.* Multisidehole catheter technique for selective over-the-wire completion angiography following renal angioplasty. *J Vasc Intervent Radiol* 1994; **5:** 387–9.
32 Trost D, Sos T. Complications of renal angioplasty and stenting. *Semin Interven Radiol* 1994; **11**(2): 150–160.
33 Trost DW, Sos TA. Palmaz stents for the treatment of ostial renal artery stenosis. Abstract presented at 19th Annual Scientific Meeting of SCVIR, San Diego, California, USA, 1994.
34 Raynaud AC, Beyssen BM, Turmel–Rodrigues LE *et al.* Renal artery stent placement: immediate and midterm technical and clinical results. *J Vasc Intervent Radiol* 1994; **5:** 849–58.
35 Kuhn FP, Malms J, Kutkuhn B *et al.* Renal stent implantation. The current indications, 2-year results and the possibilities for percutaneous stent recovery. *Rofo Fortschr Geb Rontgenstr Neuen Bildgeb Verfahr* 1992; **157**(1): 65–71.

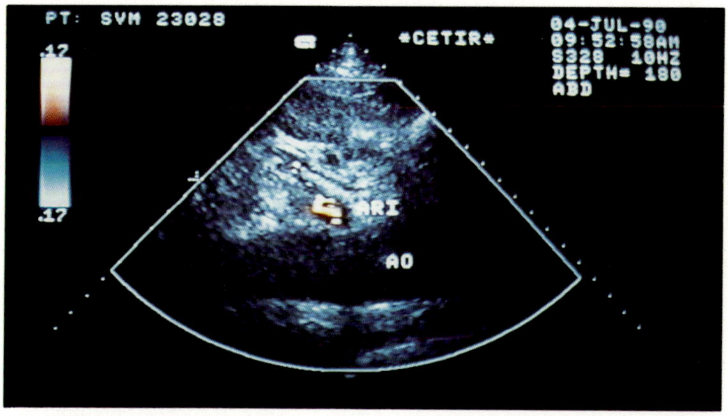

(a)

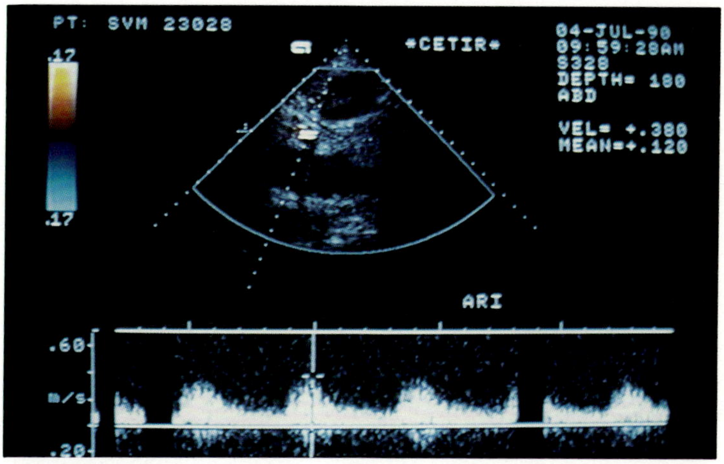

(b)

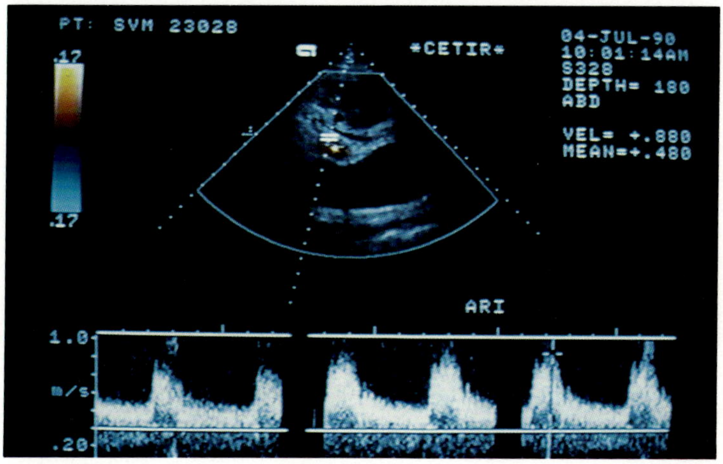

(c)

Plate 1. (a) Color duplex Doppler shows left renal artery aneurysm (ARI) and aorta (AO). (b) Doppler waveform inside the aneurysm shows slow blood flow (peak systolic velocity of 0.38 m/s). (c) Doppler waveform from post-aneurysm segment shows normalization of flow (peak systolic velocity of 0.88 m/s).

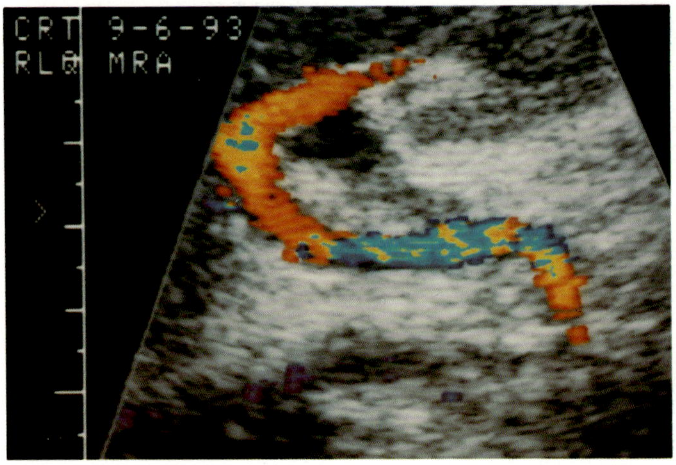

Plate 2. Color aided duplex Doppler of lesion in Figure 20.4 demonstrating focal color aliasing distal to anastomosis of main transplant renal artery (MRA) to external iliac artery.

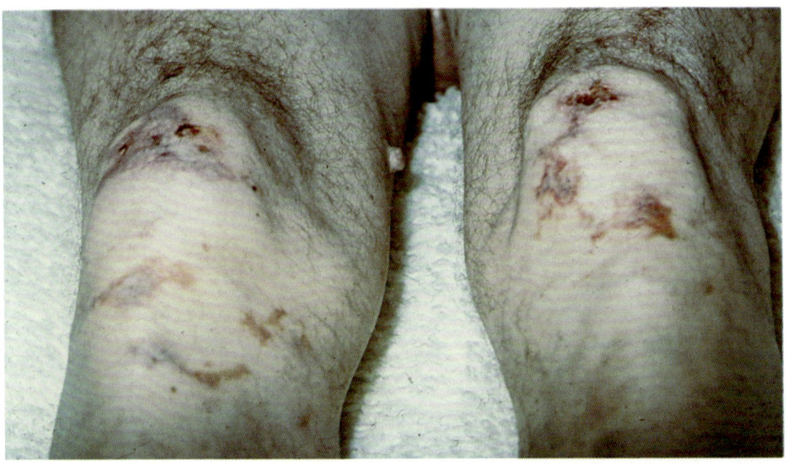

(a)

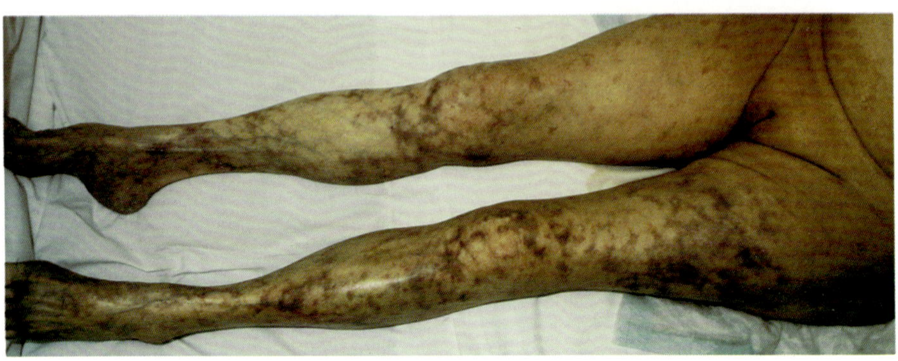

(b)

Plate 3. Cholesterol emboli: (a) light and (b) more severe, white and blue patches of the skin with painful ulceration and intact pulsations of the larger arteries.

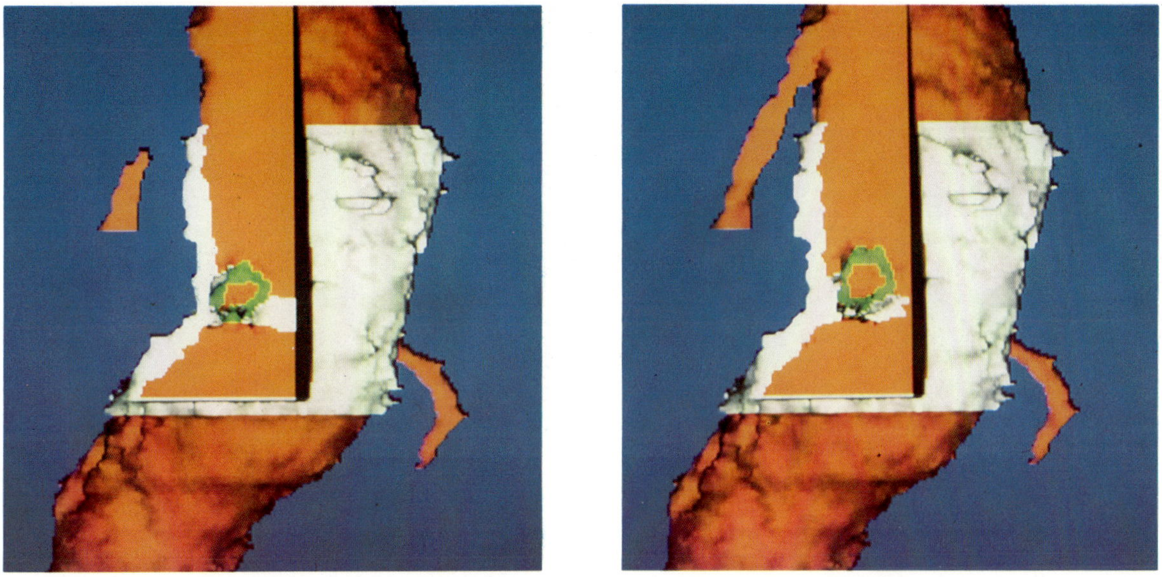

(a) (b)

Plate 4. Computer reconstructions of atheromatous renal artery stenosis dilated by PTRA with stent.

A 77-year-old woman had an acceleration of her chronic hypertension. Angiotensin converting enzyme inhibition was followed by sufficient antihypertensive response but her serum creatinine increased from 140 to 208 μmol/1. Arteriography showed right-sided stenosis of the origin of a very atheromatous aorta and occlusion of the left renal artery. PTRA was followed by reoccurrence of the stenosis, clinically shown by progression of the renal insufficiency during continued angiotensin converting enzyme inhibition. After her second reoccurrence of stenosis a Palmaz stent was placed. Computer reconstructions show additional information that can be obtained by spiral angio-CT scanning. Red: blood column; white: arterial wall with atheroma; green: the metallic Palmaz stent.

Different from angioplasty that visualizes only the blood column, spiral angio-CT scanning shows the thickness of the atheromatous wall of the aorta at the origin of the renal artery. (a) Frontal plane, just behind the origin of the right renal artery. (b) Frontal plane 5mm anterior from (a) showing the origin. (*Continued overleaf.*)

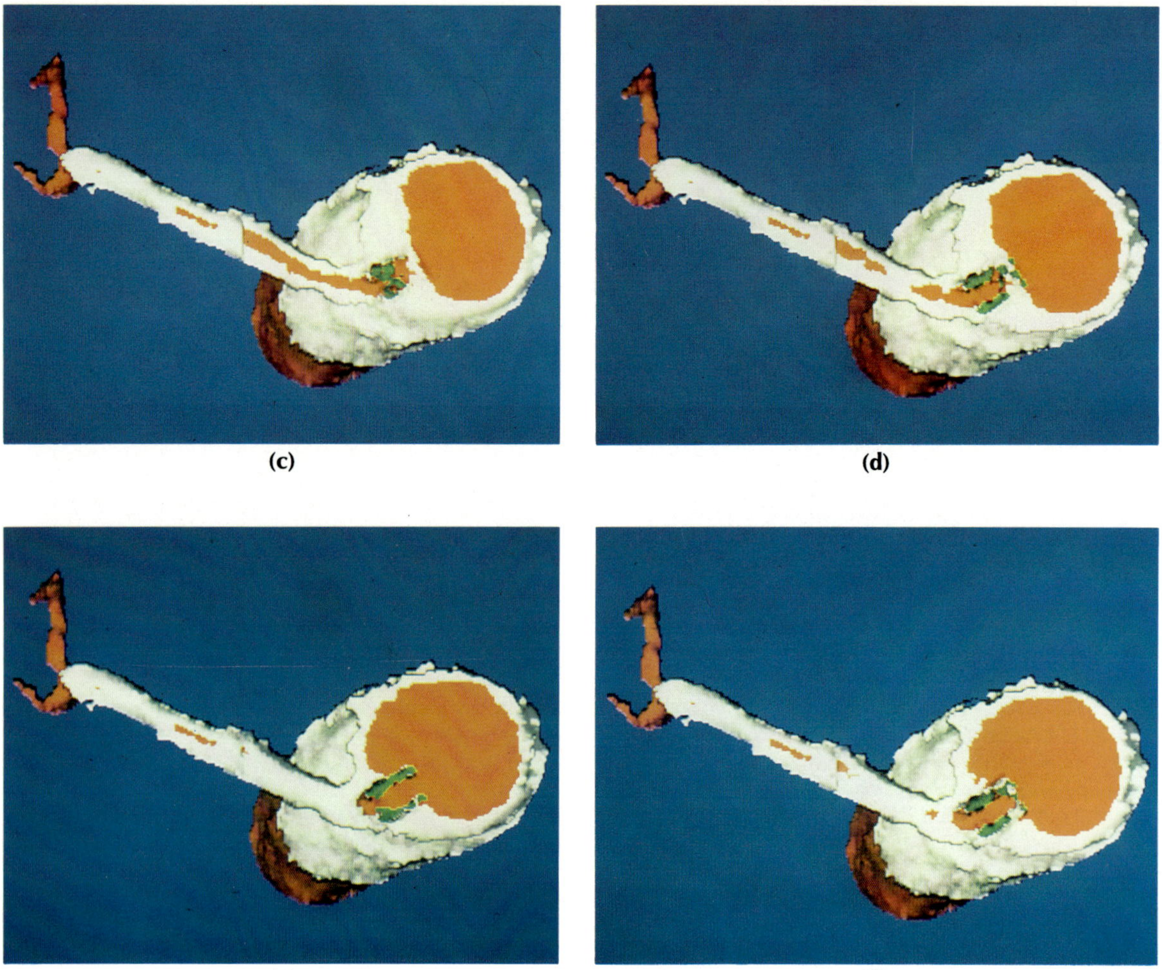

(c) (d) (e) (f)

Plate 4 *continued.* Computer reconstructions of a spiral-CT scanning of a Palmaz stent in the origin of the right renal artery (same investigation as (a) and (b)). (c)–(f) Reconstruction in different horizontal plane, showing protrusion of the stent by the atheromatous aortic wall. Red: blood column; white; arterial wall with atheroma; green: the metallic Palmaz stent.

30

Atherectomy and laser therapy in renal artery stenosis

ANDREW D PLATTS

Despite their theoretical advantages atherectomy or laser atheroablation are not frequently utilized in the treatment of renal artery stenosis (RAS) nor is their use supported by clinical trials. Anecdotal reports suggest that both atherectomy and laser atheroablation can be used alone or as an adjunct to balloon dilatation in successful treatment of renal arterial ostial or mainstem stenosis.[1–6]

Whilst balloon angioplasty provides satisfactory and sustained improvement when used in mainstem RAS it performs suboptimally in ostial stenosis. Concentric dilatation of ostial disease produces fissuring of the aortic atheroma that projects into the lumen of the renal artery but deflation of the balloon allows the atheroma to fall back with immediate recurrence of the stenosis (Fig. 30.1).

Stenting of ostial stenosis provides early success but there is a relatively high restenosis rate caused by neointimal hyperplasia. Resection of the overhanging plaque would offer a good chance of early and sustained success but none of the devices that are currently available are specifically designed to operate at the ostium of a vessel.

Two effective techniques of mechanical atherectomy are available: concentric resection or abrasion (TEC, Pullback atherectomy catheter and Rotablator) and sidecutting resection (Simpson Atherocath). Each can undeniably resect or otherwise ablate atheroma in anatomically ideal locations, that is, in relatively straight vessels. Their performance is impaired when compelled to perform in the more challenging circumstances found when operating within the renal vessels.

Though success is reported[1–4] devices that work concentrically are disadvantaged when working at the ostium of the renal artery because the guiding wire over which they work will take the widest possible radius and distort the course of the vessel. This distorts the path of the device

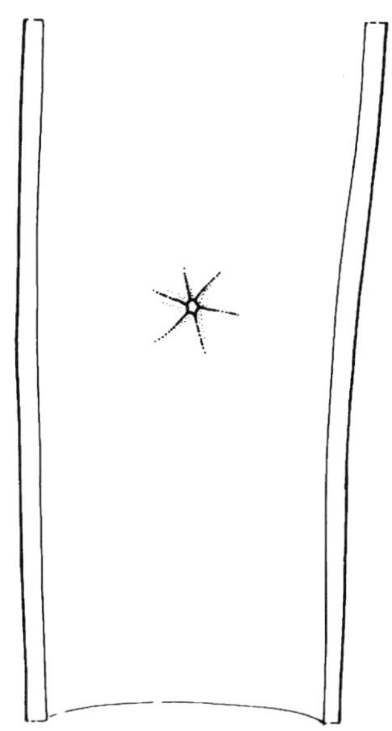

Figure 30.1. En face view of ostial RAS showing fissuring of plaque but no improvement in the lumen.

forcing it to cut an eccentric channel with the potential that it may cut out of the lumen completely (Figs 30.2 and 30.3). The sidecutting device relies on atheroma prolapsing into the cutting chamber where it is amputated by a rotating blade. The resected tissue is packed into a retaining cylinder. The cutting chamber and cylinder are rigid and cannot easily be advanced around acute angles. If the shaft of the device is angled it increases the friction on the drivewire to the blade causing it to fail. It is possible to resect plaque within the mainstem of the renal artery[4] and at the ostium of a vessel that does not leave at an acute angle,[6] but it is impossible to reliably produce an adequate lumen when operating in the ostium of a sharply angulated vessel.

If a device becomes available that can cut a concentric lumen around a centering wire perpendicular to the main axis of the delivery system it would offer enormous potential for treating ostial arterial disease.

Laser atheroablation utilizes direct laser energy to vaporize plaque or laser energy indirectly as a heat source to produce thermal ablation. Both techniques have been enthusiastically

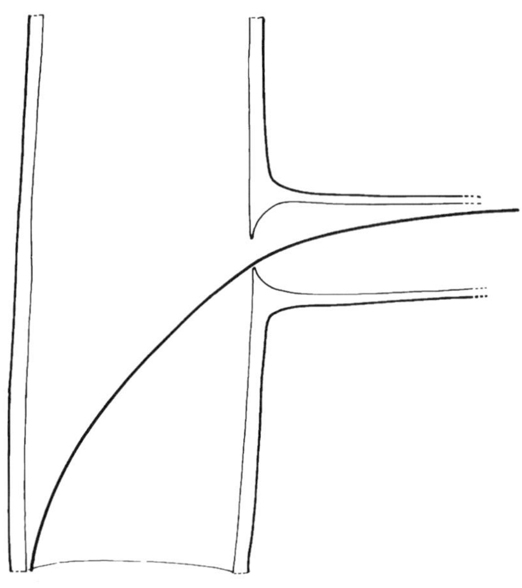

Figure 30.2. Course of a guidewire through an ostial stenosis.

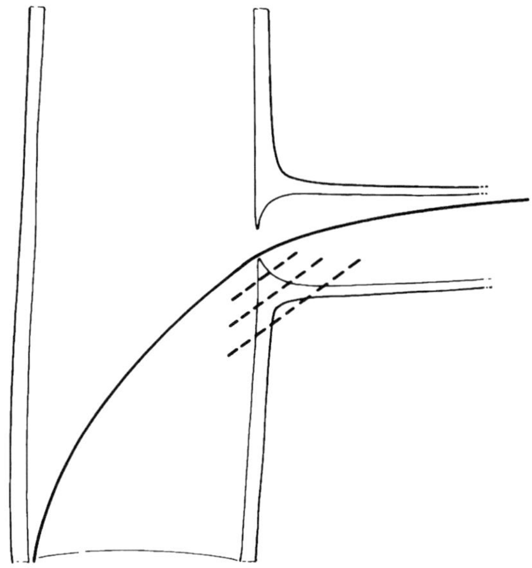

(a)

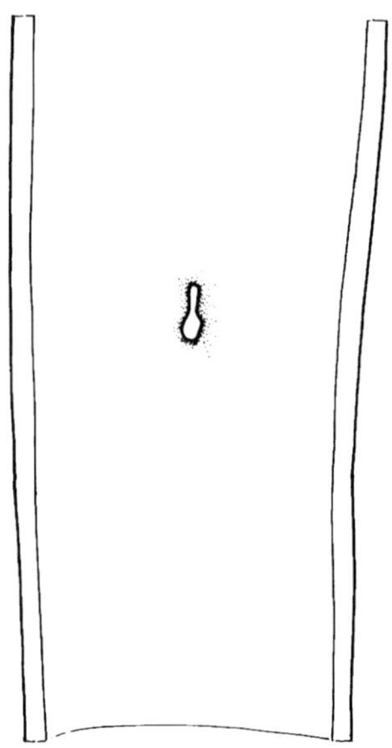

(b)

Figure 30.3. (a) Course of cuts produced by an atherectomy device may eventually cut out of the vessel wall. (b) Lumen produced by an atherectomy device seen en face.

pursued in the peripheral and coronary vasculature but with little lasting impact on clinical practice. Misgivings were voiced about the effectiveness of these devices when it became clear that success was independent of the laser energy being switched on. It has become clear that lasers cannot be used to produce a definitive lumen alone and that their role is to produce a channel through an occluded vessel prior to balloon dilatation[5, 7] Other technological innovations such as hydrophilic coated wires and low speed rotational guidewires (Rotacs) can be used to cross occlusions or stenoses when conventional wires have failed and at considerably less expense than laser devices.

Laser recanalization offers no specific benefit in the renal artery. Laser probes tend to be less flexible than conventional wires and are no more likely to find the true lumen through an occluded vessel than conventional recanalization techniques.

The promise of atheroma selectivity and sparing of undiseased vessel wall has not been shown in clinical practice. The potential for the development of useful laser atheroablative devices currently seems remote.

Hydraulic atheroablation, rheolysis, has been shown to ablate atheroma under experimental conditions.[8] Its application within small vessels suggests that it may offer potential benefit in the renal artery if the renal parenchyma can survive the release of the small particles that are inevitably produced.

References

1 Zaitoun R, Dorros G, Iyer SS, Lewin RF. Percutaneous high-speed rotational atherectomy (Rotablator) of a restenosed ostial renal artery; a case report. *Cath Cardiovasc Diagn* 1990, **20:** 254–6.
2 Dorros G, Iyer S, Zaitoun R *et al.* Acute angiographic and clinical outcome of high-speed percutaneous rotational atherectomy (Rotablator). *Cath Cardiovas Diagn* 1991, **22:** 157–66.
3 White CJ, Ramsee SR, Escobar A *et al.* High-speed rotational ablation (Rotablator) for unfavorable lesions in peripheral arteries. *Cath Cardiovasc Diagn* 1993, **30:** 115–19.
4 Kushner FG, Helm MJ. Successful directional atherectomy of eccentric renal artery stenosis using the Simpson directional coronary atherocath as a primary therapy. *Cath Cardiovasc Diagn* 1993, **29:** 128–30.
5 Tani M, Mizuno K, Midorikawa H *et al.* Thermal laser assisted angioplasty of renal artery stenosis for renovascular hypertension. *Cardiovasc Intervent Radiol* 1993; **16:** 52–4.
6 Polniz A, Hofling B. Percutaneous atherectomy of a recurrent renal transplant artery stenosis. *Transplantation* 1993; **48:** 880–3.
7 Bauer R, Pokorney E, Muckenhuber P *et al.* Is laser assisted angioplasty a real alternative to surgical treatment of occluded peripheral vessels? *Eur J Vasc Surg* 1991; **5:** 637–40.
8 Drasler WJ, Jenson ML, Wilson GJ, Thielen JM, Protonotarios EL, Dutcher RG *et al.* A rheolytic system for percutaneous coronary and peripheral plaque removal. *Angiology* 1991; **42:** 90–8.

31

Fibrinolytic therapy in renovascular disease

GEORGE HAMILTON

Introduction

Acute ischemia of the kidney is a relatively uncommon presentation of renovascular disease. Usually this results from embolic or thrombotic occlusion of the renal artery, nowadays often iatrogenic, and perhaps less commonly from aortic dissection and trauma. Unlike most manifestations of renovascular disease these conditions present acutely, requiring urgent treatment to preserve renal function. Fibrinolytic dissolution of thrombus causing acute renal ischemia is increasingly being used as an acceptable alternative to surgical intervention.

Acute renal ischemia

Trauma commonly damages the renal parenchyma with main renal artery occlusion or disruption being less frequent. Severe deceleration injury is the usual cause with a multiply injured patient presenting with loin pain, tenderness and hematuria. These signs are difficult to elicit in the presence of polytrauma but a one-shot intravenous pyelogram or contrast enhanced computerized tomography (CT) scan will confirm the diagnosis. In the presence of severe renal parenchymal laceration, probable renal arterial disruption and dissection, and a high likelihood of trauma to other organs, fibrinolytic therapy has little to offer. Indeed because of aggravation of hemorrhage and amplification of any clotting diathesis from further loss of clotting factors its use must be positively contraindicated. Treatment of traumatic renal artery occlusion is surgical where indicated although the results of the operative approach are not encouraging.[1]

Embolic renal artery occlusion is also a rare presentation of acute renal ischemia. The vast majority are cardiac in origin (>90%). Over 30% may involve both kidneys but overall only 5% of all arterial emboli will travel to the visceral vessels.[2] Major renal emboli seem to occur more commonly than clinically suspected as illustrated by a postmortem series reported in 1940 by Hoxie and Coggin. In this series of over 14 000 postmortems, 1.4% (205 patients) were found to have renal infarction secondary to embolism but a correct antemortem diagnosis of this condition was made in only 2 of these 205 cases.[3] Renal artery embolism should be suspected when there are features of acute renal ischemia in the presence of cardiac dysrrhythmia, particularly atrial fibrillation, myocardial ischemia, heart failure and less commonly in rheumatic heart disease, cardiomyopathy and prosthetic heart valves. Because the embolic occlusion is often partial, a degree of renal perfusion is maintained, which probably explains the good results of 70% renal salvage obtained by surgical treatment.[4] Mortality in this group is high at 25% whether treated surgically or conservatively, reflecting the underlying poor cardiac status of these patients. Fibrinolytic therapy is an attractive therapeutic option in this high anesthetic risk group.

The final event in progression of renal artery stenosis is thrombosis. Because of the collateral circulation which has had time to develop this event is usually clinically silent, manifesting itself as a deterioration in renal function. Consequently there is not such a degree of urgency in revascularization. However acute renal arterial thrombosis can occur in previously healthy vessels when involved in aortic disease such as aortic dissection or in the aortic thrombotic syndromes of the neonate. Renal artery dissection may also complicate fibromuscular dysplasia. Dissection can result in either partial or complete occlusion presenting variably as hypertension, deteriorating renal function, renal infarction or often as an incidental finding at angiography. In any of these conditions acute thrombosis may supervene and should be suspected in the presence of upper abdominal and flank pain, hematuria, exacerbation of pre-existent hypertension or *de novo* onset of severe hypertension.[5] Obviously treatment should be prompt in this situation in order to prevent progression to complete occlusion by thrombosis. Fibrinolytic therapy in suspected thrombosis may buy time by maintaining a degree of renal blood supply while revascularization is organized. Indeed having cleared the thrombosis, revascularization by angioplasty with or without stenting may become possible. It is worth emphasizing that operative management of renal artery dissection should be by surgeons capable of dealing with segmental artery lesions if need be by bench surgery.

The explosive increase in interventional radiological and endovascular techniques to the heart, kidney and other vessels over recent years has inevitably resulted *pari passu* in an increase in iatrogenic renal artery occlusions. Percutaneous transluminal renal angioplasty (PTRA) is widely used in treatment of renal stenoses in fibromuscular dysplasia, atherosclerosis and transplant kidney. Successful angioplasty depends on disruption not only of the plaque but also of components of the vessel wall itself. The angioplasty lesion is characterized by intimal fissuring, variable disruption of the media and dissection. It is therefore not surprising that PTRA is complicated by thrombosis of the angioplasty site resulting in reocclusion. Passage of radiological catheters across the renal artery origins for access to the heart, carotid, mesenteric and peripheral vascular circulations is rarely complicated by thrombosis. In the presence of the severely atherosclerotic 'shaggy' aorta so commonly seen in the region of the visceral vessels, atheroembolism to the renal arteries does result; indeed the kidney is the organ most commonly affected by this form of embolism. Catheterization of the renal arteries in the diffuse aortic atherosclerosis seen in 15% of vascular patients is particularly prone to this complication. The prognosis in renal failure secondary to atheroembolism is dismal with few episodes of recovery reported. Fibrinolytic therapy will be of limited value in atheroembolism adding little to the effects of heparin anticoagulation.

Acute renal ischemia in children occurs mainly in neonates with aortic thrombosis secondary to the increasing use of umbilical artery catheterization in neonatal intensive care units. Treatment has traditionally been conservative mainly in control of the severe hypertension so common when renal thrombosis supervenes. In the presence of oliguria or anuria surgical intervention to perform embolectomy and revascularization is required. This poses major problems for the anesthetist and pediatric surgeon. Fibrinolytic therapy has theoretical advantages as a much less invasive procedure not requiring general anesthesia.

Fibrinolytic therapy

The most common indication for fibrinolytic therapy is in acute coronary thrombosis where systemically administered agents have good clinical success rates. Over the last decade enthusiasm for lower dose local intra-arterial delivery of fibrinolysis has become widespread in vascular centres mainly for treatment of acute peripheral arterial occlusions. Lower limb ischemia, thrombosed popliteal aneurysms and blocked vascular grafts are now routinely and successfully treated by this method.

Fibrinolytic therapy has several theoretical advantages over more traditional methods such as anticoagulation, thrombectomy or embolectomy and emergency vascular reconstruction. Anticoagulation simply limits extension of thrombus formation, facilitating fibrinolysis by endogenous plasminogen activators. This process is slow, taking weeks to achieve complete lysis of a major clot such as that seen in a deep venous thrombosis. Embolectomy remains a valuable surgical procedure most effective in fresh occlusions (<48 h) and in true embolism into a normal artery. This technique has the disadvantage of causing stripping and denudation of vascular endothelium with subsequent stenosis and rethrombosis.[6, 7] In addition embolectomy in diseased vessels causes atheromatous plaque disruption, thus aggravating the occlusion and leading to the depressingly common outcome in our elderly populations of worsening of the degree of ischemia. In the renal circulation embolectomy is of most value in clearance of segmental emboli but will not be able to remove microemboli or distally propagated thrombus. Peroperative infusion of a fibrinolytic agent during a procedure will of course achieve distal clearance.

Clearly any operative approach carries the considerable risks of anesthesia and surgery in a patient usually very unfit from associated coronary, carotid and peripheral vascular disease. Fibrinolytic therapy does not require general anesthesia and in theory carries less risk to the patient. Perhaps more importantly successful fibrinolysis combines both therapeutic and diagnostic advantages. Once lysis has been achieved, any underlying pathology such as a shorter stenosis or occlusion than that seen originally may be revealed and treated by angioplasty if suitable or less urgent reconstruction if not. A further important benefit is clearance of thrombus in distal vessels not otherwise amenable to treatment and achieving distal reperfusion to an extent impossible to achieve by other means.

The fibrinolytic system

Clot lysis results when plasminogen produced by the liver is converted to plasmin by endogenous agents such as tissue-type plasminogen activator produced by vascular endothelial cells. Plasmin, a proteolytic enzyme, cleaves fibrin into soluble polypeptides or fibrin degradation products by hydrolysis. It will also hydrolyze circulating coagulation factors such as fibrinogen and Factors V and VII. A delicate balance exists in the normal circulation between coagulation and fibrinolysis, both systems being regulated by production of specific inhibitors. α_2-Antiplasmin is the main inhibitor of fibrinolysis in plasma but others include antithrombin III, antitrypsin and α_2-microglobulin. These factors limit both plasminogen activation and the hydrolytic effect of plasmin, and also act by instantly neutralizing free circulating plasmin. Thrombus-bound plasmin is protected from these inhibitors as long as it remains bound to fibrin within the clot. Thus an elegant system of fibrinolysis specific to thrombus with protection against fibrinolysis in the rest of the circulation is ensured (Fig. 31.1).[8]

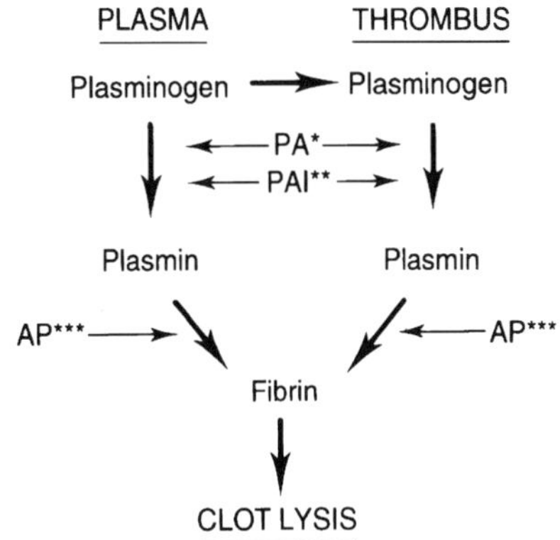

Figure 31.1. The fibrinolytic system: PA*: plasminogen activators, streptokinase, urokinase, r-tPA; PAI**: plasminogen activator inhibitors: AP***: the antiplasmins.

Fibrinolysis: agents and techniques

Three fibrinolytic agents are in common use at present, streptokinase, urokinase and recombinant tissue plasminogen activator (r-tPA). Streptokinase discovered in 1933 was first used clinically in the early 1960s. It remains the preferred and most cost-effective agent in systemic fibrinolysis for coronary thrombosis. Because of its low cost it is still used by many vascular centres for intra-arterial therapy. Streptokinase is non-enzymatic, indirectly activating plasminogen by forming an intermediate complex with plasminogen and then promoting cleavage to active plasmin.[9, 10] It is non-selective in its action binding both to thrombus-bound and circulating plasminogen. Circulating plasmin thus formed is neutralized by α_2-antiplasmin in the circulation eventually depleting levels of this inhibitor and allowing plasmin to act unopposed. When plasma levels of coagulation factors are lowered as a result, a systemic bleeding tendency can result.[11] This effect together with its relatively long half-life of 27 min explains the higher incidence of bleeding complications seen with use of streptokinase. There are further problems with this agent because of its streptococcal origin and thus a foreign bacterial protein. High levels of antistreptococcal antibodies are commonly present in most patients due to previous β-hemolytic streptococcal infection. Also after streptokinase therapy for coronary thrombosis antibody titers can remain very high for as long as 12 months; this is a problem in patients with vascular disease where coronary artery disease is so prevalent. On initial infusion streptokinase will be neutralized by formation of antigen–antibody complexes until the antistreptococcal antibodies are consumed. Since these complexes are biologicaly inert, fibrinolysis cannot begin until this has been achieved, thus explaining the slower and more variable response seen with streptokinase. Finally streptokinase has a high incidence of unpleasant side-effects: fever, nausea, hallucinations and even anaphylaxis. For these reasons streptokinase has been abandoned as a fibrinolytic agent in many vascular units.

Urokinase, originally derived from human urine in 1947[12] and now extracted from cultured human kidney cells[13] is the most widely used fibrinolytic agent in North America for arterial thrombosis.[14, 15] It is a trypsin-like serine protease capable of direct activation of fibrinolysis without antigenicity and low pyrogenicity. Like streptokinase, however, it is not clot specific acting both on circulating and fibrin-bound plasminogen, thus potentially resulting in systemic bleeding tendency.

Tissue-type plasminogen activator is a serine protease which has the advantage of being clot specific. It was first identified in 1947 and its DNA structure sequenced and cloned in 1983.[16] The activator produced by this recombinant technology, r-tPA, appears to be biologically identical to that produced by human vascular endothelial cells. This agent has a high affinity for thrombus-bound plasminogen but low affinity for plasminogen in the absence of fibrin, thus exerting a powerful effect local to clot but with little systemic action.[10] This clot specificity and sparing of the systemic fibrinolytic system results in lower hemorrhagic complication rates for low dose arterial infusions. Its non-antigenicity, lack of side-effects and short half-life of only 6 min make r-tPA an ideal fibrinolytic agent for local arterial infusion.[17] The major problem with this thrombolytic agent remains its relatively high cost.

Other activators such as pro-urokinase and acetylated streptokinase–plasminogen complex are under clinical development and evaluation, but currently the above three agents are the only ones in common use.

Protocols for intra-arterial thrombolysis

Most commonly streptokinase is infused at between 5000 to 8000 units per hour; typical infusion times are in excess of 12–24 h.[18] In many centers urokinase is currently given in an initial high dose infusion of 4000 iu/min for 2–4 h and then at a reduced rate of 1000–2000 iu/min for 6–8 h or longer if necessary.[19, 20] Tissue plasminogen activator can be given in either low or high dose regimens. Low dose r-tPA infusion is given at 0.5–1.0 mg/h while the high dose regimen is given at between 2 and 10 mg/h; lysis times are typically less than 6 h.[21, 22]

The above protocols relate more to fibrinolysis in peripheral vascular occlusions. A flexible and aggressive approach to renal thrombosis is required tailored to achieving speedy restoration of perfusion. To prevent pericatheter thrombus formation during the infusion most authors recommend heparinization throughout although this is controversial. Heparinization will have been implemented in most patients before fibrinolysis is commenced and it is convenient and safe to maintain heparin infusion before, during and most importantly after the infusion keeping the activated partial thromboplastin time (aPTT) ratio at 1.5–2.

Delivery and techniques of fibrinolytic therapy

A diagnostic angiogram must precede every consideration of fibrinolytic therapy and a decision to proceed made between the vascular surgeon, nephrologist and radiologist. With the possible exception of neonatal aortic thrombosis, intra-arterial delivery is preferable to the systemic intravenous approach. Typically, a suitable 5 French gauge or smaller catheter is introduced using the Seldinger technique via the femoral artery. Occasionally the brachial or axillary artery approach will be used according to the presence of aortic or iliac disease, or if severe angulation of the renal artery origin presents difficulty in negotiating the guidewire across the renal ostium (Fig. 31.2). Catheter technology is constantly improving with ever better variations being produced. To be recommended is the use of microcatheters or infusion guidewires which are small enough to be passed through the center of the main infusion catheter and located into distal segmental renal arteries. In this way distal delivery of the agent can be ensured at the same time as the main trunk is being perfused (Fig. 31.3). The use of an introducer sheath facilitates manipulation and changing of catheters, a real boon if for example angioplasty becomes necessary. The introducer sheath also helps to limit groin hematoma.[23]

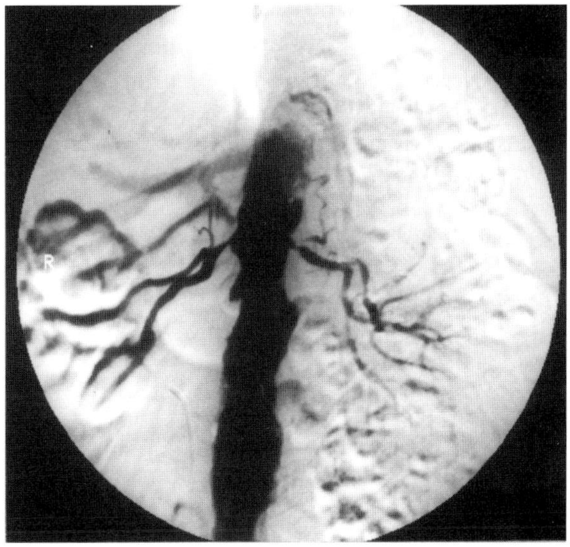

Figure 31.2. This angiogram shows severe concomitant disease of the infrarenal aorta; catheter manipulations of the renal arteries across such an aorta runs the risk of atheroembolism and ostial occlusion of main aortic branches. There is also acute angulation of the renal arteries. Complications in this situation can be avoided by use of the brachial or axillary artery for access.

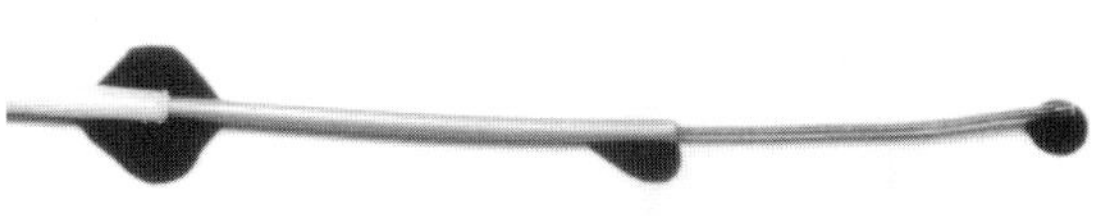

Figure 31.3. The use of coaxial catheters allows delivery of fibrinolysis to more of the thrombus; the innermost microcatheter or perfusion guidewire can be positioned to perfuse the distal renal circulation.

Several strategies to achieve efficient and speedy clot lysis are used, all directed at maximizing the interface between thrombus and lytic agent. If at all possible the occlusion should be traversed by the guidewire to agitate and break up the clot. Catheter aspiration of the clot can significantly speed up reperfusion of the kidney but is technically difficult and cannot routinely be achieved. The thrombus is laced with lytic agent throughout as much of its length as possible before embedding the catheter tip at the proximal edge of the clot. Using the microcatheters delivered coaxially, simultaneous infusion proximally and distally within the clot can be employed to achieve speedier lysis. The recent development of high pressure radial spray or 'pulse spray' catheter systems has led to quicker lysis times in peripheral vascular thrombosis. This system injects a fine high pressure spray of lytic agent through multiple holes thus breaking up and more effectively increasing the interface between clot and lytic agent. Small 3 French gauge catheters are becoming available which would be suitable for renal artery treatment (Fig. 31.4). An alternative faster method is the use of standard catheters but with high dose bolus infusions into the clot. Both methods are particularly useful in renal occlusion because of the speedier lysis of clot and reperfusion.

Thus several strategies are available to the clinician. Choice of method should involve considerations such as the viability of the kidney, the extent and nature of the clot and most importantly local expertise.

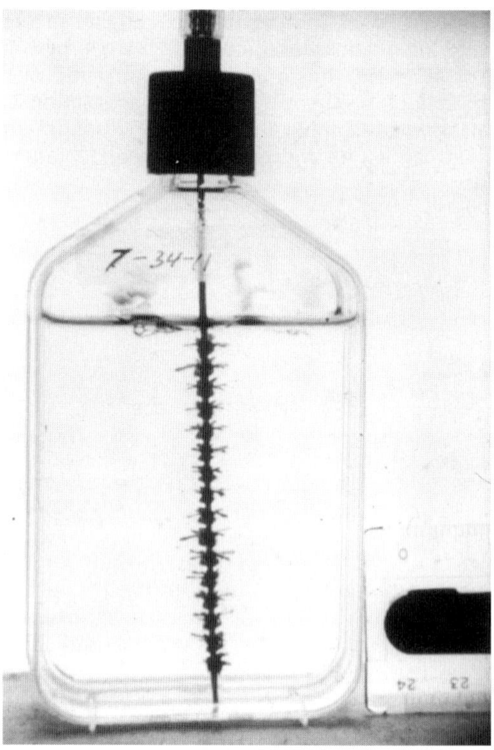

Figure 31.4. Pulse spray catheters have multiple sideholes or slits which open under pressure and force multiple sprays of fibrinolytic agent throughout the length of the catheter. This maximizes mixing of thrombus and agent. There are automated systems which will pulse at frequent intervals; otherwise this can be done by hand by catheter injection every 2 min. Illustrated is such a catheter suspended in gelatin and perfused with dye.

Close angiographic monitoring of progression of the lytic process is important. With pulse spray or high dose bolus infusion clearance may occur rapidly, perhaps within 30 min to 1 h, and the patient should remain in the angiogram suite throughout. If the other slower methods are used repeat angiography perhaps after an hour and thereafter at regular longer intervals will be necessary until sufficient lysis is shown.

Because of the long length of catheter in the aortic circulation there is a considerable risk of thrombus formation around it. This problem should be prevented by administration of heparin (5000 iu bolus then 500–1000 iu hourly to maintain aPTT ratio of 1.5–2). If there is pericatheter thrombus this will be dislodged when the catheter is removed at the end of the procedure causing a sizable embolism into the leg. This can usually be satisfactorily dealt with by directing the lytic infusion into the affected femoral artery although prevention has to be better than cure.

All of these procedures must be performed under the attendance of a vascular surgeon able to deal with complications which uncommonly happen. These patients are best managed in a high dependency area ideally within or close to the angiography suite. Specialist nursing care is of the highest importance which together with a team approach of vascular surgeon, nephrologist and interventional radiologist will lead to optimal management.

Monitoring

Patients with acute renal ischemia, invariably ill and at high risk because of severe associated cardiovascular disorders, require careful clinical monitoring of vital signs, pulse oxymetry, electrocardiography, neurological status and of course renal function.

As previously discussed, careful and regular angiography is the only reliable tool for monitoring of lysis progress and deciding when to stop the therapy. Timing of angiography will largely be determined by whether a low or high dose regimen is used.

Monitoring for hemorrhage, the major complication of fibrinolytic therapy, requires meticulous attention to catheter and puncture sites. Bleeding from these sites is usually the first warning of a developing bleeding diathesis. Laboratory monitoring of coagulation by measurement of hematocrit, prothrombin time, activated partial thromboplastin time, fibrinogen, fibrinogen degradation products, fibrin monomers and dimers and bleeding time is widely performed to varying degrees. Unfortunately the hope that detection of systemic activation of the fibrinolytic system would be possible by these methods has not been fulfilled since there is poor correlation between changes in these parameters and risk of hemorrhage.[10] The only worthwhile correlation is between risk of bleeding and serum fibrinogen levels of less than 1.2 g/l. When considered together with the general lack of easy access to these measurements out of hours, these facts have led many clinicians not to rely absolutely on investigations as predictors of hemorrhage. Similarly attempts to predict successful clot lysis by measurement of parameters such as fibrinogen degradation products and fibrin monomers and dimers have proved unsuccessful. In fibrinolytic therapy of renal artery occlusions monitoring of lytic success can only be reliably achieved by angiography.

Contraindications to fibrinolytic therapy

Patients obviously at particular risk of hemorrhage should be excluded *ab initio*. A history of recent hemorrhagic status, bleeding diathesis, major trauma or active peptic ulceration are examples. Because of the risk of lysis of hemostatic thrombus, recent major surgery, abdominal, intracranial or thoracic, would be relative contraindications. Again because of the risk of dissolution of the lining pannus, fibrinolytic therapy to blocked Dacron grafts has been described as hazardous because of the inherent porosity of many Dacron preparations. In knitted grafts in particular, major hemorrhage could result, although recent experience in aortic and iliac grafts suggests that this is not a problem.[24] Dacron is used in aortorenal bypass grafting and thus fibrinolytic therapy is best avoided until 3 months after implantation when graft incorporation by scar tissue will be maximal. There are no such problems with grafts made from expanded polytetrafluoroethylene but the reality of hemorrhage from a fresh suture line subjected to thrombolytic perfusion must be borne in mind irrespective of the graft material used.

In embolic renal artery occlusions the presence of intracardiac thrombus must be sought by echocardiography. Although a relative contraindication, the small risk of showering off of additional emboli detached because of systemic spillover during the lytic period must be considered in the choice of therapy. Obviously atheroemboli should not be treated by fibrinolysis. Finally consideration must also be given to the likely age of the thrombus and the urgency of revascularization of the kidney. A fresh thrombus will lyse quickly and totally while a more mature, adherent clot will take much longer and may not ever lyse completely. If the kidney needs revascularization urgently and within a short time period, the latter scenario becomes a contraindication to low dose fibrinolysis.

Complications

These can be considered as minor and major. Minor complications include small puncture site bleeds usually occurring later in the course of therapy and easily controlled by pressure. Puncture site bleeding early in the course of the treatment, however, is more sinister indicating a potential systemic effect and bleeding diathesis, and there should be a low threshold for cessation of therapy. Pericatheter thrombus is a problem best treated by prevention by concomitant heparin administration. Thrombus dislodged into the distal circulation can of course be successfully treated by catheter redeployment and fibrinolytic therapy, but at the cost of pain, the systemic effects of leg ischemia and the exposure to the patient of prolonged fibrinolysis. Catheters can block if the infusion is allowed to stop and can also be inappropriately removed. These problems can be best avoided by adequate training of nursing staff, good protocols and careful handling of infusion pumps and catheters. Drug-related complications have already been discussed, the major complication being anaphylaxis when streptokinase is used. Suitable facilities for recognition and prompt treatment of anaphylactic shock must be available if it is used.

The major complications are of significant hemorrhage and stroke. Major bleeding defined as that requiring cessation of therapy and/or blood transfusion, occurs in 5% of patients, even when high risk cases are excluded.[25] Duration of infusion has been associated significantly with increased bleeding complications, but this has not been so in the Royal Free Hospital experience where catheter sheaths and the use of r-tPA are routine.[26] Higher dosage infusion regimens given to promote more rapid lysis are associated however with more complications, particularly hemorrhage.[27] Internal and occult bleeding can occur as evidenced by hypotension and falling hematocrit. Intracranial hemorrhage complicates less than 2% of intra-arterial fibrinolytic treatments of all types but is usually severe. Any change in neurological status must be investigated urgently by contrast CT scan and the infusion stopped immediately signs appear. Non-hemorrhagic embolic stroke does also occur presumably due to lysed thrombus from a cardiac source. Severe hemorrhage, in addition to immediate stopping of fibrinolysis, may need administration of fresh frozen factors and clotting factors such as cryoprecipitate if the diathesis continues. Antifibrinolytic agents such as epsi-aminocaproic acid are not of value in stopping this degree of bleeding and indeed may aggravate the underlying thrombotic problem.

Indications and results

Fibrinolysis is an attractive, less invasive option than surgery in the severely ill cardiovascularly compromised patient. It still carries risks however and the decision to use fibrinolysis should not be made without due consideration. In bilaterally occluded renal arteries or where a solitary functioning kidney is affected intervention to salvage renal function is necessary. If however only one of two functioning kidneys has a vascular occlusion then in the high risk patient it may be safer to accept the loss of that kidney and avoid the risks of fibrinolysis. Fibrinolytic treatment of renal artery occlusion is not common and this is reflected in the literature. Discussion of the results obtained in the following conditions is based mainly on review of the literature over the last two decades.

Acute renal artery embolism

Just under 30 cases of acute renal artery embolism treated by intra-arterial fibrinolysis are recorded in the world literature.[28–35] Most were treated with streptokinase or urokinase with quite prolonged treatments (>12 h) being reported. In one remarkable case successful lysis with good long-term renal function was reported after 18 h treatment for a 7-day-old renal artery occlusion.[33] Technically successful clot lysis was achieved in most cases but good long-term renal function was achieved in less than half. The importance of prompt treatment is stressed by all authors. Partial or segmental renal artery occlusion and the finding of a good collateral circulation is associated with good outcome for both surgical and thrombolytic treatments.[28, 29, 36] Long-term follow-up by renal scintigraphy however revealed no improvement in function where there was complete renal artery occlusion, with only incomplete recovery in segmental occlusion even in technically successful clot lysis and reperfusion. This observation indicates that restoration of renal blood flow in acute renal artery embolism will not be successful if irreversible ischemic damage to the nephrons has already occurred. It is important to remember that the warm ischemia tolerance of the kidney *in situ* is at best 90 and probably only 50 min. Despite this sobering fact, good results have been reported with fibrinolysis. Presumably these were cases of partial embolic occlusion or perhaps not embolic at all. Surgical revascularization in this group carries a mortality of 11–25%[4, 37] and the less invasive method of fibrinolysis using one of the more rapid techniques performed expeditiously warrants further experience.

Acute renal artery thrombosis

Successful lysis of acute renal artery thrombosis with good long-term renal function has been reported by several centres.[38–46] Most treatments were by the intra-arterial route but there are three reports of successful systemic intravenous lysis of renal artery thrombosis.[43–45] Vogelzang and his colleagues report a novel use of intra-arterial fibrinolysis delivered into the left renal artery to successfully lyze a left renal vein thrombosis.[46] Most treatments have been with streptokinase but with a recent emphasis on urokinase and r-tPA. In contrast to renal embolism, renal artery thrombosis appears to respond well to lytic therapy with preservation of renal function. By and large this was a very ill group of patients with severe cardiothoracic disease commonly presenting with thrombosis of the visceral aorta and its branches. One can only presume that this pathology develops more insiduously thus allowing some scope for collateral circulation to develop. These results indicate that fibrinolytic treatment should be considered as the initial therapy for this extremely ill group of patients.

Acute thrombosis in renal artery stenosis

The final event in progression to complete occlusion of a severe atherosclerotic stenosis is usually thrombosis. In the renal artery total occlusion is often proximal with distal patency allowing bypass procedures to be performed. Such revascularizations are not only possible but successful providing the kidney is greater than 8.5 cm in length. An attractive alternative would be to dissolve the thrombus component of a total occlusion thereby revealing the underlying stenosis which could then be angioplastied. Three groups report success with this approach in a total of five patients.[47–49] This combination of clearance of propagated thrombus by thrombolysis then angioplasty of the underlying stenosis is well established in treatment of superficial femoral and popliteal occlusions. These blockages are much longer than those found in the renal circulation yet respond well to this stratagem. This method has the potential for avoiding major reconstructive surgery but obviously comparison of long-term results of both approaches would be important. Certainly fibrinolysis and angioplasty in renal arterial thromboses warrants further clinical study.

Iatrogenic renal artery occlusion

Occlusion of the renal artery as a result of angiographic manipulations or PTRA occurs infrequently – most often as a complication of ostial dilatations. The volume of these procedures is increasing, thus inevitably more iatrogenic occlusions are being encountered. In a literature review by Bergentz and Bergqvist the frequency of this complication was found to be 2.3% with distal renal embolization of 1.9%.[50] They suggest that this complication is probably underreported and therefore more common. Certainly the high clinical failure rate reported in angioplasty of renal ostial lesions must be mainly as a result of a combination of early recoil and superimposed thrombosis on the fissured vessel lumen. Fibrinolytic clearance of these occlusions will restore renal perfusion and perhaps allow another attempt at angioplasty with deployment of a stent. The classical approach remains surgical but comparison with this less invasive technique would be interesting. There is little written in the literature about fibrinolysis of PTRA-related thromboses with the exception of four cases reported from Atlanta, Georgia.[29] Most vascular radiologists now regard intra-arterial fibrinolysis as part of their armamentarium, complimentary to angioplasty and probably already in much wider use than the literature would suggest (Figs 31.5 and 31.6).

Infant aortic thrombosis

This condition complicates placement of umbilical arterial catheters in neonates requiring intensive therapy. The clinical picture is one of aortic thrombosis of variable extent usually compromising the visceral aorta and thus the renal circulation, resulting in renal failure. Fibrinolysis has been used to treat this terrible complication with

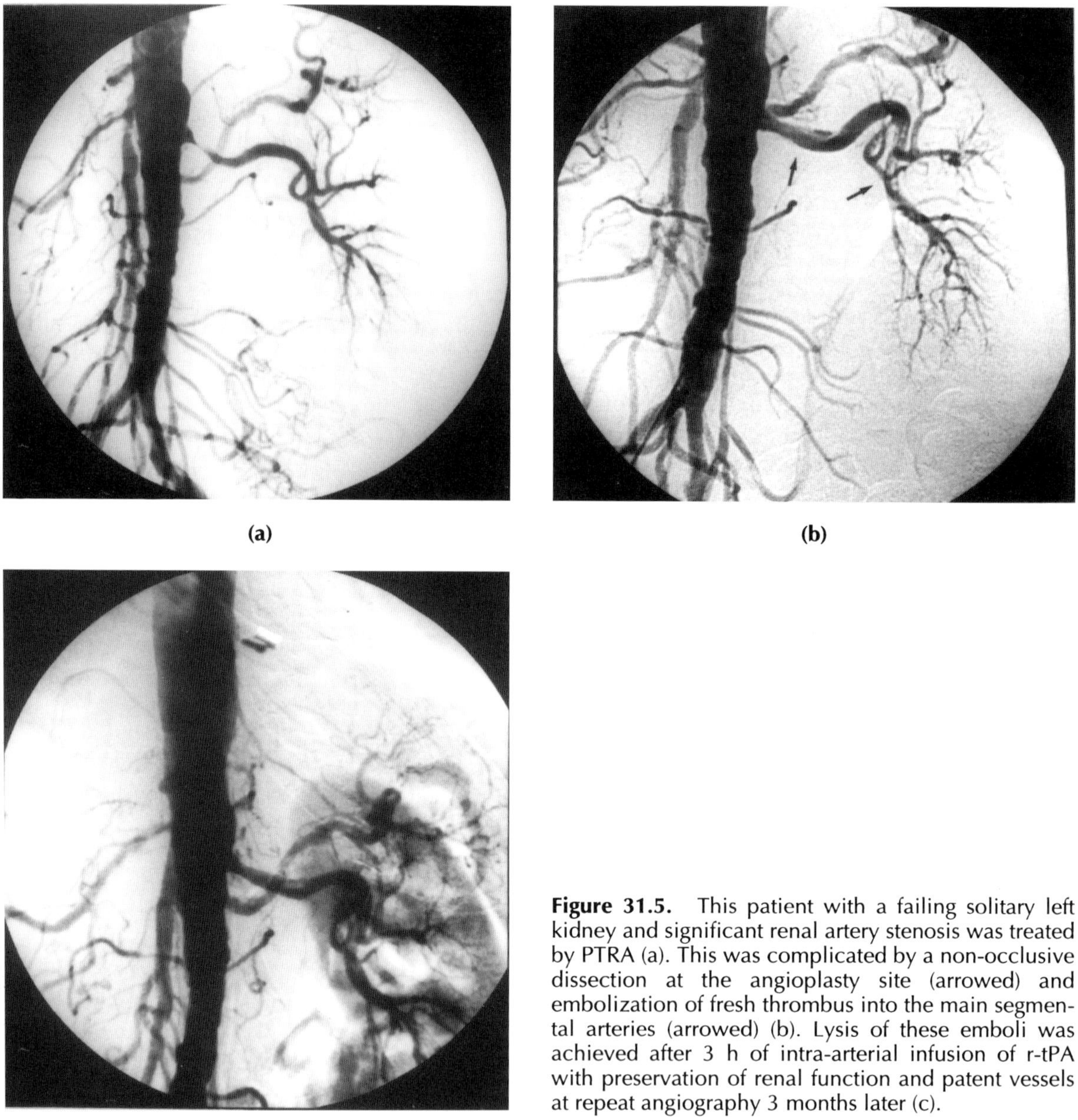

(a) (b) (c)

Figure 31.5. This patient with a failing solitary left kidney and significant renal artery stenosis was treated by PTRA (a). This was complicated by a non-occlusive dissection at the angioplasty site (arrowed) and embolization of fresh thrombus into the main segmental arteries (arrowed) (b). Lysis of these emboli was achieved after 3 h of intra-arterial infusion of r-tPA with preservation of renal function and patent vessels at repeat angiography 3 months later (c).

some success and little apparent morbidity.[51–54] A pediatric group from Wisconsin report long-term renal salvage in an infant after intra-arterial urokinase lysis of an ischemic kidney of 5 days' duration. They suggest that the neonatal kidney has remarkable powers of recovery even after days of warm ischemia and advocate an aggressive fibrinolytic approach.[52] The pediatricians from Northwestern, Chicago, however, report a series of 15 children with aortic thrombosis and renal impairment all treated without intervention but by aggressive antihypertensive therapy. At 2 years' follow-up increased renal perfusion and good renal function was found but with persistence of perfusion deficits in many.[55] Possibly the vascular reserves of the infant kidney are such that revascularization is not needed but empirically it must be better to maximize renal perfu-

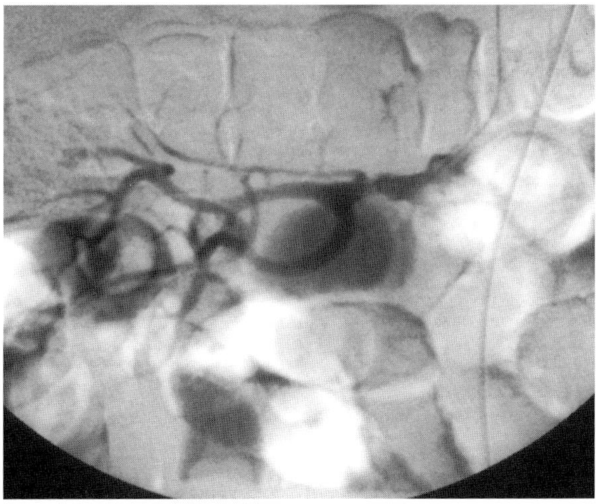

(a)

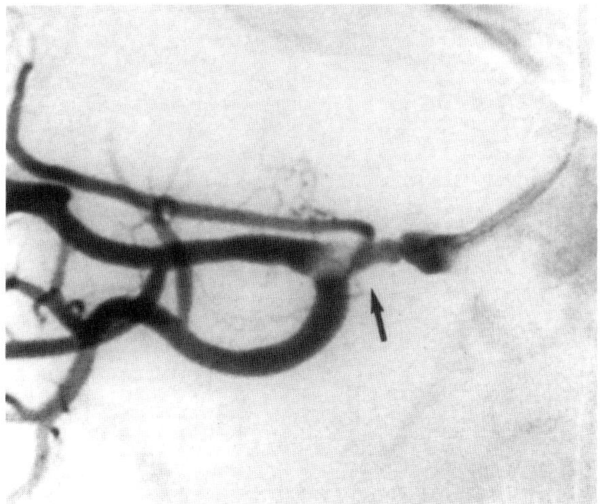

(b)

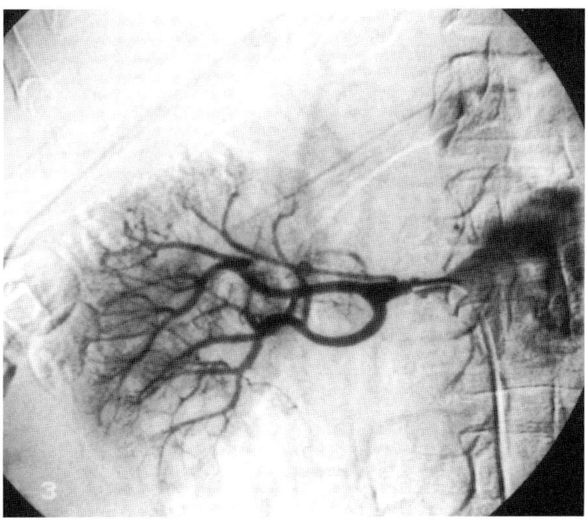

(c)

Figure 31.6. The presentation in this patient was renal failure and severe hypertension in a solitary right kidney with a peri-ostial renal artery stenosis (a); PTRA was complicated by thrombosis at the angioplasty site extending to the renal artery bifurcation (arrowed) (b). Restoration of blood flow was achieved by intra-arterial r-tPA infusion; despite no deterioration in renal function the renal artery stenosis persisted (c). Surgical revascularization by a hepatorenal bypass was performed on the next elective operating list.

sion providing that this goal can be achieved with acceptable risk. The limited experience reported in the literature reveals no deaths and only one major hemorrhage suggesting that fibrinolysis in infant aortic thrombosis is safe and effective.

Vascular complications in transplanted kidneys

Arterial stenosis in renal transplants commonly results from intimal hyperplasia most often anastomotic. This responds well to angioplasty and stenting in the case of multiple restenoses and dissection. Thrombosis can complicate these procedures but this can be usefully treated by intra-arterial thrombolysis (Fig. 31.7).[56]

Summary

Fibrinolytic therapy is now firmly established as a major treatment of thrombotic vascular occlusion. The intra-arterial approach is accept-

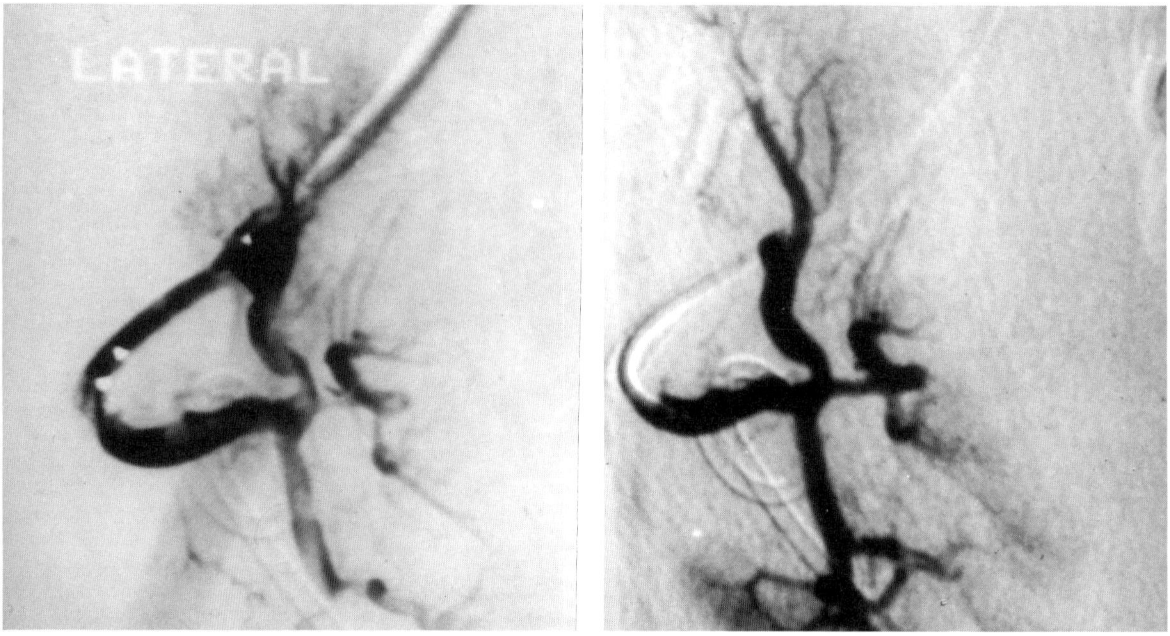

(a) (b)

Figure 31.7. Anastomotic stenosis in a transplanted kidney was treated by angioplasty and stenting. Thrombosis at the site of stenting with embolization distally complicated this procedure (a). Successful clearance with a good long-term clinical result was obtained after immediate infusion of 4 mg of r-tPA (b). (Clinical history and angiograms kindly supplied by Dr A Al-Kotouby, Consultant Radiologist, St Mary's Hospital, London, UK.)

ably safe limiting the total lytic dose required and thus hemorrhagic complications. The majority of vascular radiologists are skilled in these techniques but a proper team approach is of the utmost importance in achieving the best results. This team should consist of nephrologist, vascular surgeon, interventional radiologist and skilled nurses. Appropriate facilities for care of these patients must be available but this need not mean intensive care. Intra-arterial fibrinolytic therapy has an important and developing role to play in the management of renal artery occlusions with exceptions of those resulting from trauma and perhaps acute embolism. Iatrogenic renal thromboses will be increasingly encountered as angioplasty and stenting become more diffusely applied to the treatment of atherosclerotic renal disease. Instant use of fibrinolysis in this situation will mean more salvaged kidneys and improve the results of this developing therapy.

References

1 Clark DE, Georgitis JW, Ray FS. Renal arterial injuries caused by blunt trauma. *Surgery* 1981; **90:** 87–96.
2 Lessman RK, Johnson SF, Coburn JW *et al.* Renal artery embolism: clinical features and long-term follow-up of 17 cases. *Ann Int Med* 1978; **89:** 477–82.
3 Hoxie HJ, Coggin CB. Renal infarction: statistical study of two hundred and five cases and detailed report of an unusual case. *Arch Int Med* 1940; **65:** 587–94.
4 Lacombe M. Surgical versus medical treatment of renal artery embolism. *J Cardiovasc Surg* 1977; **18:** 281–90.
5 Smith BM, Holcomb GW III, Richie RE *et al.* Renal artery dissection. *Ann Surg* 1984; **200:** 134–46.
6 Schwarcz TH, Dobrin PB, Mrkvicka R, Skowrom L, Cole MBJ. Early myointimal hyperplasia after balloon catheter embolectomy: effect of shear forces and multiple withdrawals. *J Vasc Surg* 1988; **7:** 495–9.
7 Bowles CR, Ollcott C, Pakter RL *et al.* Diffuse arterial narrowing as a result of intimal prolifera-

tion: a delayed complication of embolectomy with the Fogerty balloon catheter. *J Vasc Surg* 1988; **7:** 487–94.

8 Francis CW, Marder VJ. Physiologic regulation and pathologic disorders of fibrinolysis. In Colman RW, Hirsh J, Marder VJ, Salzmann EW (eds) *Haemostasis and Thrombosis: Basic Principles and Clinical Practice*, 2nd edn, p. 358. Philadelphia: JB Lippencott, 1987.

9 Holden RW. Plasminogen activators: pharmacology and therapy. *Radiology* 1990; **174:** 993–1001.

10 Collen D, Stump DC, Gold HK. Thrombolytic therapy. *Ann Rev Med* 1988; **39:** 405–423.

11 Verstraete M, Collen D. Thrombolytic therapy in the eighties. *Blood* 1986; **57:** 1529–41.

12 McFarlane RG, Pilling J. Fibrinolytic activity of normal urine. *Nature* 1947; **159:** 779.

13 MacFarlane RG, Pilling J. Observations on fibrinolysis, plasminogen, plasmin and antiplasmin content of human blood. *Lancet* 1965; **ii:** 562–5.

14 Van Breda A, Katzen BJ, Deutsch AS. Urokinase versus streptokinase in local thrombolysis. *Radiology* 1987; **165:** 109–11.

15 Belkin M, Belkin B, Bucknam CA, Straub JJ, Lowe R. Intra-arterial fibrinolytic therapy: efficacy of streptokinase versus urokinase. *Arch Surg* 1986; **121:** 769–73.

16 Pennica D, Holmes WE, Kohr WJ *et al.* Cloning and expression of human tissue-type plasminogen activator c DNA in *E. coli. Nature* 1983; **301:** 214–21.

17 Berridge DC, Gregson RH, Hopkinson BR, Makin GS. Intra-arterial thrombolysis using recombinant tissue plasminogen activator (r-tPA): the optimal agent, at the optimal dose? *Eur J Vasc Surg* 1989; **3:** 327–32.

18 Mori KW, Bookstein JJ, Heeney DJ *et al.* Selective streptokinase infusion: Clinical and laboratory correlates. *Radiology* 1983; **148:** 677–82.

19 McNamara TO, Fischer JR. Thrombolysis of peripheral arterial and graft occlusions: Improved results using high dose urokinase. *Am J Radiol* 1985; **144:** 769–75.

20 McNamara T. Technique and results of 'higher dose' infusion. *Cardiovasc Intervent Radiol* 1988; **11:** S48–S57.

21 Earnshaw JJ, Westby JC, Gregson RH, Makin GS, Hopkinson BR. Local thrombolytic therapy of acute peripheral arterial ischaemia with tissue plasminogen activator: a dose ranging study. *Br J Surg* 1988; **75:** 1196–200.

22 Risius B, Graor RA, Geisinger MA *et al.* Thrombolytic therapy with recombinant human tissue-type plasminogen activator: a comparison of two doses. *Radiology* 1987; **164:** 465–8.

23 Dawson K, Dex E, Platts A, Hamilton G. Groin haemorrhage complicating intra-arterial thrombolytic therapy: choice of technique and agent. *Br J Surg* 1991; **78:** 362–4.

24 Hamilton G, Dawson K. Thrombolytic therapy for acute vascular emergencies. In Greenhalgh RM, Hollier LH (eds) *Emergency Vascular Surgery*, pp. 37–54. London: WB Saunders, 1992.

25 Berridge DC, Makin GS, Hopkinson BR. Local low-dose intra-arterial thrombolytic therapy: the risk of stroke or major haemorrhage. *Br J Surg* 1989; **76:** 1230–3.

26 Dawson KJ, Reddy K, Platts AD, Hamilton G. Results of a recently instituted programme of thrombolytic therapy in acute lower limb ischaemia. *Br J Surg* 1990; **77:** 179–82.

27 Dawson KJ, Hamilton G. Recombinant tissue-type plasminogen activator versus urokinase in peripheral arterial occlusions. *Radiology* 1991; **178:** 283–4.

28 Blum V, Billman P, Krause T, Gabelmann A, Keller E, Moser E *et al.* Effect of local low-dose thrombolysis on clinical outcome in acute embolic renal artery occlusion. *Radiology* 1993; **189:** 549–54.

29 Salam TA, Lumsden AB, Martin LG. Local infusion of fibrinolytic agents for acute renal artery thromboembolism: report of ten cases. *Ann Vasc Surg* 1993; **7:** 21–6.

30 Gasparini M, Hofmann R, Stoller M. Renal artery embolism: clinical features and therapeutic options. *J Urol* 1992; **147:** 567–72.

31 Mugge A, Gulba DC, Frei U, Wagenbrath I, Grote R, Daniel WG *et al.* Renal artery embolism: thrombolysis with recombinant tissue-type plasminogen activator. *J Intern Med* 1990; **228:** 279–86.

32 Skinner RE, Hefty T, Long TD, Rosch J, Forsyth M. Recovery of function in a solitary kidney after intra-arterial thrombolytic therapy. *J Urol* 1989; **141:** 108–10.

33 Fischer P, Konnak JW, Cho KJ *et al.* Renal artery embolism: therapy with intra-arterial streptokinase infusion. *J Urol* 1981; **125:** 402–4.

34 Frey FJ, Stirnemann P, Fritschi P, Mahler F. Renal artery embolism treated with intra-arterial streptokinase infusion results in patent but small renal arteries. *Am J Nephrol* 1986; **6:** 214–16.

35 Gagnon RF, Horosko F, Herba MJ. Local infusion of low-dose streptokinase for renal artery thromboembolism. *Can Med Assoc J* 1984; **131:** 1089–91.

36 Bouttier S, Valverde J–P, Lacombe M, Nussaume O, Andreassian B. Renal artery emboli: the role of surgical treatment. *Ann Vasc Surg* 1988; **2:** 161–8.

37 Nicholas GC, De Muth WE. Treatment of renal artery embolism. *Arch Surg* 1984; **119:** 278–81.

38 Pilmore HL, Walker RJ, Solomon C, Packer S, Wood D. Acute bilateral renal artery occlusion: successful revascularisation. *Am J Nephro* 1995; **15:** 90–1.

39 Fu GY, Candela RJ, Mishkind M, Obarski T, Yakubov SJ. Bilateral renal artery occlusion: an unusual presentation of atrial fibrillation and

hypertrophic cardiomyopathy. *Clin Cardiol* 1994; **17:** 631–3.

40 Takeda M, Katayama Y, Takahashi H, Saito K, Tsutsui T, Komeyama T. Successful fibrinolitis therapy using tissue plasminogen activator in acute renal failure due to acute thrombosis of bilateral renal arteries. *Urol Int* 1993; **51:** 177–80.

41 Morag B, Rubinstein Z, Schneiderman J. Renal artery occlusion: intra-arterial thrombolytic therapy. *J Intervent Radiol* 1988; **3:** 77–80.

42 Cronan JJ Jr, Dorfman GS. Low-dose thrombolysis: a non-operative approach to renal artery occlusion. *J Urol* 1983; **130:** 757–9.

43 Francois D, Delgrange B. A case of acute renal failure caused by thrombosis of both renal arteries. *Acta Clin Belg* 1994; **49:** 177–82.

44 Guinda-Sevillano C, Fernandez-Rosaenz J, Arnaiz-Esteban F, Mainar-Turon A, Perez-Arbej JA, Martinez-Parez E *et al.* Repermeabolisation of renal artery thrombosis through systemic fibrinolysis. *Actas Urol Españ* **17:** 680–682.

45 Mandelbaum JA, Henry ML, Summer BG, Smead WL, Ferguson RM. Streptokinase lysis of arterial thrombus threatening renal allograft – a case report. *Vasc Surg* 1987; **21:** 431–5.

46 Vogelzang RL, Moel DI, Cohn RA, Donaldson JS, Langman CB, Memcek AA Jr. Acute renal vein thrombosis: successful treatment with intra-arterial urokinase. *Radiology* 1988; **169:** 681–2.

47 Schlanger LE, Haire HM, Zukerman AM, Loscalzo CE, Mitch WE. Reversible renal failure in an elderly woman with renal artery stenosis. *Am J Kidney Dis* 1994; **23:** 123–6.

48 Adler J, Ibrahim IM, Goldman M, Thomashow DF. Combined thrombolysis with low-dose streptokinase and angioplasty in the treatment of renal artery occlusion. *Urol Radiol* 1983; **5:** 113–16.

49 Dardik H, Sussman BC, Kahn M, Greweldinger J, Adler J, Mendes D *et al.* Lysis of arterial clot by intravenous or intra-arterial administration of streptokinase. *Surg Gynecol Obstet* 1984; **158:** 137–40.

50 Bergentz S-E, Bergqvist D. *Iatrogenic Vascular Injuries*. Berlin: Springer Verlag, 1989.

51 Berger C, Fancoise M, Durand C, Sandre D, Gouyon JB. Treatment of neonatal aortic thrombosis with recombinant tissue plasminogen activator (tPA). *Arch Paediatr* 1994; **1:** 1014–18.

52 Molteni KH, George J, Messersmith R, Puppala BL, Mangurten HH, Kallen RJ. Intrathrombic urokinase reverses neonatal renal artery thrombosis. *Paediatr Nephrol* 1993; **7:** 413–15.

53 LeBlanc JG, Culham JA, Chan KW, Patterson MW, Tipple M, Sandor GG. Treatment of grafts and major vessel thrombosis with low-dose streptokinase in children. *Ann Thoracic Surg* 1986; **41:** 630–5.

54 Smith PK, Miller DA, Lail S, Mehta AV. Urokinase treatment of neonatal aortoiliac thrombosis caused by umbilical artery catheterisation: a case report. *J Vasc Surg* 1991; **14:** 684–7.

55 Caplan MS, Cohn RA, Langman CB, Conway J, Shkolnik A, Brouillette RT. Favourable outcome of neonatal aortic thrombosis and renovascular hypertension. *J Paediatr* 1989; **115:** 291–5.

56 Fays J, Hennequin L. Techniques and complications of interventional radiology for vascular problems after kidney transplantations. *J Radiol* 1994; **75:** 77–80.

32

Perioperative management of patients with renal vascular disease

BARRIE D HIGGS

Introduction

In the presurgical or anesthetic assessment of patients with atherosclerotic renal artery disease there are three main areas that need to be considered by the anesthetist when planning the anesthetic management: renal pathology and pathophysiology; associated pathology and pathophysiology; and allied pathology and problems arising.

The coordinated approach involving the departments of surgery, medicine and anesthesia ensure that all patients presented for surgery are appropriately and fully investigated. It is not realistic to describe all of the problems likely to be encountered, so only those that are peculiar or important to the management of these patients will be described.

Renal pathology and pathophysiology

Renal failure and compromised renal function

Fluid and electrolyte balance

Dehydrated patients require careful rehydration, with measurement of central venous pressure if indicated. If there is significant cardiac disease then left and right heart pressures will need to be monitored with a flow-directed pulmonary artery catheter.

An overhydrated patient may or may not be edematous. If renal function is so compromised that response to diuretics is severely limited then preoperative dialysis should be arranged. Cerebral and/or pulmonary edema may need to be treated as well. Overhydration usually occurs as a result of overzealous fluid replacement.

Hyponatremia is often associated with overhydration. This should respond to dialysis. It should be remembered that hyponatremic patients are often edematous although that edema may not be obvious. Cerebral edema may present as confusion and pulmonary edema may present as tachypnea with or without hypoxia.

Treatment for hyperkalemia should be considered and steps taken to reduce it – because of the effects on cardiac rhythm (high peaked T-waves, decreased amplitude of R-wave, widened QRS complex and progressive diminution of the amplitude of the P-wave). Glucose/insulin infusions, resonium enemas, and/or dialysis should be considered. Levels of potassium up to 5.5 mmol/l are acceptable. Rarely hypokalemia can present.[1]

Hypermagnesemia can lead to muscle weakness with respiratory and/or cardiac failure.[2] Non-depolarizing muscle relaxants are potentiated.

Altered drug distribution/elimination

Hypoalbuminemia may result in reduced binding of acidic drugs. Binding sites, in addition, may be partly or wholly occupied by drug metabolites or endogenous substances. Uremia may result in the alteration of the conformation of some plasma and tissue proteins and consequently alter the ability to bind drug molecules at receptor sites.[3] Water-soluble metabolites which are normally excreted via the kidney may accumulate and occupy binding sites or prolong elimination of parent drugs by hepatic endproduct inhibition and/or by the law of mass action.

It is of interest to note that although the half-life of many commonly used drugs is only slightly prolonged as long as the creatinine clearance is greater than 20 ml/min, but because of the variability it is important to be aware of the effect of altered renal function on all drugs used. For example, the half-life of many cephalosporins is prolonged significantly with renal failure[4] while the half-life of pentamidine is unaffected.[5]

Acid base status

Acid metabolites accumulate because of the failure to excrete. The result is metabolic acidosis, reduced plasma bicarbonate concentration, hyponatremia, hyperchloremia and hyperkalemia. Most changes can be reversed by hemodialysis or hemofiltration.

Associated pathology and pathophysiology

Atherosclerosis and hypertension

The combination of these two features present the greatest threat to the patient's well-being during anesthesia/surgery. All patients should be thoroughly examined and further tests should be ordered (see below) in the light of the history and examination. In a large number of patients the renal pathology will not be isolated, and although the patient may perhaps be asymptomatic, other systems will be involved.

Many patients with renal artery atherosclerosis are likely to have widely distributed atherosclerosis. The main areas affected, that can present problems to the anesthetist, are the heart, the brain, the gut and the periphery. Patients on hemodialysis may be prone to accelerated atherosclerosis and changes in lipoproteins have been recently suggested as a possible cause.[6]

Hypertension is one of the most common consequences of atherosclerotic renal disease, although it is not a sensitive indicator of this disease.[7] The effect is far reaching and the implications for the heart and cerebral circulation are of great clinical significance.

It is in the management of a patient with significant degree of atherosclerosis and hypertension that the anesthetist, with an appropriate understanding of the physiology and an anesthetic conducted accordingly, can make a significant contribution to the reduction in morbidity/mortality associated with the surgery and anesthesia.

Coronary artery atherosclerosis may result in myocardial ischemia and/or infarction. This should be elicited either in the history with pain, particularly on exertion, but while remembering that many patients will be immobile and may be unable to exert themselves and consequently will deny any history of chest pain. An ECG may detect ischemia, but a stress test ECG may be of more use where doubt persists. In addition, uremic cardiomyopathy may be present.[8] Valve and wall motion, performance and ejection fraction may need to be assessed.

Hypertension associated with renal artery stenosis will result in changes in the vascular tree that alter the way in which the already hypertensive patient will respond to various stresses. Thickening of the arterial wall will result in a narrower lumen and any given shortening of the vascular wall smooth muscle will result in a greater narrowing of the internal lumen and an exaggerated hypertensive response.[9] This is seen as exaggerated swings in blood pressure and can be more marked during anesthesia when changes in sympathetic tone can occur. These patients present something of a dilemma, because the renal function, albeit reduced, is often 'dependent' on the high blood pressure but the consequences of this high blood pressure on the heart and cerebral circulation can be catastrophic.

It is therefore important to consider the effect of hypertension on the heart whose blood supply may already be compromised by atherosclerosis.

A heart where the blood supply is compromised because of narrowed atherosclerotic arteries, is emptying against a high vascular resistance (afterload) and developing a high pressure. It is working hard generating a high wall tension and high end-diastolic pressure. However, the heart is being asked to work hard in spite of the fixed or limited blood supply and the end result of this imbalance between supply and demand can only be myocardial ischemia.

In addition to the increased afterload, and limited blood supply there is a further problem associated with endocardial perfusion. The increased afterload results in a raised end-diastolic pressure. Normally myocardial and endocardial circulation is completed during diastole. With the raised end-diastolic pressure there is physical compression of the endocardium that may limit perfusion of muscle that should be relaxed during diastole, this can severely restrict the blood supply to the endocardium. Changes in the ECG associated with endocardial ischemia can be seen during acute rises in blood pressure. Shortened diastole associated with tachycardia in response to the stress will further reduce myocardial blood supply. It is not unusual for these effects to be compounded by the disturbances in cardiovascular autonomic function.[10]

This contrasts with the heart emptying against a low/normal vascular resistance which generates a low wall tension and empties with ease. A slow heart rate and less heart work may help to minimize the effects on the heart muscle of limited blood supply associated with atheroma.

The anesthetist's technique must aim to prevent hypertension and tachycardia, but not to precipitate hypotension.

In the light of the risk of severe myocardial ischemia associated with atherosclerosis and hypertension and autonomic disturbances, the presurgical assessment must include full examination and investigation of the cardiovascular system. ECG and chest X-ray will obviously be required, this will help to detect left ventricular hypertrophy in response to the hypertension and ischemia may also be evident. As mentioned earlier a stress ECG may be appropriate to elicit ischemia that was not apparent at rest. Ultrasound and scanning of the heart may reveal abnormal wall motion and valvular disorders.

Cerebral blood flow is autoregulated so that blood flow to the brain is almost constant over a varying range of systemic blood pressures. In the normotensive individual this constant flow is maintained over a mean blood pressure of between approximately 50 mmHg and 150 mmHg.[11] In the chronically hypertensive patient the level of autoregulation is reset at higher levels to protect the brain from the higher pressures and to maintain a constant cerebral blood flow in the face of this increased systemic blood pressures. In patients with severe atherosclerosis this cerebral autoregulation may be blunted by atherosclerotic deposits in the cerebral circulation. Thus the cerebral perfusion of a patient with hypertension may be very vulnerable to 'swings' in blood pressure. Hypotension in these individuals (normotension for normotensive patients) may result in markedly reduced cerebral blood flow, and atherosclerosis may further complicate the matter. In addition the systemic vascular changes that predispose these individuals to episodes of hypertension may similarly cause severely raised cerebral blood pressure/flow rates above the level of autoregulation, and cerebral bleeding in weakened atherosclerotic cerebral blood vessels is possible.

The hypertension must be controlled, and all management should be directed toward maintaining an acceptable blood pressure and minimizing the hypertensive response to various stimuli. Medical treatment (antiarrhythmics, antihypertensives and β-blockers) may be indicated and in some instances it will be appropriate to take steps to improve the blood supply to the myocardium (CABG) before the renovascular surgery. The use of angiotensin converting enzyme inhibitors should be used with caution as they may lead to a deterioration in renal function,[12] and calcium antagonists are often used.[13]

Atherosclerotic disease involving the blood supply to the gut may only become significant if any degree of hypotension or manipulation and clamping occur during surgery/anesthesia.

Peripheral vascular disease is often associated with generalized atherosclerosis. Leg pain associated with exercise may restrict activity such that angina is never experienced. Any alteration in blood flow or perfusion pressure to a diseased limb may result in deterioration.

Uremia

The effects of uremia are many and varied and each effect must be considered when assessing the patient preoperatively.

Uremic cardiomyopathy[8] and/or pericarditis can occur and may severely limit cardiac output and restrict the ability to respond to stress (e.g. hemorrhage). The presence of hypertension and autonomic disturbances compound the stress. The patient may well complain of breathlessness on exertion but chest pain will not be a prominent feature.

Urea has both direct and indirect (osmotic) effects on the brain and nervous tissue, resulting in tiredness and compromised mental ability, although anemia can play a significant contributory role.[14] In severe cases it may proceed to fitting, coma and death. Peripheral neuropathies occur and it has been suggested that hemodiafiltration might prevent the worsening of electroneurographic indices occurring during hemodialysis treatment.[15] The autonomic nervous system may be affected, but may be vague and unspecific, but can usually be detected if tested for .[16]

Urea can affect the gastrointestinal system in a number of ways. Central nervous effects may result in anorexia and protein wasting,[17] and clotting/bleeding abnormalities may result in gastrointestinal bleeding. In addition patients may complain of hiccoughs, diarrhea, nausea and vomiting.[18] Esophageal reflux[19] and the increased risk of inhalation of gastric contents occur due to associated increased resting gastric volume and lowered pH. The anesthetist will need to minimize the risk of inhalation of gastric contents during anesthesia.

It has been suggested that uremic patients have a depressed immune system.[20] Great care must be taken in minimizing the risk of infection with preoperative investigations and treatments.

Coagulation

Platelet dysfunction associated with poor renal function and accumulation of urea and metabolites may result in abnormalities of the clotting mechanism.[21] The platelets are not so adhesive and bleeding time is prolonged. Hemodialysis will improve platelet function and the preoperative management may necessitate the use of platelet concentrate and/or cryoprecipitate. DDAVP has also been shown to improve the bleeding time.[22] It is known that erythropoeitin will correct the coagulopathy[21] and it has been shown that recombinant human erythropoeitin can induce thrombosis in hemodialyzed patients.[23]

Effective dialysis should restore clotting as the metabolites and urea are removed and platelet function recovers. However, the use of heparin to facilitate hemodialysis may be associated with bleeding. Laboratory studies of the clotting/bleeding profile may suggest that treatment, either with clotting factors or protamine may be appropriate. We have yet to evaluate the thromboelastograph[24] (± heparinase) for use in these patients but preliminary studies are encouraging.

Anemia

Renal failure is associated with anemia to varying degrees. In the days prior to regular and effective hemodialysis it was not uncommon to anesthetize patients with potassium 'values' approximately double those of their hemoglobin (6–8 mmol/l vs 3–4 g/100 ml)! This should not occur now, and with the advent of synthetic erythropoeitin (rHuEPO) it should be unusual to see such low hemoglobin levels. Treatment with either erythropoeitin or by transfusion may result in a period of increased thrombotic sequelae.

Other causes of anaemia are bone marrow depression with uremia; iron, folate, vitamin B_6 and/or B_{12} deficiency and a decreased red cell lifespan and repeated blood loss during hemodialysis.

The consequence of anemia is a reduced capacity to deliver oxygen to the tissues. The amount of oxygen delivered to the tissues is a function of the hemoglobin (each gram of hemoglobin will carry 1.34 ml of oxygen), arterial oxygen saturation, blood flow to the tissues (a function of cardiac output, vascular tone and blood viscosity) and the small amount of oxygen dissolved in plasma. Changes in acid base status (acidosis) will cause a shift of the oxygen dissociation curve to the right and may help oxygen unloading, but this may be outweighed by the negative inotropic effect on the heart.

An otherwise fit healthy anemic individual will maintain oxygen delivery to the tissues and vital organs by increasing cardiac output while maintaining good oxygen saturation. In concert with the lowered blood viscosity and low vascular tone, the blood flow to tissues and vital organs is well maintained, as long as the circulating volume is maintained. Patients with anemia and hypertensive and atherosclerotic changes in the vascular tree and myocardium strive to maintain oxygen delivery, but the system is stressed (increased cardiac output, increased vascular tone) and any further stresses associated with anesthesia/surgery may result in myocardial ischemia and/or reduced oxygen delivery.

The fatigue and lethargy associated with uremia have a biochemical and physiological basis, which is only partly due to anemia.[25]

Allied problems and pathology

Age

Many patients with significant renal artery atherosclerotic disease will be old. Any assessment of their fitness for anesthesia/surgery must, therefore, take into account the general condition of the patient. The effects that must be considered vary from the obvious (limited respiratory and cardiovascular reserve) to the more obscure (limited movement with postoperative venous stasis and possible deep vein thrombosis)

Elderly individuals may also be in a poor state of nutrition and this must be noted and corrected if morbidity is to be minimized.

When we assess elderly individuals we adopt a team assessment approach involving physicians (general, old age and renal), anesthetists and surgeons. We consider quality of life in the assessment.

Concomitant drug therapy

Many patients presenting for assessment are taking drugs that may influence the technique and choice of anesthetic.

Antihypertensive drugs and regimes should be discussed and a system that will enable control to be maintained, as regimes change from oral to intravenous or intramuscular, should be devised.

Antiarrhythmic and/or other cardiac drugs should be managed jointly with the cardiologists. It must be remembered that many drugs now used reduce afterload and may therefore reduce blood pressure. β-Blocking drugs may increase airway tone and reduce airway calibre.

Analgesia may present a problem, particularly if renal function is compromised. We now like to consider epidural analgesia, combined with general anesthesia during operation and for postoperative pain relief we use a continuous infusion of a weak solution of local anesthetic (bupivacaine) and an opiate (fentanyl), for up to 1 week. The benefits are that renal and gut blood flow is maintained following sympathetic blockade, afterload is reduced, the requirement for general anesthetic is reduced and postoperative analgesia is excellent with all the attendant benefits (good ventilatory excursion, etc.).

Clotting and bleeding problems are always examined and epidural is not performed if the risks of epidural hematoma are thought to outweigh the advantages of good analgesia and sympathetic block. In these cases postoperative analgesia is obtained with titrated doses and an intravenous infusion of opiates.

Dialysis

Patients who are dialyzed should all have clotting/bleeding studies performed before anesthesia/surgery. Abnormalities include the so-called 'rebound heparinization' where bleeding may occur up to 12 h postdialysis.

Rapid fluid and electrolyte shifts may occur and are associated with weakness, nausea and vomiting. In addition the individual may be relatively dehydrated and hypotensive.

Accelerated atherosclerosis can occur in some dialyzed patients.[6]

HIV and hepatitis

The pool of dialysed patients at risk in a system where scrupulous attention is paid to sterility, is much smaller than in other areas where equipment is often reused.[26] However, all staff should take all precautions and treat all patients as potentially infected. The risk of both hepatitis and HIV infections are increased, and increasing. It is my opinion that all patients should be screened for HIV and hepatitis.

Anemic patients who have been transfused with blood and/or red cells, and those with abnormal clotting who have been given clotting factors and other blood products are also at increased risk of carrying the infection.

Monitoring

Preoperative monitoring must include regular recording of blood pressure and not just outpatient and admission blood pressures, so that true resting blood pressure can be determined. Great care should be taken to protect any fistula or shunt.

Intravenous infusions should be sited in the free arm, but it is wasteful to site intravenous cannulae in the larger veins that may be required during surgery. If continuous venous access is required then a central venous cannula should be sited aseptically with local anesthetic. Infusions should all be warmed, as should the patient.

Intraoperative monitoring is restricted by the presence of a shunt or fistula. All patients undergoing surgery have venous access and invasive arterial pressure monitoring, and depending on their preoperative assessment of renal, fluid, electrolyte, clotting and cardiovascular and respiratory status they may require central venous or pulmonary artery monitoring lines. If a pulmonary artery catheter is inserted we always monitor mixed venous oxygen saturation, cardiac output and when possible right heart ejection fraction.

Summary of preoperative investigations

Non-invasive
Blood pressure (serial)
ECG (± exercise)
Chest X-ray
Nutrition/dietetics
(Neurological assessment)
(Heart wall motion/ejection fraction)
Invasive
Full blood count
Urea and electrolytes
Clotting/bleeding
Plasma proteins
Blood gas and acid base
(Angiography ± heart catheter studies)
(Hepatitis/HIV)
Bracketed investigations () if indicated
Correction
Electrolyte/water
Anemia
Clotting
Nutrition
Prioritize vascular problems (CABG)
Hypertensive control

References

1 Ruby ST, Burch A, White WB. Unilateral renal artery stenosis seen initially as severe and symptomatic hypokalemia. Pathophysiologic assessment and effects of surgical revascularization. *Arch Surg* 1993; **128**(3): 346–48.
2 Hashizume N, Mori M. An analysis of hypermagnesemia and hypomagnesemia. *Jpn J Med* 1990; **29**(4): 368–72.
3 Calvo R, Suarez E, Rodriguez-Sasiain JM, Martinez I. The influence of renal failure on the kinetics of intravenous midazolam: an '*in vitro*' and '*in vivo*' study. *Res Commun Chem Pathol Pharmacol* 1992; **78**(3): 311–20.
4 Lameire N, Malerczyk V, Drees B *et al.* Single-dose pharmacokinetics of cefpirome in patients with renal impairment. *Clin Pharmacol Ther* 1992; **52**(1): 24–30.
5 Conte JE Jr. Pharmacokinetics of intravenous pentamidine in patients with normal renal function or receiving hemodialysis. *J Infect Dis* 1991; **163**(1): 169–75.
6 Maggi E, Bellazzi R, Falaschi F *et al.* Enhanced LDL oxidation in uremic patients: an additional mechanism for accelerated atherosclerosis? *Kidney Int* 1994; **45**(3): 876–83.

7 Rimmer JM, Gennari FJ. Atherosclerotic renovascular disease and progressive renal failure. *Ann Int Med* 1993; **118**(9): 712–19.

8 Parfrey PS, Griffiths SM, Harnett JD *et al.* Outcome of congestive heart failure, dilated cardiomyopathy, hypertrophic hyperkinetic disease, and ischemic heart disease in dialysis patients. *Am J Nephrol* 1990; **10**(3): 213–21.

9 Kolkow B. The haemodynamic consequences of adaptive structural changes in the resistance vessels in hypertension. *Clin Sci* 1971; **41:** 1–12.

10 Chu TS, Tsai TJ, Lee SH, Yen TS. Evaluation of cardiovascular autonomic function tests in dialysis patients. *J Formosan Med Assoc* 1993; **92**(3): 237–40.

11 Walters JM, Ingram GS, Jenkinson JL. *Anaesthesia and Intensive care for the Neurosurgical Patient*, 2nd edn. Oxford: Blackwell Scientific Publications, 1994.

12 Rosenthal T. Drug therapy of renovascular hypertension. *Drugs* 1993; **45**(6): 895–909.

13 Klaus D. The role of calcium antagonists in the treatment of hypertension. *J Cardiovasc Pharmacol* 1992; **20** (Suppl. 6): S5–14.

14 Nissenson AR. Epoetin and cognitive function. *Am J Kidney Dis* 1992; **20** (Suppl. 1): 21–4.

15 Malberti F, Surian M, Farina M, *et al.* Effect of hemodialysis and hemodiafiltration on uremic neuropathy. *Blood Purif* 1991; **9**(5–6): 285–95.

16 Vita G, Messina C, Savica V, Bellinghieri G. Uraemic autonomic neuropathy. *J Autonom Nerv Sys* 1990; **30** (Suppl.): S179–84.

17 Mitch WE, Jurkovitz C, England BK. Mechanisms that cause protein and amino acid catabolism in uremia. *Am J Kidney Dis* 1993; **21**(1): 91–5.

18 Kang JY. The gastrointestinal tract in uremia. *Digest Dis Sci* 1993; **38**(2): 257–68.

19 Ravelli AM, Ledermann SE, Bisset WM *et al.* Foregut motor function in chronic renal failure. *Arch Dis Child* 1992; **67**(11): 1343–7.

20 Haag-Weber M, Horl WH. Altered cellular host defence in malnutrition and uremia. *Contrib Nephrol* 1992; **98:** 105–11.

21 Zachee P, Vermylen J, Boogaerts MA. Hematologic aspects of end-stage renal failure. *Ann Hematol* 1994; **69**(1): 33–40.

22 Soslau G, Schwartz AB, Putatunda B *et al.* Desmopressin-induced improvement in bleeding times in chronic renal failure patients correlates with platelet serotonin uptake and ATP release. *Am J Med Sci* 1990; **300**(6): 372–9.

23 Zirkman DM, Zeigler ZR, Fraley DS *et al.* Evaluation of platelet hyperfunction in hemodialysis patients receiving recombinant human erythropoietin. *Am J Kidney Dis* 1993; **21**(1): 31–7.

24 Mallett SV, Coc DJA. Thromboelastography. *Br J Anaesthes* 1992; **69:** 307–13.

25 Thompson CH, Kemp GJ, Taylor DJ *et al.* Effect of chronic uraemia on skeletal muscle metabolism in man. *Nephrol Dial Transplant* 1993; **8**(3): 218–22.

26 Dyer E. Argentinian doctors accused of spreading AIDS (news). *Br Med J* 1993; **307**(6904): 584.

33

Aortorenal bypass and renal artery aneurysmectomy

J HAJO VAN BOCKEL, JOHAN L TERPSTRA

Introduction

Interventional therapy is the most rational therapy for renovascular disease associated with hypertension or impaired renal function. Among intervention, percutaneous transluminal renal angioplasty (PTRA) has taken a significant place in its treatment.[1–3] However, the long-term results of surgical repair are still the gold standard to which other therapies should be compared. Currently, there are virtually no prospective randomized studies comparing the various treatment options.

A variety of techniques are available for surgical reconstruction of the renal artery. Many of these techniques are tailored to a specific type or location of the disease. Aortorenal bypass is probably the most popular of all these renal revascularization procedures. One of the reasons is that it can be utilized for repair of a variety of lesions, including stenosis and aneurysms caused by atherosclerotic and fibrodysplastic disease both proximal in the renal artery and more distally. Another advantage is that dissection of the juxtarenal aorta, as required, for example, for endarterectomy, is not necessary.

Normal anatomy and anatomical variations

Usually there is one single left and right renal artery. In the horizontal plane, the angle of the renal arteries with the aorta is 72° (±13) for the right and 81° (±13) for the left renal artery. In the sagittal plane the angle has a mean of 45°.[4] The right renal artery is situated in 96% caudal to the caval vein and is longer (mean 6–7 cm) than the left one (4–5 cm).[5] Single renal arteries always originate from the aorta. However, occasionally, there is an ectopic origin of the main renal artery originating from the distal thoracic aorta,[6] the splenic artery[7] and the celiac axis.[8] However, in 20–25% there are accessory renal arteries.[9] In one series it appeared that less than one-half of the patients, who were studied angiographically as potential renal allograft donors, demonstrated the simplest vascular pedicle, namely, one single artery and vein bilaterally, prehilar and premature segmental branching occurred in 17% of the cases.[10] These variations, in particular prehilar branching, and accessory renal arteries are relevant for surgical therapy and may require adaptation of the standard surgical procedure.

Collateral circulation is important to preserve renal tissue from infarction in chronic occlusive disease of the renal artery. Collateral pathways include ganglionar, capsular, suprarenal, inferior mesenteric, ureteral, gonadal and diaphragmatic arteries.[11–13] These branches contribute to an extrarenal collateral network[14] which may preserve viability of the kidney even if a renal artery becomes totally occluded. During the operation as many collaterals as possible should be preserved.

Aortorenal bypass

Indications

The main indications for reconstruction are renovascular disease associated with hypertension and/or impaired function. Renovascular hypertension is defined retrospectively as arterial hypertension which responds favorably to operative or angioplastic repair of a renovascular stenosis or occlusion.[15] Ischemic nephropathy is characterized by a clinically significant reduction in glomerular filtration rate in patients with hemodynamically significant renal artery stenosis.[16]

The diagnosis is a retrospective diagnosis by definition and surgical reconstruction and angioplasty are a means of defining the disease.[17, 18] Unfortunately, there is currently still no single test or combination of tests available that can accurately predict either the blood pressure response or retrieval of renal function to surgical reconstruction or PTRA.[19] In particular, diagnosis in bilateral renovascular disease is difficult because most tests are based on lateralization. Therefore we have always relied on the clinical characteristics rather than on the outcome of functional tests. However, the currently available tests are helpful in selecting hypertensive patients for intervention, particularly when used in combination with clinical evaluation. Popular tests with relatively high sensitivities and specificities are the captopril test with a sensitivity of around 75% and a specificity of about 90%, and captopril renography with a sensitivity of 93% and a specificity of 95%. Some have found much lower sensitivities and specificities and conclude that the usefulness of these tests is very limited.[20] A critical overview with an evaluation of the tests currently available has been published recently.[21]

With the availability of new drugs most patients' hypertension can be satisfactorily treated medically and the main indication for intervention is changing to preservation or retrieval of renal function.[22, 23] Also for ischemic nephropathy there are no clearcut criteria for surgical repair. Obviously, the best candidates for intervention are those patients in whom the complete renal mass is involved such as bilateral disease or when a single kidney is involved, in the absence of parenchymal disease and end-stage renal disease.[24, 25]

Contraindications

The risk of surgical reconstruction in the younger patients, like those with fibrodysplastic disease is considered very low. Operative mortality is limited to patients with atherosclerosis. Patients without manifestations of extrarenal atherosclerosis can be operated with a low mortality rate around 1–2%.[26] On the other hand, the surgical risk in older patients, and particularly in those with azotemia or with generalized atherosclerosis including cerebrovascular disease and heart disease, is universally considered much higher. However, low morbidity and mortality rates around 2% can be also obtained in these patients with generalized atherosclerosis by careful analysis of coronary artery and cerebrovascular disease. If present, significant and symptomatic coronary and carotid artery stenosis should be repaired before the renovascular procedure.[27] It is important to avoid aortic reconstruction if possible, e.g. replacing a badly diseased but patent aorta by a prosthesis to have a point for takeoff of a renal bypass, because it is associated with increased mortality rates around 8–10%.[26, 28–30] In these situations the surgical risk can be decreased by selecting alternative procedures not involving clamping of the aorta such as: splenorenal anastomosis,[31, 32] hepatorenal anastomosis[33] or using a bypass which originates from the iliac artery instead of the aorta.[34]

Preoperative preparation

Blood pressure is brought under control as much as possible. Although uncontrolled hypertension seems not to be a factor significantly associated with operative mortality, such patients experience a greater relative intraoperative blood pressure decrease than controlled hypertensives which may contribute to myocardial ischemia.[35] Occasionally intravenous nitroprusside is required if the diastolic blood pressure is over 120 mmHg. Most antihypertensive agents can be continued to the moment of the operation. Among the antihypertensive medication, reserpine (currently not widely used anymore) and β-blockers do not interfere with a safe anesthesia. Guanethidine is abandoned preoperatively because of its interference with circulatory reflexes. Abrupt discontinuation of clonidine may occasionally precipitate a withdrawal syndrome with hypertension and tachycardia. Angiotensin converting enzyme inhibitors can be safely continued until surgery.[35]

Dehydration, commonly associated with the use of diuretics and contributing to deterioration of renal function, is corrected. Approximately one-third of the patients have a deficit in blood volume of about 1 l, ranging from 504 to 1740 ml.[36] This deficit should be replaced early during the operation to guarantee adequate hydration to prevent renal, cerebral and cardiac perfusion complications.

Studies on prevention of acute tubular necrosis in kidney transplantation have indicated that adequate hydration[37] and the use of mannitol[38, 39] have a beneficial effect on this complication. In this respect it is important to realize that mannitol is only effective in adequately hydrated patients. Mannitol induces an increase in intravascular volume due to an increased osmotic pressure gradient, as well as a systemic and renal afferent arteriolar vasodilatation. The potential beneficial effect of the administration of furosemide has never been clearly demonstrated. Therefore, 10–15 min before clamping the renal artery we slowly administer mannitol (200 ml mannitol 20%) intravenously after adequate hydration.

Finally, after angiography the operation should be postponed until renal dysfunction due to nephrotoxic contrast agents, and associated with the use of antihypertensive drugs and impaired renal function, has recovered.[40]

Surgical technique

The patient is placed in the supine position with arms at sides. A Foley catheter is introduced in the bladder to monitor urine output. During operation, adequate filling pressures are monitored by central venous pressure measurement, or occasionally by a pulmonary artery (Swann–Ganz) catheter if the patient tends to left ventricular dysfunction. An arterial line is introduced in the radial artery to monitor the blood pressure contiously.

The skin of the chest, abdomen and both legs is prepared and draped so that the circulation of the lower extremities can be monitored and procurement of the saphenous vein in the upper part of the thigh is possible.

Exposure

Various incisions have been proposed according to the personal preference of the surgeon. The choice of the incision is dependent on the surgical technique and graft material used. A midline incision is preferred if an autogenous arterial graft from the internal iliac artery is used and a bilateral reconstruction with or without autotransplantation has been planned. A transverse incision provides excellent exposure for unilateral or bilateral repair. For a unilateral bypass procedure we prefer a transverse abdominal incision from the lateral border of the contralateral rectus muscle extending across the midline into the ipsilateral flank between the 11th and 12th rib. A retroperitoneal approach can be used for unilateral extracorporeal repair and autotransplantation. In all cases an automated retractor, such as the Omni–Tract (Minnesota Scientific, Inc., Minneapolis, MN.), is used which greatly simplifies the exposure.[41, 42]

For access to the right renal artery, the right colon and duodenum are reflected medially. Complete mobilization of the ascending colon and the radix of the small bowel is very helpful for access to both renal arteries in obese patients.

Mobilization of the renal veins is required for a adequate exposure of the renal arteries. On the right side the short renal vein is mobilized. If the caval vein has to be mobilized it is often necessary to ligate and divide one or two pairs of lumbar veins. To the left the renal vein is exposed by a transverse incision in the left mesocolon preserving the intestinal circulation in the mesocolon. The left renal vein is mobilized by transecting its tributaries. During reconstruction, the renal vein can be retracted by vessel loops which can be temporarily attached to the frame of the retractor. Before mobilization of the left renal vein by ligation of adrenal, gonadal and lumbar veins one should decide on transection of the left renal vein. Transection of the left renal vein has the advantage of a better exposure of the origin of the renal arteries. This may be an advantage if an endarterectomy is planned but is rarely required for a renal bypass. The disadvantage of dividing the renal vein is that this maneuver results in increased venous pressure in the left retroperitoneum. This usually produces troublesome venous bleeding during subsequent dissection of the renal artery. In addition, transection of the renal vein may have an adverse effect on renal function.[43] Therefore we usually reanastomose the left renal vein after the arterial repair has been completed.

Subsequently, the aorta is dissected to allow for cross-clamping of the aorta rather than partial clamping with a Satinsky vascular clamp because the infrarenal aorta is often diseased and thick walled. In patients with a healthy aorta a side-biting clamp may be used. Occasionally, it is impossible for a bypass to originate from the infrarenal aorta. In older patients such a diseased, slightly dilated, aorta with a thickened wall may introduce several problems. First, mural thrombus may be present which has to be removed partially and is associated with the risk of distal embolization. Second, it is necessary to create a relatively wide opening in the diseased aorta for the anastomosis with the bypass graft. It is often difficult to anastomose a thin-walled venous graft to a thick-walled diseased aorta. In these cases alternative techniques such as a splenorenal[31, 32] or hepatorenal bypass,[33] the iliac artery or the aorta at the level of diaphragm,[44–46] are much more preferable (Fig. 33.1).

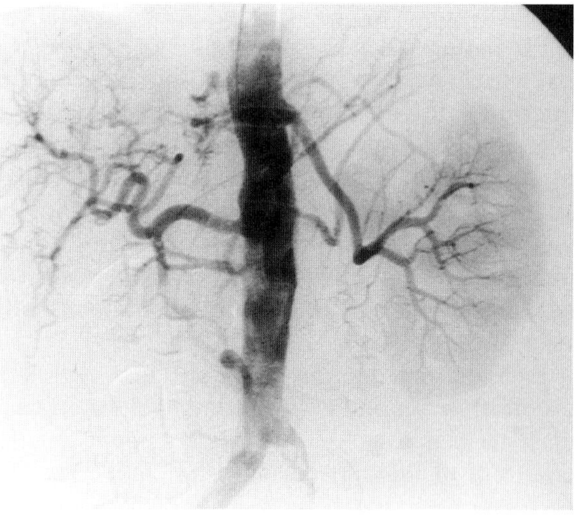

Figure 33.1. Venous bypass to the left renal artery originating from the thoracic aorta.

Graft material

An autogenous arterial graft is preferred for a bypass graft to avoid the problems of stenosis and dilatation inherent with venous bypass grafts. In younger patients the internal iliac artery can be used (Fig. 33.2). Unilateral utilization of one internal iliac artery with a normal contralateral artery does not result in erectile disorders in the male patient. Alternatively, we use the superficial femoral artery which is subsequently replaced by the greater saphenous vein. In older patients with atherosclerotic disease it is often impossible to find a suitable arterial graft. Alternatively a segment of the occluded superficial femoral artery can be used after eversion endarterectomy under direct vision. The core can easily be removed by everting the adventitia and media, subsequently, the endarterectomized segment can be reversed.[47] If no suitable arterial segment is available, the saphenous vein is preferred. We prefer to use the vein in the normal, not reversed, position. To this end we excise or destroy the valves. Often there is only one valve at the origin of the greater saphenous vein which can be removed with a fine pair of scissors. After checking the destruction of the valves, the vein is anastomosed in the normal, not reversed, position. All these autologous grafts are preferably preserved in heparinized blood.[48, 49] Finally, if an autologous vein is also not available, a prosthesis can be used. Regarding the choice of prosthetic material there has never been a comparative study between Dacron and polytetrafluoroethylene. Currently, the most popular bypass material is manufactured from polytetrafluoroethylene and has been used with satisfactory results.[50, 51]

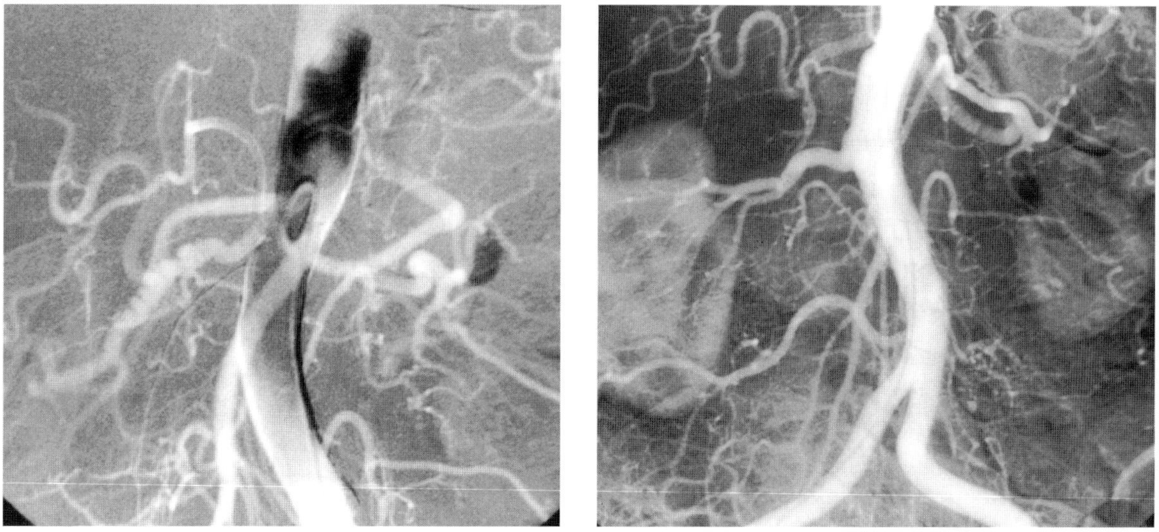

(a) (b)

Figure 33.2. Fibrodysplasic disease of the right renal artery (a). Autologous arterial bypass obtained from the internal iliac artery for *in situ* reconstruction of extensive fibrodysplastic disease (b).

Reconstructive technique

The atherosclerotic lesion is usually localized at the origin of the renal artery but fibrodysplastic stenosis can easily extend into the distal renal artery and its branches. In these cases extracorporeal reconstruction and autotransplantation should be considered, as will be discussed in Chapter 37. The renal artery is gently dissected free of its surrounding adventitial tissue from about 1 cm from the origin to a point well beyond the lesion(s) and time is allowed to recover from spasm. The patient receives 50–70 mg heparin intravenously, a dose which does not require reversal by protamine sulfate after completion of the reconstruction.

For the end-to-side anastomosis of the bypass with the aorta an arteriotomy is made of about two to three times the diameter of the graft. To this end an oval opening is cut with a knife or a commercially available aortic punch instrument is used. If a venous bypass is used a side branch may be incised and included in the anastomosis to enlarge the proximal anastomosis.[52] The anastomosis is made with a running 5–0 Prolene suture starting cranially from inside the anastomosis. To prevent suture line stenosis caused by a pursestring effect, the anastomosis is allowed to expand by carefully removing the clamp before the suture has been completely tied. After removal of the aortic clamps a atraumatic bulldog clamp is placed at the graft near the aortic anastomosis. Kinking of the graft may occur if too long an anastomosis has been constructed, or if the anastomosis is located on the anterior rather than lateral side of the aorta. If the anastomosis is too long, the position of the graft is parallel to the aorta resulting in kinking if the graft is carried upward and laterally to the renal artery.

The distal anastomosis is performed in an end-to-end rather than end-to-side configuration. An end-to-end anastomosis has better flow characteristics and avoids competitive flow. The proximal renal artery is ligated and the mobilized distal renal artery is clamped with an atraumatic mini vascular clamp. The graft is straightened and cut at the appropriate length to avoid kinking. At the right side, the graft is usually located anterior to the vena cava although the graft may also be tunneled under the vena cava if kinking seems to occur in the other position. To obtain a spatulated distal anastomosis at least two to three times the diameter of the graft, the artery is incised ventrally and the graft dorsally. The oblique anastomosis is performed under loupe magnification with two sutures Prolene 6–0 one starting at the heel and the other starting at the toe of the anastomosis. In children both anastomoses are performed, at least partially, with interrupted sutures to allow for future growth of the vessels. Again, after removal of the clamps the anastomosis is allowed to expand before the sutures are tied.

An alternative method for bilateral renal bypass has been described using a side-to-side bridging aortic-saphenous vein graft followed by bilateral end-to-end saphenous vein to renal arterial anastomosis.[53, 54] However, we have never favored this technique because in our experience this technique is associated with an increased incidence of kinking and stenosis, probably due to excessive turbulence, compared to the standard aortorenal bypass.

Evaluation of patency

After blood flow has been restored, the patency of the reconstruction is evaluated. The reconstruction is palpated, however, palpation alone is not sufficient. Angiography has been used by some but intraoperative renal angiography is difficult and awkward. It is also not without risk because it requires reclamping of the aorta and the injection of contrast agents. We, among others, prefer the use of duplex ultrasound which appears to have a sensitivity of 89% and a sensitivity of 77% to identify major defects.[55–57] A 7.5 MHz probe is wrapped in a long sterile sleeve. The distal part is covered in a gynecological condom filled with ultrasonic gel. Care is taken to exclude air bubbles. If necessary, a standoff can be easily made using a sterile rubber glove filled with saline and removing all air bubbles. The probe is positioned on the graft and both the B-mode image and the flow velocity signals are evaluated along the anastomoses, the graft and the distal renal artery. Currently criteria for intraoperative evaluation of patency are being developed and it appears that a peak systolic flow over 3.0 m/s is indicative for a significant residual stenosis. Comparing the flow velocities of the graft to the aorta, we found that the systolic peak velocity in the aorta during anesthesia is significantly less than in the conscious patient. Therefore the aortorenal ratio rather than the absolute blood flow velocity is probably a better criterium. The B-mode image is particularly helpful to evaluate residual defects. Significant defects in the reconstruction should be repaired immediately. Minor defects can probably left without reintervention.

Complications

Significant intraoperative complications include bleeding and a stenosis or thrombosis of the reconstruction. Bleeding usually involves the vena cava or the left renal vein and its branches. Bleeding from the left renal vein or its tributaries can be easily controlled. Bleeding from the vena cava can be more difficult if caused by a torn lumbar vein. In this situation, an atraumatic Allis clamp can usually be temporarily applied directly to the bleeding vein. After the vena cava has been mobilized the lesions can be repaired. Occasionally, bleeding is caused when a severely atherosclerotic aorta has been clamped and sutures torn out. If the infrarenal aorta is severely atherosclerotic, the aorta cannot be used as a place of takeoff for a renal bypass. We prefer to use other techniques such as a splenorenal bypass or the use of the suprarenal aorta rather than to replace the aorta with a Dacron graft. Simultaneous aortic graft replacement and renal artery reconstruction carry a significant higher mortality 7–10% than renal bypass surgery alone.[28–30, 58] However, results of others suggests that simultaneous aortic and renal artery surgery can be performed with low morbidity and mortality rates equal to those of aortic reconstruction alone.[59–61] These differences in the results between the various studies are most likely due to differences in patient selection.

Early occlusion of an aortorenal bypass may occur because of errors in the surgical technique, usually at the distal anastomosis. Failures of surgical technique include: distal anastomosis to a thick-walled diseased renal artery, anastomotic stenosis due to a pursestring effect caused by using one single prolene suture tied before the clamps have been removed, distal clamp lesion and kinking or twisting due to excessive length and malalignment of the bypass.

Results

Anatomic results

Anatomic results of reconstructive surgery have been satisfactory. Using angiographic evaluation, the early failure rate appeared to be equal to or less than 5% in experienced hands.[62–64] Our results with arterial autografts have been superior to those with venous autografts.[64, 65] In addition, results are clearly improved with increased surgical expertise and better patient selection, e.g. selecting those with distal branch lesions for extracorporeal reconstruction and autotransplantation.[64]

Late complications of the venous aortorenal bypass graft include: suture line stenosis, graft dilatation and, very occasionally, anastomotic aneurysm formation. Stenoses may be caused by intimal hyperplasia due to turbulent flow at the anastomotic sites or due to trauma of an autologous graft, in particular vein graft. Angiographic follow-up has demonstrated that vein graft stenosis may in occur in 8–41%.[63, 66] In an arterial graft, late stenosis is rare.[65, 67] Dilatation of a venous autograft is not uncommon (Fig. 33.3). Again, this complication seems to be limited to venous autografts and may occur in 20–45%[66, 68] usually within the first years after the operation. This complication appears to be not very progressive: progression to a renal aneurysm (defined as an increase in diameter of 50%) is less than 5–8% and reoperation for dilatation is rarely indicated (Fig. 33.4).

In one series of mostly autogenous saphenous aortorenal bypass grafts, the overall reoperation rate was 15.5% (58 of 373 patients) which fell to 9.7% during the last decade. Most reoperations were performed within the first year after the primary operation. Reoperation typically followed persistent or recurrent hypertension caused by graft thrombosis, perianastomotic graft narrowing, or progressive non-anastomotic graft stenosis. Reoperation was associated with a high nephrectomy rate of 43% (31 of 72 procedures). Aneurysmal deterioration of vein grafts was an uncommon reason for reoperation.[69] Finally, the formation of an anastomotic aneurysm may be a rare late complication of an aortorenal bypass which requires repair (Fig. 33.5).

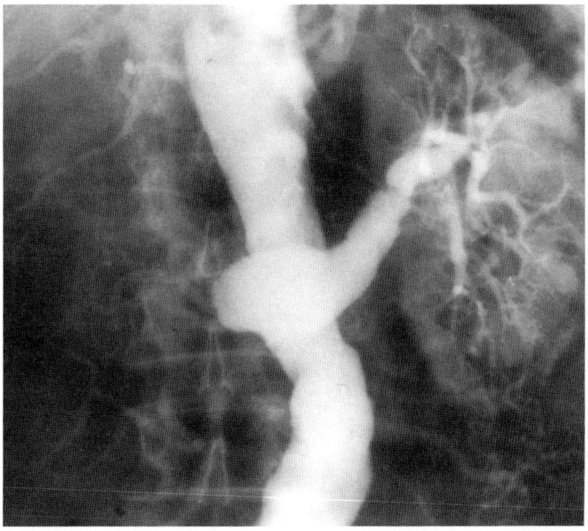

Figure 33.3. Bilateral venous bypass 23 years after the operation. The bypass has dilated and occluded on the right side. On the left side there is a severe stenosis at the anastomotic side. The patient presented with severe hypertension and impaired renal function. Successful reconstruction was performed with a left renal bypass using an arterial autograft. From ref. 100, with permission

Functional results

Functional results of aortorenal bypass operations exclusively are not available; most series report on combined results of various surgical techniques. Moreover, the patients with renovascular disease are a heterogeneous group with variations in age and type of disease and the functional result is not influenced by the surgical technique applied. Finally, functional results are related to patient selection. Strict patient selection on the basis of functional tests will on the one hand result in higher beneficial blood pressure response rates but on the other hand a chance for a beneficial response will be denied in others. Generally, the combined cure and improved rates are not much different between patients with atherosclerotic disease and fibrodysplastic disease. However, most series report high cure rates up to 50–60% in patients with fibrodysplastic disease, whereas cure is usually obtained in only 20–35% of the patients with atherosclerosis.

Regarding overall results when patient selec-

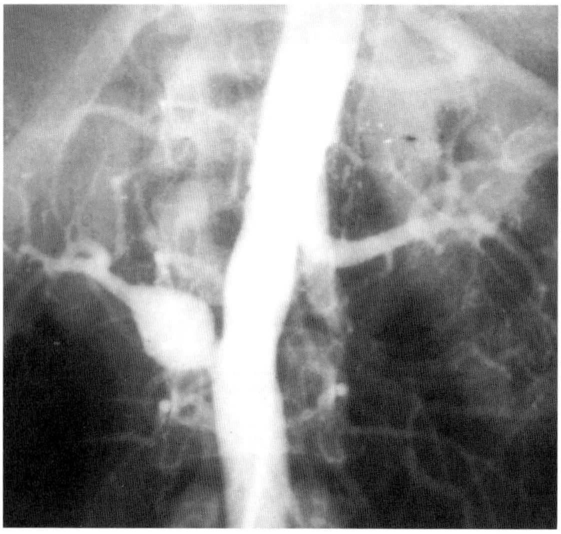

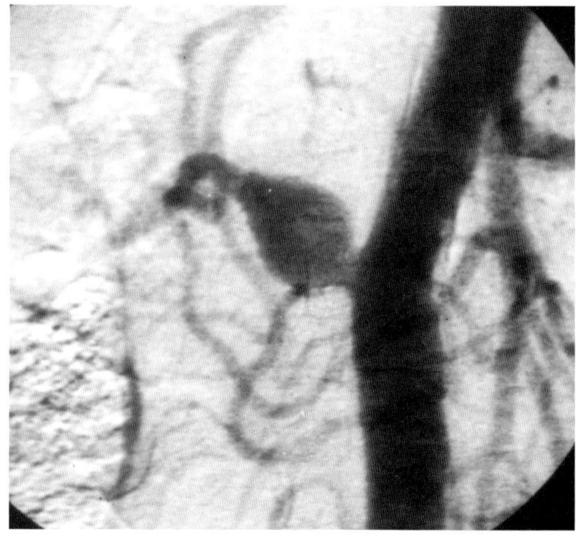

(a) **(b)**

Figure 33.4. Venous bypass with aneurysmal dilatation already within 2 years after the operation (a). The patient refused operation and follow-up angiography 16 years later showed no progression of the aneurysmal dilatation (b).

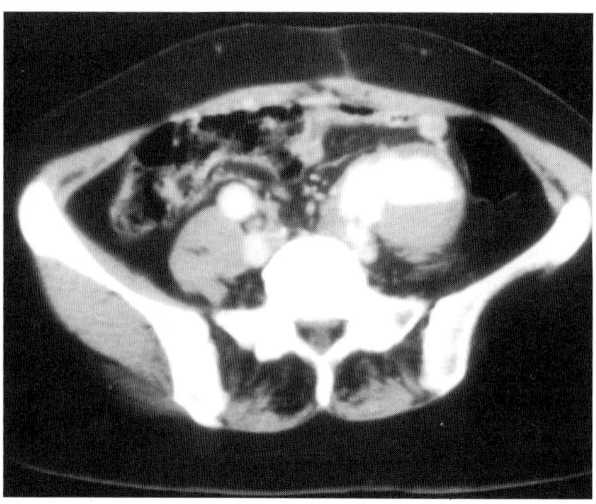

(a)

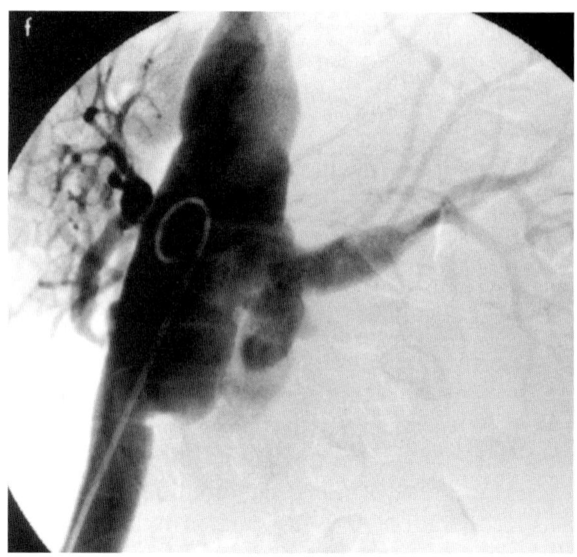

(b)

Figure 33.5. Large false aneurysm containing thrombus at the anastomosis of a venous bypass to an aortic Dacron graft 11 years after the initial operation (a: CT scan; b: angiogram). The initial operation, performed because of an mid-aortic syndrome, consisted of bilateral renal venous bypass and mesenteric bypass anastomosed to the body of a bifurcated Dacron aortoiliac bypass. The patient presented with multiple anastomotic aneurysms and clinical signs of rupture (same patient as in Fig. 33.1).

tion was based on clinical characteristics, we obtained a combined cure and improved response rate of 83% which was maintained during long-term follow-up of 1–24 years (mean: 9 years).[70, 71] Surprisingly, the results in patients with overt generalized atherosclerosis were not significantly different from those with focal atherosclerosis.[72, 73] Importantly, in patients with atherosclerosis a beneficial blood pressure response was associated with an improved life expectancy.[72] This beneficial response rate is similar to the 80% obtained in comparable series followed during a similar interval[73] and to the 80% calculated for 2430 patients from 25 series published between 1961 and 1983 and reviewed by Mackay *et al.*[74] However, it is less favorable when compared with the 90–95% rates reported currently by several specialized centers (where the tertiary referral center is already an important selection) using functional tests for the selection of patients.[27, 75]

Renal aneurysmectomy

Indications

An aneurysm of the main renal artery is a rare condition. Usually, it is a coincidental finding on an angiogram made for an other indication. Most patients are asymptomatic since a renal aneurysm usually does not interfere with renal blood flow.[76] Although it is sometimes believed that a renal aneurysm can contribute to a renovascular cause of hypertension, this has never been made plausible and is possible due to selection of hypertensive patients for angiography. Occasionally, an arterial kink caused by a renal artery aneurysm and not apparent with angiography, may be the cause for hypertension.[77] Also, renal infarction caused by embolization from a thrombus-containing aneurysm, may be a rare cause of hypertension.[78] Small aneurysms can be caused by systemic diseases such as periarteritis nodosa.[79] However, most aneurysms, and in particular macroaneurysms, are associated with fibrodysplastic disease or atherosclerosis.[80] Neurofibromatosis has also been associated with abnormalities in the media as a rare cause for a renal aneurysm.[81, 82]

The prevalence of renal aneurysms is unknown. In one postmortem angiographic study saccular aneurysms were found in 9.7%, many aneurysms being very small.[83] In a more recent report on 8500 patients subjected to angiography for non-renal disease, the prevalence for macroaneurysms was 0.9%.[78] Swedish investigators estimated the prevalence from an autopsy study to be about 0.7–0.9%. This study also indicated that the natural history of a renal aneurysm is usually benign and that rupture rarely occurs.[84] These authors have classified aneurysms into: (1) saccular (Fig. 33.6) (2) fusiform (Fig. 33.7), (3) dissecting (Fig. 33.8) and (4) intrarenal aneurysms. Most aneurysms are saccular with an average size of 1.3 cm. Three-quarters of these aneurysms are located at the primary or secondary renal bifurcations.[83]

The great majority of renal aneurysms are asymptomatic. The indication for surgical correction is the risk of complications including: distal embolization, thrombosis, dissection and rupture. Distal embolization is a rare complication and can be deduced from the angiogram if renal infarcts are present.[85] The risk of rupture and exsanguinating hemorrhage is considered

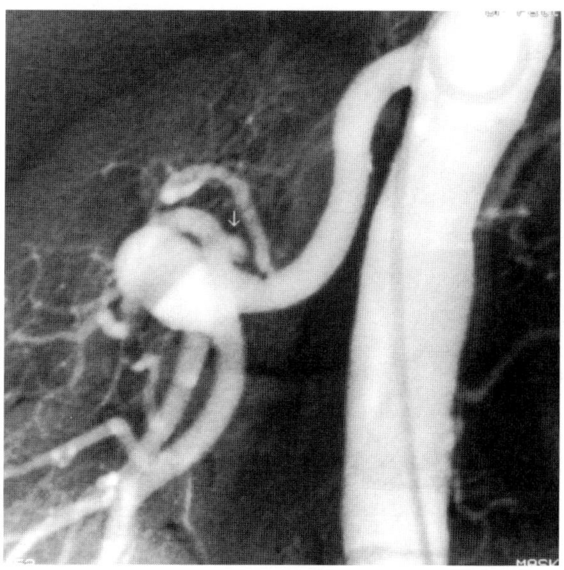

Figure 33.6. Saccular macroaneurysm of the right renal artery in a female patient with a single kidney. Extracorporeal reconstruction was successfully performed using a branched internal artery iliac autograft.

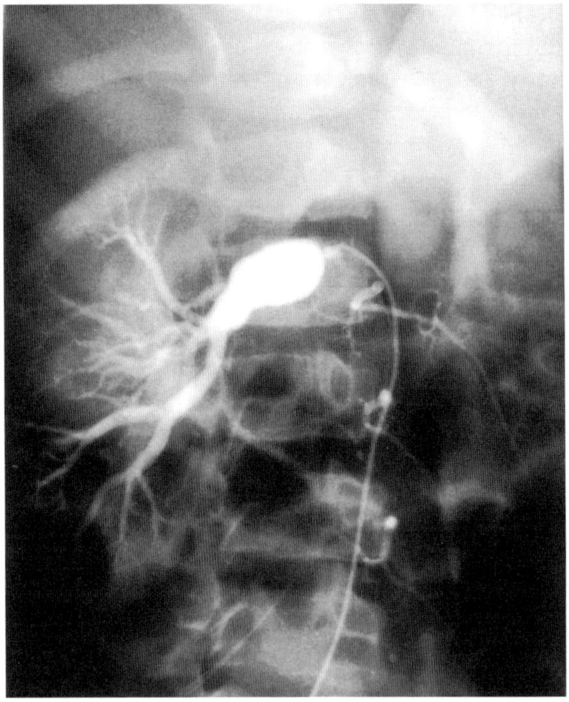

Figure 33.7. Fusiform aneurysm of the right renal artery associated with a stenosis in a pediatric patient. *In situ* reconstruction was successfully performed with arterial autograft.

the major risk. Rupture is considered to be increased in aneurysms of 1.5–2.0 cm and greater, in particular in females of child-bearing age (Fig. 33.9).[86–88] Although rupture occurred in 2.8% of the Michigan experience, rupture never occurred among those patients followed conservatively. Dissection of the renal artery is usually symptomatic and presents with flank pain, hematuria, acute onset of often severe hypertension and/or impaired renal function. Dissection may occasionally be associated with fibrodysplastic disease.

Surgical technique

If the aneurysm is located in the main renal artery, *in situ* reconstruction can be performed. In these cases the surgical technique can be used as outlined above. It is important to use autologous autografts in young patients. However, most aneurysms, apart from those associated with medial dysplasia appearing as a 'string of beads', occur in the distal part of the renal artery, in the renal bifurcation or its hilar branches. In those cases, and in particular when

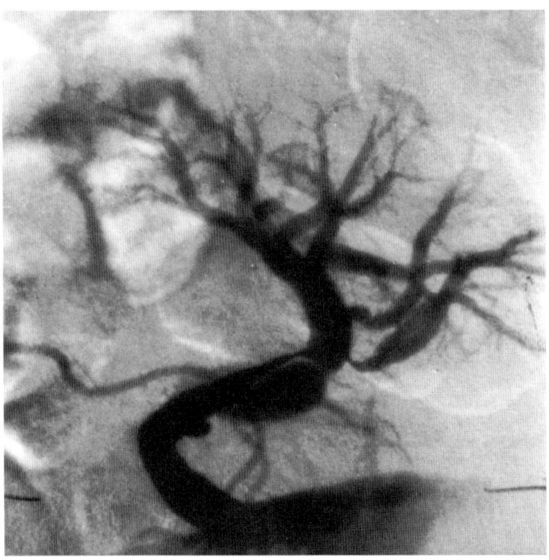

(a)

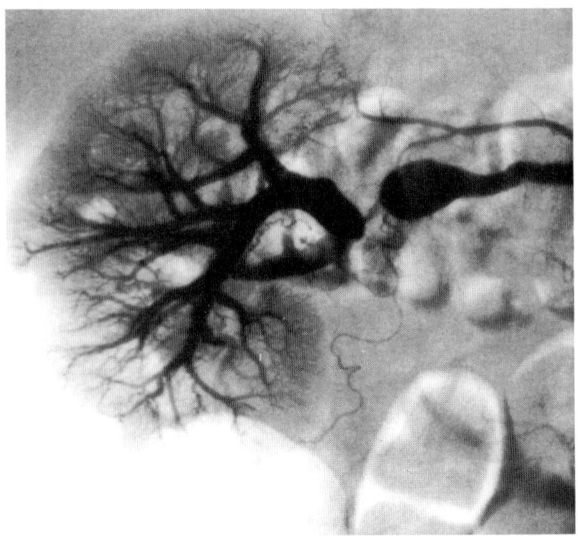

(b)

Figure 33.8. Bilateral dissection into the renal branches in a 40-year-old male patient (a: left renal artery; b: right renal artery). Presentation with severe acute onset of hypertension and impaired function. Repaired by bilateral simultaneous extracorporeal reconstruction and autotransplantation (same patient as in Fig. 33.12). From ref. 98, with permission

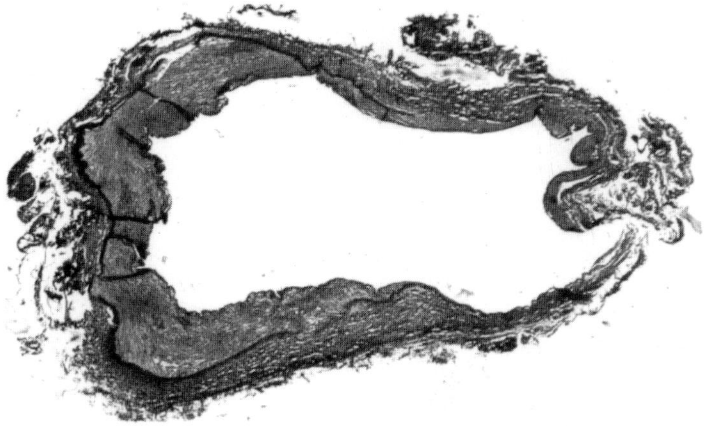

Figure 33.9. Renal artery aneurysm caused by medial fibroplasia. The aneurysm ruptured in the first trimester of the pregnancy of a 38-year-old woman. Successful repair with resection and end to end anastomosis resulted in salvage of the patient and the kidney. From ref. 99, with permission

a distal dissection is present, extracorporeal reconstruction and autotransplantation rather than *in situ* repair is the optimal technique to reconstruct these lesions.

Our technique has been described previously.[89] Intravenous fluids are liberally infused to ensure adequate hydration and urine production. The kidney involved is freed avoiding unnecessary manipulation and traction to prevent renal vasospasm which interferes with optimal renal preservation. Significant collateral circulation is interrupted only after dissection had been completed and renal preservation can be started immediately. Subsequently, the ureter is dissected free while preserving the ureteral collateral circulation to the kidney. As soon as hydration is adequate mannitol is infused 5–10 min prior to arterial occlusion to promote renal perfusion and diuresis. The ureter is clamped with a tourniquet for the period of preservation and extracorporeal repair. Subsequently, the kidney is removed and placed on melting ice-slush in a flat basin on top of the patient's pubic bone. The artery(ies) are cannulated and flushed with approximately 300 ml of Collins' solution at 4°C until the venous effluent becomes clear. The renal artery branches are dissected and all aneurysmal lesions are removed. For reconstruction of branches we have preferably applied two techniques. The first is joining two or more branches (Fig. 33.10). Joining two or more branches creates a wide ostium and occasionally obviates the need for an interposition graft. This technique is preferable to anastomosing thin-walled renal branches end-to-side to a relatively thick-walled hypogastric artery graft, since such a technique may easily produce a stenosis.[90] Alternatively, adjacent branches are joined and subsequently

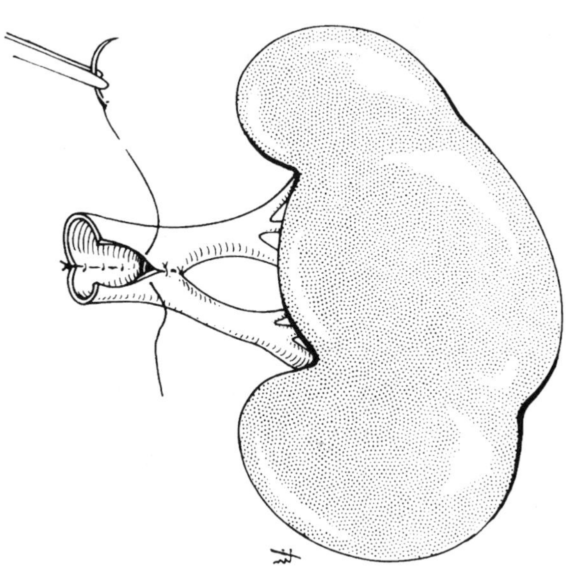

Figure 33.10. Technique of joining branches to a common ostium.

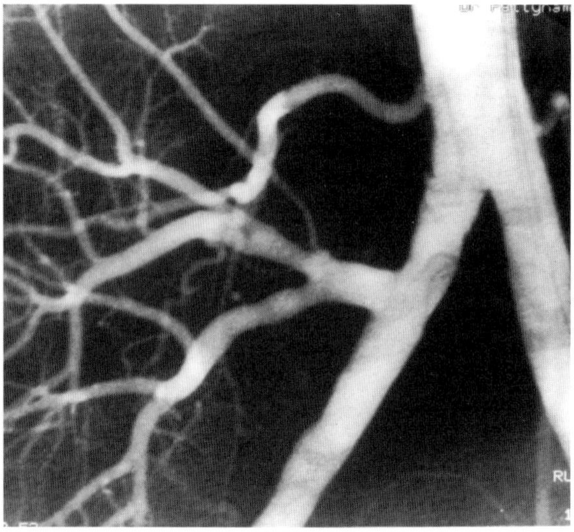

Figure 33.11. Extracorporeal reconstruction and autotransplantation for a renal artery aneurysm of the renal hilar branches (same patient as in Fig. 33.6).

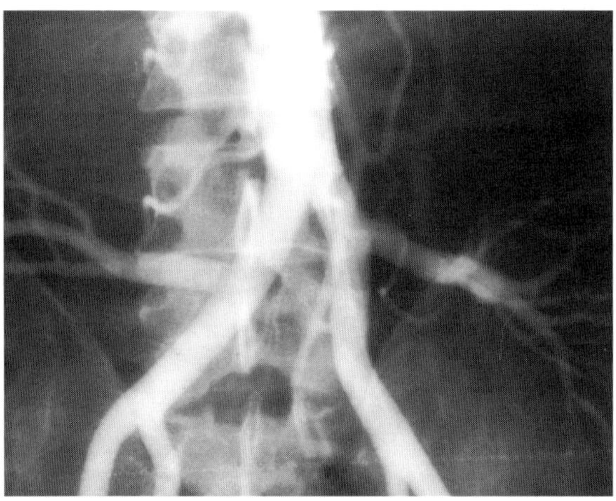

(a)

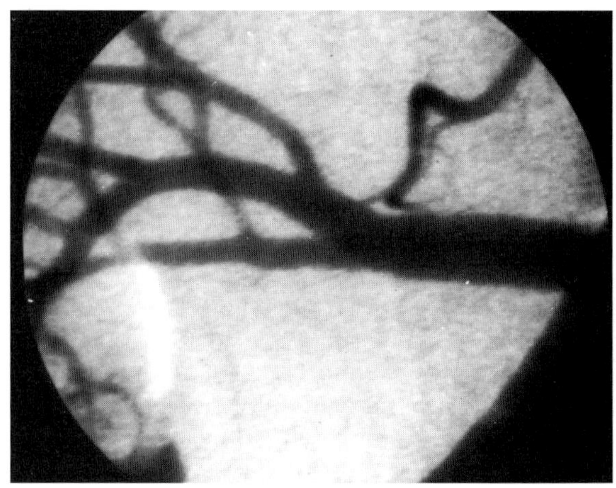

(b)

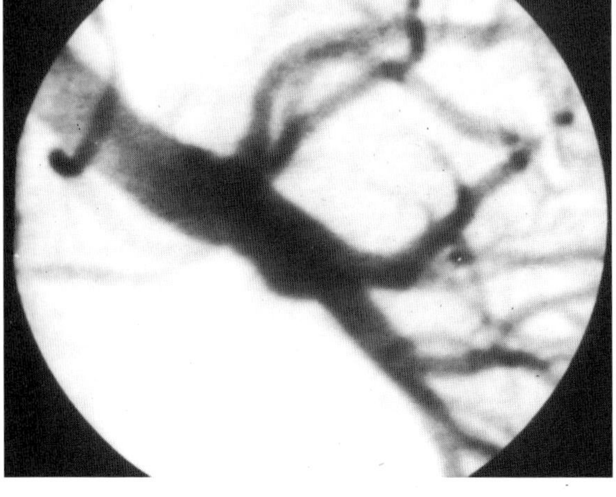

(c)

Figure 33.12. (a) Simultaneous extracorporeal reconstruction with arterial autografts and autotransplantation of a dissecting aneurysm of the right and left renal artery (same patient as in Fig. 33.8). (b) Left detail. (c) Right detail. From ref. 98, with permission anastomosed in an end-to-end fashion to a single limb of a branched graft. The second is an oblique end-to-end anastomosis of branches to a hypogastric arterial autograft (Figs 33.11 and 33.12). Very small polar arteries, that supply only about 1 cm^2 of the upper pole, can be ligated. Finally, the arterial tree is examined for leakage with Collins' solution and the procedure is completed by anastomosing the renal vessels in an end-to-side fashion to the distal aorta and vena cava or common iliac artery and vein using standard renal transplant techniques.

Results

Results of reconstruction of renal macroaneurysms are satisfactory, in particular after the introduction of extracorporeal repair and autotransplantation. In one of the largest series, treatment in 97 patients with 101 aneurysms consisted of 16 nephrectomies and 85 arterial repairs; 16 of the repairs were performed by *ex situ* surgery.[91] In a number of contemporary series employing extracorporeal reconstruction and autotransplantation for complex renovascular lesions including renal aneurysm repair, the nephrectomy rate appeared to be very low.[89, 92–97]

Conclusion

Renal bypass can be considered as the standard method for reconstruction of lesions of the renal artery. The method can be used for reconstruction of uncomplicated lesions of the main renal artery but can also be easily adapted to the repair of more complicated lesions in the distal renal artery or its branches. The most durable results are obtained with autologous bypasses. In the young patient with fibrodysplasia an arterial autograft is used because of its excellent long-term results. In the older patient with atherosclerosis a venous bypass is an excellent alternative if endarterectomy is technically not feasible or advisable. Currently, in skilled hands the operative mortality is less than 2%, the postoperative occlusion less than 5% and the beneficial response rate 80–95%.

References

1 Ramsay LE, Waller PC. Blood pressure response to percutaneous transluminal angioplasty for renovascular hypertension: an overview of published series. *Br Med J* 1990; **300:** 569–72.

2 Sos TA. Angioplasty for the treatment of azotemia and renovascular hypertension in atherosclerotic renal artery disease. *Circulation* 1991; **83:** 1162–6.

3 Tegtmeyer CJ, Selby JB, Hartwell GD, *et al.* Results and complications of angioplasty in fibromuscular disease. *Circulation* 1991; **83:** 1155–61.

4 Keen EH. Origin of renal arteries from the aorta. *Acta Anat* 1981; **110:** 285–6.

5 Benoit G, Delmas V, Gillot C, Hureau J. Anatomical bases of kidney transplantation in man. *Anat Clin* 1984; **6:** 239–45.

6 Van Baalen JM, Van Bockel JH, Overbosch EH. Thoracic origin of right renal artery. *J Vasc Surg* 1994; **19:** 762–63.

7 Kruyt RH. Vascularization of left kidney by single vessel originating from splenic artery. *Urology* 1992; **39:** 487–9.

8 Garti I, Meiraz D. Ectopic origin of main renal artery. *Urology* 1980; **15:** 627–9.

9 Sykes D. The arterial supply of the human kidney with special reference to accessory renal arteries. *Br J Surg* 1963; **50:** 368–74.

10 Harrison LH, Flye MW, Seigler HF. Incidence of anatomical variants in renal vasculature in the presence of normal renal function. *Ann Surg* 1978; **188:** 83–9.

11 Merklin RP, Michaels NA. The variant renal and suprarenal blood supply with data on the inferior phrenic, ureteral and gonadal arteries. *J Int Coll Surg* 1958; **29:** 41–6.

12 Edsman G. Angionephrography and supra-renal angiography. *Acta Radiol* 1957; **155:** 5–141.

13 Kahn PC. Selective angiography of the inferior phrenic arteries. *Radiology* 1967; **88:** 1–8.

14 Wilkins RA, Sandin B, Price A, Twomey B. Extrarenal arterial connections of the normal renal artery. *Cardiovasc Intervent Radiol* 1986; **9:** 119–22.

15 Maxwell MH, Waks AU. Application of diagnostic procedures in patient management. In Van Schilfgaarde R, Stanley JC, Van Brummelen P, Overbosch EH (eds) *Clinical aspects of Renovascular Hypertension*, pp. 75–94. Boston and the Hague: Martinus Nijhoff, 1983.

16 Jacobson HR. Ischemic renal disease: an overlooked clinical entity? *Kidney Int* 1988; **34:** 729–43.

17 Maxwell MH, Bleiffer KH, Franklin SS, Varady PD. Cooperative study of renovascular hypertension. Demographic analysis of the study. *JAMA* 1972; **220**: 1195–204.

18 Maxwell MH, Waks AU. Evaluation of patients with renovascular hypertension. *Hypertension* 1984; **6**: 589–92.
19 Stanley JC. The evolution of surgery for renovascular occusive disease. *Cardiovasc Surg* 1994; **2**: 195–202.
20 Postma CT, van Oijen AH, Barentsz JO, *et al.* The value of tests predicting renovascular hypertension in patients with renal artery stenosis treated by angioplasty. *Arch Int Med* 1991; **151**: 1531–5.
21 Mann SJ, Pickering TG. Detection of renovascular hypertension. State of the art: 1992. *Ann Int Med* 1992; **117**: 845–53.
22 Libertino JA, Flam TA, Zinman LN, *et al.* Changing concepts in surgical management of renovascular hypertension. *Arch Int Med* 1988; **148**: 357–9.
23 Bergentz SE, Bergqvist D, Weibull H. Changing concepts in renovascular surgery. *Br J Surg* 1989; **76**: 429–30.
24 Dean RH, Englund R, Dupont WD, *et al.* Retrieval of renal function by revascularization. Study of preoperative outcome predictors. *Ann Surg* 1985; **202**: 367–75.
25 Dean RH, Tribble RW, Hansen KJ, *et al.* Evolution of renal insufficiency in ischemic nephropathy. *Ann Surg* 1991; **213**: 446–55.
26 Van Bockel JH, Van Schilfgaarde R, Felthuis W, *et al.* Influence of preoperative risk factors and the surgical procedure on surgical mortality in renovascular hypertension. *Am J Surg* 1988; **155**: 770–5.
27 Novick AC, Straffon RA, Stewart BH, *et al.* Diminished operative morbidity and mortality in renal revascularization. *JAMA* 1981; **246**: 749–53.
28 Dean RH, Keyser JE, DuPont WD, *et al.* Aortic and renal vascular disease. Factors affecting the value of combined procedures. *Ann Surg* 1984; **200**: 336–44.
29 Tarazi RY, Hertzer NR, Beven EG, *et al.* Simultaneous aortic reconstruction and renal revascularization: risk factors and late results in eighty-nine patients. *J Vasc Surg* 1987; **5**: 707–14.
30 Atnip RG, Neumyer MM, Healy DA, Thiele BL. Combined aortic and visceral arterial reconstruction: risks and results. *J Vasc Surg* 1990; **12**: 705–14.
31 Khauli RB, Novick AC, Ziegelbaum M. Splenorenal bypass in the treatment of renal artery stenosis: experience with sixty-nine cases. *J Vasc Surg* 1985; **2**: 547–51
32 Moncure AC, Brewster DC, Darling RC, *et al.* Use of the splenic and hepatic arteries for renal revascularization. *J Vasc Surg* 1986; **3**: 196–203.
33 Chibaro EA, Libertino JA, Novick AC. Use of the hepatic circulation for renal revascularization. *Ann Surg* 1984; **199**: 406–11.
34 Fichelle JM, Colacchio G, Farkas JC, *et al.* Renal revascularization in high-risk patients: the role of iliac renal bypass. *Ann Vasc Surg* 1992; **6**: 403–7.
35 Gross RJ, Kern DE. Cardiovascular disease and hypertension. In Kammerer WS, Gross RJ (eds) *Medical Consultation. The Internist on Surgical, Obstetric and Psychiatric Services*, 2nd edn, pp. 117–22. Baltimore: Williams and Wilkins, 1990.
36 Foster JH, Dean RH, Pinkerton JA, Rhamy RK. Ten years' experience with the surgical management of renovascular hypertension. *Ann Surg* 1973; **177**: 755–66.
37 Luciani J, Frantz Ph, Thibault Ph *et al.* Early anuria prevention in human kidney transplantation. Advantage of fluid load under pulmonary arterial pressure monitoring during surgical procedure. *Transplantation* 1979; **28**: 308–12.
38 Collins GM, Green RD, Boyer D, Halasz NA. Protection of kidneys from warm ischemic injury. Dosage and timing of mannitol administration. *Transplantation* 1980; **29**: 83–4.
39 Tiggeler RGWL, Berden JHM, Hoitsma AJ, Koene RAP. Prevention of acute tubular necrosis in cadaveric kidney transplantation by the combined use of mannitol and moderate hydration. *Ann Surg* 1985; **201**: 246–51.
40 Gussenhoven MJ, Ravensbergen J, Van Bockel JH, *et al.* Renal dysfunction after angiography; a risk factor analysis in patients with peripheral vascular disease. *J Cardiovasc Surg* 1991; **32**: 81–6.
41 Wengerter KR, Veith FJ. Self-retaining retraction techniques for vascular surgery: use of a mechanical robot arm. *J Vasc Surg* 1988; **8**: 14–20.
42 Veith FJ, Stoney RJ. Self-retaining retraction in vascular surgery. *J Vasc Surg* 1986; **3**: 824.
43 Huber D, Harris JP, Walker PJ, *et al.* Does division of the left renal vein during aortic surgery adversely affect renal function? *Ann Vasc Surg* 1991; **5**: 74–9.
44 Fry RE, Fry WJ. Supraceliac aortorenal bypass with saphenous vein for renovascular hypertension. *Surg Gynecol Obstet* 1989; **168**: 180–2.
45 Beebe HG, MacFarlane SD. Antegrade aortorenal bypass graft: a new alternative. *Am J Surg* 1988; **155**: 647–50.
46 Novick AC, Stewart R, Hodge EE, Goldfarb D. Use of the thoracic aorta for renal arterial reconstruction. *J Vasc Surg* 1994; **19**: 605–9.
47 Wylie EJ, Stoney RJ, Ehrenfeld WK. *Manual of Vascular Surgery*, p. 32. New York Springer–Verlag, 1980.
48 Adcock OT Jr, Adcock GL, Wheeler JR, *et al.* Optimal techniques for harvesting and preparation of reversed autogenous vein grafts for use as arterial substitutes: a review. *Surgery* 1984; 96: 886–94.
49 Wagner R. Intimal protection of bypass-veins during intraoperative storage in blood or Euro–

Collins-solution: the role of medium, temperature, and time. *J Thoracic Cardiovasc Surg* 1990; **38:** 151–6.

50 Lagneau P, Michel JB, Charrat JM. Use of polytetrafluoroethylene grafts for renal bypass. *J Vasc Surg* 1987; **5:** 738–42.

51 Cormier JM, Fichelle JM, Laurian C, *et al.* Renal artery revascularization with polytetrafluoroethylene bypass graft. *Ann Vasc Surg* 1990; **4:** 471–8.

52 Royle JP. Autogenous vein bypass: an improved technique. *Surgery* 1966; **60:** 795–6.

53 Van Dongen RJ. Renal and intestinal artery occlusive disease. *World J Surg* 1988; **12:** 777–87.

54 Dugoni WE Jr, Bartlett ST, Ward RE. A simplified method for bilateral aortorenal bypass. *Surg Gynecol Obstet* 1990; **170:** 159–60.

55 Okuhn SP, Reilly LM, Bennett JB, *et al.* Intraoperative assessment of renal and visceral artery reconstruction: the role of duplex scanning and spectral analysis. *J Vasc Surg* 1987, **5:** 137–47.

56 Hansen KJ, O'Neil EA, Reavis SW, *et al.* Intraoperative duplex sonography during renal artery reconstruction. *J Vasc Surg* 1991; **14:** 364–74.

57 Dougherty MJ, Hallett JW Jr, Naessens JM, *et al.* Optimizing technical success of renal revascularization: the impact of intraoperative color-flow duplex ultrasonography. *J Vasc Surg* 1993; **17:** 849–56.

58 Piquet P, Ocana J, Verdon E, *et al.* Atherosclerotic lesions of the aorta and renal arteries: results of simultaneous surgical treatment. *Ann Vasc Surg* 1988; **2:** 319–25.

59 Stewart MT, Smith RB III, Fulenwider JT, *et al.* Concomitant renal revascularization in patients undergoing aortic surgery. *J Vasc Surg* 1985; **2:** 400–5.

60 De Rose G, Harris KA, Jamieson WG. Are simultaneous aortic reconstruction and renal revascularization safe and effective? *J Cardiovasc Surg* 1991; **32:** 648–51.

61 O'Mara CS, Maples MD, Kilgore TL Jr *et al.* Simultaneous aortic reconstruction and bilateral renal revascularization. Is this a safe and effective procedure? *J Vasc Surg* 1988; **8:** 357–66.

62 Ernst CB, Stanley JC, Marshall FF, Fry WJ. Autogenous saphenous vein aortorenal grafts. A ten-year experience. *Arch Surg* 1972; **105:** 855–64.

63 Ekelund L, Gerlock J Jr, Goncharenko V, Foster JH. Angiographic findings following surgical treatment for renovascular hypertension. *Radiology* 1978; **126:** 345–9.

64 Van Bockel JH, Van Schilfgaarde R, Felthuis W, *et al.* The influence of the surgical technique upon the short term and long term anatomic results in reconstructive operation for renovascular hypertension. *Surg Gynecol Obstet* 1988; **166:** 402–8.

65 Van Bockel JH, Van Schilfgaarde R, Van Brummelen P, Terpstra JL. Long term results of renal artery reconstruction with autogenous artery in patients with renovascular hypertension. *Eur J Vasc Surg* 1989; **3:** 515–21.

66 Stanley JC, Ernst CB, Fry WJ. Fate of 100 aortorenal vein grafts: characteristics of late graft expansion, aneurysmal dilatation, and stenosis. *Surgery* 1973; **74:** 931–44.

67 Stoney RJ, Olofsson PA. Aortorenal arterial autografts: the last two decades. *Ann Vasc Surg* 1988; **2:** 169–73.

68 Dean RH, Wilson JP, Burko H, Foster JH. Saphenous vein aortorenal bypass grafts: serial arteriographic study. *Ann Surg* 1974; **130:** 469–78.

69 Stanley JC, Whitehouse WM Jr, Zelenock GB, Graham LM, Cronenwett JL, Lindenauer SM. Reoperation for complications of renal artery reconstructive surgery undertaken for treatment of renovascular hypertension. *J Vasc Surg* 1985; **2:** 133–44.

70 Van Bockel JH, Van Schilfgaarde R, Felthuis W, *et al.* Reconstructive surgery for renovascular hypertension. II. Influence of patient selection and anatomical result on the blood pressure response after operation. *Quart J Med* 1988; 66 (251): 259–68.

71 Van Bockel JH, Van Schilfgaarde R, Felthuis W, *et al.* Surgical treatment of renovascular hypertension caused by arteriosclerosis. I. Influence of preoperative factors on the blood pressure control early and late after reconstructive surgery. *Surgery* 1987; **101:** 698–705.

72 Van Bockel JH, Van Schilfgaarde R, Felthuis W, *et al.* Surgical treatment of renovascular hypertension caused by arteriosclerosis. II. Influence of preoperative risk factors and postoperative blood pressure response on late patient survival. *Surgery* 1987; **101:** 468–77.

73 Dean RH, Krueger TC, Whiteneck JM, *et al.* Operative management of renovascular hypertension. Results after a follow-up of fifteen to twenty-three years. *J Vasc Surg* 1984; **1:** 234–42.

74 Mackay A, Brown JJ, Lever AF, *et al.* Unilateral renal disease in hypertension. In JIS Robertson, (ed.) *Handbook of Hypertension*, Vol 2: *Clinical Aspects of Secondary Hypertension*, pp. 33–79. Amsterdam: Elsevier, 1983.

75 Stanley JC, Whitehouse WM, Graham LM, *et al.* Operative therapy of renovascular hypertension. *Br J Surg* 1982; **69:** S63–6.

76 Stanley JC, Whitehouse WM Jr. Occlusive and aneurysmal disease of the renal arterial circulation. *Dis Mon* (US) 1984; **30**(7): 51–62.

77 Youkey JR, Collins GJ Jr, Orecchia PM, *et al.* Saccular renal artery aneurysm as a cause of hypertension. *Surgery* 1985; **97:** 498–501.

78 Stanley JC, Rhodes EL, Gewertz BL, *et al.* Renal artery aneurysms: significance of macroa-

neurysms exclusive of dissections and fibrodysplastic mural dilatations. *Arch Surg* 1975; **110:** 1327–33.
79 Smith DL, Wernick R. Spontaneous rupture of a renal artery aneurysm in polyarteritis nodosa: critical review of the literature and report of a case. *Am J Med* 1989; **87:** 464–7.
80 Bulbul MA, Farrow GA. Renal artery aneurysms. *Urology* 1992; **40:** 124–6.
81 Sharma AK. Renal artery aneurysm, hypertension and neurofibromatosis. *J Royal Soc Med* 1991; **84:** 373–4.
82 Faggioli GL, Gargiulo M, Bertoni F, *et al.* Hypertension due to an aneurysm of the left renal artery in a patient with neurofibromatosis. *Ann Vasc Surg* 1992; **6:** 456–9.
83 Schwartz CJ, White RA. Aneurysm of the renal artery. *J Pathol Bacteriol* 1965; **89:** 349–56.
84 Tham G, Ekelund L, Herrlin K, *et al.* Renal artery aneurysms. Natural history and prognosis. *Ann Surg* 1983; **197:** 348–52.
85 Hupp T, Allenberg JR, Post K, *et al.* Renal artery aneurysm: surgical indications and results. *Eur J Vasc Surg* 1992; **6:** 477–86.
86 Cohen JR, Shamash FS. Ruptured renal artery aneurysms during pregnancy. *J Vasc Surg* 1987; **6:** 51–9.
87 Schoon IM, Seeman T, Niemand D, *et al.* Rupture of renal arterial aneurysm in pregnancy. Case report. *Acta Chir Scand* 1988; **154:** 593–7.
88 Dayton B, Helgerson RB, Sollinger HW, Acher CW. Ruptured renal artery aneurysm in a pregnant uninephric patient: successful *ex vivo* repair and autotransplantation. *Surgery* 1990; **107:** 708–11.
89 Van Bockel JH, Van den Akker PJ, Chang PC, *et al.* Extracorporeal renal artery reconstruction for renovascular hypertension. *J Vasc Surg*, 1991; **13:** 101–10.
90 Belzer FO, Schweizer RT, Kountz SL. Management of multiple vessels in renal transplantation. *Transplant Proc* 1972; **4:** 639–44.
91 Lacombe M. Les anevrismes de l'artere renale. Experience personnelle de 101 cas. *Chirurgie* 1989; **115** (Suppl. 1): 28–33.
92 Novick AC. Management of intrarenal branch arterial lesions with extracorporeal microvascular reconstruction and autotransplantation. *J Urol* 1981; **126:** 150–4.
93 Belzer FO, Raczkowski A. *Ex vivo* renal artery reconstruction with autotransplantation. *Surgery* 1982; **92:** 642–5.
94 Dubernard JM, Martin X, Mongin D, *et al.* Extracorporeal replacement of the renal artery: techniques, indications and long-term results. *J Urol* 1985; **133:** 13–16.
95 Kent KC, Salvatierra O, Reilly LM, *et al.* Evolving strategies for the repair of complex renovascular lesions. *Ann Surg* 1987; **206:** 272–8.
96 Barral X, Gournier J-P, Frering V, *et al.* Dysplastic lesions of renal artery branches: late results of *ex vivo* repair. *Ann Vasc Surg* 1992; **3:** 225–31.
97 Brekke IB, Sodal G, Jakobson A, *et al.* Fibromuscular renal artery disease treated by extracorporeal vascular reconstruction and renal autotransplantation: short- and long-term results. *Eur J Vasc Surg* 1992; **6:** 471–6.
98 Van Bockel JH, Van Baalen JM, Chang PC *et al.* The role of extracorporeal renal artery reconstruction and autotransplantation for complex renovascular and renal problems. A critical review. *J Nephrol* 1994; **7:** 200–207.
99 Van Bockel JH. Fibromusculaire dysplasie, een zeldame afwijking? *Ned T Geneesk* 1979; **123:** 276–82.
100 Van Bockel JH, Van Baalen JM, Chang PC *et al.* Resultats anatomiques et fonctionels de la chirugie artérielle rénale pour hypertension réno-vasculaire. In Kieffer E (ed.) *Chirugie des Artères Rénales*, pp. 113–29. Paris: AERCV, 1993.

34

Renal artery endarterectomy

SVEN-ERIK BERGENTZ, HENRIK WEIBULL

Introduction

Atherosclerosis is by far the most common cause of renal artery stenosis and occlusion, and its importance in vascular surgery is increasing. It has usually a distinct localization to the ostium of the renal artery, extending 1–2 cm into the artery with a distal tapering. In the majority of patients the aortic wall is more or less affected by the atherosclerotic process. Sometimes it is actually limited to the aortic wall and overhanging the ostium of the renal artery, thereby compromising the renal artery flow.[1]

Endarterectomy is now for many surgeons the preferred surgical method for treating atherosclerotic renal artery stenosis. We and others have used alternative methods such as aortorenal bypass, but found this technique more difficult and less durable.[2] There are, however, some contraindications against using the endarterectomy technique. The most important is the finding of an extremely hard and incompressible aorta, making it impossible to apply an occlusive clamp, or an aorta filled with debris with a risk for massive embolization during manipulation. In these situations extra-anatomical reconstructions can be used, such as splenorenal or hepaticorenal shunt or bypass from the gastroduodenal or iliac artery.[2] Other alternatives are a mesenterorenal bypass or an aortorenal bypass, originating from the supraceliac aorta where the atherosclerosis usually is less severe than in the abdominal aorta.[3,4]

Indications for surgery

The general indication for surgical intervention is a hemodynamically significant renal artery stenosis, causing an elevated blood pressure (renovascular hypertension) with or without impairment of the renal function (ischemic nephropathy). Since most patients are in the age group above 60–70 years and suffer from more or less generalized atherosclerosis it is usually required that the hypertension is severe and difficult to treat with antihypertensive drugs. Many physicians have a very restrictive attitude to renovascular surgery for hypertension, enhanced by the fact that we now have available highly effective antihypertensive drugs, which make it relatively easy to control the blood pressure in the majority of patients. It is, however, important to remember that a symptomatic atherosclerotic renal artery stenosis is a progressive condition, with an occlusion of the affected vessels as the potential endpoint, and that blood pressure control, although valuable, does not stop the progression of the disease.[5] If both the renal arteries occlude, or if one occludes and the contralateral kidney is absent or damaged or has a severely stenotic renal artery, the patients become uremic.[6] Studies from the UK indicate that about 14% of the patients above 50 years of age in need of dialysis suffer from ischemic nephropathy as the cause for their uremia and might be treated with renal vascularization.[7] Uremia and threatening uremia rather than hypertension alone has therefore become a most important indication for surgical reconstruction of the renal arteries.[8, 9]

How should we handle an occluded renal artery? If the occlusion is caused by atherosclerosis it is usually 'acute upon chronic', i.e. it comes as the end-result of a renal artery stenosis. Due to the pre-existing collateral circulation there is usually no renal infarction, and if the patient has a functioning contralateral kidney the signs and symptoms are mostly mild. They are characterized by a slight elevation of serum creatinine, a tendency to fluid retention, increasing difficulty to control blood pressure and minor pain over the affected kidney, but in most cases they are so modest that they pass unnoticed.[10] The occluded artery can often be reconstructed if angiography shows that the kidney is not too small (exceeding about 9–9.5 cm in length), that the renal artery can be visualized behind the occlusion (indicating a patent artery) and that there is a reasonable nephrographic phase.[10, 11] The fact that it may be technically possible to reconstruct the artery is not in itself an indication to do it. If the contralateral kidney is normal and the contralateral renal artery is patent and without stenosis it is usually not justified to undertake reconstructive surgery of an occluded renal artery in this elderly patient group with a high operative risk and a relatively short life expectancy. A nephrectomy may be indicated if the hypertension is severe and difficult to control.

In the majority of patients with atherosclerotic renovascular hypertension or ischemic nephropathy there is a bilateral stenosis, but hemodynamically significant usually only on one side. Should we then aim at a uni- or bilateral reconstruction? This is a difficult question and the answer varies considerably among surgeons. Our general philosophy is not to reconstruct a stenotic artery prophylactically, i.e. if it is not hemodynamically significant and therefore not contributing to the hypertensive state. This attitude is favored by the fact that our preferred technique is aortorenal rather than transaortic endarterectomy (see below). Because of our restrictive attitude we sometimes have to treat the contralateral side separately one or several years later if we find that a significant and symtomatic stenosis has developed there, but we think that this is acceptable. In the uremic patient we tend to be more active since we think it is important to save as much renal parenchyma as possible, a policy also supported by data from the literature.[12] Surgeons who favor transaortic endarterectomy often prefer to reconstruct the renal arteries bilaterally for technical reason even if one of the stenoses is insignificant.[13]

Patients undergoing surgery for aneurysmatic or stenotic disease in the aorta very often have stenosis of one or more renal arteries as seen on angiography. This is actually a common finding in patients with atherosclerotic peripheral vascular disease.[14] Again we do not think that a reconstruction is indicated just because of this anatomical finding alone. We have no knowledge about the natural course of these asymtomatic lesions and a renal reconstruction certainly increases the risk with aortic surgery.[15, 16] A symtomatic renal artery stenosis may, however, be reconstructed in combination with the aortic surgery.

Preparation for surgery

Patients with atherosclerotic renal artery stenosis represent a high risk group for coronary, cerebrovascular and peripheral vascular disease. They should therefore be evaluated in cooperation with the internist–cardiologist according to the same principles as used for other elderly, atherosclerotic patients undergoing major surgery. Associated coronary artery disease is initially identified on the basis of history of myocardial infarction or angina pectoris, and electrocardiographic findings. Occasionally coronary angiography should be performed and, if indicated, subsequent cardiac revascularization carried out before the renal artery surgery, which probably results in a lower postoperative mortality.[3] Symptomatic carotid artery stenosis is operated upon before the renovascular surgery. We have not found it necessary to operate on patients with an asymtomatic carotid artery stenosis, but it might be recommended if the stenosis is very tight.

Before surgery the hypertension should be as well controlled as possible, and the antihypertensive drugs should be continued until the day of surgery. A modest impairment of the kidney function, causing a slight elevation of the serum creatinine value, is not unusual and does not require any special attention. A severe impairment of the kidney function can be chronic or 'acute upon chronic'. In addition to the elevated serum creatinine these patients often have a severe fluid retention, which is difficult or impossible to treat with diuretics, and often is misinterpreted as a sign of cardiac insufficiency. In this situation it is important to have the patient dialyzed before surgery. Note that in the 'acute upon chronic' [4] situation there is usually no renal infarction, only a progressive but relatively slow decrease in kidney size following the occlusion.[10] We have therefore plenty of time (days, not hours) to plan the operation and to evaluate and prepare the patient for surgery. The situation is completely different when there is an acute traumatic or embolic occlusion of a previously normal renal artery. This usually results in a renal infarction, and must be handled within hours if the renal parenchyma is to be saved.

Surgical technique

There are three different ways to perform an endarterectomy of the renal artery: Aortorenal, transaortic with longitudinal incision and transaortic with transection of aorta.

Aortorenal endarterectomy

Aortorenal endarterectomy has been our standard technique for more than 15 years, particularly when only one side is going to be reconstructed. With the patient placed in a position with the affected side elevated about 30° and tilting the table under the patient's flank we use a unilateral transverse, subcostal incision to the midline. The table can be rotated and the incision extended to the contralateral side if a bilateral repair is found to be necessary. A transverse incision is well tolerated by the patient and gives a good exposure of the entire renal artery on that side. The *left* renal artery and kidney are exposed by translocating the intestine, stomach, colon and spleen and dividing the inferior mesenteric vein. It is important to mobilize the renal vein by dividing the adrenal and genital veins as well as one or sometimes more lumbar veins entering the renal vein from below or from the back (Fig. 34.1). The renal vein must be dissected free all the way to its entry in the vena cava. These steps are very important in order to make the renal vein mobile and get a good exposure of the renal artery, lying behind the vein. To expose the *right* kidney and renal artery the ascending colon and duodenum are reflected to the left. The anterior side of the kidneys is visualized and inspected. The short right renal vein (or veins) is identified and dissected free. The vena cava is mobilized around the entry of both renal veins and 2–3 cm above and below. It is important to free the vena cava completely, which usually requires division of one or more of the lumbar veins (Fig. 34.2). The right renal artery is now visualized behind the renal vein and vena cava all the way to its origin from aorta, and should be encircled on each side of the vena cava.

The next step, either the operation is carried out on the right or on the left side, is to mobilize

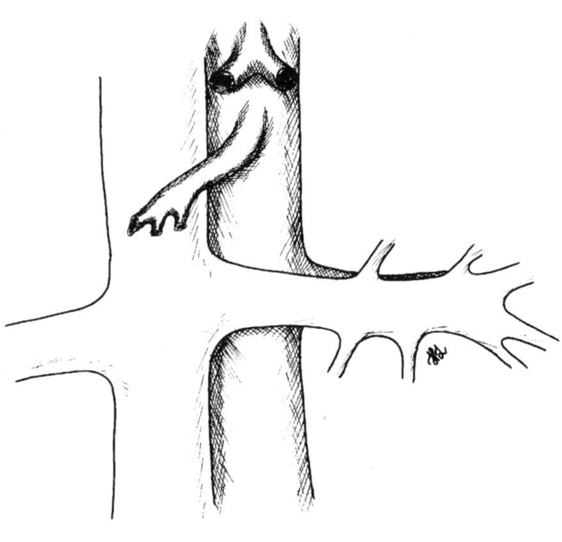

Figure 34.1. The left renal artery is localized behind the left renal vein. To get access to the artery it is necessary to divide the adrenal vein, the genital vein, and one or more lumbar veins.

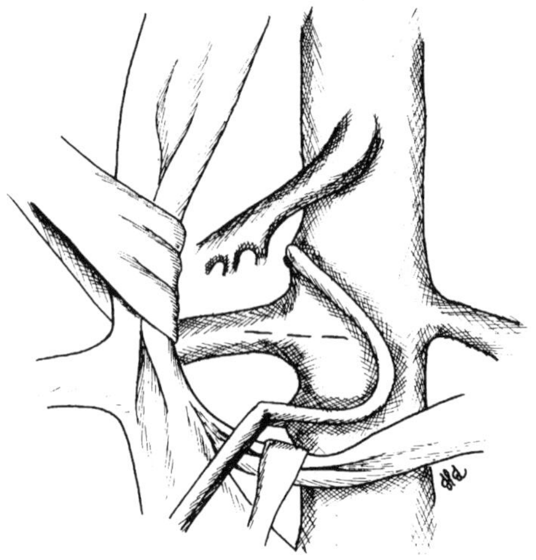

Figure 34.2. To get access to the right renal artery it is necessary to mobilize the vena cava extensively, as well as the proximal parts of each renal vein.

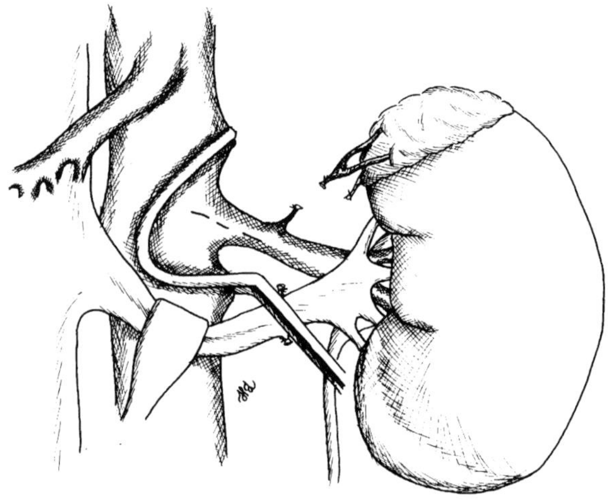

Figure 34.3. To perform a renal artery endarterectomy it is necessary to mobilize aorta extensively enough to apply a U-clamp occluding about half of the aortic lumen. Sometimes a branch from the renal artery to the adrenal gland has to be divided.

aorta generously about 2 cm above and below the origins of the respective renal artery. At least half of the circumference of aorta must be dissected completely free, which often makes it necessary to divide a lumbar artery. Fibrous, hard bands from the crura of diaphragm are found on each side of aorta, sometimes lifting the origin of respective renal artery anteriorly. These bands should be divided. The extensive mobilization of aorta makes it possible to place a side-clamp that can encompass about half of the aorta (Figs 34.2 and 34.3). This is necessary to avoid slipping of the clamp, leaving too small a segment of the thickened aortic wall for the endarterectomy.

The atherosclerotic plaque at the origin of the renal artery can now be palpated. An incision is made longitudinal to the renal artery and transverse to aorta, dividing the stenosing atherosclerotic plaque. It is important that the incision goes far enough into aorta to reach a free aortic lumen (Fig. 34.4). Between 20 and 40 ml of heparinized saline (5000 units of heparin in 500 ml saline) is injected into the renal artery to dilute the blood and decrease the risk for clotting. An endarterectomy (or thromboendarterectomy if applicable) is now performed. The proximal, intra-aortic part of the plaque is always thick and has to be cut off. The distal part of the plaque in the renal artery is tapered in the same manner as the plaques in the internal carotid artery, and here it is usually relatively easy to get a clean break. Occasionally, however, it is necessary to tackle the distal intima. The aortorenal incision is then closed, using a Dacron double-velour patch (Fig. 34.5).

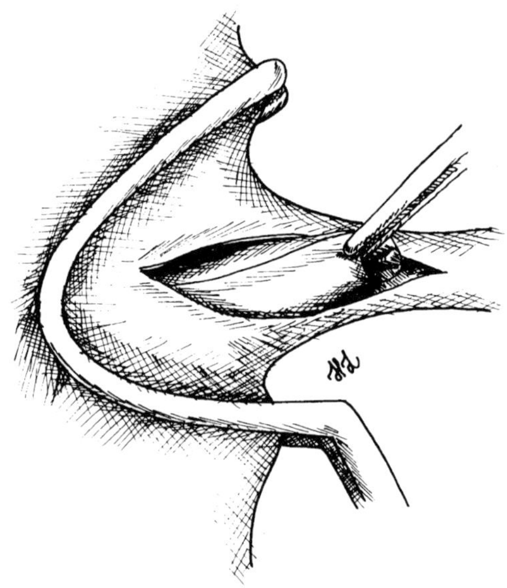

Figure 34.4. Endarterectomy of the left renal artery.

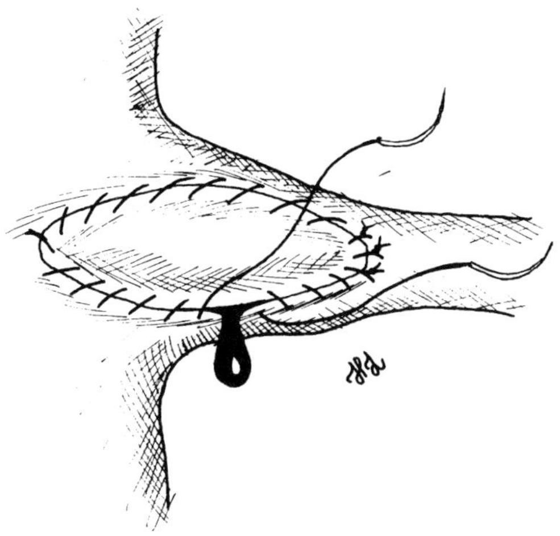

Figure 34.5. Patch closure after the renal artery endarterectomy. Note the interrupted stitches at the distal end of the patch to diminish the risk for stricture.

There are two critical points in this suture. The first is in the aortic wall where a dissection of the thickened intima may occur distally. This is avoided by taking big bites with the suture needle in the aortic wall, including the thickened intima and thereby tackling it. The second critical point is at the distal end of the patch, where a stenosis may occur. To avoid this it is important to make a rounded end of the patch and to place a few interrupted stitches longitudinal and not transverse to the renal artery. For the remaining part of the anastomosis either continuous or interrupted sutures can be used (Fig. 34.5). We prefer not to use a vein patch, which is more difficult to handle than a Dacron patch and has a tendency to dilate and blow out.

Intraoperative control

It is essential to control the result of the reconstruction intraoperatively. We have previously used an electromagnetic flow meter and are currently using a transit time flow meter. The blood flow in the main renal artery should exceed 300 ml/min after the reconstruction. A duplex scanner may be used in addition or alternatively.

Transaortic endarterectomy using a longitudinal incision

This technique was first described by Wylie[17] and is particularly recommended by Stoney and co-workers in San Fransisco.[13] For exposure the San Fransisco group recommends a longitudinal incision from xiphoid to pubis, which may be acceptable for the thin, leptosome patient. Particularly in the fat, pyknic patient we prefer a bilateral subcostal transverse incision, which we think is better tolerated and also gives a more satisfactory exposure of both the renal arteries and the kidneys, although the opening and closure may take a longer time.

Aorta is exposed from a few centimeters below the origin of the renal arteries up to and including the origin of the superior mesenteric artery. It is dissected free from all lymphatic and neural tissue which is particularly abundant in its proximal parts at the level of the superior mesenteric artery. The renal veins and the vena cava are mobilized as described above, exposing the origins and first parts of each renal artery. The crura of diaphragm are also dissected free from aorta and divided if necessary. The patient is then heparinized and the aorta is clamped 3–4 cm below the renal arteries, and just above or just below the superior mesenteric artery. The second alternative is preferred if there is a relatively long distance from the renal arteries to the superior mesenteric artery, and if the aortosclerotic process disappears or is considerably diminished below this level. Otherwise the endarterectomy has to be extended above the superior mesenteric artery. The renal arteries are then clamped bilaterally, and a longitudinal incision made in aorta, starting about 3 cm below the renal arteries and extending to the same distance above, turning to the left of the superior mesenteric artery. The aortic lumen is flushed and the renal arteries perfused with Ringer's lactate or heparinized saline. A core of the thickened intima of the pararenal aorta is then dissected free and cut at the distal and proximal ends (Fig. 34.6). Gentle traction is applied to the intima core while the media of the renal arteries is pushed away with a dissector to avoid prolapse of the renal arteries into the lumen. The intima core then usually separates at the distal endpoint

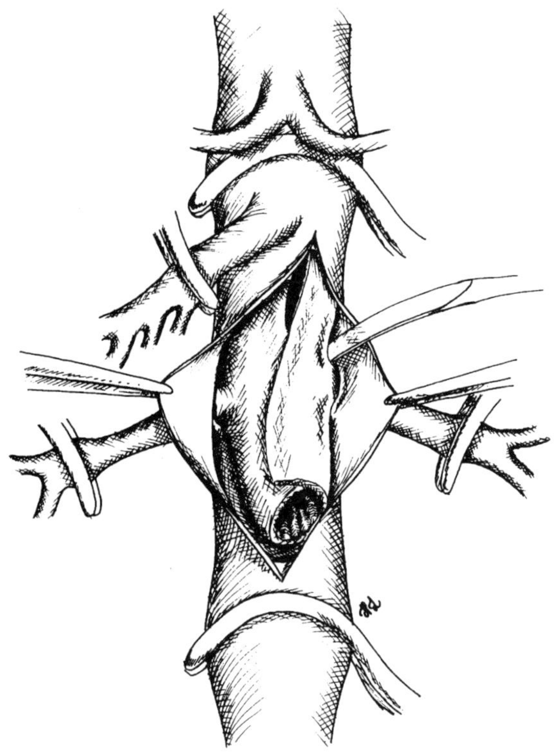

Figure 34.6. Dissection of the atherosclerotic core of the aorta in transaortic longitudinal endarterectomy.

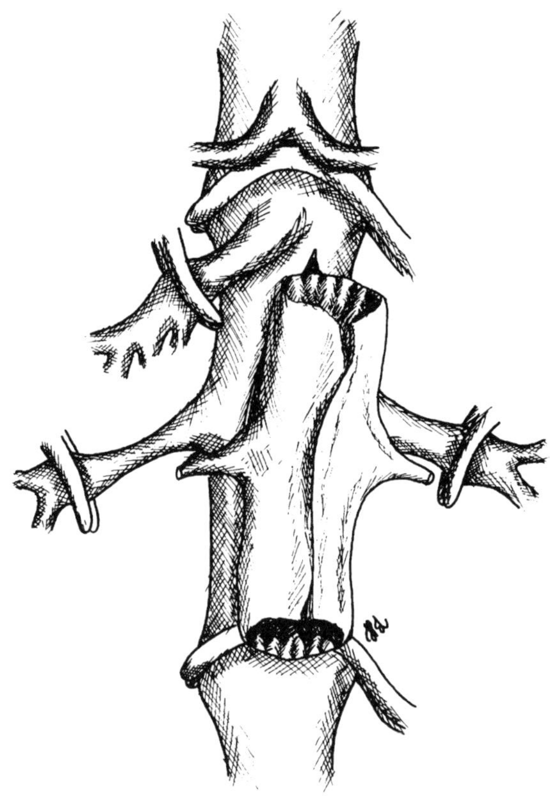

Figure 34.7. Removal of the atherosclerotic core, including the plaques in the origins of both renal arteries.

of the atherosclerotic plaque in the renal artery (Fig 34.7). With this technique it is often difficult to visualize the endpoint of the atherosclerotic plaque. It is therefore important, after closure of the arteriotomy, to evaluate the result intraoperatively. Using an intraoperative probe and duplex scanner it is possible to see aorta and the renal arteries in transverse sections from their origin to beyond the end point of the endarterectomy. In addition, the blood flow in the renal arteries may be measured. If there is suspicion of a persistent stenosing lesion or an intima flap a side-occluding clamp (U-clamp) is applied on aorta at the origin of the renal artery. The artery is opened over the lesion and the lesion is removed. If this is done via a longitudinal incision in the renal artery it is usually necessary to use a patch for closure. Jicha *et al.* recommend a transverse incision just distal to the site of the lesion, which then can be closed without a patch.[13]

Aortic endarterectomy by transection of aorta

This technique was described in 1989 by Stoney *et al.*[18] and is particularly designed to be used for treatment of renal artery stenosis combined with stenosing or aneurysmatic disease in aorta, making it necessary to replace the abdominal aorta with a graft (Fig. 34.8) After exposure and encircling of the aorta, vena cava, the renal veins and renal arteries as just described, the aorta is clamped proximally at the level of the superior mesenteric artery, and distally at the site for the planned aortic reconstruction. The aorta is then transected about 1 cm below the renal arteries. The proximal stump is mobilized by dividing any lumbar arteries, and everted anteriorly, permitting a direct view into the aortic lumen. The

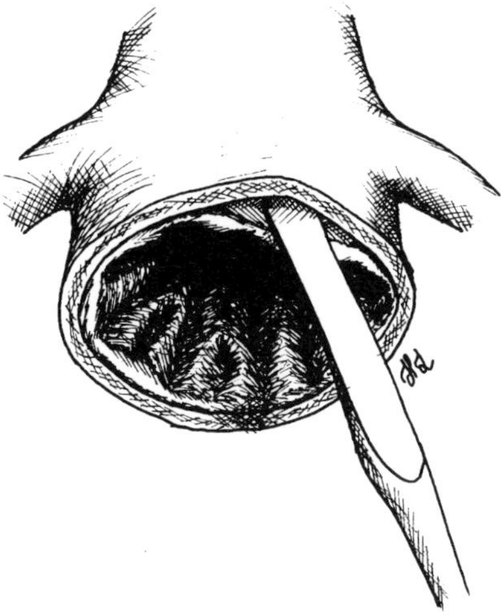

Figure 34.8. Transaortic endarterectomy by transection of aorta.

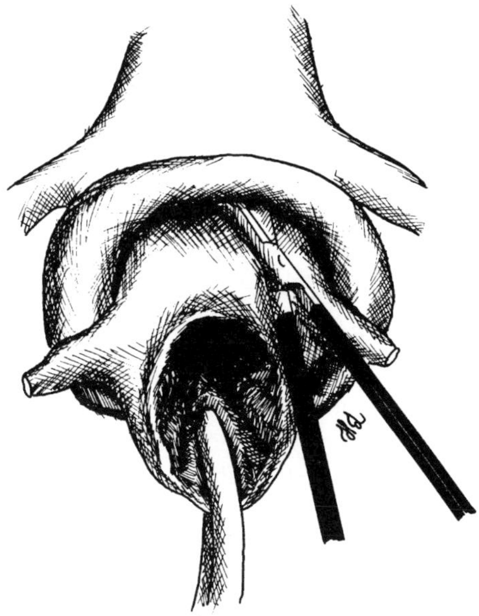

Figure 34.9. The atherosclerotic core is being removed, including the origins of the plaques in both renal arteries.

atherosclerotic plaque is dissected circumferentially, usually up to a level just above or below the superior mesenteric artery, where in most cases it becomes thin. The renal endarterectomy is performed as described above by gentle traction on the large atherosclerotic plaque (Fig. 34.9). The plaque is then divided at the level of the superior mesenteric artery. Aorta and the renal arteries are flushed with heparinized saline. An end-to-end anastomosis is performed to an aortic graft. After that the aortic clamp is replaced with a clamp distal to the anastomosis and the renal perfusion therefore restored.

Postoperative care

The patient should spend at least the first 24 postoperative hours in an intensive care ward with strict control of blood pressure and diuresis. After a successful vascularization of an ischemic kidney there is often a temporary *rise* in blood pressure which may last for a few hours and be due to a renin washout. A short-acting antihypertensive drug may be necessary during this time. The risk for occlusion of the reconstructed renal artery is small if the intraoperative control has shown a good patency and good blood flow. The risk is increased if there has been a chronic renal artery occlusion preoperatively, probably due to a lower flow through the small, sometimes fibrotic or nephrosclerotic kidney. We have no experience of the use of Doppler, renal scan or other non-invasive techniques to diagnose a postoperative renal artery occlusion. If indicated from persistent oliguria, hematuria or blood pressure elevation we may perform a renal angiography but are anxious to use as low volume of the contrast medium as possible to diminish the nephrotoxic damage of the kidneys.

During the first postoperative week it is important to monitor the blood pressure carefully and give the patients antihypertensive drugs if needed. Before the patient leaves the hospital a control of the renal artery patency should be done using angiography or Doppler. The blood pressure contol must continue on an outpatient basis. It often takes weeks, sometimes longer, before blood pressure is stabilized on a new level. A modest increase of blood pressure is not unusual when the patient comes back to active life. If the increase is marked and progressive a new angiography is indicated.

Results

The results must be evaluated with regard to surgical complications, early and late mortality, the short- and long-term renal artery patency (technical success), effects on blood pressure and on kidney function.

Surgical technical complications include ischemic feet, caused by multiple atheromatous embolizations from a severely atherosclerotic and ulcerated aorta. Such embolization may also occur into the kidney. The only way to avoid these complications is to choose extra-anatomical techniques when the aorta appears to be too unattractive. We have also seen once a total occlusion of aorta from a distal intimal flap. This complication is rare, as is pancreatitis, probably caused by mechanical trauma to the pancreas upon surgery of the left renal artery.[19]

The postoperative (30 days) mortality is generally relatively high (2–5%, or even higher) but varies considerably with the type of patient, the indication for surgery and the type of procedure. Most postoperative deaths are related to the patients' generalized atherosclerosis, particularly in the coronary arteries. Hansen *et al.* have demonstrated a considerable difference in mortality between patients with a limited atherosclerotic disease (which only were 12% in their series) and patients with diffuse and extreme atherosclerosis.[12] Bilateral renal artery disease is always a bad sign, indicating a more generalized atherosclerosis and therefore a higher mortality and complication rate. Preoperative uremia or impaired renal function also increases the mortality.[12] Simultaneous reconstruction of aorta for aneurysmatic or stenosing disease has been reported to be connected with an exceedingly high mortality, but recent reports are more favorable.[15]

Also the 5-year mortality is high (30–40%) and related to the patients' generalized atherosclerotic disease.[12]

The most reliable method to evaluate technical results with regard to reocclusion and restenosis is conventional angiography, which should be used when there is any doubt. In experienced hands the endarterectomy technique seems to give a 5-year patency of about 90%.[20,21]

With regard to blood pressure the patients are usually reported as cured, improved or failures according to the criteria recommended by the US Cooperative Study of Surgery for Renovascular Hypertension. A patient is considered cured if the diastolic pressure is 90 mmHg or less in the absence of antihypertensive medication. If there is a decrease in diastolic pressure of at least 15%, but medication still is required, the patient is considered improved. A failure means no or a smaller fall in blood pressure. Several authors have modified these criteria in different ways. Furthermore blood pressure is often not controlled in a standardized fashion or for a reasonably long time, making it difficult to draw reliable conclusions from published data and to compare different techniques. In most reports relatively few (about 20%) in this group of patients are actually cured. The largest group, 50–70%, is characterized as improved. In most series there are 10–20% failures, which can be due either to error in selection of the patient (i.e. insufficient or inaccurate diagnosis of the hypertension) or sometimes to failure to correct the renal ischemia.[2]

The effect of the renal artery reconstruction on renal function is even more difficult to evaluate from the literature.[22] Preoperative impairment of renal function may be due to renal parenchymal damage (such as nephrosclerosis), to ischemic nephropathy, or to a combination of both. It is necessary to have a more severe flow disturbance to cause an impairment of the renal function than to cause hypertension. Therefore clinicians have a tendency to make the diagnosis of renovascular uremia too often. On the other hand it is important not to underdiagnose this condition, which also happens. In particular it is often not realized that a patient who has renal parenchymal damage in addition may develop a severe renal artery stenosis which is worth repairing. The best chances to improve renal function by renovascular surgery is seen in patients with a sudden or rapidly progressing uremia in combination with oliguria and clinical signs of severe fluid retention. These patients may have a bilateral renal artery occlusion, or occlusion of a single kidney, or an occlusion on one side and severe renal artery stenosis or parenchymal damage on the other side. A stable renal function is much more difficult to influence by renovascular surgery, even if the function is more or less impaired.[23]

Which is the optimal reconstruction?

Of the three techniques described we have used the aortorenal reconstruction most frequently. It is technically a very reliable and durable procedure.[2, 20, 21] It is well tolerated by the patient since it is done through a one-sided subcostal incision, not requiring complete occlusion of aorta at any time. The technical complications are few. The technique is particularly suitable for unilateral surgery. If we think the patients should be operated on both sides we either stage the procedure or use the transaortic longitudinal technique. This technique is in our experience more demanding, and carries a higher risk for postoperative renal artery occlusion or restenosis, since the critical first centimeters of the renal arteries are not clearly visualized. It has the advantage of allowing bilateral reconstruction in one setting, but this also means a major operation, requiring clamping of the aorta at the level of the superior mesenteric artery, and therefore heparinization of the patient. The technique with transection of aorta should be used only when simultaneous reconstruction of aorta is indicated. Also this technique is demanding, and requires an experienced team to achieve acceptable results.

Percutaneous transluminal angioplasty (PTA) has during the last decade been used more and more frequently in the treatment of patients with renovascular hypertension or ischemic nephropathy. We have recently in a prospective, randomized fashion evaluated PTA vs surgical reconstruction with endarterectomy in the treatment of symtomatic atherosclerotic renal artery stenosis.[21] The patients were followed carefully with regard to blood pressure, kidney function and patency of the reconstruction according to repeated postoperative angiographies. Of the 29 patients initially allotted to PTA four had to undergo surgery because of technical failure or repeated restenosis, and one of the patients initially treated surgically had to later undergo PTA because of restenosis. After 3 years the secondary patency was almost equal in the two groups, and so was the blood pressure and the renal function. We concluded from this study that PTA can be used for inital treatment of atherosclerotic renovascular hypertension, provided it is combined with intensive follow-up, particularly during the first year, and active reintervention with surgery and re-PTA when indicated.[21] It is important to point out that a number of patients were excluded from randomization and treated surgically. These were patients not suitable for PTA due to occlusion of the renal artery, patients with a stenosis close to a branch, or with a severe occlusive disease in the aorta and/or the iliac arteries. Our results show that by using PTA in selected patients it is possible to spare a number of patients from a surgical intervention. The health care costs do, however, not diminish significantly in spite of the lower number of operations, because of higher costs for the intensive follow-up, re-evaluations and reinterventions in the PTA group.[24]

References

1 Cicuto KP, McLean GK, Oleaga JA *et al.* Renal artery stenosis: anatomical classification for transluminal angioplasty. *Am J Radiol* 1981; **137:** 599–601.
2 Bergentz SE, Bergqvist D, Weibull H. Optimal reconstruction of the renal arteries. *Acta Chir Scan* 1990; (Suppl.) **555** 227–35.
3 Novick AC, Straffon RA, Stewart BH *et al.* Diminished operative morbidity and mortality in renal revascularization. *JAMA* 1981; **246:** 749–53.
4 Inderbir SG, Novick AC, Hodge EE. Extra-anatomic renal revascularization in patients with renal artery stenosis and abdominal aortic occlusion. *Urology* 1993; **42:** 630–4.
5 Bergentz SE. Natural history of renal artery stenosis. *Ann Chir Gynaecol* 1992; **81:** 98–101.
6 Bengtsson U, Bergentz SE, Norback B Surgical treatment of renal artery stenosis with impending uremia. *Clin Nephrol* 1974; 2: 222–7.
7 Scoble JE, Maher ER, Hamilton *et al.* Atherosclerotic renovascular disease causing renal impairment – a case for treatment. *Clin Nephrol* 1989; **31:** 119–22.
8 Jacobsson HR Ischemic renal disease: an overlooked clinical entity? *Kidney Int* **34:** 729–43.
9 Bergentz SE, Bergqvist D, Weibull H Changing concepts in renovascular surgery. *Br J Surg* 1989; **76:** 429–30.

10 Weibull H, Bergqvist D, Andersson *et al.* Symptoms and signs of thrombotic occlusion of atherosclerotic renal artery stenosis. *Eur J Vasc Surg* 1990; **4:** 159–65.
11 Novick AC Percutaneous transluminal angioplasty and surgery of the renal artery. *Eur J Vasc Surg* 1994; **8:** 1–9.
12 Hansen KJ, Starr SM, Sands E *et al.* Contemporary surgical management of renovascular disease. *J Vasc Surg* 1992; **16:** 319–31.
13 Jicha DL, Ehrenfeld WK, Stoney RJ. Surgical techniques for renal revascularization. In Greenhalgh R (ed.) *Vascular and Endovascular Surgical Techniques*, pp. 189–202. London: WB Saunders, 1994.
14 Missouris CG, Buckenham T, Cappucio F, MacGregor G. Renal artery stenosis: a common and important problem in patients with peripheral vascular disease *Am J Med* 1994; **96:** 10–14.
15 Dean RH, Keyser JE, Dupont WD *et al.* Aortic renal vascular disease. *Ann Surg* 1984; **200:** 336–44.
16 Tarazi RY, Hertzer NR, Beven EG *et al.* Simultaneous aortic reconstruction and renal revascularization: risk factors and late results in eighty-nine patients. *J Vasc Surg* 1987; **5:** 708–14.
17 Wylie EJ, Perloff DL, Stoney RJ. Autogenous tissue revascularization techniques in surgery for renovascular hypertension. *Ann Surg* 1969; **170:** 416–28.
18 Stoney RJ, Messina LM, Goldstone J Reilly LM. Renal endarterectomy through the transected aorta: a new technique for combined aortorenal atherosclerosis – a preliminary report. *J Vasc Surg* 1989; **9:** 224–33.
19 Bergqvist D, Weibull H, Bergentz SE. Acute necrotizing pancreatitis complicating surgery for renovascular hypertension. *Acta Chir Scand* 1989; **155:** 492–8.
20 Bergentz SE, Weibull H, Bergqvist D. Long-term patency after reconstructive surgery and PTA for renal artery senosis. In Greenhalgh RM, Hollier L (eds) *The Maintenance of Arterial Reconstruction*, pp 384–96. London: WB Saunders, 1991.
21 Weibull, H, Bergqvist D, Bergentz SE *et al.* Percutaneous transluminal renal angioplasty versus surgical reconstruction of atherosclerotic renal artery stenosis: a prospective randomized study. *J Vas Surg* **18:** 841–52.
22 Rimmer JM, Gennan J. Atherosclerotic renovascular disease and progressive renal failure. *Ann Int Med* 1993; **118:** 712–19.
23 Dean RH, Tribble RW, Hansen KJ *et al.* Evolution of renal insufficiency in ischemic nephropathy. *Ann Surg* 1991; **213:** 446–56.
24 Weibull H, Bergqvist D, Jendteg S *et al.* Clinical outcome and health care costs in renal revascularization – percutaneous transluminal renal angioplasty versus reconstructive surgery. *Br J Surg* 1991; **78:** 620–4.

35

Alternative bypass techniques for renal revacularization

ANDREW C NOVICK

Introduction

A variety of surgical revascularization techniques are available for treating patients with hypertension or renal insufficiency due to renal artery disease.[1] Aortorenal bypass with a free graft of autogenous hypogastric artery or saphenous vein remain a popular method in patients with a non-diseased abdominal aorta.[2, 3] Polytetrafluoroethylene aortorenal bypass grafts have been successfully employed by some investigators, usually when an autogenous graft is not available.[4, 5] Renal endarterectomy also continues to be utilized to treat atherosclerotic renal artery disease.

In older patients with renal artery disease, involvement of the abdominal aorta with severe atherosclerosis, aneurysmal disease or dense fibrosis from a prior operation may render an aortorenal bypass or endarterectomy technically difficult and potentially hazardous to perform. Simultaneous aortic replacement and renal revascularization are associated with operative mortality rates of 5–30%[6–9] compared with rates of 2–6%[10, 11] for renal revascularization without aortic replacement. Dean *et al.* analyzed various risk factors to identify patients at greatest risk from a combined aortic and renal operation.[9] The most significant risk factors were myocardial infarction, existing myocardial ischemia or ventricular hypertrophy, a serum creatinine level >3 mg/dl, diffuse peripheral vascular disease and revascularization of both renal arteries at the time of aortic replacement. While operative mortality was zero if none of these risk factors was present, it increased to 63% if three or more were present. Therefore, simultaneous aortic replacement and renal revascularization should be considered only in patients with a significant aortic aneurysm or symptomatic aortoiliac occlusive disease. In the absence of a definite indication for aortic replacement, alternate bypass techniques are preferable since they can safely and effectively restore renal arterial blood flow while avoiding the need for a more hazardous operation. These alternate bypass operations include hepatorenal bypass, splenorenal bypass, iliorenal bypass, thoracic aortorenal bypass and mesenterorenal bypass. The relative indications, surgical technique and efficacy of these approaches are reviewed in this chapter.

Preoperative evaluation

In considering patient eligibility for alternate visceral renal arterial bypass operations, the absence of occlusive disease involving the donor artery must be verified by preliminary arteriography. Candidates for hepatorenal or splenorenal bypass must be evaluated with both anteroposterior and lateral abdominal aortography to ensure that the celiac artery and its branches are unobstructed. Pelvic arteriography is a requisite study in patients considered for an iliorenal bypass. If thoracic aortorenal revascularization is contemplated, lower thoracic aortography must be obtained.

In recent years, surgical revascularization has been performed more often to preserve renal function in patients with ischemic nephropathy from atherosclerotic renal artery disease.[12] Such patients are generally older with ostial renal artery lesions and diffuse atherosclerosis involving other major abdominal vessels. Significant atherosclerotic occlusive disease involving the celiac and iliac arteries may preclude use of these vessels for renal revascularization. In a recent study from our center, abdominal aortographic findings were reviewed in 254 patients with atherosclerotic renal artery disease to document the prevalence of associated abdominal aortic and visceral arterial atherosclerosis.[13] All patients were evaluated with both anteroposterior and lateral aortography. The renal, celiac, superior mesenteric and common iliac arteries were evaluated for the presence and severity of stenosis. The incidence of moderate (50–75%) or severe (>75%) visceral artery stenosis was determined in patients with varying degrees of renal artery stenosis (Table 35.1).

In the overall group of 254 patients with atherosclerotic renal artery stenosis, the incidence of significant celiac and iliac artery stenosis was 54% and 50%, respectively. Patients with severe renal artery stenosis bilaterally or in a solitary kidney are of greatest interest since they comprise the most common candidate group for revascularization to preserve renal function. In this group, the incidence of significant celiac and iliac artery stenosis was 59% and 58%, respectively. Patients with severe unilateral renal artery stenosis also occasionally require revascularization to treat poorly controlled hypertension. In this group, the incidence of significant celiac and iliac stenosis was 52 and 30%, respectively. A majority (75–81%) of patients in both of the above groups had significant abdominal aortic atherosclerosis which would preclude abdominal aortorenal revascularization. Our findings underscore the prevalence of celiac and iliac arterial occlusive disease in these patients which, if present, obviates use of these vessels for renal revascularization. The only other published study bearing on this issue is from Valentine *et al.* who noted celiac artery stenosis in 17 of 50 patients (34%) with >50% renal artery stenosis, and in 10 of 20% (50%) with >75% renal artery stenosis.[14]

In patients with atherosclerotic renal vascular disease, the preoperative evaluation should include a thorough search for coronary artery disease, because this has been the leading cause of operative death following surgical revascularization.[15] In addition to a careful history, a physical examination and an electrocardiogram, all operative candidates in this category undergo a thallium cardiac stress test in our program. If any of the latter assessments suggests the presence of coronary artery disease, our policy is to perform coronary cine angiography and left-sided ventriculography. Myocardial revascularization is recommended for patients with significant correctable coronary artery disease prior to renal revascularization.

Cerebrovascular accident has also been a significant cause of death after renal revascularization in patients with atherosclerosis, albeit a less common complication than myocardial infarction. The approach to patients whose history or

Table 35.1 Incidence of significant aortic disease and visceral artery stenosis in patients with renal artery stenosis

Renal artery status	Aortic disease (%)	Celiac stenosis (%)	SMA stenosis (%)	Iliac stenosis (%)
Unilateral mild or moderate stenosis (*N*=45)	89	53	31	48
Unilateral severe stenosis (*N*=44)	75	52	20	30
Bilateral mild or moderate stenosis (*N*=36)	72	39	25	47
Severe stenosis bilaterally or in a solitary kidney (*N*=129)	81	59	29	58

SMA: Superior mesenteric artery.

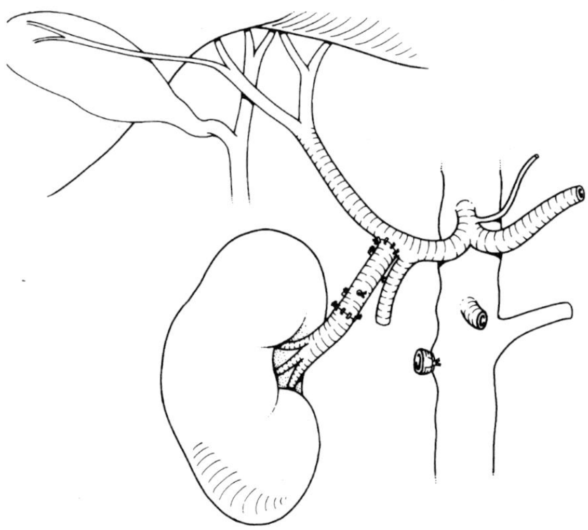

Figure 35.9. The most common method of performing hepatorenal bypass with an interposition saphenous vein graft anastomosed end-to-side to the common hepatic artery and end-to-end to the right renal artery. From ref. 26, with permission.

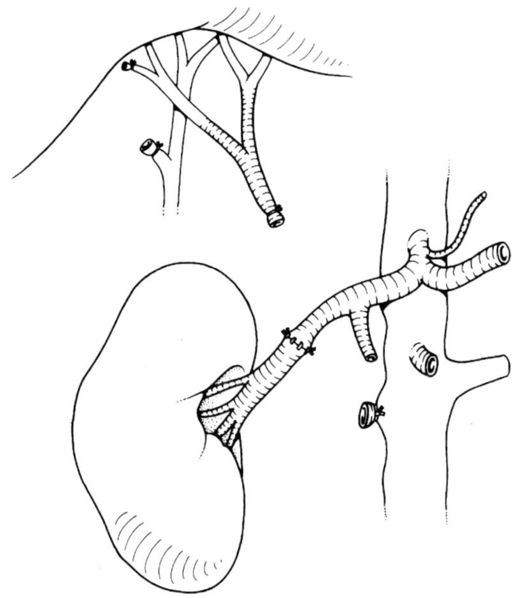

Figure 35.10. Performance of hepatorenal bypass by direct end-to-end anastomosis of the common hepatic artery to the right renal artery. From ref. 26, with permission.

origin. In these situations, the available major hepatic arteries are generally all of insufficient caliber to maintain adequate blood flow both to the liver and the right kidney. It is then preferable to perform end-to-end anastomosis of either the common, right, or left hepatic arteries to the right renal artery (Fig. 35.10).[19] In some patients, a direct tension-free anastomosis of these vessels can be done; otherwise, an interposition saphenous vein graft is needed. Despite the resulting total or segmental hepatic dearterialization in these patients, postoperative liver function studies have remained normal. However, the gall bladder is more susceptible to ischemic damage and may undergo necrosis when its blood supply from the right hepatic artery is interrupted.

There are three available strategies to avoid the complication of gall bladder ischemia in patients undergoing end-to-end hepatorenal revascularization. First, when separate right and left hepatic arteries are present, the left hepatic artery should be used preferentially for anastomosis with the renal artery (Fig. 35.11). Second, if it is necessary to use the common or right

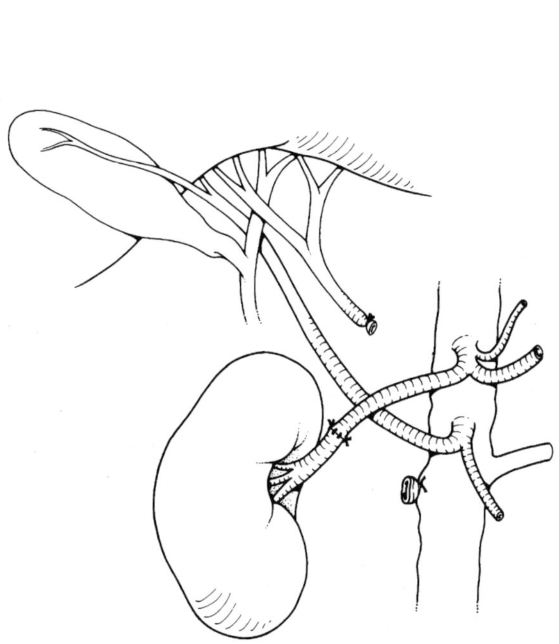

Figure 35.11. A method of hepatorenal revascularization when the right and left hepatic arteries have a separate origin. Here, the left hepatic artery is anastomosed end-to-end to the right renal artery. From ref. 26, with permission.

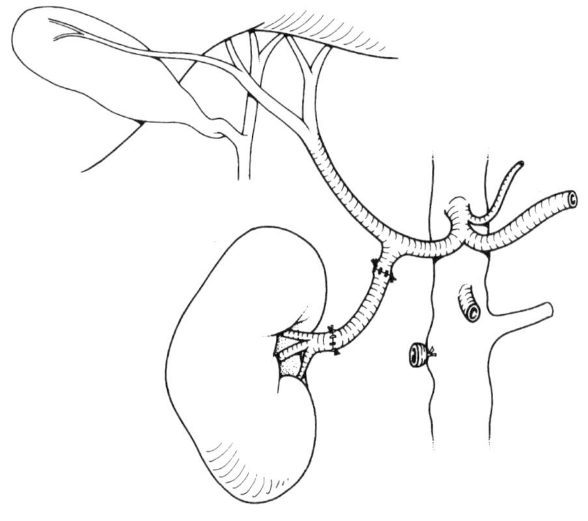

Figure 35.12. Use of the gastroduodenal artery to perform hepatorenal revascularization with a saphenous vein graft interposed between the gastroduodenal and right renal arteries. From ref. 26, with permission.

hepatic arteries in this manner, an adjunctive cholecystectomy should be performed. A third option is to perform end-to-end anastomosis of the gastroduodenal and renal arteries, with an interposition saphenous vein graft if necessary (Fig. 35.12). However, the origin and course of the gastroduodenal artery must be such that proximal kinking does not occur when this vessel is rotated toward the right kidney. It is also somewhat more difficult to mobilize an adequate length of this artery, and care must be taken to avoid damage to the duodenum or pancreas. This technique is not as widely applicable as other methods of hepatorenal revascularization but it does offer the advantage of preserving hepatic arterial flow.

The results of hepatorenal bypass for right renal arterial occlusive disease have been excellent and indicate that this is a safe and effective operative approach in properly selected patients with a diseased abdominal aorta (Fig. 35.13).[20]

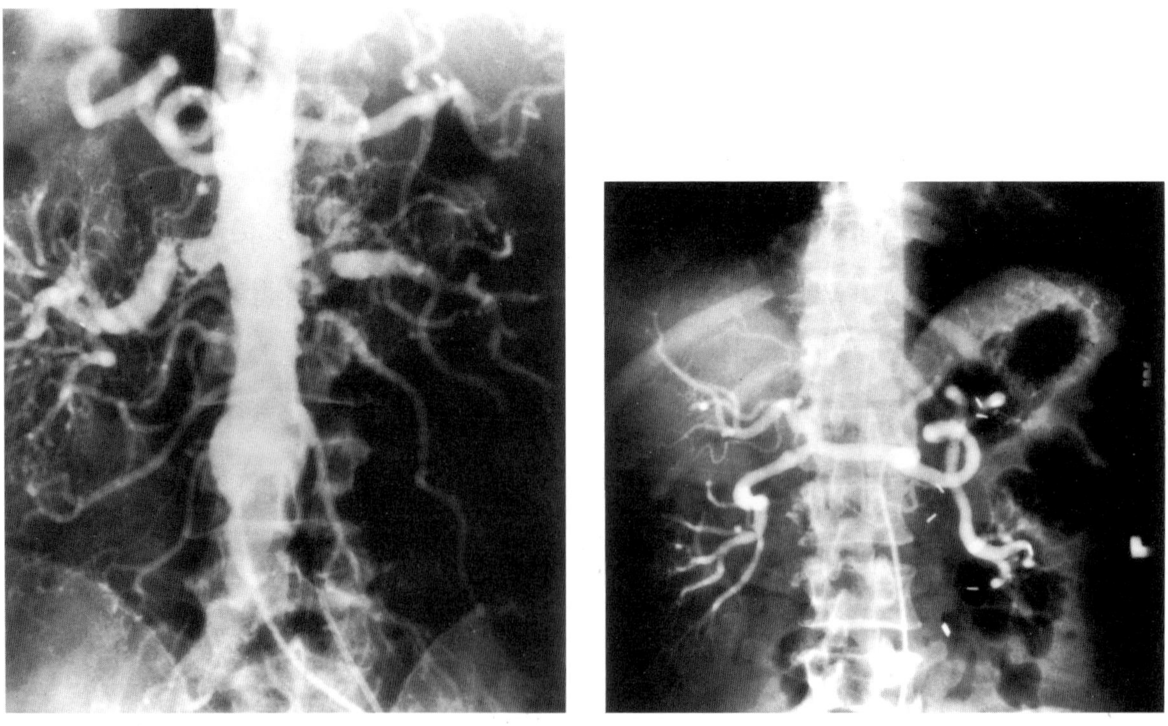

(a) (b)

Figure 35.13. (a) Abdominal aortogram demonstrates highgrade bilateral renal artery stenosis and severe aortic atherosclerosis. (b) Following staged bilateral splenorenal and hepatorenal bypass operations, a selective celiac arteriogram demonstrates excellent flow to both kidney.

Thoracic aortorenal bypass

Use of the thoracic aorta for renal revascularization is a new surgical alternative for patients with significant abdominal aortic atherosclerosis, celiac artery stenosis and no primary indication to replace the abdominal aorta. The subdiaphragmatic supraceliac and descending thoracic aorta are often relatively free of disease in such patients and can be used to achieve renal vascular reconstruction with an interposition saphenous vein graft.[21, 22] Preoperative angiographic evaluation should include views of the supraceliac and thoracic aorta to verify their disease-free status.

For left renal revascularization, we have employed the descending thoracic aorta as a donor site because we believe that it is more readily accessible than the subdiaphragmatic supraceliac aorta. A left thoracoabdominal incision is made below the 8th rib and extended medially across the midline. This incision provides excellent simultaneous exposure of the thoracic aorta and renal artery with no need for extensive abdominal visceral mobilization. The left colon is reflected medially to expose the kidney and renal artery. The descending thoracic aorta is exposed above the diaphragm and is partially occluded laterally with a DeBakey clamp (Fig. 35.14). A small aortotomy is made, a reversed saphenous vein graft is anastomosed end-to-side to the aorta, and the aortic clamp is then removed (Fig. 35.15). During performance

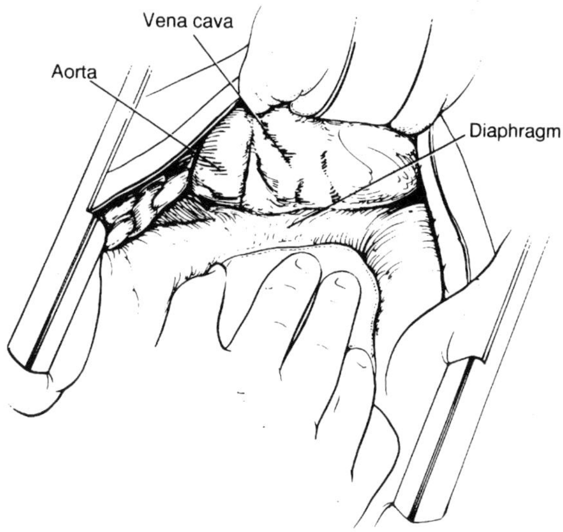

Figure 35.14. The lower descending thoracic aorta is exposed above the diaphragm, through a left thoracoabdominal incision. From ref. 27, with permission.

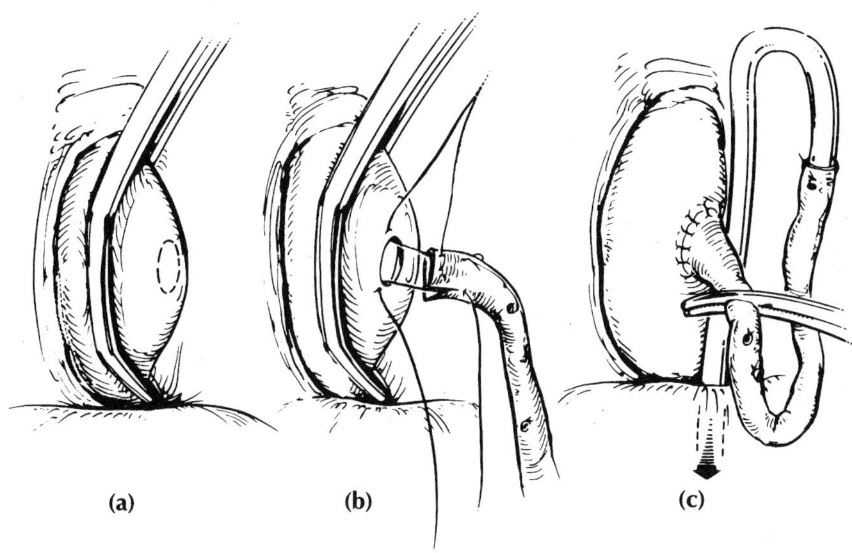

Figure 35.15. After partial aortic occlusion (a) an oval aortotomy is made. A saphenous vein graft is anastomosed end-to-side to the thoracic aorta (b and c). The graft is then passed through the aortic diaphragmatic hiatus into the retroperitoneum (c). From ref. 27, with permission.

of the proximal anastomosis, distal aortic flow is preserved and systemic heparinization is therefore not employed. A 2 cm incision is then made in the diaphragm just lateral to the aorta to enlarge the hiatus. The saphenous vein graft is passed alongside the aorta, through the diaphragmatic hiatus, posterior to the pancreas and into the left retroperitoneum. End-to-end anastomosis of the vein graft and distal left renal artery are performed to complete the operation (Fig. 35.16). On the right side, the subdiaphragmatic supraceliac or lower thoracic aorta are equally accessible through an anterior bilateral subcostal incision. The technique of thoracic aortorenal bypass is otherwise analogous to that described on the left side.

We reported our initial results with thoracic aortorenal bypass in 23 patients with hypertension, abdominal aortic atherosclerosis and celiac artery stenosis; in 21 patients, renal artery stenosis was present bilaterally or in a solitary kidney.[22] There was one operative death due to myocardial infarction. Postoperatively, among the remaining 22 patients, hypertension was cured or improved in 19 (86%) and renal function was stable or improved in 21 (95%) (Fig. 35.17).

Thoracic aortorenal revascularization is an attractive approach for several reasons. The thoracic aorta provides an excellent inflow source and the proximal end-to-side vein graft anastomosis yields an antegrade acute angle that is hemodynamically advantageous. Since the thoracic aorta is only partially occluded during performance of the proximal anastomosis, distal aortic flow is preserved and systemic heparinization is unnecessary. The potential morbidity of aortic cross-clamping which includes the risk of spinal cord ischemia is avoided. The period of renal ischemia is also minimal and is limited to the time required for completion of the distal anastomosis which is 15–20 min. Revascularization of the kidney is achieved with an auto-

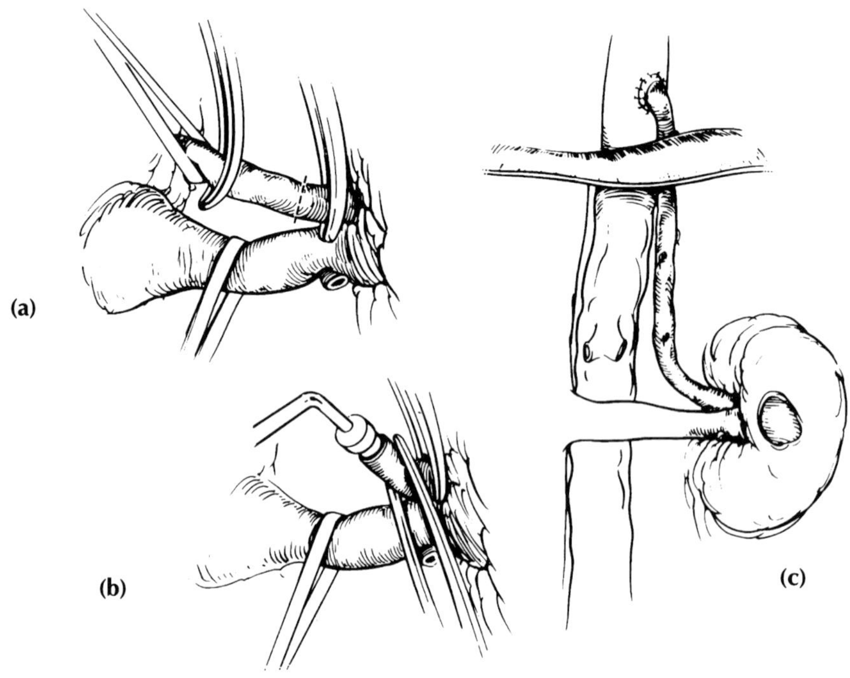

Figure 35.16. The saphenous vein graft is anastomosed end-to-end to the distal left renal artery to complete the thoracic aortorenal bypass. From ref. 27, with permission.

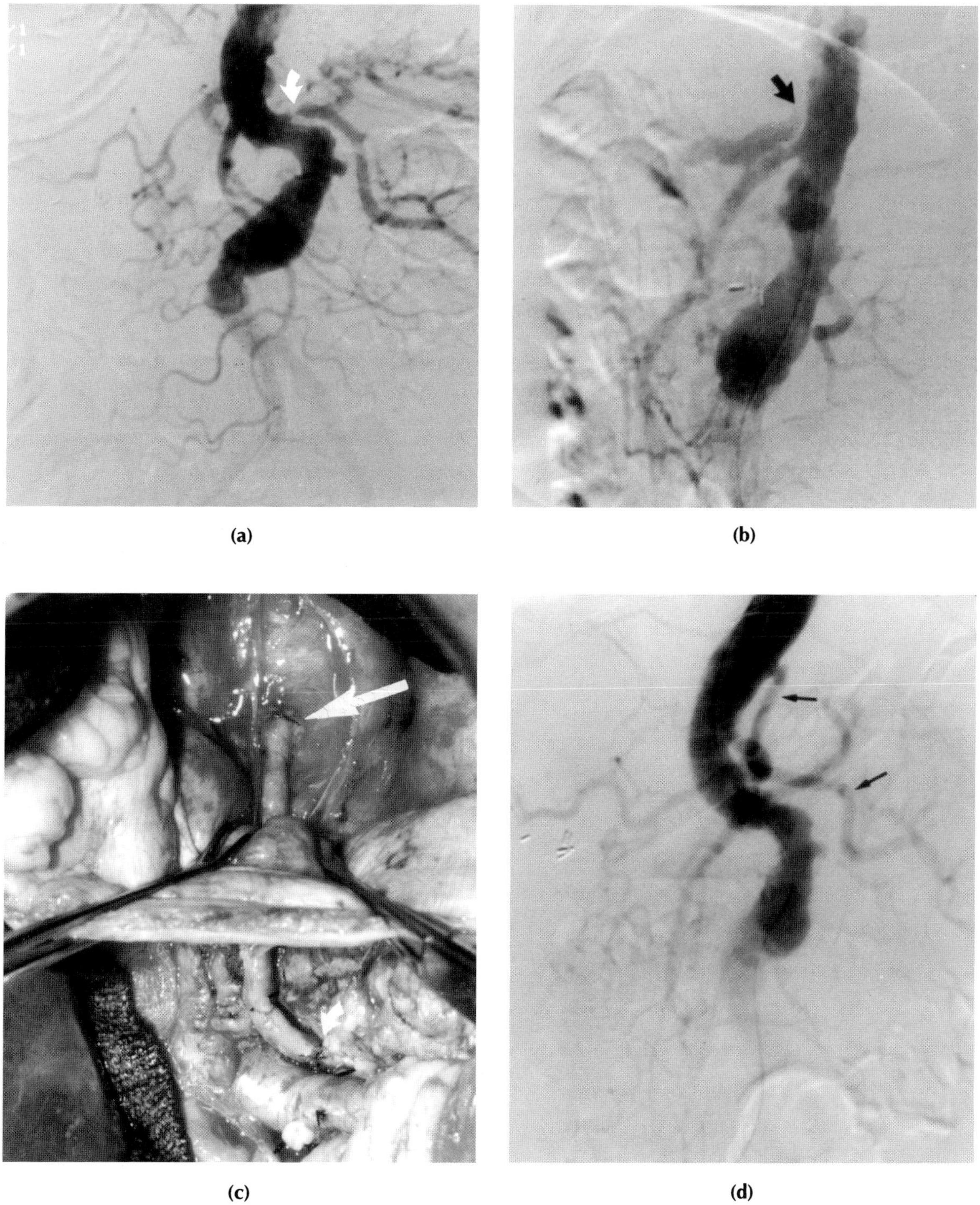

Figure 35.17. (a) Preoperative aortogram shows solitary left kidney with high grade arterial stenosis. (b) Lateral aortography shows high grade stenosis of the celiac artery. (c) Operative photograph of completed thoracic-aortorenal revascularization. Long and short arrows indicate proximal and distal graft anastomoses, respectively. (d) Postoperative aortogram shows patent thoracic aortorenal saphenous vein bypass graft. From ref. 17, with permission.

genous vascular graft which represents the optimum material for renal artery replacement. Finally, use of the invariably healthy thoracic aorta minimizes the risk of peripheral embolization.

Iliorenal bypass

Iliorenal bypass is an occasionally useful technique for revascularization in patients with severe aortic atherosclerosis, provided there is satisfactory flow through the diseased aorta and absence of significant iliac disease (Fig. 35.18).[23, 24] The author's current approach is to consider this operation only when a splenorenal, hepatorenal or thoracic aortorenal bypass cannot be done. This preference is based on the fact that aortic atherosclerosis may continue to progress in these patients, and if so, this process is most likely to involve the inrarenal aorta. Such a development might then compromise flow to a revascularized kidney whose blood supply is derived exclusively from one of the iliac arteries. The suprarenal and supraceliac aorta are more often spared from progressive atherosclerosis, hence, our preference for bypass procedures originating from these locations.

In generally, iliorenal bypass is performed using the ipsilateral iliac artery because this simplifies exposure of the operative field. This is a relatively minor consideration and use of the contralateral common iliac artery is also satisfactory, particularly if this is less diseased than the ipsilateral counterpart. Iliorenal bypass is performed through a midline transperitoneal incision after harvesting a long saphenous vein graft. The colon is reflected medially to obtain simultaneous exposure of the ipsilateral common iliac and renal arteries. The common iliac artery is occluded proximally and distally with bulldog clamps. An oval arteriotomy is made on the anterolateral aspect of the common iliac artery. The distal clamp is temporarily released to enable 20 ml of dilute heparin solution to be instilled into the distal iliac and femoral arteries. Systemic heparinization is not routinely employed.

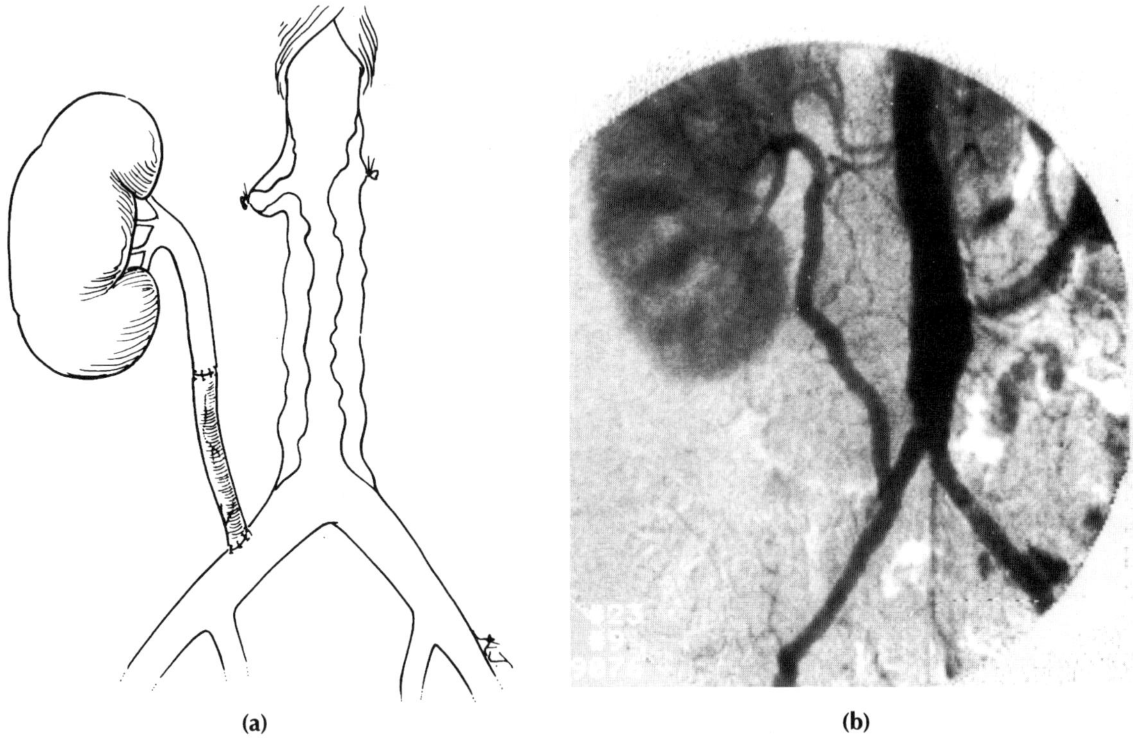

(a) (b)

Figure 35.18. (a) Technique of iliorenal bypass with a saphenous vein graft. (b) Digital subtraction angiogram in a patient who underwent a successful right iliorenal bypass operation. From ref. 26, with permission

The proximal end of the saphenous vein graft is spatulated and the apex of the spatulation is placed at the cephalic end of the arteriotomy. Stay sutures are placed in both cephalic and caudal margins of the anastomosis, which is then completed with interrupted 6–0 arterial sutures. A bulldog clamp is placed across the proximal portion of the vein graft and the iliac clamps are removed restoring circulation to the lower extremity. The saphenous vein graft follows a direct cephalad course toward the ipsilateral renal artery between the aorta medially and the ureter laterally. An end-to-end anastomosis of the saphenous vein graft to the distal disease-free renal artery is then performed with interrupted 6–0 arterial sutures. The graft is positioned to allow a tension-free distal anastomosis while avoiding angulation or kinking of the renal artery.

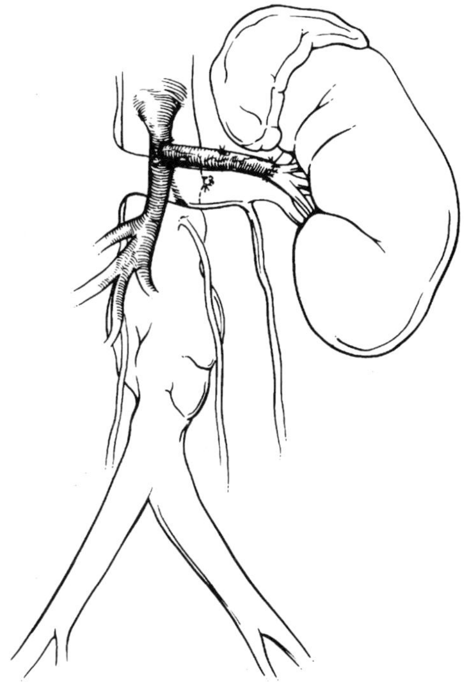

Figure 35.19. The technique of superior mesenterorenal bypass to the left kidney with a saphenous vein graft. From ref. 24, with permission.

Mesenterorenal bypass

In unusual cases, aortography reveals an enlarged superior mesenteric artery (SMA) that may then be employed for visceral arterial bypass to either kidney (Fig. 35.19). We have employed the superior mesenterorenal bypass technique in occasional patients with a troublesome aorta in whom a bypass to the kidney from the celiac or iliac arteries is not possible.[24, 25] The finding of an enlarged and widely patent SMA is most often observed in patients with total occlusion of the infrarenal aorta. In such cases, the SMA has a wider caliber than normal because it is supplying collateral vessels to areas ordinarily vascularized from the infrarenal aorta, i.e. the large bowel, pelvis and lower extremities. Use of such an enlarged SMA for performance of a mesenterorenal bypass has been well tolerated with no compromise of intestinal blood flow. We have not used this approach in patients with normal-sized SMA and cannot comment on its efficacy in this setting.

To perform mesenterorenal bypass the abdomen is entered through a midline incision. During revascularization of the left kidney, the descending colon and splenic flexure are reflected medially and a plane of dissection is developed between the pancreas and Gerota's fascia. Exposure of the suprarenal aorta is obtained by gentle retraction of the pancreas and first portion of jejunum cephalad, while the mesocolon is reflected medially. If necessary, additional exposure may be obtained by mobilization and evisceration of the right colon and small bowel, as is done commonly for retroperitoneal lymphadenectomy. The SMA can be palpated readily at its origin from the aorta approximately 1–2 cm above the level of the renal arteries. The vessel lies against the neck of the pancreas as it courses between the neck and the uncinate process. The artery then crosses the third part of the duodenum to enter the large bowel mesentery, where it lies posterior and to the left of the superior mesenteric vein. The SMA is mobilized for a distance of 2–3 cm beyond its origin, where it is most accessible and without branches. The left renal artery then is exposed and isolated similarly. A reversed segment of saphenous vein is anastomosed end-to-side to the lateral aspect of the SMA with interrupted 6–0 vascular sutures. After completion of this anastomosis, which generally takes 15–20 min, blood flow through the SMA is restored immediately and the saphenous vein graft is occluded temporarily. End-to-end anastomosis

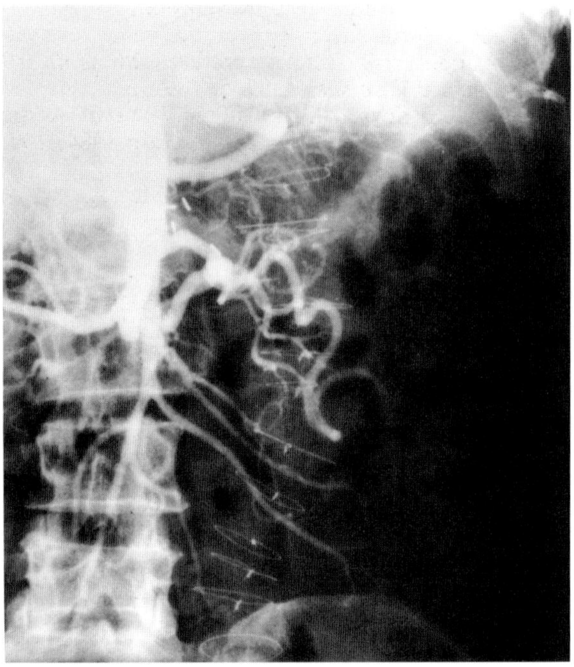

Figure 35.20. Aortagram in a patient who underwent left mesenterorenal saphenous vein bypass shows excellent flow to the left kidney.

of the vein graft to the left renal artery then is done with interrupted 6–0 vascular sutures (Fig. 35.20).

During revascularization of the right kidney the ascending colon and duodenum are reflected medially to gain exposure of the aorta and right renal artery. The ascending colon and small bowel are then rotated back to their normal position and the SMA is palpated where it crosses the third portion of the duodenum. The SMA is mobilized and isolated in this location for a distance of 3–4 cm. A saphenous vein graft is sutured end-to-side to this portion of the SMA and the graft is then passed through a tunnel in the root of the small bowel mesentery, following a gentle curve as it crosses the third portion of the duodenum to enter the right retroperitoneum. End-to-end anastomosis of the graft to the right renal artery is performed to complete the operation.

Postoperative care

Patients undergoing surgical renal revascularization may experience wide fluctuations in blood pressure in the early postoperative period, with either hypotensive or hypertensive episodes, which may predispose to graft thrombosis or bleeding from vascular anastomotic sites, respectively. Therefore, these patients are placed in the intensive care unit for monitoring of the central venous pressure, urine output, pulse rat and serum levels of hemoglobin and creatinine. During this period, the diastolic blood pressure is maintained at approximately 90 mmHg to ensure satisfactory renal perfusion. If hypertensive episodes occur, they are managed with intravenous infusion of sodium nitroprusside. Within the first 24 h postoperatively, a technetium-99 m renal scan is obtained to verify perfusion of the revascularized kidney. If clear evidence of perfusion is not present, then arteriography should be done immediately to examine the repaired renal artery.

If the patient's condition is stable, the nasogastric tube, central venous line, arterial line and urethral catheter are removed 48 h postoperatively, and intensive care monitoring is discontinued. Most patients are discharged from the hospital 1 week postoperatively. Subsequent follow-up is performed by periodic evaluation of the blood pressure, serum creatinine level and technetium-99 m renal scanning.

Clinical results

We recently analyzed our experience with alternate bypass techniques for renal revascularization at the Cleveland Clinic from January 1980 to December 1992.[13] A total of 175 revascularization operations were performed in 171 patients. In all patients, alternate bypass techniques were employed due to severe abdominal aortic atherosclerosis or previous aortic surgery. The revascularization operations comprised hepatorenal bypass (N=59), splenorenal bypass (N=54), iliorenal bypass (N=37), thoracic aortorenal bypass (N=23), renal autotransplantation (N=1) and superior mesenterorenal bypass (N=1). Surgical renal revascularization was indicated to treat poorly controlled hypertension in 13 patients and to treat ischemic nephropathy in 158 patients; all patients in the latter group had severe renal artery stenosis bilaterally or in a solitary kidney.

There were five patient deaths within the first postoperative month for an overall operative mortality rate of 2.9%. Postoperative thrombosis of the repaired renal artery occurred after 7 of 175 revascularization operations (4%). In the 13 patients with severe hypertension, the mean preoperative blood pressure was 176/101 mmHg, and the mean postoperative blood pressure was 142/78 mmHg. The mean preoperative and postoperative serum creatinine levels in this group were 1.2 mg/dl and 1.0 mg/dl, respectively.

In patients with ischemic nephropathy, postoperative renal function was improved in 41%, stable in 44% and deteriorated in 15%. The best results were obtained in patients with a preoperative serum creatinine level <2 mg/dl where 90% experienced postoperative improvement or stabilization of renal function. While preservation of renal function was the predominant indication for intervention in the ischemic nephropathy group, all of these patients also had hypertension which was controlled with medical therapy. Postoperatively, hypertension was cured in 14%, improved in 63% and unchanged in 23%. The results of this study affirm the efficacy of alternate bypass techniques for renal revascularization when the prerequisite conditions for their use are present.

References

1 Novick AC. Surgical correction of renovascular hypertension. *Surg Clin North Am* 1988; **68:** 1007–25.
2 Ernst CB, Stanley JC, Marshall FF *et al.* Autogenous saphenous vein aortorenal autografts: a ten-year experience. *Arch Surg* 1972; **105:** 855–64.
3 Stoney RJ, Olofsson P. Aortorenal arterial autografts: the last two decades. *Ann Vasc Surg* 1988; **2:** 169–73.
4 Khauli RB, Novick AC, Coseriu CV. Renal revascularization and polytetrafluoroethylene grafts. *Cleve Clin Quart* 1984; **51:** 365–9.
5 Cormier JM, Fichelle JM, Laurian C *et al.* Renal artery revascularization with polytetrafluoroethylene bypass graft. *Ann Vasc Surg* 1990; **4:** 471–8.
6 Brewster DC, Buth J, Darling RC. Austen WG. Combined aortic and renal reconstruction. *Am J Surg* 1976; **131:** 457–63.
7 Shahian DM, Najafi H, Javid H *et al.* Simultaneous aortic and renal artery reconstruction. *Arch Surg* 1980; **115:** 149–7.
8 Tarazi RY, Hertzer NR, Beven EG *et al.* Simultaneous aortic reconstruction and renal revascularization: risk factors and late results in 89 patients. *J Vasc Surg* 1987; **5:** 709–15.
9 Dean RH, Keyser JE III, DuPont WD *et al.* Aortic and renal vascular disease. *Ann Surg* 1984; **200:** 336–44.
10 Novick AC, Ziegelbaum M, Vidt DG *et al.* Trends in surgical revascularization for renal artery disease: ten years' experience. *JAMA* 1987; **257:** 498–501.
11 Libertino JA, Bosco PJ, Ying CY *et al.* Renal revascularization to preserve and restore renal function. *J Urol* 1992; **147:** 1485–7.
12 Novick AC. Atherosclerotic ischemic nephropathy: epidemiology and clinical considerations. *Urol Clin North Am* 1994; **21:** 195–200.
13 Fergany A, Kolettis P, Novick AC. The contemporary role of extra-anatomic surgical renal revascularization in patients with atherosclerotic renal artery disease. *J Urol* 1995; **153:** 1798–802.
14 Valentine RJ, Martin JD, Myers SI *et al.* Asymptomatic celiac and superior mesenteric artery stenoses are more prevalent among patients with unsuspected renal artery stenoses. *J Vasc Surg* 1991; **14:** 195–9.
15 Novick AC, Straffon RA, Stewart BH *et al.* Diminished operative morbidity and mortality in renal revascularization. *JAMA* 1981; **246:** 749–53.
16 Khauli R, Novick AC, Ziegelbaum W. Splenorenal bypass in the treatment of renal artery stenosis: experience with 69 cases. *J Vasc Surg* 1985; **2:** 547–51.
17 Brewster DC, Darling RC. Splenorenal arterial anastomosis for renovascular hypertension. *Ann Surg* 1979; **189:** 353–8.
18 Novick AC, Palleschi J, Straffon RA, Beven E. Experimental and clinical hepatorenal bypass as a means of revascularization of the right renal artery. *Surg Gynecol Obstet* 1979; **148:** 557–62.
19 Novick AC, McElroy J. Renal revascularization by end-to-end anastomosis of the hepatic and renal arteries. *J Urol* 1985; **134:** 1089–93.
20 Chibaro EA, Libertino JA, Novick AC. Use of hepatic circulation for renal revascularization. *Ann Surg* 1984; **199:** 406–11.
21 Fry RE, Fry WJ. Supraceliac aortorenal bypass with saphenous vein for renovascular hypertension. *Surg Gynecol Obstet* 1989; **168:** 181–2.
22 Novick AC. Use of the thoracic aorta for renal arterial reconstruction. *J Vasc Surg* 1994; **19:** 605–9.
23 Novick AC, Banowsky LH. Iliorenal saphenous vein bypass: alternative for renal revascularization in patients with surgically difficult aorta. *J Urol* 1979; **122:** 243–5.
24 Novick AC, Iliorenal and mesenterorenal bypass. In Novick AC, Streem SB, Pontes J *Stewart's Operative Urology*. (eds) Baltimore: Williams and Wilkins, 1989.

25 Khauli RB, Novick AC, Coseriu GV *et al.* Superior mesenterorenal bypass for renal revascularization with infrarenal aortic occlusion. *J Urol* 1985; **133:** 188–90.
26 Novick AC, Khauli R, Vidt D *et al.* Diminished operative risk and improved results following revascularization for atherosclerotic renovascular disease. *Urol Clin North Am* 1984; **11:** 435.
27 Novick AC. Use of the thoracic aorta for renal revascularization. *Urol Clin North Am.* 1994; **21:** 355.

36

Aortic replacement and renal revascularization

WILHELM SANDMANN, GIOVANNI TORSELLO

Etiology and incidence of combined disease

The natural incidence of combined aortic and renal artery disease is unknown. Although almost half of the patients undergoing repair for infrarenal aortic aneurysm are hypertensive, only a minority is suspected of having coexisting significant renal artery occlusive disease.[1] In centers with special interest in renovascular diseases patients with combined lesions probably appear more often (Table 36.1). Angiographical studies in patients undergoing abdominal aortic surgery have shown coexisting significant renovascular disease in 19%.[2] In Europe more patients undergo aortic replacement with selective use of angiography, while in the United States angiography in most centers is thought to be inevitable. However, it can be assumed that 20% of patients with abdominal aortic disease have artherosclerotic occlusive disease of one or more renal arteries and there is virtually no difference if aortic aneurysmal disease is compared to occlusive disease (Table 36.2).[3] It is our experience that if the degenerative disease extends into the suprarenal or the thoracoabdominal part of the aorta the renal arteries are involved more often. For example, the calcified thrombus of a coral reef aorta usually extends into the renal and visceral arteries as well and in patients with a thoracoabdominal aortic aneurysm renal and visceral arterial occlusive disease was found in almost 30% of our patients. In chronic aortic dissection renal perfusion is often reduced unilaterally, because the dissecting membrane extends into the renal artery (Fig. 36.1).

Besides the degenerative causes of combined aorto-renal vascular disease other etiologies are rather rare. Aortic coarctation involving segment IV and V of the descending aorta usually causes renal hypoperfusion and arterial hypertension, not because the collateral circulation cannot compen-

Table 36.1. Renal artery occlusive disease: simultaneous aortic replacement and renal artery reconstruction, 1974–1994 at the Heinrich-Heine University, Düsseldorf.

Patients	502
Renal arteries	808
Age (years)	64.3
Bilateral	310 (61.7%)
with AAA	163 (32.5%)
with aortoiliac OD	193 (38.4%)

AAA: abdominal aortic aneurysm; OD: occlusive disease

Table 36.2. Simultaneous aortic and renal artery reconstruction: epidemiologic data in 356 patients operated from 1974 to 1994 at the Heinrich Heine University, Düsseldorf.

8.8% of all patients operated upon for AAA (163/1850)
9.8% of all patients operated upon for aortoiliac OD (193/1720)
32.5% of all patients with renal artery OD (AAA)
38.4% of all patients with renal artery OD (aortoiliac OD)
70.9% of all patients with renal artery OD (overall 356/502)

Patients who required treatment for thoracoabdominal aortic aneurysm are not included.

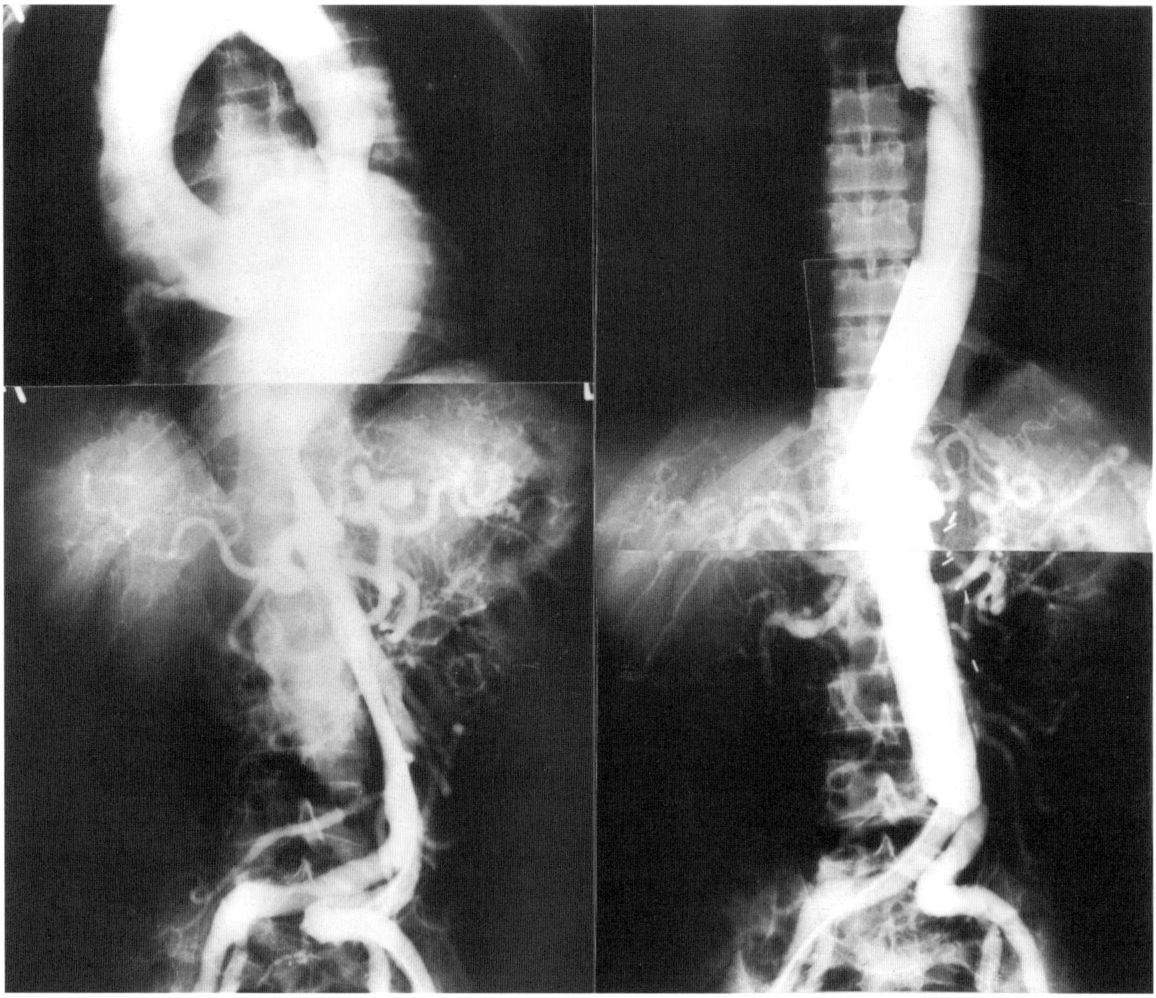

(a) (b)

Figure 36.1. Thoracoabdominal angiogram of a 59-year-old patient suffering from chronic dissection and severe hypertension. The dissecting membrane extended in both renal arteries (a) which had to be endarterectomized before normal renal circulation by implantation into the thoracoabdominal aortic graft could be performed (b).

sate the aortic stenosis but because the hypoplasia involves the origin of the renal arteries.

Very rare conditions of combined aortic and renovascular involvement may be present in patients with Takayasu's disease, giant cell arteritis, Behçet's disease and Marfan's syndrome. Typically these patients are between 15 and 30 years old and much younger than those with artherosclerotic disease.

Takayasu's disease has been described to involve the supra-aortic branches and the neck arteries in Caucasian women mainly, but involvement of the descending aorta and visceral branches has been described as well and has been found in non-Caucasian natives also.[4] The other inflammatory diseases may be described as aneurysmosis, because of multiple aneurysmal formation of the peripheral arterial system. Behçet's disease is an immunologically explained inflammatory disease, predominantly found in people from the Near East countries presenting with multiple aneurysms of the aorta and its branches. Despite the aneurysmal enlargement the vessel wall is thickened enormously like in patients with inflammatory aneurysms of the aorta (Fig. 36.2). Giant cell arteritis in its late burned

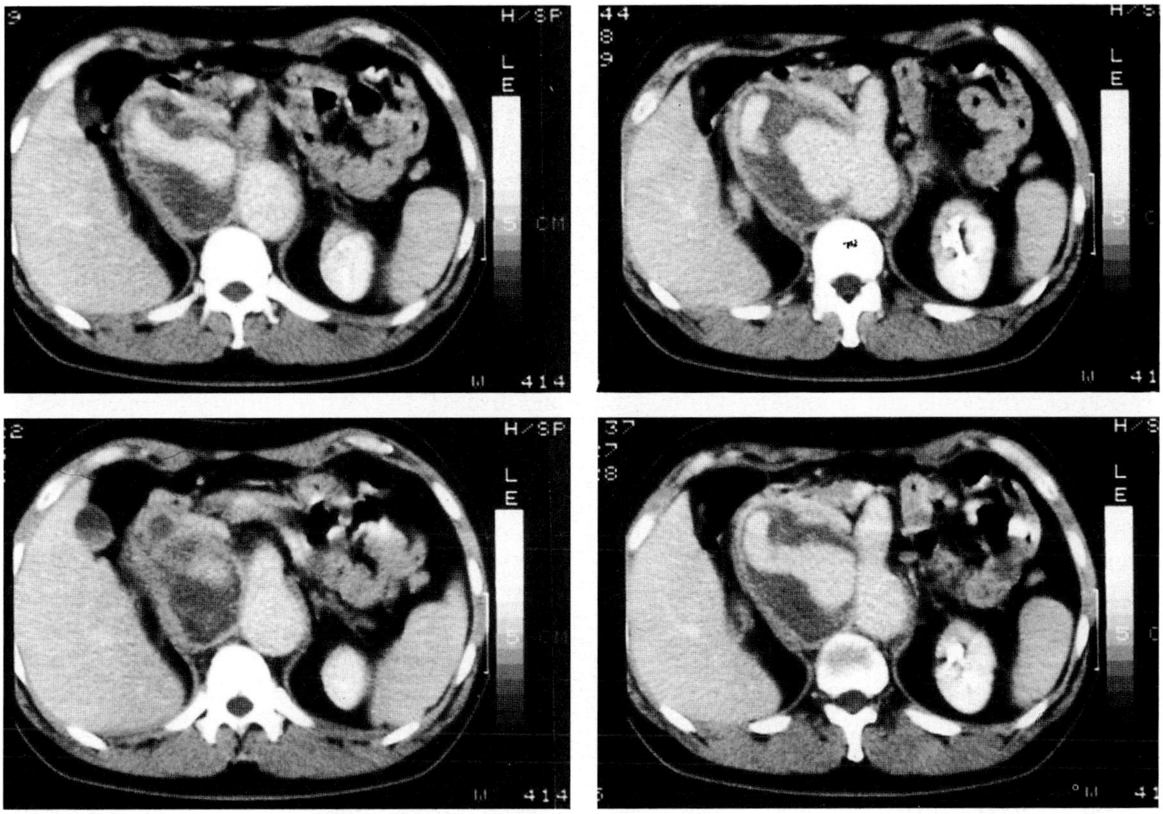

(a)

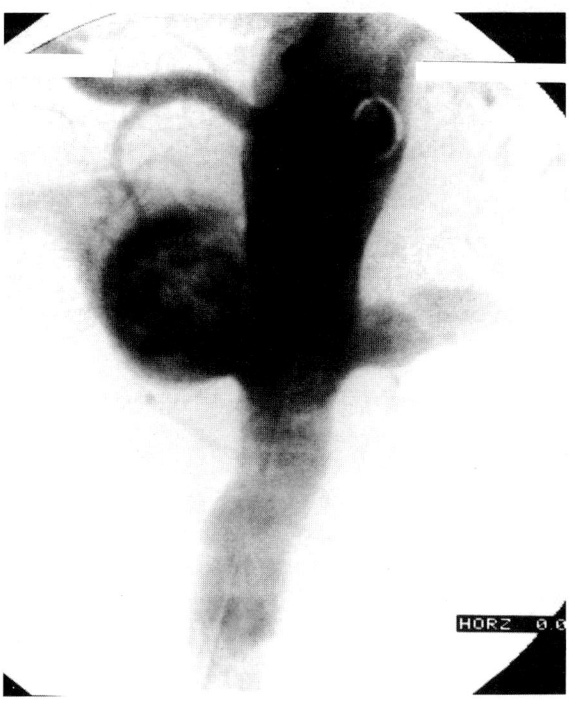

(b)

Figure 36.2. Inflammatory thoracoabdominal aortic aneurysm in a 28-year-old Persian man with additional aneurysms in all visceral arteries. CT scanning shows the significant thickening of the renal and mesenteric arterial wall (a). The angiogram understates the real severity of the disease (b).

out phase can cause multiple aneurysms, predominantly in the mesenteric and renal arteries. In one of our patients we removed 9 of 11 aneurysms from the visceral and renal arteries during the same operation.

Patients with Marfan's syndrome typically present between the age of 15 and 25 years. Overdistensibility of elastic and fibrotic tissue leads to aortic valvular incompetence, abnormal movement of the lenses, hemorrhoids and hernias. Instability of the joints may appear. Although in patients with Marfan's syndrome the proximal aorta is mainly involved, in rare instances the disease involves the peripheral part of the aorta and its branches only.

Diagnostic essentials

The diagnostic armamentarium today offers every possibility to evaluate kidney function and to study the morphology of aorta and renal arteries in patients with coexistent disease.

However, in daily practice all patients with aortic occlusive disease and many patients with abdominal aortic aneurysms are quickly scheduled for aortography, by which coexistent renal artery disease is detected. There is no argument against this routine except in cases with hypertension or symptoms and laboratory findings of renal insufficiency. These patients should first have evaluation of kidney function and non-invasive studies to measure size and function of the kidneys, before contrast material is injected. Contrast computerized tomography (CT) and sequential angiography may cause impairment of already reduced renal function directly related to the amount of contrast medium. This is most important in patients who require aortic clamping above the renal arteries or longer periods of renal ischemia for reconstruction thereafter. In general, clamping ischemia adds to pre-existing renal damage possibly leading to cardiac, circulatory and respiratory problems and eventually to hemodialysis; this can be avoided if less contrast material is used or if surgery is postponed. Waterloading and forced diuresis either by application of furosemide or mannitol have been shown to protect the kidneys.[5] As many patients with aneurysmal aortic disease may require surgery soon after the diagnostic procedures, protection of the kidney before and during surgery is essential.

If possible, angiotensin converting enzyme blocking agents should be replaced by other drugs to avoid renal artery occlusion before vascular surgery. However, in urgent situations CF scanning and/or aortography must be performed and the preoperative medication must be continued without regard to kidney function. In these cases preoperative volume loading, infusion of 100–250 ml of 20% mannitol and increased diuresis should be started before the diagnostic workup whenever possible.

In an emergency case of a ruptured aortic aneurysm there is usually no time for preoperative evaluation of the renal vasculature, so that simultaneous reconstruction of the renal arteries at the time of aortic replacement is performed more or less accidentally. From our own experience, especially from reimplantation and reconstruction of renal arteries, which surprisingly were found to originate from the aortic aneurysm or found by inspection and palpation to be diseased during aneurysm repair, we have learned that renal arteriography is not an indispensable prerequisite for successful renal artery reconstruction in aortic surgery, if the surgeon is aware of possible renal vascular abnormalities and disease. In elective surgery preoperative CT scans sometimes show calcified stenoses at the origin of the renal arteries with or without parechymal signs of chronic hypoperfusion, so that ostial or near ostium stenosis of the renal artery can be anticipated. Patients with a juxtarenal aortic aneurysm will require suprarenal clamping anyhow, so that we might prefer to examine the lumen of the renal arteries during surgery instead of performing preoperative aortorenography. Even in patients with highly suspected atherosclerotic ostial and near ostium lesions presenting with hypertension and reduced kidney function we sometimes try to avoid preoperative arteriography, because after suprarenal clamping transaortic thromboendarterectomy can be performed easily on one or both renal arteries. However, this concept should be the exception and performed in carefully selected cases, and the surgeon must be familiar with intraoperative measures to protect the kidney and intraoperative diagnostic tools must be used which ensure unrestricted renal circulation at the end of the combined procedure section on adjunctive measures below).

Indications for simultaneous repair

Symptomatic disease of the aorta and both renal arteries, i.e. the coexistence of renal failure from occlusive disease and a painful infrarenal aortic aneurysm, presents an absolute indication for simultaneous reconstruction. There is convincing evidence that to leave out the repair of one or the other disease will expose the patient to substantial risk in the postoperative period. Only simultaneous reconstruction offers the possibility of an uncomplicated postoperative course and a normal life afterwards. Slightly reduced kidney function and renovascular hypertension in patients with an asymptomatic aortic aneurysm are currently the most common indications for simultaneous management. In these patients simultaneous surgery is more or less prophylactic. However, hypertension is a well-known risk factor for aneurysm rupture and should be treated, and it does not make sense to wait until kidney function deteriorates. Epidemiologic data show that the risk of aneurysm rupture increases after the maximum diameter has exceeded 5 cm.[6–9] Hypertension is an additional risk factor for growth and rupture of aneurysms. Patients with excentric or without mural thrombosis of the aneurysm sac probably have a higher risk of rupture than those with a concentric thrombus. In patients with large aneurysms the hypertension is sometimes not very impressive because the aneurysm seems to cause a pressure leak, but after aneurysm repair without renal artery reconstruction the hypertensive values will be exceedingly higher.

Symptomatic aortic and renal occlusive disease likewise are felt to be appropriate conditions for simultaneous repair although prospective studies to support this concept have not been performed. We mention this point because theoretically infrarenal aortic occlusion could be treated by an extra-anatomic axillo-femoral graft and renal vascular hypertension could be managed conservatively. However, if the patient seems to tolerate the direct anatomic approach to the aorta, the chance to repair the renal arteries at the same time and improve the patient's overall prognosis should be taken (Table 36.3).

Technical considerations play an important role when deciding on simultaneous repair. If the aortic disease extends to or involves the renal arteries, the possible extent of aortic cross-clamping and the anatomic approach necessary to allow complete restoration of the vascular system are of major importance. In patients with additional involvement of the mesenteric arteries, especially the indication for simultaneous renal reconstruction is affected by the surgical tactics. For example, in patients with an infrarenal aortic aneurysm and coexisting combined renal and mesenteric occlusive disease it might be considered dangerous to normalize renal perfusion without reconstruction of the mesenteric arteries, because as a result of success of the renal revascularization the blood pressure will probably drop to normal causing intestinal ischemia. This is especially the case in patients in whom the inferior mesenteric artery is ligated during aneurysm repair. Crawford *et al.*[4] have summarized their experiences and pointed out that 'in all patients with renal artery disease with bilateral lesions and in those with recent onset of hypertension and in all patients with partial superior mesenteric artery obstruction and in those with symptoms of mesenteric artery insufficiency regardless of the extent of obstruction, operative correction is indicated at the time of aortic replacement'. In the San Francisco series reported by Qvarfordt *et al.*[10] the perioperative mortality rate was 1.3% and the perioperative morbidity rate 28%, which demonstrated that combined repair can be performed with results similar to those of simple infrarenal replacement. The severity of renal artery disease and the extent of the renal artery reconstruction were the limiting factors determining postoperative morbidity, which is a fact well known from reconstructive procedures in patients with renovascular occlusive disease alone. To summarize, if significant obstruction of one renal artery (>70%) or of both renal arteries (>50%) has been detected, simultaneous repair at the time of

Table 36.3. Surgical management in 356 patients undergoing simultaneous repair for aortic disease and renovascular occlusive disease from 1974 to 1994 at the Heinrich-Heine University, Düsseldorf

Renal artery reconstruction		
Transortic endarterectomy	199	55.9%
Conventional endarterectomy	13	3.6%
Bypass graft	15	4.2%
Reimplantation	69	19.4%
Combined techniques	60	16.9%
Total	356	
Aortic reconstruction		
Graft implantation		
aortoiliac	29	
aortofemoral	94	
aortic	140	
Aortoiliac thromboendarterectomy	93	

aortic replacement can be recommended. This appears justified in centers where surgical expertise in dealing with problems in both parts of the circulation has shown low morbidity and mortality results.

In about 10% of patients with coexistent disease the stenotic plaque extends into the distal renal and sometimes into the segmental arteries and will require distal thromboendarterectomy or aorto to distal renal artery bypass, which makes reconstruction more difficult. The indication for simultaneous repair in this subgroup is relative. It may be prudent to reconstruct the aorta only and to deal with the renal artery problem by a separate incision during a second operation, but in experienced hands simultaneous reconstruction may be both feasible and safe, sparing the patient a second operation.

In patients with less common etiologies like Takayasu's disease, giant cell arteritis, aortic dissection, Behçet's disease and Marfan's syndrome simultaneous reconstruction is only necessary if the diseased renal artery originates from the aortic segment to be replaced. Reconstruction of the renal arteries will most probably require replacement or bypass techniques.

Incisions, approach, exposures

Exposure of the infrarenal aorta together with the proximal segments of the renal arteries is usually achieved through a transperitoneal approach using a midline incision from the sternum to the symphysis. In patients with renal arteries originating high at the level of L1 vertebral body and in obese patients, it is helpful to extend the incision around the xiphoid. Even in patients with distal renal artery lesions at the hilus and within the segmental arteries, the midline laparotomy gives sufficient view of the anatomic structures. However, besides incision of the retroperitoneum along the aorta a lateral retroperitoneal incision for mobilization of the colon and on the right side of the duodenum is required to expose the hilus of the kidney. In patients with suprarenal and visceral artery disease an oblique intercostal combined with a midline incision or a totally oblique thoracoabdominal incision on the left side through the 8th or 9th interspace can be used to facilitate medial visceral rotation, which has been described by Stoney *et al.*[11] This approach is not purely retroperitoneal, because the peritoneal sac is opened. As the proximal aortic clamp may be close to the visceral arteries or the diaphragm in order to allow simultaneous revascularization of the visceral arteries as well, it is of major importance that the circulation of the viscera can be assessed at the end of the procedure by inspection and palpation of the intestinal circulation. It is not necessary to open the pleura, but most likely this will occur accidentally requiring chest drainage at the end of the procedure.

Adjuncts

Autotransfusion has been proven to be helpful and sometimes lifesaving in aneurysm repair. We have been using the cell saver principle for almost 20 years and it has helped us to avoid homologous transfusion, even in patients with simultaneous aortorenal repair, in over 90% of cases.

Protecting the kidneys against ischemia is of major importance during the reconstructive procedure. Intravenously infused mannitol before interruption of renal inflow has shown to prevent anuria following release of the clamp in dogs.[12] Although the mechanism of its beneficial action is not completely understood, its use is recommended to prevent renal failure.[13]

If aortic clamping above the renal arteries is unavoidable we prefer to flush and cool one kidney while reconstructing the other. A double lumen 9 French balloon catheter is used. The applied pressure in the perfusion bag should not exceed 160 mmHg. If both renal arteries are severely obstructed, flush perfusion is started after one side has been reconstructed, 500 ml Ringer's lactate cold solution (4°C) containing 40 μg prostaglandin E1 and 1250 units of heparin are flushed per kidney. Prostaglandin E1 has been evaluated and found to increase ischemic tolerance time significantly.[14] In the same study similarly good results in dogs were obtained by the use of diltiazem, which has been shown to be protective in kidney transplantation as well,[15] so that in centers not permitted to use prostaglandin E1 the administration of diltiazem is a good alternative. One might argue that in experienced surgical hands renal ischemia time rarely exceeds 30 min, which should cause no significant damage. However, surgeons tend to forget that there are exceptions to the rule. In teaching institutions especially it is a great advantage to have a longer ischemic tolerance time. In patients with poorly functioning kidneys any additional damage will lead towards hemofiltration and hemodialysis, which unnecessarily complicates postoperative management. Furthermore, some of the elder patients might develop septic complications which add to ischemic renal damage and can finally end up in multiorgan failure; this can be avoided by a simple protective method during the surgical procedure.

The completeness of the renal artery reconstruction must be checked before closure. Angiography on the table has been used in earlier years, but was replaced by duplex studies and ultrasound spectral analysis.[16] We have used duplex scanning as well but have found it difficult to view both renal arteries adequately. In patients undergoing transortic endarterectomy we are currently using angioscopy, which helps to detect intima-media flaps, residual stenosis and dissection which can then be immediately.[17] After the clamps have been released, renal arterial flow and velocity spectrum are measured by ultrasound to detect any obstructing lesion. Correction is achieved by cutting the renal artery transversly, removing the remaining obstruction, and doing an end-to-end anastomosis. In this way an eventual distal dissection can be repaired at the same time. In our studies, out of 289 renal arteries reconstructed for stenosis or occlusion in patients undergoing simultaneous replacement, 254 (87.9%) were patent on postoperative angiography within the first year after surgery, 19 (6.6%) became reoccluded, 5 (1.7%) showed recurrence and 7 (2.4%) and 4 (1.4%) had a residual stenosis of >50% and <50% diameter reduction respectively.

Graft material

The preferred graft material for aortic replacement is polyester (Dacron). Because of greater flexibility and convenient suturing knitted grafts are preferred in the abdominal segment, while woven grafts are used for replacement of the thoracic aorta because of less distensibility. For renal artery replacement the greater saphenous vein is our first choice, because prosthetic grafts due to compliance mismatch are more likely to cause late stenosis at the renal site and graft thrombosis in cases of low flow (Fig. 36.3). We have limited experience with polytetrafluoroethylene grafts, but expect them to function better than Dacron grafts. Autogenous arteries (internal iliac, splenic, femoral, external iliac) have been described to be optimal replacement material for renal arteries and homologous veins can be helpful and durable in patients without available autogenous veins.

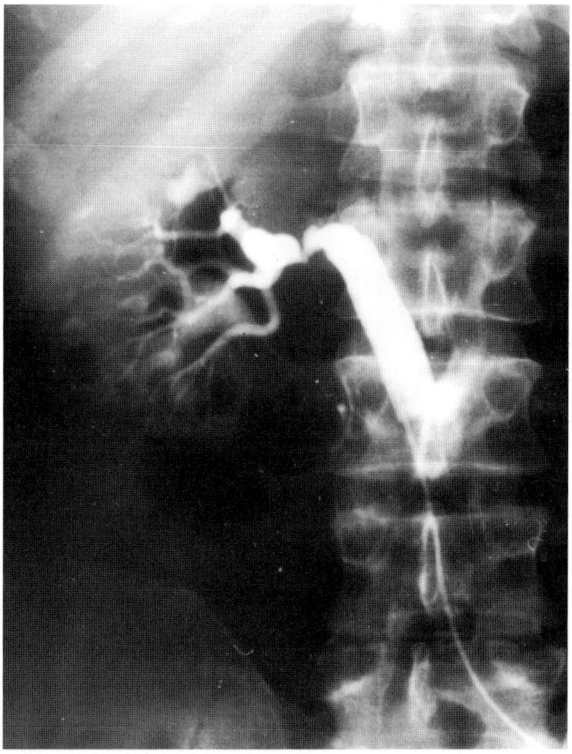

Figure 36.3. Aortorenal Dacron graft, which was implanted 5 years earlier. Significant stenosis at the distal anastomosis can be seen. Embolizing thrombotic material was found at the distal anastomosis causing thromboembolism into the segmenterial arteries of the upper pole.

Operative tactics

Infrarenal aortic aneurysm and proximal renal artery stenosis

Infrarenal aortic aneurysm and proximal renal artery stenosis is the most commonly observed combination of pathologies. The retroperitoneal incision should be placed on the right side of the aneurysm or along the inferior vena cava to preserve sexual function. It is helpful to dissect the tissue along the diseased parts of the renal arteries in order to facilitate the 'pulling out' maneuver during transortic endarterectomy. It is not necessary to dissect the inferior mesenteric artery, which can be blocked with a Fogarty catheter after the aneurysm sac has been opened. Usually the plane for renal endarterectomy is within the lamina elastica externa, because the media is diseased as well, which gives a clean cleavage plane. Care must be taken not to pull too hard because this will cause distal medio-intimal dissection. The plaque should be gently removed by pulling the aortic and renal artery wall aside like peeling a banana (Fig. 36.4). For control of the transition zone, the endarterectomized renal

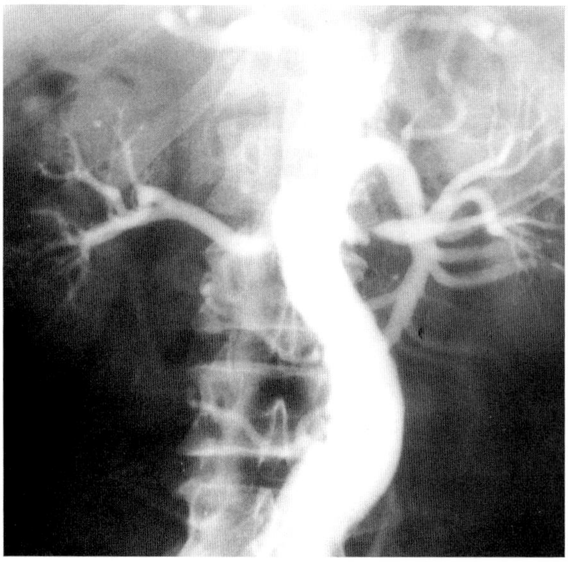

(a)

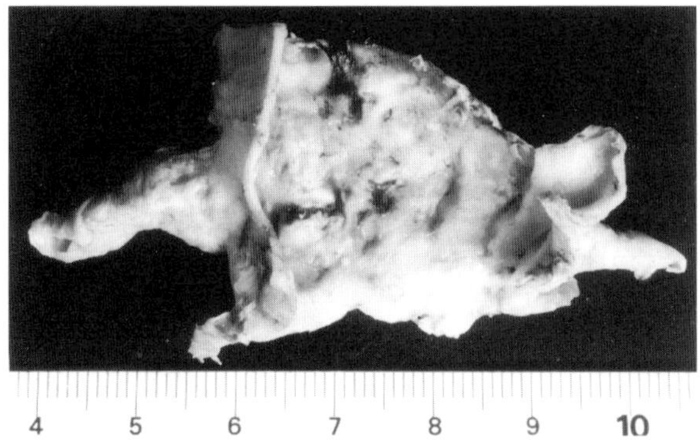

(b)

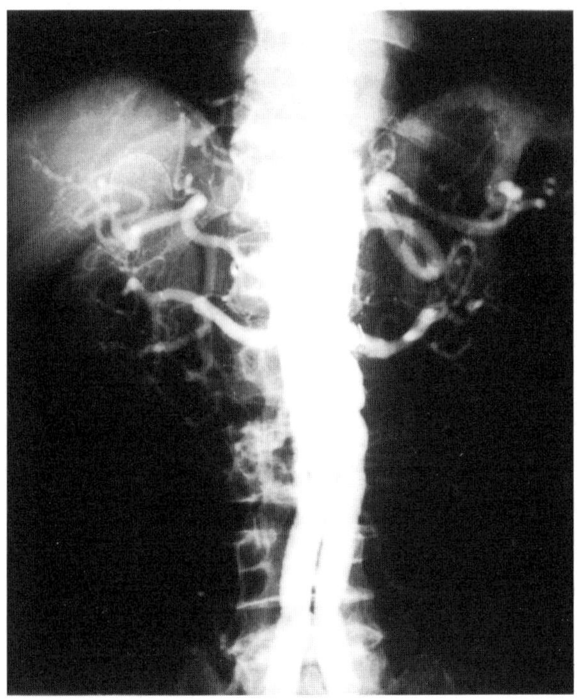

(c)

Figure 36.4. Bilateral renal artery stenosis in a 62-year-old man presenting with infrarenal aortic aneurysm and renovascular hypertension. Although the angiography shows only a tight stenosis on the left side (a), during surgery both renal arteries were found to be involved (b). After thromboendarterectomy aortobiiliac aneurysm was replaced by an aortobiiliac interposition graft (c).

artery can be pushed and everted towards the lumen of the aorta which allows a better insight into the renal artery for 1 or 2 cm. If this maneuver is impossible, we have found endoscopy to be a helpful tool for control after thromboendarterectomy. In about 10% of the cases it is necessary to perform additional distal endarterectomy and fixation of the distal step or to bridge the defect with an aorto-prosthetic renal graft (Fig. 36.5). However this can be done after the aorta has been replaced, either by a tube or an aortoiliac bifurcation graft, as blood flow first should be released into the other renal artery as promptly as possible. Without endoscopy incomplete thromboendarterectomy will be most probably noticed after the clamps have been released because the dissection can be felt and seen through the thin renal artery wall. Intraoperative angiography, duplex scanning or measurement of flow quality and velocity can be used for quality control.

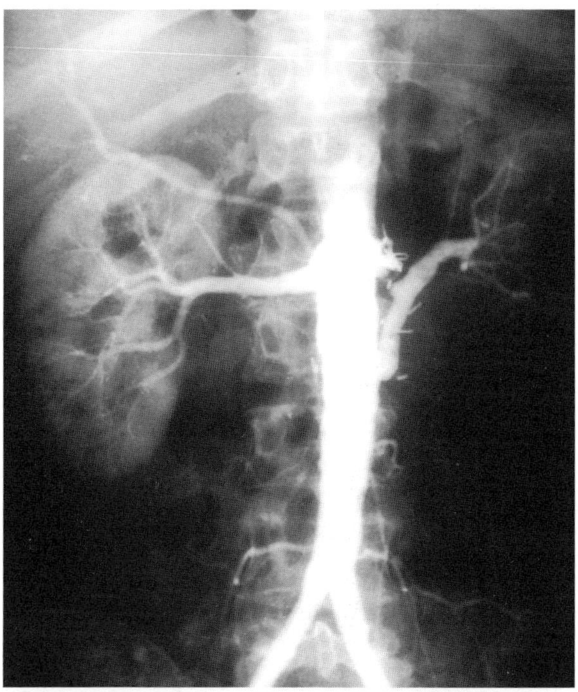

Figure 36.5. A 61-year-old patient after thromboendarterectomy of both renal arteries and aortoiliac tract. As was noticed during surgery, reconstruction of the totally occluded left renal artery by transaortic thromboendarterectomy failed, so that an aortorenal venous bypass was performed.

Suprarenal aortic aneurysms and renal artery occlusive disease

With the exception of the extended exposure of the aorta, the principles applied to aortic replacement are not different from infrarenal aneurysms. In patients with aneurysms including the renal arteries only, the transabdominal midline approach is used. The level of aortic clamping depends on the anatomy. If placing the clamp just above the renal arteries is difficult because of limited space, the minor omentum and the crura of the diaphragm should be incised to allow supramesenteric clamping. The left kidney can either be left in place[18] or rotated to the right.[11] If clamping ischemia to the mesenteric arteries is to be avoided, it is sometimes helpful to divide the left renal vein between clamps, which can be reanastomosed after renal and aortic reconstruction have been performed. In patients with aneurysms involving the mesenteric arteries as well, the thoracoabdominal approach is highly recommended (Fig. 36.6). Retrograde flow from the mesenteric arteries is blocked by balloon catheters while transaortic endarterectomy of the renal arteries is performed. The left renal artery is easy to reconstruct if the plaque extends far distally, but the right side can cause trouble. It may be helpful to perform a circumcision in the aortic wall, place holding sutures and pull the right renal artery towards the surgeon to facilitate eversion thromboendarterectomy. However, if the disease cannot be removed completely, an iliorenal graft should be implanted after aortic and left renal flow has been restored.

Aortic and renal artery occlusive disease

In many European centers aortic thromboendarterectomy is preferred over graft replacement, in patients with occlusive disease of both aorta and renal arteries if the disease is limited to the aorta and the proximal iliac arteries (Fig. 36.7). The plane for disobliteration is usually found between the media and the adventita. The strength of the remaining aortic wall tolerates arterial pressure without aneurysmal development. Care should be taken to preserve the

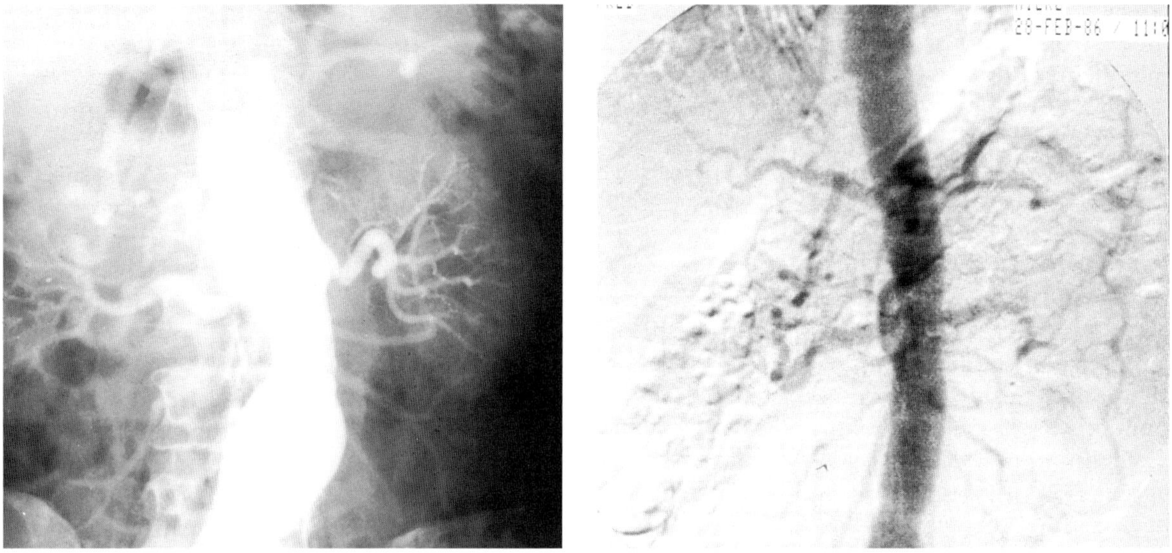

(a) (b)

Figure 36.6. Thoracoabdominal aneurysm extending from the diaphragm to the aortic bifurcation. (a) The angiogram demonstrated bilateral renal artery stenosis. (b) The control angiography 4 months after thromboendarterectomy of both renal arteries and reimplantation into the thoracoabdominal Dacron prosthesis together with the visceral arteries shows unrestricted circulation. The patient was operated on almost 10 years ago at the age of 57 and is still living a normal life.

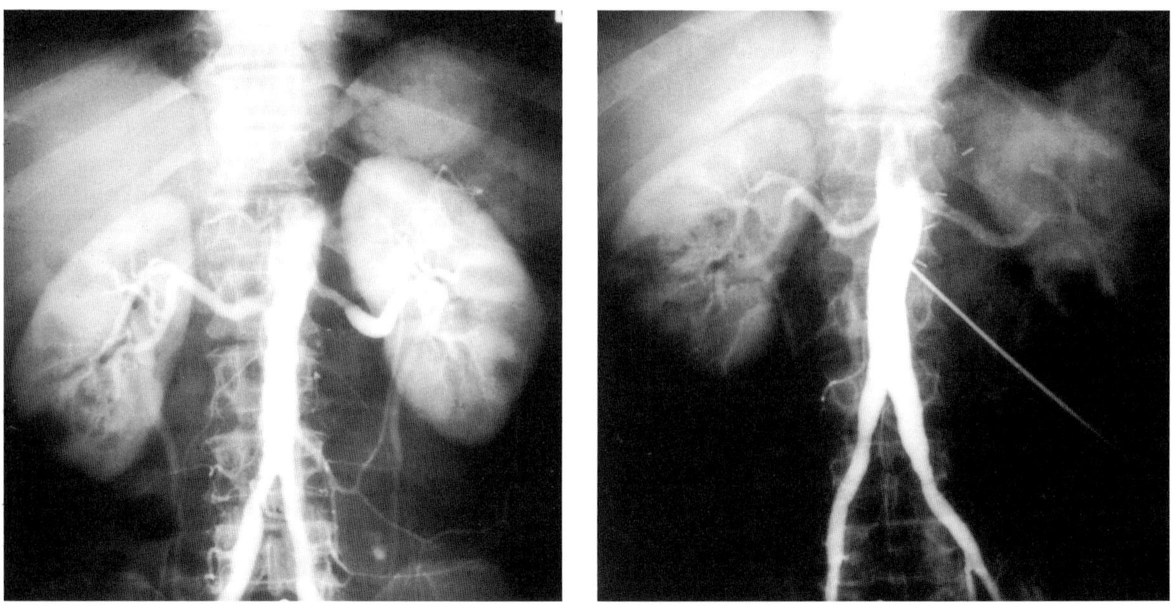

(a) (b)

Figure 36.7. Bilateral renal artery stenosis in a 72-year-old man with aortobiiliac occlusive disease (a). One year later control arteriography after bilateral renal and aortobiiliac thromboendarterectomy shows a smooth and unrestricted lumen of the reconstructed arteries (b).

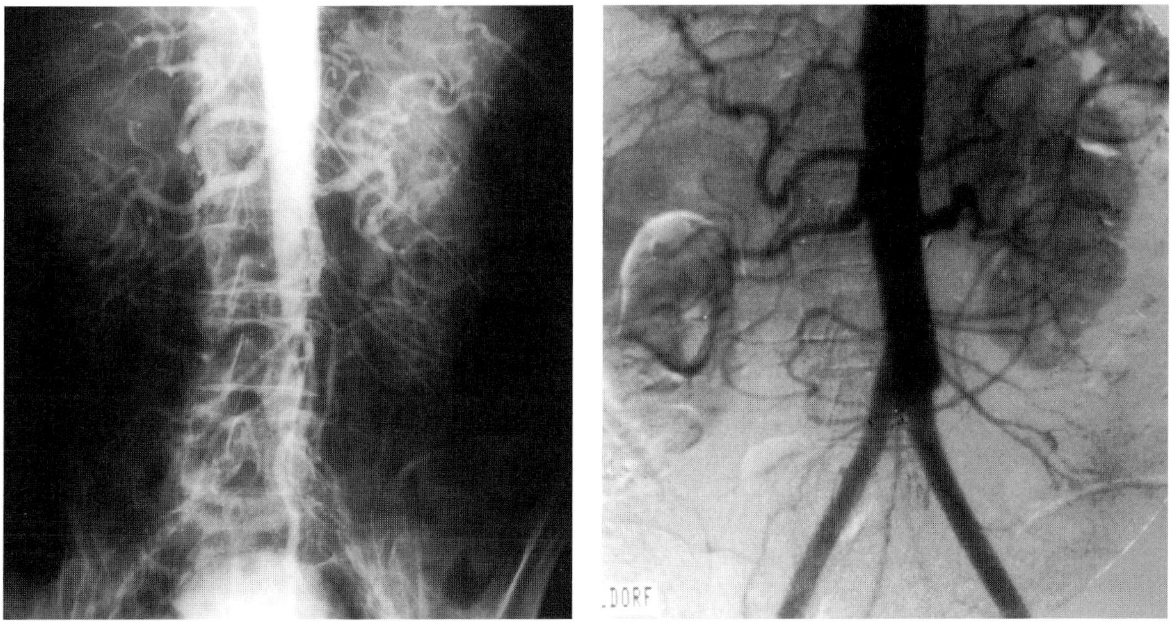

(a) (b)

Figure 36.8. A 52-year-old patient who presented with severe claudication and significant hypertension. The angiogram shows complete occlusion of the distal aorta and both common iliac arteries. The distal circulation on the lower extremities was maintained through the inferior mesenteric artery. The patient suffered from primary hypertension, which had caused bilateral renal artery stenosis and renal insufficiency (a). An aorto-bifemoral Dacron graft was implanted. Both renal arteries where thromboendarterectomized with the left renal artery being implanted into the prosthesis (b).

inferior mesenteric artery to avoid left colon ischemia. Aberrant renal arteries originating from the lower lumbar aorta can be endarterectomized and protected by flush perfusion using a smaller double-lumen catheter. If endarterectomy fails to restore the renal artery lumen completely, the endarterectomized aorta or the common iliac artery can be used as an inflow source for a bypass to the renal artery. If a bifurcated graft has to be implanted, the endarterectomized renal arteries can be directly implanted or an interposition graft can be used (Fig. 36.8).

Rare conditions of aortic replacement and renal artery reconstruction

Abdominal aortic coarctation with renal artery stenosis

Abdominal aortic coarctation causes fibrotic stenosis of both aorta and renal arteries (Fig. 36.9). Often the visceral arteries are involved. A variety of reconstructive methods can be used depending on the individual malformation. If the aorta has to be replaced due to ischemia of the lower extremities, the renal arteries can be attached to the aortic prosthesis using either vein graft or prosthetic material. We prefer the greater saphenous vein for replacement, because prosthetic material becomes occluded more often.

Marfan's syndrome

The abdominal aorta is not the typical site of aneurysm formation in patients with Marfan's syndrome, but five such patients have been treated at our institution. In one female patient the aorta and the iliac arteries had been replaced by a bifurcated graft. The left renal artery developed a large aneurysm, penetrating into the kidney, which was subsequently removed. Multiple peripheral arterial aneurysms in the femoro-popliteal, brachial and carotid segments had to be replaced with vein

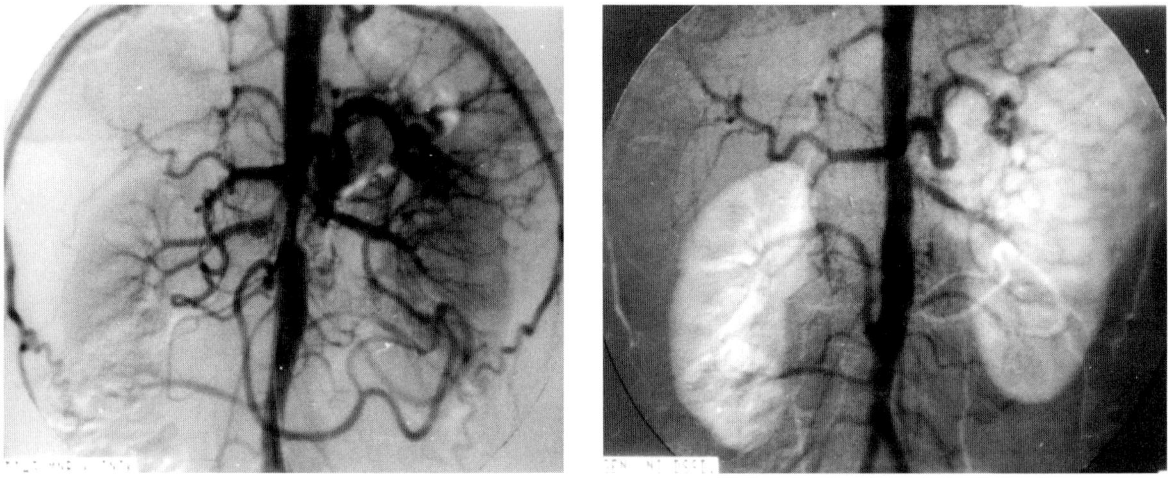

(a) (b)

Figure 36.9. A 21-year-old man suffering 5 years from severe hypertension. The aortogram shows subtotal stenosis of the right renal artery, a slight stenosis of the left renal artery and a typical abdominal coarctation. Due to excellent collateralization the patient's life was unrestricted (a). The operative procedure consisted of aortic patch angioplasty and implantation of the right renal artery using a greater saphenous interposition graft. The angiogram 7 days after surgery shows significant reduction of the diameter of the collateral vessels and normal perfusion of the kidneys. Blood pressure was immediately normalized (b).

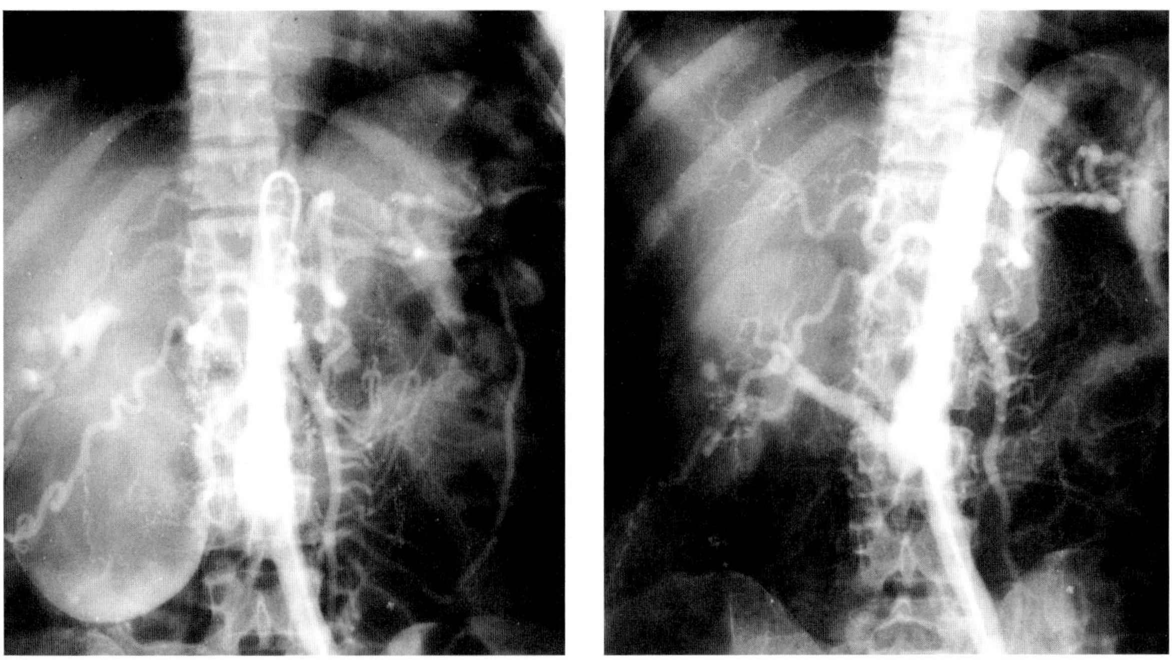

(a) (b)

Figure 36.10. Huge aneurysm of the right renal artery in a 27-year-old woman, in which multiple peripheral aneuysms had been replaced due to Marfan's syndrome (a). Preservation of the right kidney was possible by the use of a fresh venous homograft, which was implanted into the aortic prosthesis (b).

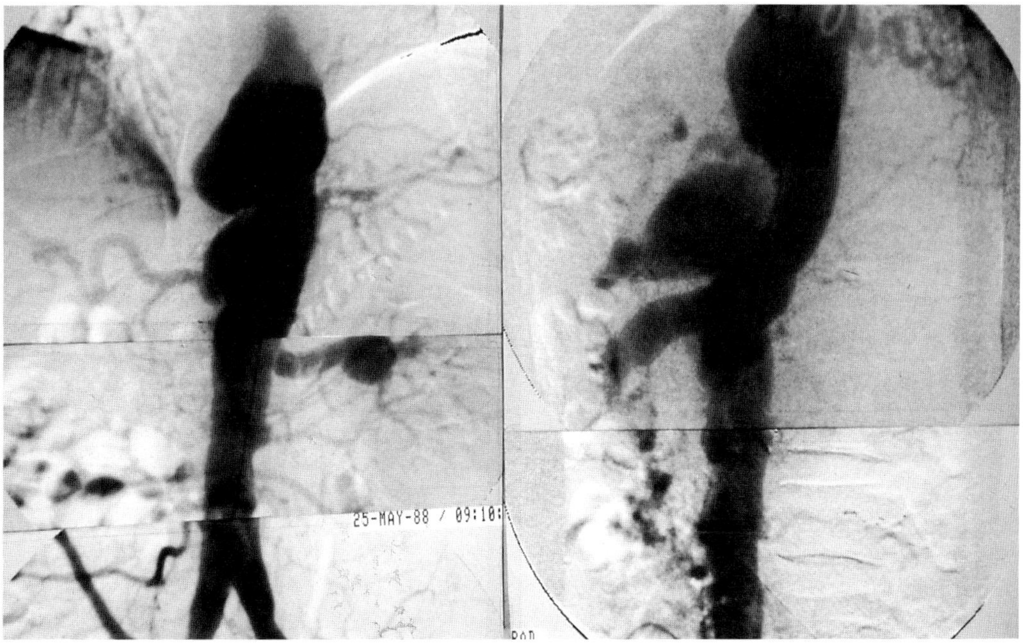

(a)

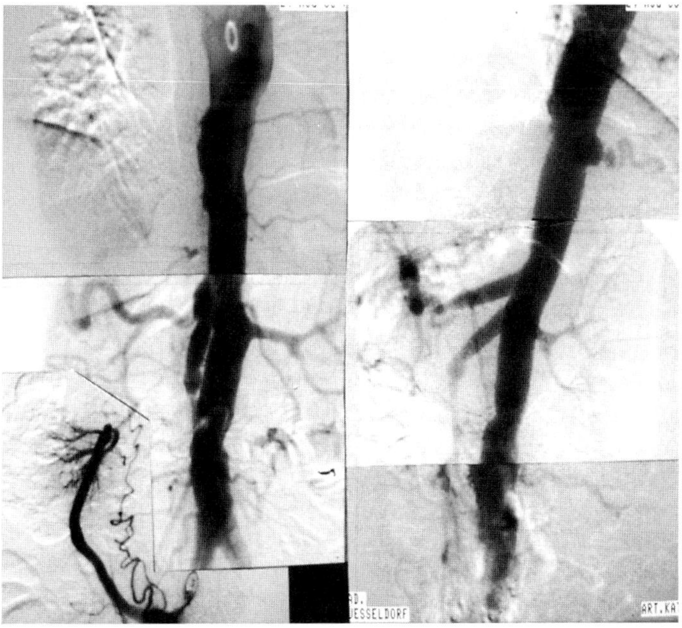

(b)

Figure 36.11. Recurrent thoracoabdominal aneurysm involving the visceral arteries in a 29-year-old patient, who had undergone thoracoabdominal aortic replacement and partial replacement of the visceral arteries (same patient as in Fig. 36.2). The right renal artery aneurysm has been treated previously by iliorenal venous grafting (a). The definitive treatment consisted in extended thoracoabdominal aortic replacement, reimplantation of intercostal arteries and replacement of the left renal and both mesenteric arteries using Dacron grafts. The operation was performed in 1988, the patient is still free from recurrence and living a normal life including sporting activities (b).

material. When the patient, who was still young, was readmitted with a large aneurysm of the right renal artery, autogenous graft material was no longer available, so we used a segment of homologous greater saphenous vein, which remained patent for 15 years without aneurysmal deformation until the patient died from intracranial hemorrhage (Fig. 36.10).

Inflammatory aortorenal aneurysms

Inflammation of the aortic wall is reported to be usually limited to the infrarenal aorta and not to involve the renal arteries. Operation is performed to relieve pain, to prevent rupture – which does occur despite the thickened wall – and because the ureter is often compressed adjacent to or within the inflammatory mass. In some patients not only the aorta but also the renal and visceral arteries are aneurysmal and encased in inflammatory tissue requiring complete reconstruction. The principal strategy for replacement is no different from the management of patients with atherosclerotic aneurysms including the fact that anastomotic aneurysms will occur if the graft is not sutured to the undiseased arterial wall (Fig. 36.11). The ureter, the duodenum, the colon and other adjacent structures should not be dissected from the aneurysmal wall, to avoid damage to those organs. Therefore, clamping must be performed far outside the inflammatory process.

In summary simultaneous aortic replacement and reconstruction for coexisting renal artery disease has become a routine procedure with results similar to infrarenal aortic reconstruction alone as long as the aortic disease does not involve the thoracoabdominal segment and the mesenteric arteries. Although improvement of renal perfusion after thromboendarterectomy or bypass procedure will improve the patient's condition in the long run, transient impairment of renal function from clamping ischemia is not completely avoidable, although with the use of pre- and intraoperative protective measures renal failure requiring hemodialysis has become very rare in our center. Proper planning of the operation, meticulous preparation of the patient, avoiding drugs which might reduce renal perfusion pressure or could be toxic for the ischemic kidney all help to get the patient prepared for and successfully through the operation and to achieve the best possible result.

References

1 Tarazi RY, Hertzer NR, Beven EG, O'Hara PJ, Anton GE, Krajewski LP. Simultaneous aortic reconstruction and renal revascularization: risk factors and late results in eighty-nine patients. *J Vasc Surg* 1987; **7:** 707.
2 Brewster DC, Retana A, Waltman AC, Darling RC. Angiography in the management of aneurysms of the abdominal aorta: its value and safety. *N Engl J Med* 1975; **292:** 822.
3 Torsello G, Sandmann W, Kniemeyer W. Revaskularisation der Nierenarterien in der Chirurgie des Bauchaortenaneurysma. *Angio* 1986; **8**(2): 95–100.
4 Crawford ES, Crawford JL. *Diseases of the Aorta*. London: Williams and Wilkins, 1984.
5 Abbott WM, Austen WG. The reversal of renal cortical ischemia during aortic occlusion by mannitol. *J Surg Res* 1974; **16:** 482.
6 Nevitt MP, Ballard DJ, Hallett JW Jr. Prognosis of abdominal aortic aneurysms. *N Engl J Med* 1989; **321:** 1009–14.
7 Katz DA, Littenberg B, Cronenwett JL. Management of small abdominal aortic aneurysms: early surgery versus watchful waiting. *JAMA* 1992; **268:** 2678–86.
8 Cronenwett JL, Sargent SK, Wall MH, Hawkes ML, Freeman DH, Dain BJ *et al.* Variables that affect the expansion rate and outcome of small abdominal aortic aneurysms. *J Vasc Surg* 1990; **11:** 260–9.
9 Cronenwett JL, Katz DA. When should infrarenal abdominal aortic aneurysms be repaired: what are the critical risk factors and dimensions? In Veith FJ (ed.) *Current Critical Problems in Vascular Surgery*, pp. 256–63. St Louis: Quality Medical Publishing, 1993.
10 Qvarfordt PG, Stoney RJ, Reilly LM, Skioldebrand CG, Goldstone J, Ehrenfeld WK. Management of pararenal aneurysms of the abdominal aorta. *J Vasc Surg* 1986; **3**(1): 84–91.
11 Stoney RJ, Sauer L, Cunningham C. Transabdominal exposure of the pararenal and suprarenal aorta by medial visceral rotation. In Veith FJ (ed.) *Current Critical Problems in Vascular Surgery*, pp. 207–11. St Louis: Quality Medical Publishing, 1993.
12 Selkurt EE. Changes in renal clearance following complete ischemia of the kidney. *Am J Physiol* 1945; **144:** 395.
13 Levinsky NG, Bernard DB, Johnston PA. Mannitol and loop diuretics in acute renal failure. In Brenner BM, Lazarus JM (eds) *Acute Renal*

Failure, pp. 712–20. London: WB Saunders, 1983.

14 Torsello G, Schrör K, Szabo Z, Kutkuhn B, Strobach H, Godehardt E *et al.* Effects of prostaglandin E1 (PGE1) on experimental renal ischemia. *Eur J Vasc Surg* 1989; **3:** 5–13.

15 Neumayer HH, Wagner K. Prevention of delayed graft function in cadaver kidney transplants by diltiazem: outcome of two prospective, randomized clinical trials. *J Cardiovasc Pharmacol* 1987; **10:** 170.

16 Okuhn SP, Reilly LM, Bennett JB, Hughes L, Goldstone J, Ehrenfeld WK *et al.* Intraoperative assessment of renal and visceral artery reconstruction: the role of duplex scanning and spectral analysis. *J Vasc Surg* 1987; **5**(1): 137–47.

17 Reiher L, Sandmann W. Die Angioskopie als intraoperative Erfolgskontrolle nach rekonstruktiver Chirurgie der Nierenarterien: Vorstellung einer neuen Methode. *Der Chirurg* in press.

18 Cooley DA, Wukasch DC. *Techniques in Vascular Surgery*. London: WB Saunders, 1979.

37

Extracorporeal microvascular reconstruction and autotransplantation for branch renal artery disease

ANDREW C NOVICK

Introduction

Transfer of a kidney from one site to another in the same patient evolved as a logical extension of the field of renal allotransplantation. The first successful autotransplant was performed in 1962 by Hardy in a patient whose ureter had been severely damaged by previous aortic surgery. In 1963, Woodruff achieved the first successful autotransplant for renovascular hypertension. Effective methods of renal preservation and microvascular surgical techniques subsequently resulted in the advent of extracorporeal (bench) renal surgery for selected patients with branch renal artery disease.

In patients with vascular disease involving the branches of the renal artery, the task of renovascular reconstruction is considerably more complicated because this necessitates multiple vascular anastomoses to branches that may be difficult to expose and are small in caliber. For these reasons, many patients in this category formerly were considered either inoperable or candidates for total or partial nephrectomy. However, technical advances during the past 15 years have improved this outlook and successful vascular reconstruction is now possible in most patients. This evolution has been primarily due to the incorporation of microvascular and extracorporeal techniques into the armamentarium of the renovascular surgeon.

Causes of branch renal artery disease

Fibrous dysplasia

Branch renal artery disease is most often due to one of the fibrous dysplasias; namely, intimal, medial or perimedial fibroplasia.[1] The typical clinical presentation for most of these disorders is in children or young adults with recently discovered hypertension. Bilateral renovascular involvement is frequently observed, and extrarenal vascular lesions may also be present.[2] A decision favoring medical or surgical treatment in such cases is made after evaluating the functional significance of renal artery disease and with regard for the natural history of the particular lesion. The most common indication for undertaking renal revascularization in these younger patients is the presence of significant associated hypertension, although preservation of renal function may be of equal concern with diseases that are known to cause progressive vascular obstruction, such as intimal or perimedial fibroplasia (Fig. 37.1).

Renal artery aneurysm

Renal artery aneurysms are classified as saccular, fusiform, dissecting or intrarenal.[3] Saccular aneurysms are the most common type, comprising about 75% of renal artery aneurysms. They

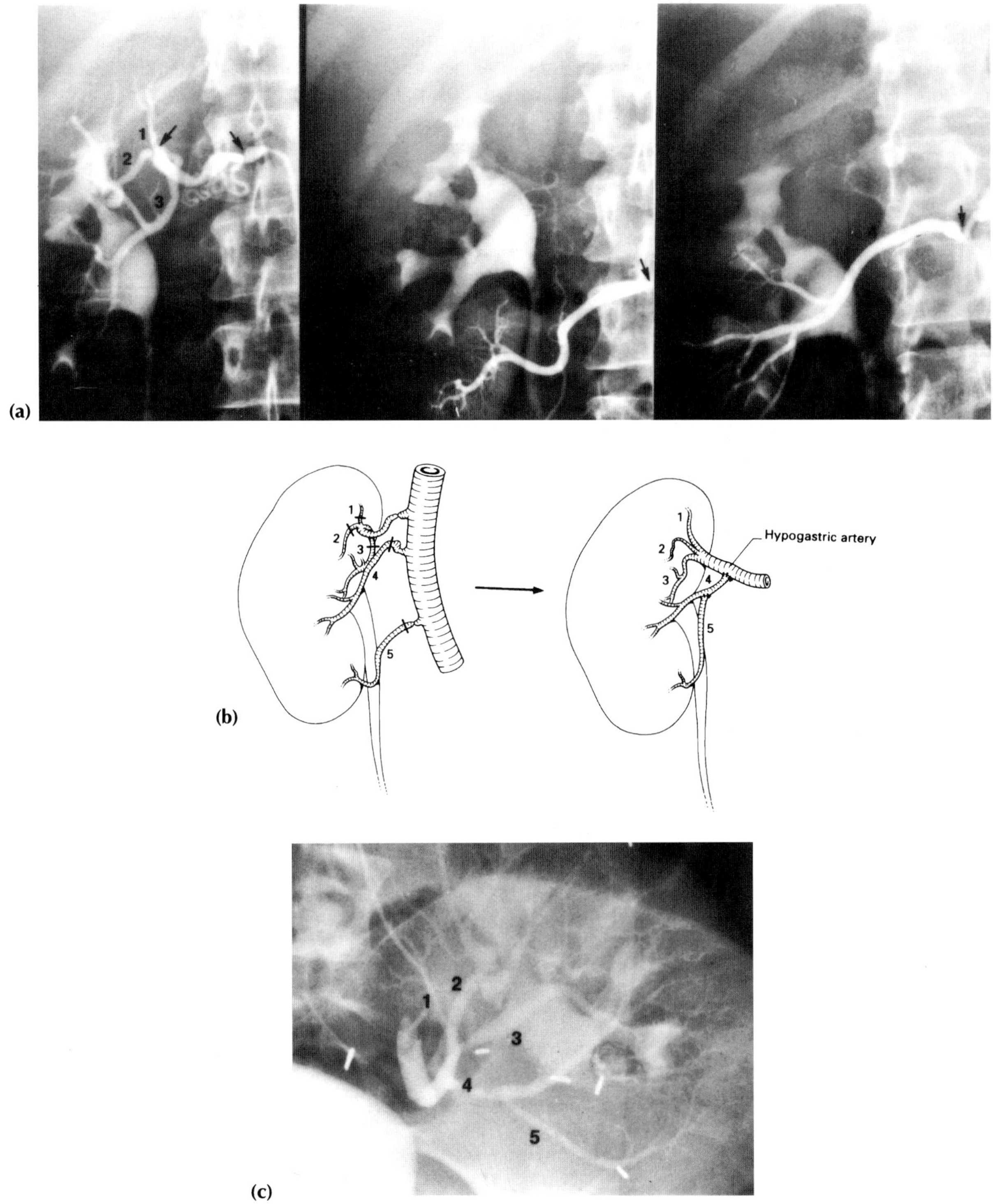

Figure 37.1. (a) Selective arteriography demonstrates three arteries supplying the right kidney, each with proximal high grade stenosis from fibrous dysplasia. Vascular disease in the most superior artery extends into three intrarenal branches. (b) Sketch illustrating the technique of extracorporeal branch arterial reconstruction with a hypogastric arterial autograft. (c) Following autotransplantation into the left iliac fossa, arteriography demonstrates excellent flow through all of the revascularized renal arterial branches. a, b, c From ref. 16, with permission.

generally occur at the bifurcation of the renal artery, perhaps due to an inherent weakness in the wall of the artery at this point. Because of this location, branch arterial involvement is common. Surgical excision of a renal artery aneurysm is indicated if it is the cause of significant hypertension or to obviate the risk of rupture (Fig. 37.2). The latter is of greatest concern with aneurysms that are larger than 2 cm in diameter and non-calcified, particularly when they occur in premenopausal women because of the predisposition for aneurysmal rupture during pregnancy. Renal

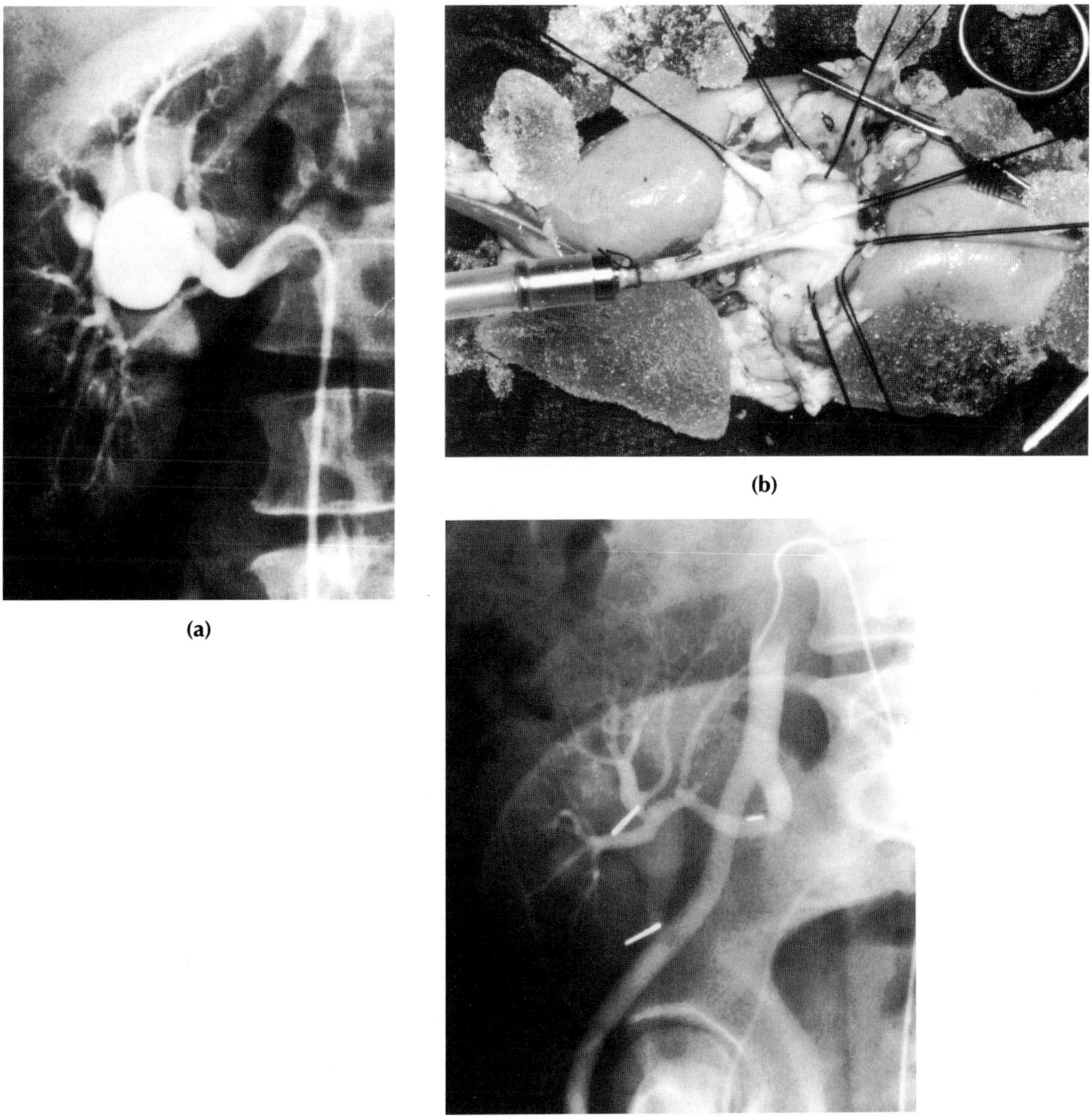

(a) (b) (c)

Figure 37.2. (a) Selective right renal arteriogram demonstrates a non-calcified 4 cm expanding arterial aneurysm. (b) Operative photograph of the removed flushed kidney demonstrates seven arterial branches originating from the aneurysm, each encircled by a ligature. (c) Following extracorporeal aneurysmectomy with branch arterial reconstruction and autotransplantation into the right iliac fossa, arteriography demonstrates normal arterial flow to the kidney. a, b, c From ref. 16, with permission.

artery aneurysmectomy may also be indicated for complicating events such as flank pain, hematuria or distal renal embolization.

Renal arteriovenous fistulas

Renal arteriovenous fistulas are relatively uncommon lesions that are generally discovered during the course of an angiographic evaluation for suspected renal or renovascular disease.[4] The most common clinical symptoms, when present, are hematuria, high output cardiac failure and diastolic hypertension. Congenital or cirsoid fistulas comprise approximately 25% of these lesions and are the result of a developmental anomaly of the involved renal vessels. Acquired fistulas are the most common type, accounting for 70–75% of all such lesions, and may be due to needle biopsy of the kidney, blunt or penetrating trauma, tumor, inflammation or prior renal surgery. Branch arterial involvement with these lesions is very common. Treatment of a renal arteriovenous fistula is indicated for patients with associated hypertension, heart failure, severe hematuria, serial angiographic evidence of an expanding lesion, rupture or progressive renal failure (Fig. 37.3). Transcatheter angiographic segmental renal arterial occlusion is a non-surgical therapeutic option for some patients. If this is not possible without sacrificing a major portion of the involved kidney, surgical excision of the fistula with renal vascular reconstruction is indicated.

Primary renal artery dissection

Dissection of the renal artery is most commonly secondary to an aortic dissection and isolated renal artery dissections are relatively rare. The causes of the latter include blunt trauma, selective renal arteriography, percutaneous transluminal renal angioplasty and underlying primary renal artery diseases such as atherosclerosis and intimal fibroplasia.[5] Surgical revascularization is indicated in patients with associated hypertension or local symptoms such as hematuria and flank pain (Fig. 37.4). The task of renal vascular reconstruction is often rendered more difficult by branch arterial involvement and perivascular scarring of the diseased arterial segments.

Recurrent renal artery stenosis following surgical revascularization

The incidence of stenosis of a surgically repaired renal artery is less than 10% with current techniques.[6] This is typically a late complication occurring weeks, months or even years following revascularization. If the involved kidney is functionally salvageable, then an attempt to restore normal renal arterial flow is indicated. Secondary surgical revascularization in such cases may be technically complicated. Reoperation often entails dissection in a surgical field obliterated by fibrous scar tissue, which may be particularly problematic when attempting to mobilize the renal artery distal to the primary revascularization site. With extensive renal hilar fibrosis or branch arterial involvement, extracorporeal revascularization may provide the optimum approach for mobilizing and repairing the distal renal arterial circulation (Fig. 37.5).

Renal artery pseudo-aneurysm

Renal artery pseudo-aneurysm formation is a potentially devastating and fortunately rare complication of renal vascular surgery.[7] Pseudoaneurysms may result from infection, mechanical injury to the renal artery, ischemic damage from excessive stripping of the artery and its vaso vasorum, faulty suture technique or external traumatic injury. These mechanisms produce disruption of the arterial wall, usually at the site of arterial anastomosis, leading to the development of a communicating sac lined by fibrous and adventitial tissue. There is usually extensive fibrosis around the pseudo-aneurysm encompassing the distal renal arterial and venous circulation (Fig. 37.6).

Other causes

Atherosclerosis is the most common cause of renal artery disease and invariably occurs in the

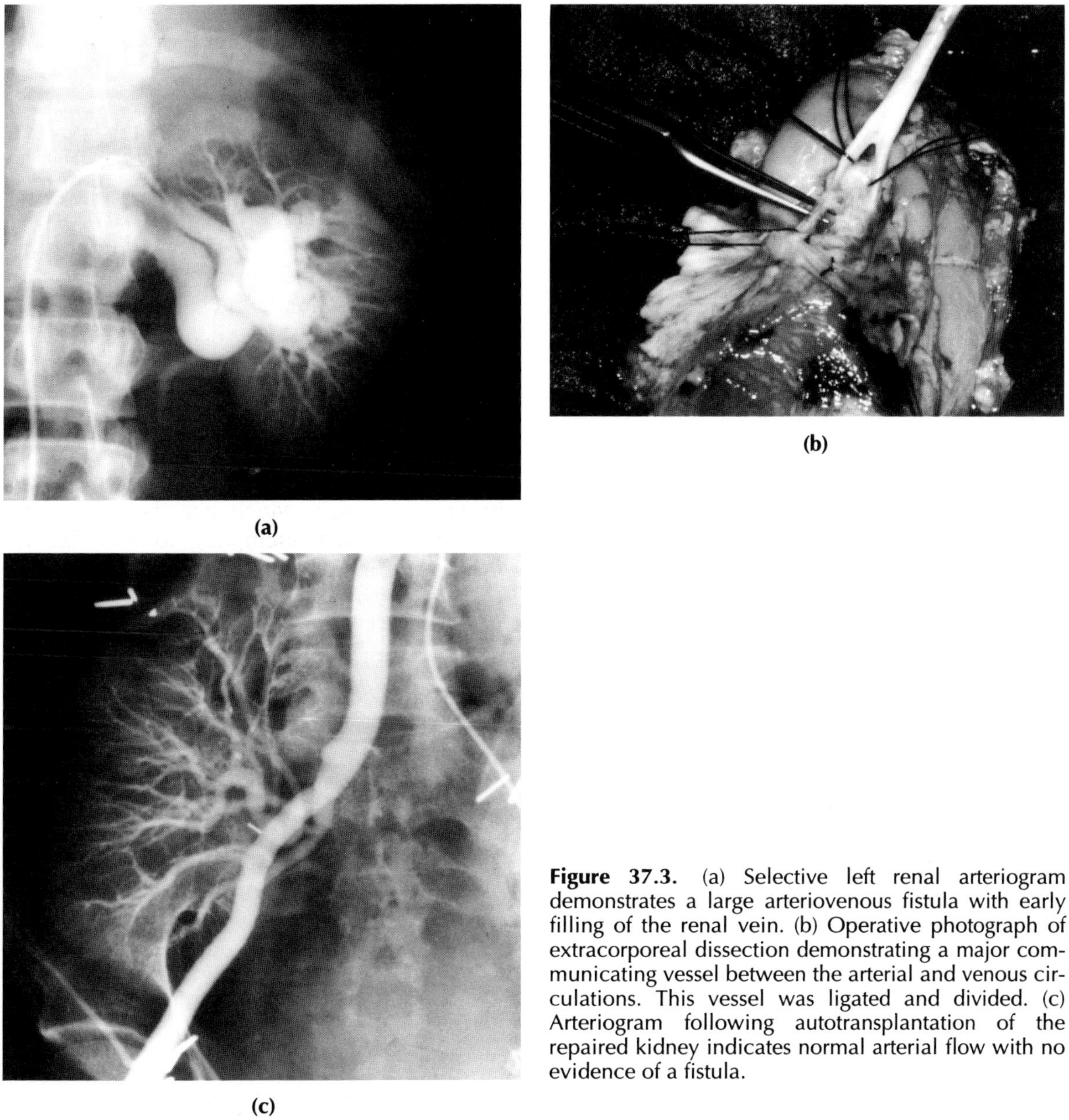

Figure 37.3. (a) Selective left renal arteriogram demonstrates a large arteriovenous fistula with early filling of the renal vein. (b) Operative photograph of extracorporeal dissection demonstrating a major communicating vessel between the arterial and venous circulations. This vessel was ligated and divided. (c) Arteriogram following autotransplantation of the repaired kidney indicates normal arterial flow with no evidence of a fistula.

proximal 2 cm of the renal artery. Branch arterial involvement is distinctly uncommon and occurs in less than 5% of patients. The latter may be due to primary atheromatous involvement of renal artery branches but is more often a consequence of complicating intramural dissection.

Takayasu's arteritis is an inflammatory disease affecting the abdominal aorta and the renal arteries.[8] Perivascular scarring eventuates in stenosis of the main renal artery and, occasionally, the renal artery branches. This disorder is most commonly encountered in children and can cause significant hypertension.

Neurofibromatosis is a congenital hereditary disorder characterized by 'cafe-au-lait' cutaneous pigmentation, cutaneous neurofibromas, tumors of the central nervous system, skeletal disorders and occasional gigantism.[9] This disorder is also associated with pheochromocytoma and renal artery stenosis. Vascular pathology consists of fibrosis and thickening of the intima,

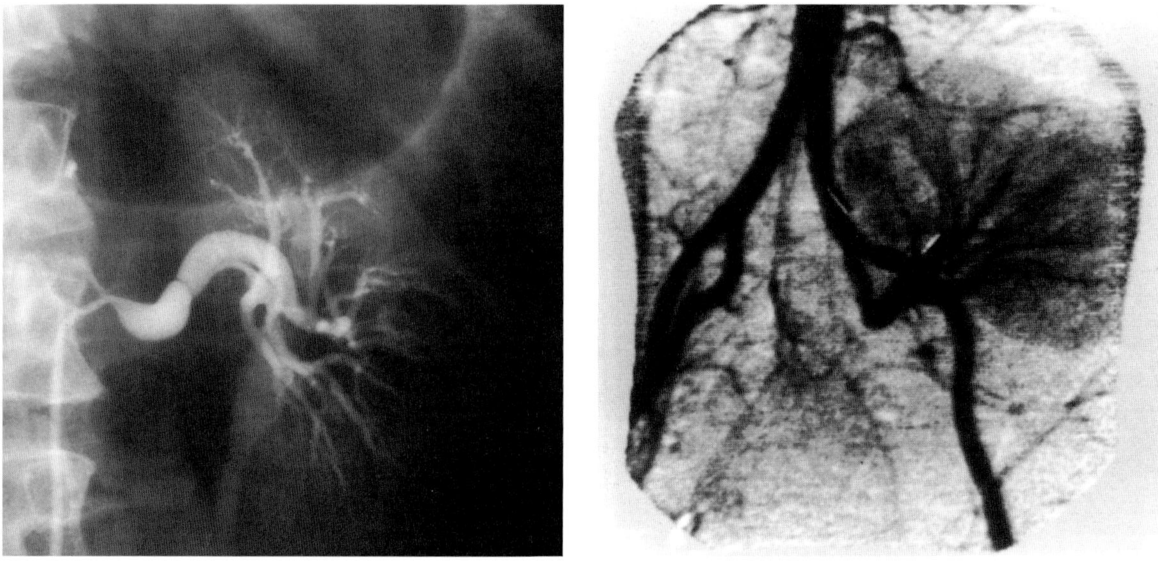

(a) (b)

Figure 37.4. (a) Selective left renal arteriogram following blunt traumatic injury demonstrates intramural dissection beginning in the mid-renal artery and extending distally. (b) Following extracorporeal revascularization, arteriogram demonstrates normal flow to the repaired kidney.

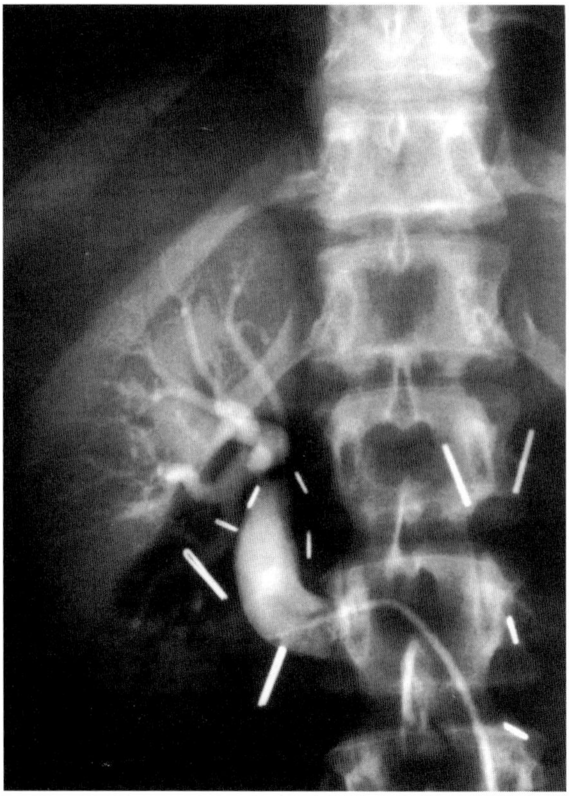

(a)

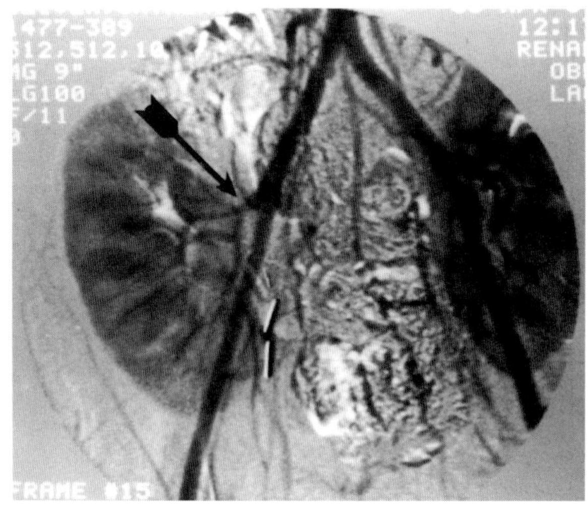

(b)

Figure 37.5. (a) Several years following a right aortorenal saphenous vein bypass operation, arteriography shows severe stenosis at the distal anastomosis of the graft. (b) Following extracorporeal revascularization of the right kidney with autotransplantation into the right iliac fossa, a digital subtraction angiogram shows normal renal arterial flow (arrow). Note that the left kidney has previously been autotransplanted into the left iliac fossa.

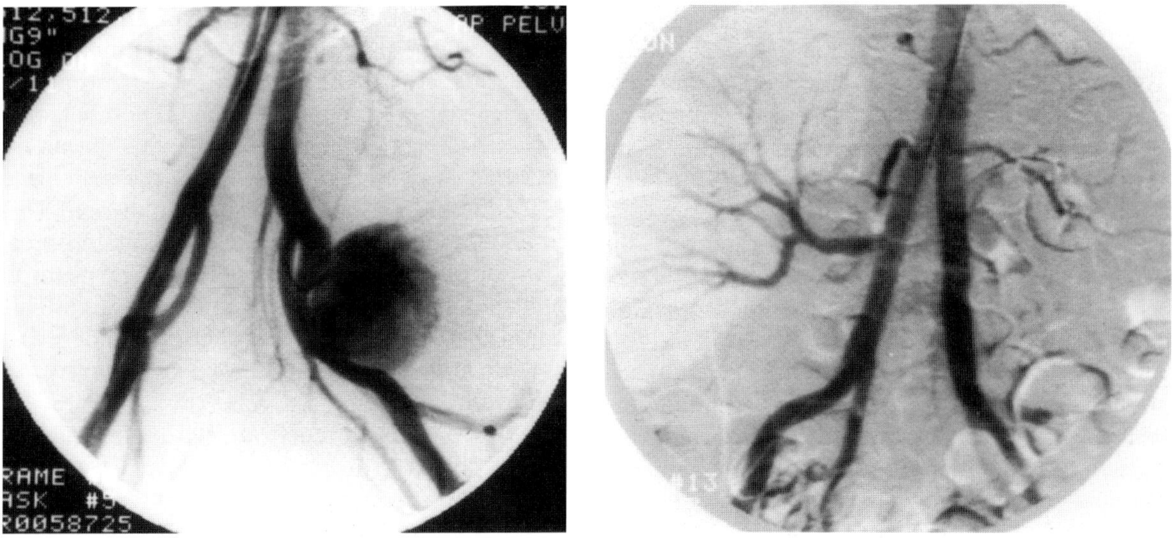

(a) **(b)**

Figure 37.6. (a) Arteriogram reveals large pseudo-aneurysm arising near arterial anastomosis between renal artery and left external iliac artery following renal allotransplantation. (b) Following extracorporeal revascularization of the left renal allograft with autotransplantation into the right iliac fossa, arteriogram shows normal arterial flow to the repaired kidney. a, b From ref. 7, with permission.

proliferation of neural tissue within the arterial wall, perivascular nodular proliferations, and occasional aneurysmal dilatation. Renal artery stenosis usually involves the proximal third of the main renal artery but may extend into arterial branches.

Patient selection and preparation

Branch renal artery lesions can occasionally be surgically repaired *in situ* with an aortorenal bypass when distal branches free of disease are present outside the renal hilus.[10, 11] Extracorporeal branch arterial repair and autotransplantation are indicated primarily when preoperative arteriography, with oblique views, demonstrates intrarenal extension of renovascular disease.[12–15] The advantages of employing an extracorporeal surgical approach include optimum exposure and illumination, a bloodless surgical field, greater protection of the kidney from ischemia, and more facile employment of microvascular techniques and optical magnification. Removing and flushing the kidney also causes it to contract in size, thereby enabling more peripheral dissection in the renal sinus for mobilization of distal arterial branches. Finally, the completed branch anastomoses can be tested for patency and integrity before autotransplantation.

In evaluating patients for extracorporeal revascularization and autotransplantation, preoperative renal and pelvic arteriography should be performed to define renal arterial anatomy, to ensure disease-free iliac vessels, and to assess the hypogastric artery and its branches for use as a reconstructive graft. Assuming the presence of a viable functioning kidney, the only absolute contraindication to this approach is such severe aortoiliac vascular disease as to preclude renal autotransplantation. It is also best to avoid autotransplantation of kidneys involved by severe renal parenchymal or small vessel disease. Such kidneys generally flush poorly after their removal, often leading to irreversible ischemic damage and non-function postoperatively.

Operative technique

Extracorporeal revascularization and autotransplantation are generally performed through an anterior subcostal transperitoneal incision combined with a separate lower quadrant transverse semi-lunar incision. For non-obese patients, a single midline incision extending from the xiphoid process to the symphysis pubis may be used. The same intraoperative measures are taken as in live donor nephrectomy for allotransplantation to ensure minimal renal ischemic and immediate function after revascularization. These include prevention of hypotension during anesthesia, administration of mannitol, minimal surgical manipulation of the kidney and rapid flushing and cooling of the kidney after its removal. Systemic heparinization before nephrectomy is unnecessary.

Immediately after its removal, the kidney is flushed intra-arterially with 500 ml of a chilled intracellular electrolyte solution and is then submerged in a basin of ice-slush saline to maintain hypothermia (Fig. 37.7). The extracorporeal operation is completed under ice-slush surface hypothermia and, if there has been minimal warm renal ischemia, the kidney can be safely preserved in this manner for many more hours than are needed to perform even the most complex renal repair. In performing extracorporeal revascularization, we have found it cumbersome to work on the abdominal wall with the ureter attached. It is preferable to divide the ureter and place the kidney on a separate workbench. This provides better exposure for the extracorporeal operation and allows a second surgical team to prepare the iliac fossa simultaneously. This approach is also justified by the low incidence of complications after ureteroneocystostomy in renal allotransplantation.

Extracorporeal branch arterial reconstruction is performed with microvascular instruments, 7–0 to 9–0 suture material, and optical magnification with loupes (3.5 × or 6.0 ×) or an operating microscope. The basic instruments required for microvascular surgery include a microneedle holder, microscissors, fine jeweler's forceps, small vessel dilators, microvascular clamps, and a 10 ml syringe with a 27 gauge blunt needle for irrigation.

After removal and flushing of the kidney, and with maintenance of surface hypothermia, the renal artery branches are mobilized distally in the renal sinus beyond the area of vascular

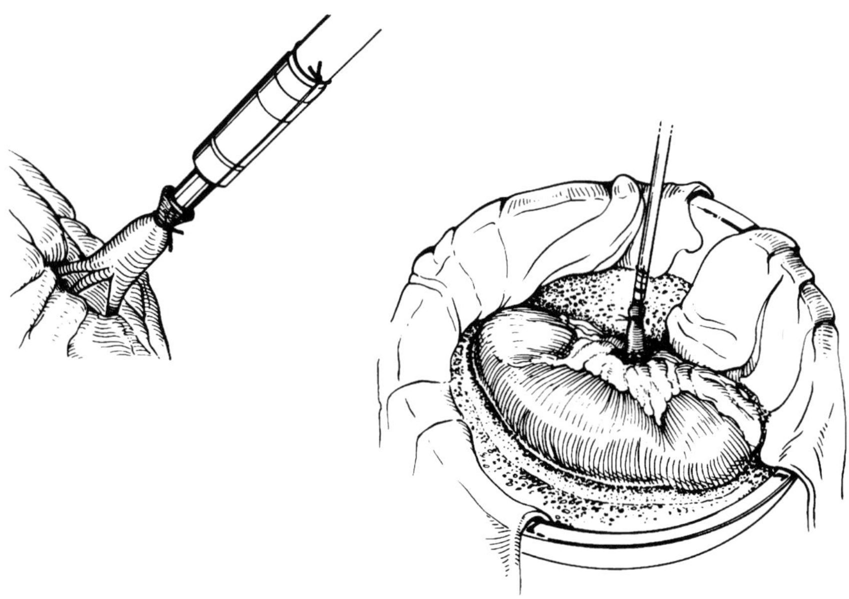

Figure 37.7. The removed kidney is flushed intra-arterially with a cold electrolyte solution and is placed in a basin of ice-slush saline to maintain hypothermia. From ref. 18, with permission.

disease (Fig. 37.8). During this dissection, care is taken not to interfere with ureteral or renal pelvic blood supply. When the diseased renal artery branches are completely exposed, an appropriate technique for vascular reconstruction is selected.

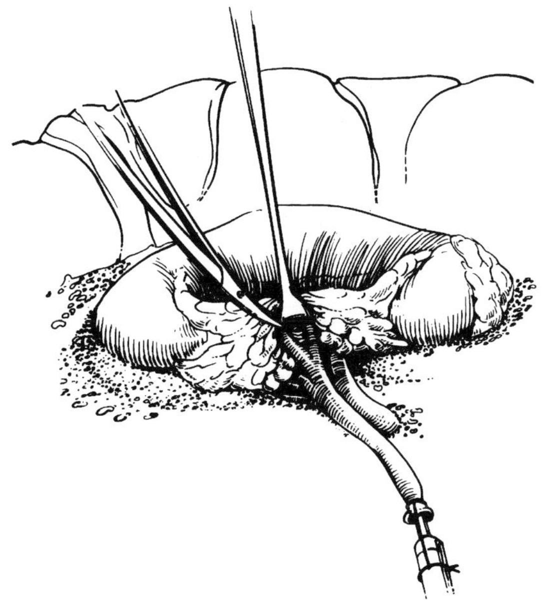

Figure 37.8. Under surface hypothermia, the diseased renal artery branches are mobilized in the renal sinus. From ref. 18, with permission.

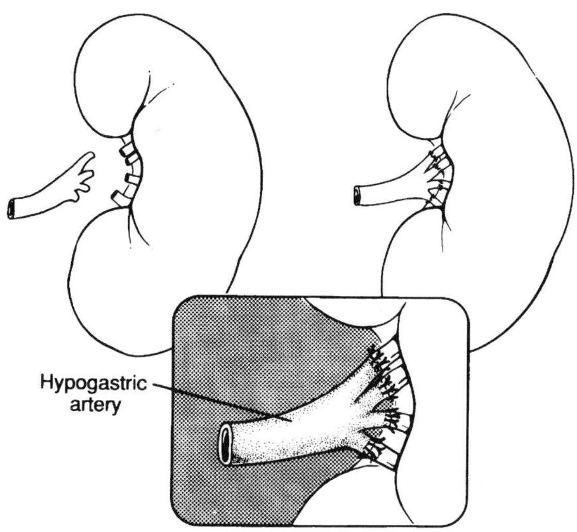

Figure 37.9. Extracorporeal repair with a branched hypogastric arterial autograft. From ref. 18, with permission.

The optimum method for extracorporeal branch renal artery repair involves the use of a branched autogenous vascular graft.[16] This technique permits separate end-to-end microvascular anastomosis of each graft branch to a distal renal artery branch (Fig. 37.9). A hypogastric arterial autograft is the preferred material for vascular reconstruction because this vessel may be obtained intact with several of its branches (Fig. 37.10).

Occasionally, the hypogastric artery is not suitable for use as a reconstructive graft because of atherosclerotic degeneration. When this occurs, a long segment of saphenous vein can be harvested and, employing sequential end-to-side microvascular anastomoses, a branched graft can be fashioned from this vessel (Fig. 37.11).

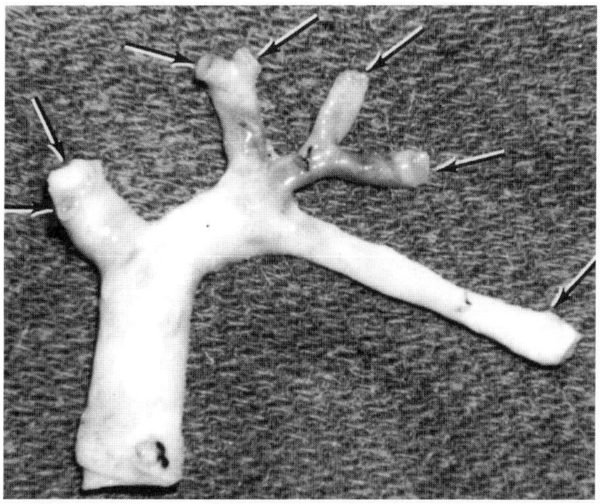

Figure 37.10. Operative photograph of the hypogastric artery removed intact with its branches (arrows).

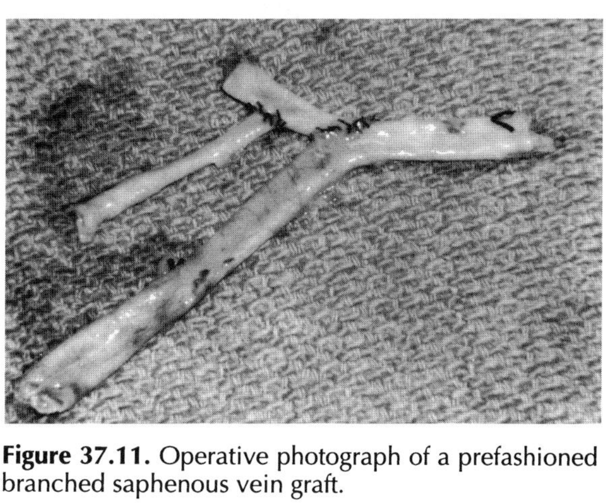

Figure 37.11. Operative photograph of a prefashioned branched saphenous vein graft.

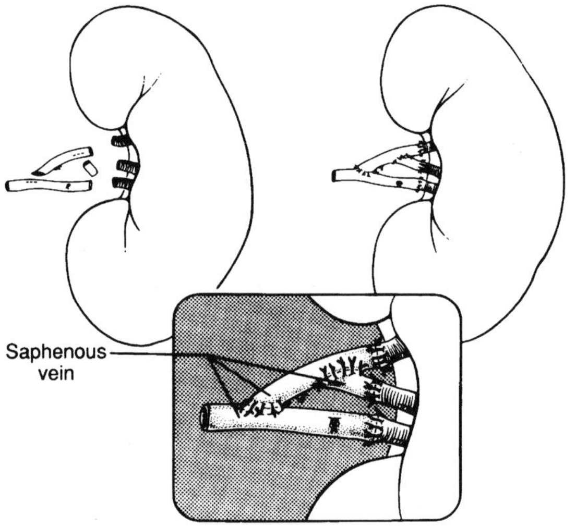

Figure 37.12. Extracorporeal repair with a branched saphenous vein graft. From ref. 18, with permission.

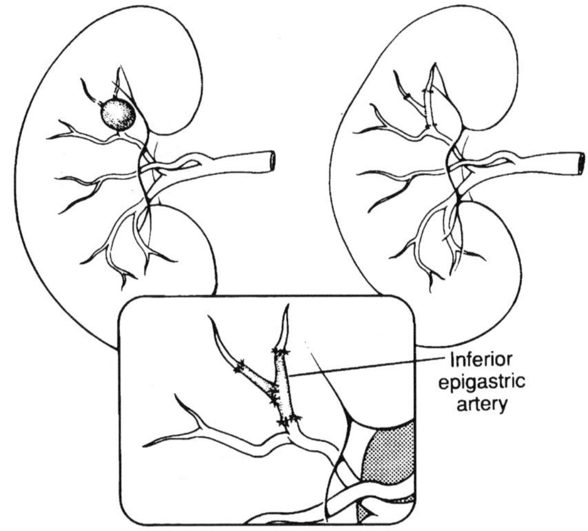

Figure 37.13. Extracorporeal repair with a branched graft of the inferior epigastric artery. From ref. 18, with permission.

This branched graft is then used in a similar manner to achieve reconstruction of the diseased renal artery branches (Fig. 37.12).

Branched grafts of the hypogastric artery and saphenous vein may occasionally prove too large in caliber for anastomosis to small secondary or tertiary renal arterial branches. In these cases, the inferior epigastric artery provides an excellent alternative free graft for extracorporeal microvascular repair.[17] This artery measures 1.5–2.0 mm in diameter, is rarely diseased and coapts nicely in caliber and thickness to small renal artery branches (Fig. 37.13). The inferior epigastric artery may also be employed as a branched graft, either individually or in conjunction with a segment of saphenous vein (Fig. 37.14).

Although use of a branched autogenous vascular graft provides a simple, versatile and effective method for branch renal arterial reconstruction, other techniques occasionally are preferable depending upon the extent of vascular disease. In some patients with localized segmental intrarenal branch lesions, there may be other arterial branches that are either uninvolved or have more proximally located vascular disease.

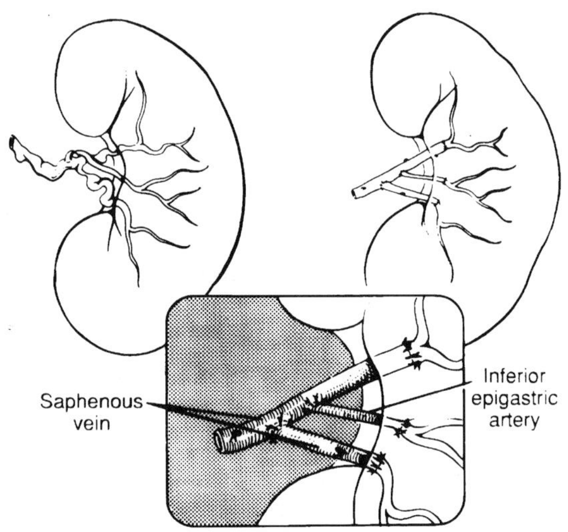

Figure 37.14. Extracorporeal repair with a branched autogenous graft of the saphenous vein and inferior epigastric artery. From ref. 18, with permission.

Such branches with longer disease-free distal segments may be anastomosed end-to-side either into a larger arterial branch or into the reconstructive vascular graft (Fig. 37.15).

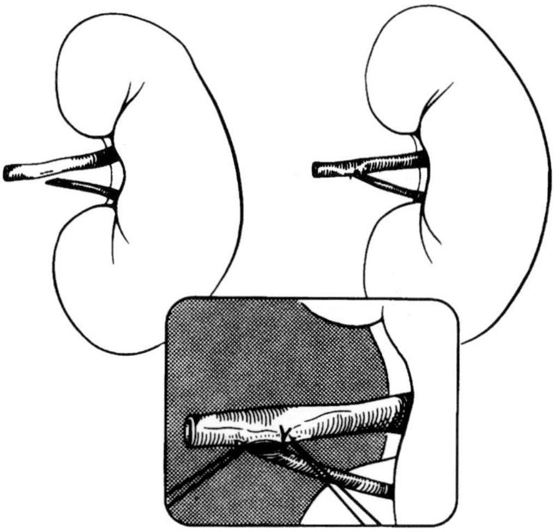

Figure 37.15. End-to-side reimplantation of a small renal artery branch into a larger one. From ref. 18, with permission.

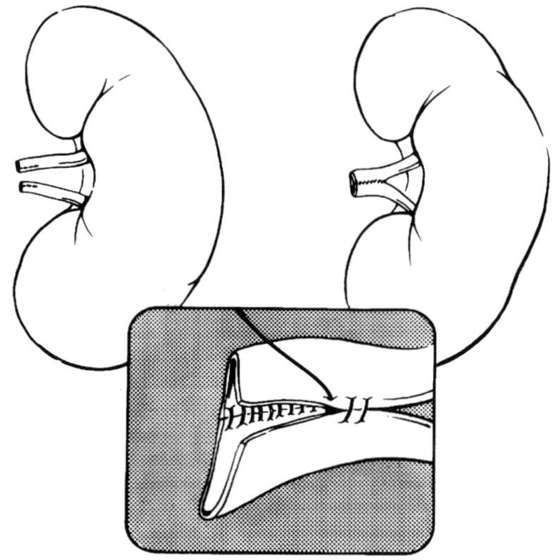

Figure 37.16. Side-to-side (conjoined) anastomosis of equal caliber renal artery branches. From ref. 18, with permission.

Occasionally, two distal arterial branches of similar diameter and free of disease are found adjacent to one another. When this occurs, the two adjacent branches can be conjoined and then anastomosed end-to-end to a single limb of the branched graft (Fig. 37.16).

Renal artery aneurysms have a variable presentation and the method of extracorporeal repair is determined by whether renovascular involvement is focal or diffuse. If the renal artery wall at the base of an aneurysm is intact, aneurysmectomy with patch angioplasty can be performed.

Aneurysms with short focal involvement of renal artery branches may also be simply resected with end-to-side branch re-anastomosis or end-to-side reimplantation into an adjacent branch. In other cases, with more extensive vascular disease, aneurysmectomy and revascularization with a branched autogenous graft are indicated (Fig. 37.17).

These extracorporeal vascular techniques are all performed with interrupted sutures, except for the conjoined anastomosis where a continuous suture is used. When revascularizing multiple arterial branches, one must anticipate the position that the various branches will assume in relation to one another upon completion of the repair. Individual branch anastomoses are then done with careful attention to avoid subsequent malrotation, angulation or tension. In all cases, extracorporeal repair leads to creation of a single main renal artery so that autotransplantation may be performed with one arterial anastomosis and no increase in the revascularization time. When extracorporeal revascularization has been completed, the kidney is either reflushed or placed on the hypothermic pulsatile perfusion unit to verify patency and integrity of the repaired branches. Renal autotransplantation into the iliac fossa is then performed, with anastomosis of the renal vessels to the iliac vessels and restoration of urinary continuity by ureteroneocystostomy.

Clinical results

From 1976 to 1991, extracorporeal microvascular reconstruction and autotransplantation were performed in 66 patients with complex branch renal artery disease at the Cleveland Clinic. This series includes 50 females and 16 males ranging in age from 4 to 62 years. Renovascular disease

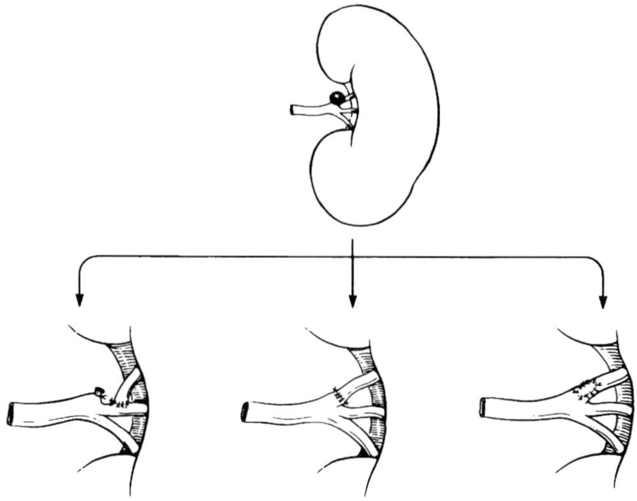

Figure 37.17. Technique for renal artery aneurysmectomy with patch angioplasty (right), resection and reanastomosis (middle), or end-to-side reimplantation (left). From ref. 18, with permission.

was caused by fibrous dysplasia in 42 patients, an arterial aneurysm in 13 patients, atherosclerosis in seven patients, a primary dissection in two patients, arteriovenous fistula in one patient and arteritis in one patient. Eighteen patients presented with branch disease in a solitary kidney, 27 patients had bilateral renovascular disease and 21 patients had unilateral branch disease with a normal contralateral kidney. Renal revascularization was indicated to treat renovascular hypertension in 58 patients, to prevent rupture of an arterial aneurysm in seven patients and to treat an asymptomatic arteriovenous fistula in one patient.

In the 66 patients who underwent extracorporeal branch reconstruction and autotransplantation (including one bilateral autotransplantation), a total of 187 diseased renal artery branches were repaired (mean 2.8 branches per operation). The period of cold renal ischemia needed to perform extracorporeal microvascular repair ranged from 1 to 3.5 h. All patients have been studied postoperatively with isotope renography and, in many cases, with arteriography as well. Postoperative follow-up in these cases ranges from 1 to 15 years. In 64 patients, branch arterial reconstruction was technically successful, while two patients suffered postoperative occlusion of the repaired renal artery. Fortunately, in both of the latter patients, a normal contralateral kidney was present. Currently, all 66 patients are normotensive, including 11 patients who continue to require low dose antihypertensive medication. The current level of renal function is stable or improved in all patients. These results attest the efficacy of extracorporeal microvascular reconstruction in enabling revascularization with preservation of renal parenchyma to be achieved in patients with complex branch arterial lesions.

References

1 Stanley JC, Gewertz BL, Bove EL *et al.* Arterial fibrodysplasia. Histopathologic character and current etiology concepts. *Arch Surg* 1975; **110:** 561–6.

2 Rybka SJ, Novick AC. Concomitant carotid, mesenteric and renal artery stenosis due to intimal fibroplasia. *J Urol* 1983; **129:** 798–800.

3 Poutasse EF. Renal artery aneurysms. *J Urol* 1976; **113:** 443–9.

4 Novick AC. Renal artery aneurysms and arteriovenous fistulas. In Novick AC, Straffon RA (eds) *Vascular Problems in Urologic Surgery*, pp. 189–204. Philadelphia: WB Saunders, 1982.

5 Slavis SA, Hodge EE, Novick AC, Maatman T. Surgical treatment for isolated dissection of the renal artery. *J Urol* 1990; **144:** 233–7.

6 Novick AC. Secondary renal vascular reconstruction for arterial disease in the native and transplant kidney. *Urol Clin North Am* 1994; **21:** 255–63.
7 Campbell SC, Gill I, Novick AC. Delayed allograft autotransplantation after excision of a large symptomatic renal artery pseudoaneurysm. *J Urol* 1993; **149:** 361–3.
8 Ishikawa K. Natural history and classification of occlusive thromboaortopathy (Takayasu's disease): *Circulation* 1978; **57:** 27–35.
9 Grad E, Rance CP. Bilateral renal artery stenosis in association with neurofibrosis (Recklinghausen's disease): report of two cases. *J Pediatr* 1972; **80:** 804–8.
10 Novick AC, Straffon RA, Stewart BH. Surgical management of branch renal artery disease: *in situ* versus extracorporeal methods of repair. *J Urol* 1980; **123:** 311–16.
11 Streem SB, Novick AC. Aortorenal bypass with a branched saphenous vein graft for *in situ* repair of multiple segmental renal arteries. *Surg Gynecol Obstet* 1982; **155:** 855–9.
12 Novick AC, Jackson CL, Straffon RA. The role of renal autotransplantation in complex urologic reconstruction. *J Urol* 1990; **143:** 452–7.
13 Dean RH, Meacham PW, Weaver FA. *Ex vivo* renal artery reconstructions: indications and techniques. *J Vasc Surg* 1986; **49:** 546–52.
14 Dubernard JM, Martin X, Mongin D *et al.* Extracorporeal replacement of the renal artery: techniques, indications and long-term results. *J Urol* 1985; **133:** 13–16.
15 Salvatierra O Jr, Olcott C, IV, Stoney RJ. *Ex vivo* renal artery reconstruction using perfusion preservation. *J Urol* 1978; **119:** 16–19.
16 Novick AC. Management of intrarenal branch arterial lesions with extracorporeal microvascular reconstruction and autotransplantation. *J Urol* 1981; **126:** 150–4.
17 Novick AC. Use of inferior epigastric artery for extracorporeal microvascular branch renal artery reconstruction. *Surgery* 1981; **89:** 513–17.
18 Novick AC, Streem S, Pontes J (eds) *Stewart's Operatime Urology*. Baltimore: Williams and Wilkins, 1989.

38

Secondary revascularization of renal vascular disease

GEORGE HAMILTON

Introduction

Lasting success in renal revascularization cannot be guaranteed since there is an intrinsic tendency toward failure of all vascular reconstructions with time. This fact of life is well recognized by vascular surgeons who, for example, employ lower limb graft surveillance programs to identify impending graft failure and by its timely treatment, pre-empt occlusion. Careful follow-up of renal revascularization by whatever method reveals a variable but significant incidence of restenosis or reocclusion. Secondary revascularization is technically possible and clinically successful in the majority of these events. The principles of management of secondary revascularization compared with the primary approach will be discussed.

Mechanisms of reocclusion

Balloon angioplasty achieves its effect in atherosclerotic lesions mainly by extensive intimal fissuring, partial shearing of atherosclerotic plaque from the media and disruption of the internal elastic lamina.[1] This constitutes not only a major injury to the structures of the media, but results in extensive denudation of endothelium and exposure of the underlying thrombogenic layers. Similar changes result after angioplasty in fibromuscular dysplasia with endothelial denudation and medial stretching. The initial event in healing of this lesion is platelet deposition and thrombosis within the intimal fissures, usually within 30 min of the injury. A neointima begins to form after 1 week with re-endothelialization completed after 1–2 months.[2] Thus reocclusion, may be an early phenomenon from thrombosis at the angioplasty site, or occurs later from excessive intimal hyperplasia. Dissection of the diseased intima is a not uncommon immediate complication of angioplasty which also can result in partial or complete occlusion. Unlike postangioplasty thrombosis which is usually localized to the area of endothelial damage, dissection can extend along the main renal artery stem into the segmental branches and be complicated by superimposed thrombosis.

More commonly, failure of angioplasty occurs in the ostial renal artery lesion which usually is aortic atherosclerotic plaque involving the renal artery origin rather than intrinsic disease[3] (Fig. 38.1). Reocclusion occurs by recoil of the extensive aortic atheroma to its original position sometime after balloon deflation and is not usually accompanied by thrombosis.

Surgical revascularization can fail for many reasons best considered as early, intermediate or late. Early failures usually occur in the postoperative period (within 30 days) and are due mainly to technical problems. These can be poor surgical and anastomotic technique, inadequate arterial inflow or outflow, a vein graft of poor condition, or kinking occurring in a long unsupported graft. In the presence of a thrombogenic

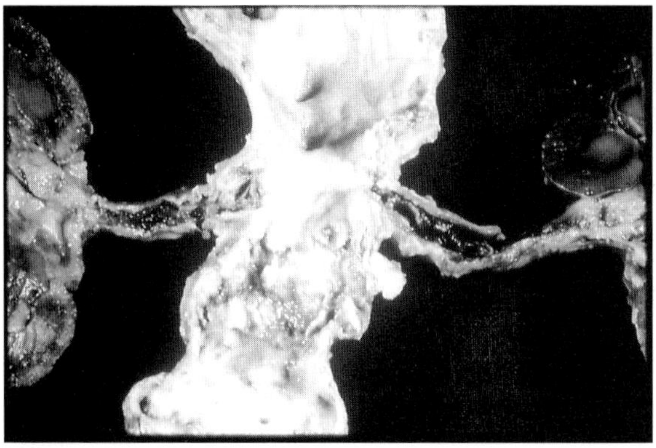

Figure 38.1 This postmortem specimen of an aorta with renal artery origins vividly illustrates the problem of ostial renal artery stenosis. As can be seen in this specimen the renal artery lesion is of complex atherosclerotic plaque of the aortic wall and not of the mainstem artery. In this case bilaterally severe renal artery stenoses were complicated by acute thrombosis secondary to an episode of hypotension.

prosthetic graft, particularly Dacron, severe postoperative hypotension such as may occur in septic shock or during a cardiorespiratory arrest, can result in spontaneous occlusion by thrombosis. Renal revascularization may be clinically unsuccessful even in the presence of a technically satisfactory procedure where the end organ is irreversibly diseased due to insufficient renal mass or to severe unrecognized stenosis of the intrarenal arterial tree. These failures can be attributed to poor preoperative assessment and selection.

Intermediate and late failures may be due to progression of disease either proximal or distal to the reconstruction (i.e. within the aortic wall or in the segmental renal arteries), or due to problems developing at the anastomosis or within the graft itself. Intimal hyperplasia commonly complicates both angioplasty and surgical reconstruction, particularly where there is extensive endothelial denudation and trauma to the arterial wall. Endarterectomy is a surgical procedure which is associated with significant stenosis from severe intimal hyperplasia, a process well described after carotid endarterectomy, but apparently less common after renal endarterectomy. Vein grafts develop stenoses along their length, often due to a combination of intimal hyperplasia and fibrosis and perhaps secondary to trauma sustained during preparation and implantation; the cause is not fully understood (Fig. 38.2). These stenoses can develop

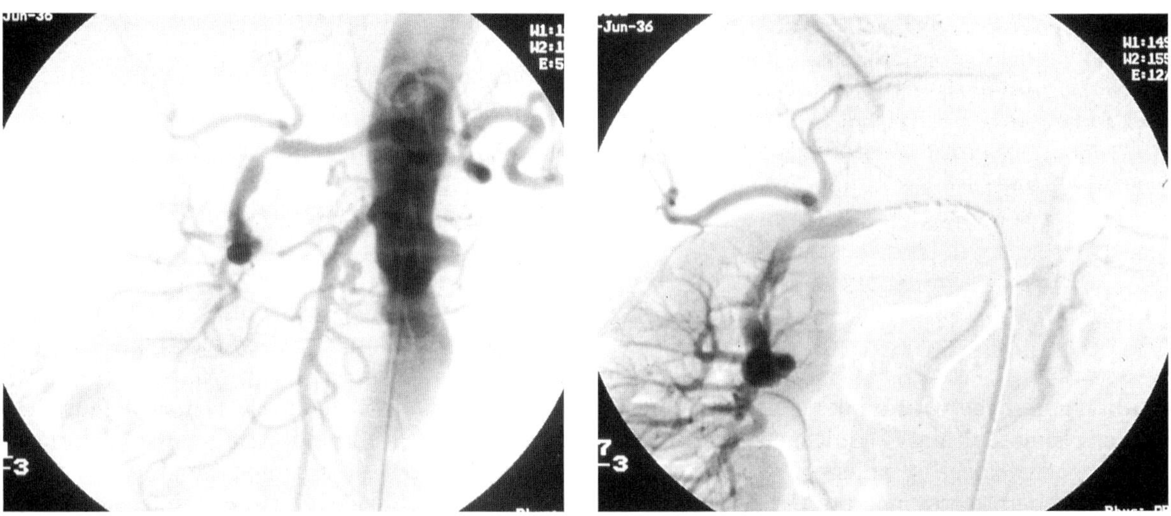

(a) (b)

Figure 38.2 (a) The distal subtraction angiogram (DSA) of a hepatorenal bypass graft performed with interposition saphenous vein 8 months after implantation. Routine postsurgical monitoring had demonstrated deterioration in hypertension control and a small deterioration in renal function. This DSA shows the development of a stenosis within the proximal few centimeters of the saphenous vein just beyond the anastomosis with the common hepatic artery. (b) The DSA shows a satisfactory appearance immediately after angioplasty for this lesion. Good function is maintained in this graft 9 months after this angioplasty.

anywhere along the length of the graft complicating 10–20% of reversed or *in situ* saphenous vein grafts in lower limb reconstructions within the first 18 months.[4, 5] These intrinsic stenoses are also extremely common in coronary artery bypass grafting with thrombosis rates of up to 50% being reported.[6] Similar high rates of saphenous vein graft stenosis have been reported in saphenous vein aortorenal bypass grafting.[7, 8] Intimal hyperplasia frequently develops a few millimeters downstream of the distal anastomosis in any graft and less commonly within the native artery just before the inflow anastomosis. A further cause of anastomotic stenosis is as a result of poor technique, most commonly found with the use of a continuous suture method.

Progression of arteriosclerosis in the inflow or outflow circulation can develop years after the original reconstruction and may even involve the vein graft itself. In prosthetic grafts significant intimal thickening may develop around the distal anastomosis.[9] A further disadvantage of prosthetic grafts is the inability to cover the luminal surface with endothelial cells beyond the first 2 cm at either end.[10] These grafts are lined by a thrombotically active pannus of fibrin and platelets which may stimulate development of downstream intimal hyperplasia by continuous release of mitogenic growth factors. This surface is obviously much more thrombogenic than an endothelial cell layer and therefore these grafts are more prone to thrombosis than arterial or venous conduits.

Dilatation of venous aortorenal grafts

Late dilatation of vein grafts is well described in aortorenal grafting with frank aneurysmal development reported in 2% of adults and 20% of children.[7, 11] Despite the potential for thrombus formation, embolism and rupture, few cases of reconstruction for this indication have been reported, perhaps suggesting that this is a stable complication which rarely requires intervention[12] (Fig. 38.3). Pseudo-aneurysms, although rare, can complicate renal vascular reconstruction. These lesions can develop at anastomotic dehiscences resulting from either poor technique, or as a result of trauma, but perhaps more commonly as a result of infection around the anastomosis site. This is a particularly feared complication in renal artery transplants.

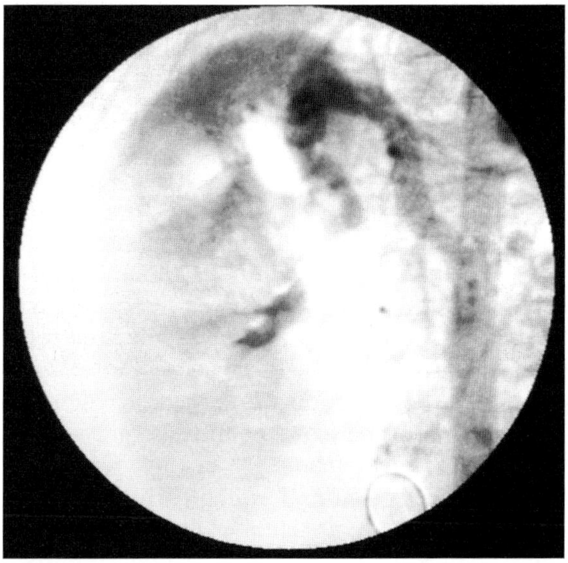

Figure 38.3 This intravenous DSA image demonstrates aneurysmal dilatation of a saphenous vein aortorenal graft in a 34-year-old woman treated for a symptomatic renal artery aneurysm associated with neurofibromatosis. Despite this alarming appearance, the graft continues to function well some 6 years after its implantation.

Incidence of restenosis or reocclusion

Documentation of the incidence of restenosis after percutaneous transluminal renal angioplasty has been rather patchy in the literature since the emphasis has been on clinical rather than radiological endpoints in follow-up. More recent studies employing regular angiographic follow-up, report restenosis rates of 8 and 9% in mainstem and branch fibromuscular dysplasia.[13, 14] In atherosclerotic disease the recurrence rates are higher with initial reports ranging from 10 to 90%,[15] but more recently lower recurrence rates of 8–42% have been reported.[16–18] Ostial lesions are more likely to restenose, particularly in the presence of aortic atherosclerosis and ectasia.[17] Balloon angioplasty with stenting shows improved patency rates for ostial lesions but with a significant restenosis rate within the stent of approximately 40% in the preliminary reports (see Chapter 29).

Restenosis after surgical reconstruction occurs to varying degrees largely according to the method used. Presentation can be within months but is most typically within the first year after reconstruction. Novick reports a stenosis rate of less than 10% in surgically revascularized renal arteries during recent experience.[19] Certainly in the hands of experienced surgeons restenosis after renal artery endarterectomy is rare with 5-year patency rates of 90% being reported.[20] Stenosis occurs more frequently in transplant renal arteries, usually at the anastomosis with rates typically of 11–20% being reported. Recurrence rates after angioplasty of this lesion of 4–18% are reported (see Chapter 39). In aortorenal bypass grafting, the most commonly performed reconstructive procedure, there is an early failure rate of less than 5%,[8, 21, 22] and a later stenosis rate of 8–41%.[7, 8] Similar to the situation in coronary artery bypass grafting, stenosis is a rare occurrence in renal grafts of arterial origin.[23] Extracorporeal reconstruction in the hands of experts has remarkably low reported restenosis rates (see Chapter 37).

Evaluation and selection of patients for secondary revascularization

After renal revascularization, by whatever method, regular follow-up of renal function is of vital importance, and ideally performed at least every 6 months. Measurement of serum creatinine, urea and creatinine clearance provide a baseline estimate of renal function. Estimation of renal mass by ultrasound measurement is of value since revascularization of a kidney with a length less than 8–9 cm is unlikely to result in a good outcome. Radioisotope renography [(mercaptoacetyltriglycine MAG_3] or diethylenetriaminepentaacetic acid [DTPA] scans) will provide assessment of perfusion and differential function where there are two functioning kidneys present. In the clinical situation of acute thrombosis of a bypass graft, the question of the underlying renal viability is of importance and isotope renography is of great value in this situation providing information regarding the degree of perfusion present. Often, however, this information is only obtained at surgical exploration.

Where there is evidence of deterioration in renal function, angiography should be performed if the patient is considered a suitable candidate for secondary revascularization. The radiologist should be requested to demonstrate not only the renal vasculature, but should also be asked to demonstrate the lower descending aorta, the supraceliac and aortoiliac components, and normal and oblique views of the celiac and superior mesenteric arterial origins (Fig. 38.4 and 38.5). In addition, views of the distal renal

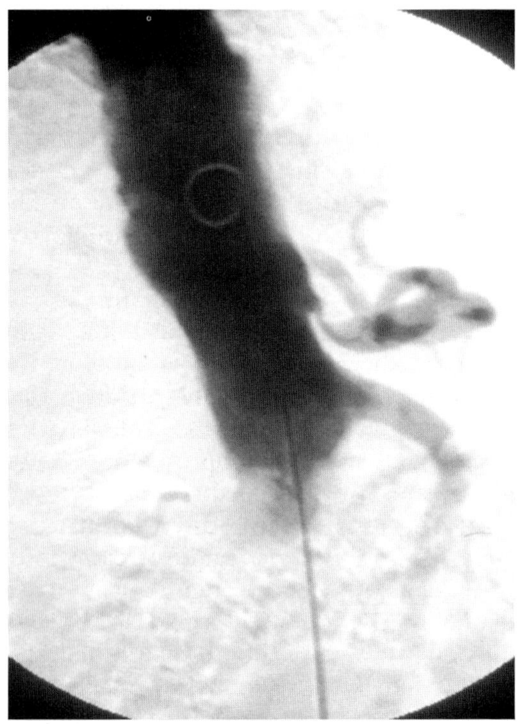

Figure 38.4 This is an oblique view of the celiac and superior mesenteric artery origins in a patient being considered for a hepatorenal bypass in treatment of right renal artery ischemia. A very tight stenosis at the origin of the celiac artery is very clearly demonstrated. The superior mesenteric artery is shown to be large with no stenosis within it, thus making this a suitable possible inflow site for a bypass on to the right renal artery.

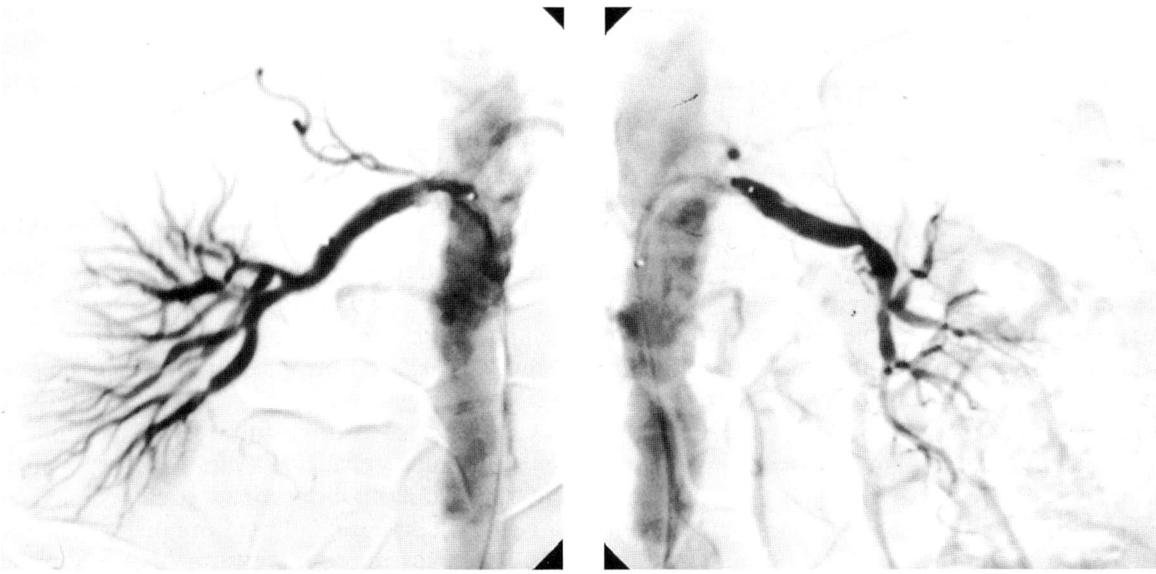

Figure 38.5 These are selective angiograms of the renal arteries of a patient treated by angioplasty for bilateral ostial stenoses. There was no improvement after these angioplasties and these selective studies clearly demonstrate multiple stenoses throughout the segmental and distal branch arteries within the kidney.

circulation, particularly of the segmental arterial branches should be obtained; by digital subtraction angiography even in the presence of complete occlusion. The demonstration of a collateral circulation is of course a favorable prognostic feature.

The general condition of the patient must be taken into consideration when planning any revascularization. This group of patients have a high incidence of associated coronary and cerebrovascular disease and any workup must include a full carotid and cardiovascular assessment. In chronic secondary renal disease there is time to optimize the patient's general status with correction of significant coronary or carotid lesions if indicated. Obviously in acute occlusion this measured approach is not possible and good cardiological support together with anesthetic expertise will be of paramount importance in securing a successful outcome to emergency surgery. Patients undergoing repeat angioplasty or fibrinolytic therapy should receive the same workup since emergency surgical intervention may be necessary in the event of a complication from these interventional procedures.

Postangioplasty restenosis or reocclusion

In a recent review of almost 700 procedures the overall complication rate of percutaneous transluminal renal angioplasty (PTRA) was about 10%. Specific renal artery complications were dissection in 2%, acute occlusion or thrombosis in 1.5% and segmental renal infarction in 1%.[24] Thus the need for intervention in the immediate post-PTRA period is small. Late recurrence is more common, indeed it has been suggested that its incidence is directly proportional to the length of follow-up.[25] These recurrences can be treated successfully by repeat dilatation, particularly in cases of non-ostial atherosclerotic, fibromuscular dysplastic and renal transplant stenoses. Where thrombosis and complete occlusion have occurred, consideration should be given to the use of intra-arterial fibrinolytic therapy to lyze the clot, reperfuse the kidney parenchyma and perhaps allow repeat angioplasty to be performed. The contribution of stenting as an adjunct remains to be determined.

Angioplasty will not always be technically

possible, however, and perhaps in ostial and para-ostial lesions this approach may not even be desirable. In the only prospectively studied series of PTRA in comparison with surgery, there was a 25% restenosis rate during the first year of follow-up (6 out of 24 PTRA procedures) with only one patient out of this group requiring surgical reconstruction. The others were successfully treated by redo angioplasty.[26] Most lesions in this study were within 1 cm of the renal artery origin. The indication for treatment was renovascular hypertension and renal function was in fact very good in this group of patients. There continues to be great debate over the management of atherosclerotic ostial lesions by PTRA with more centers reporting a high primary recurrence and complication rate.[16, 17, 28] In a recent review of 20 patients with moderate to severe renal failure treated by PTRA at the Royal Free Hospital, poor clinical outcome in terms of preservation of renal function was found in the elderly patient with an ostial stenosis in a solitary kidney. Despite a technical success rate of greater than 90%, early restenosis was common in this sick and elderly group of patients.[27] Consequently recurrent ostial renal artery stenoses should be treated by a surgical approach until such time as there is proper evaluation of the long-term patency of PTRA with stenting (Fig. 38.6).

With the widespread use of PTRA, vascular surgeons have been confronted increasingly with the problem of reconstruction of a renal artery traumatized by the angioplasty balloon. Several centers have reported increased technical problems in surgical dissection of the renal artery after this procedure.[28, 29] Retrospective reviews from Duke University and the Cleveland Clinic, however, contradict these previous findings.[30, 31] Out of a combined total of 63 patients (22 with fibromuscular dysplasia and 49 with atherosclerotic renal vascular disease) operated on after one or more PTRA treatments, only one kidney was lost and this was because of its small size. Only one patient (from the Cleveland Clinic series) was judged to have undergone a more complicated vascular reconstruction as a result of the PTRA. This patient required an extracorporeal vascular reconstruction because of branch artery involvement in a PTRA-induced dissection. Neither group observed any inflammatory or fibrotic change around the renal artery origin. The Royal Free experience in a smaller group of patients concurs with these observations (Fig. 38.7).

Unfortunately this is not the case when a stent has been placed in the renal artery. Stents become rapidly incorporated into the vessel wall and they are extremely difficult to remove without causing considerable trauma to the intima and media. Despite being metal, stents are remarkably difficult to palpate intraoperatively because of their springiness. Stent deployment across the renal artery ostium will make surgery on the renal artery origin technically more difficult. For example, a decision to treat by aortorenal endarterectomy will mandate opening of the renal artery with full exposure of the stent so that its safe removal can be achieved. Stent removal from within the aortic lumen using the classical transaortic approach without opening of the renal artery will be not only difficult but dangerous without the ability to inspect and correct the resultant damage. The use of a bypass procedure in this situation would be technically more straightforward and perhaps safer, but even in this situation ligation and division of the renal artery origin with its indwelling stent will be difficult. There are no reports as yet of surgical renal artery reconstruction after stent deployment, but this new development in treatment of renal artery disease poses an interesting surgical problem to be resolved.

Secondary revascularization

Anatomical dissection in secondary renal revascularization is always difficult. The operative field may be affected by varying degrees of obliteration of tissue planes by scar tissue. Particularly difficult is mobilization of the renal artery where a primary procedure has taken place. Basic vascular surgical technique dictates mobilization of the unoperated segments of the vessel proximal and distal to the primary reconstruction before it too is mobilized. There are particular problems with the anatomy of the renal artery, this being a short vessel close to the aorta and on the right side covered almost entirely by

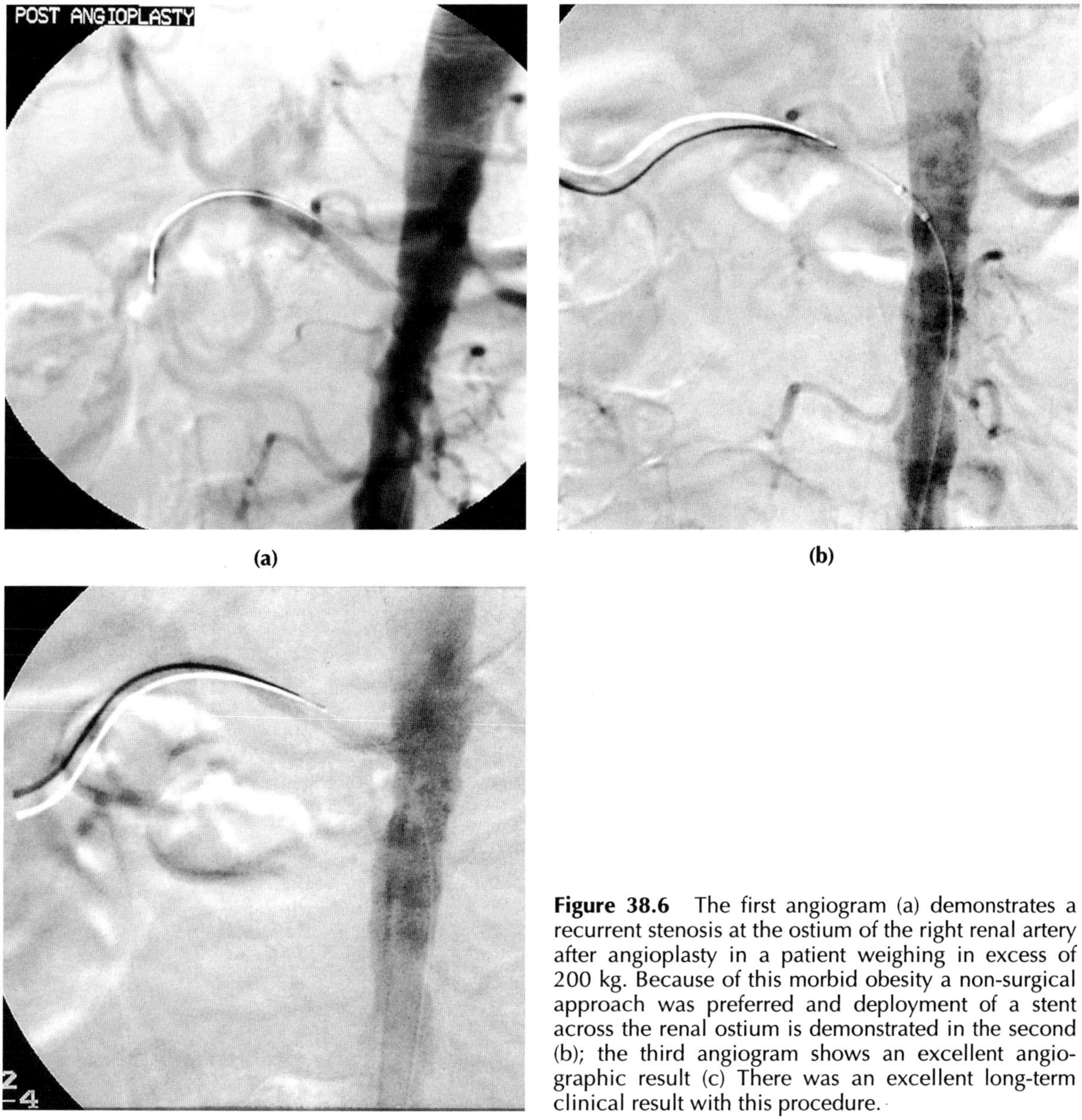

(a) (b) (c)

Figure 38.6 The first angiogram (a) demonstrates a recurrent stenosis at the ostium of the right renal artery after angioplasty in a patient weighing in excess of 200 kg. Because of this morbid obesity a non-surgical approach was preferred and deployment of a stent across the renal ostium is demonstrated in the second (b); the third angiogram shows an excellent angiographic result (c) There was an excellent long-term clinical result with this procedure.

the inferior vena cava and renal veins. The safest resolution of this technical problem is to completely avoid the scarred operative field by the use of alternative approaches. In all cases distal 'healthy' renal artery has to be found and dissection usually involves mobilization of the segmental branches in order to achieve this.

The most commonly performed primary revascularization procedures involve surgery to the aorta, i.e. aortorenal bypass, aortic replacement with bypass or aortorenal endarterectomy. Extra-anatomic bypasses are particularly useful in this situation completely avoiding the need to dissect or cross-clamp the aorta. Thus hepatorenal bypass to the right kidney and splenorenal to the left are reliable procedures which can be achieved through a subcostal incision. If these procedures are being considered biplanar

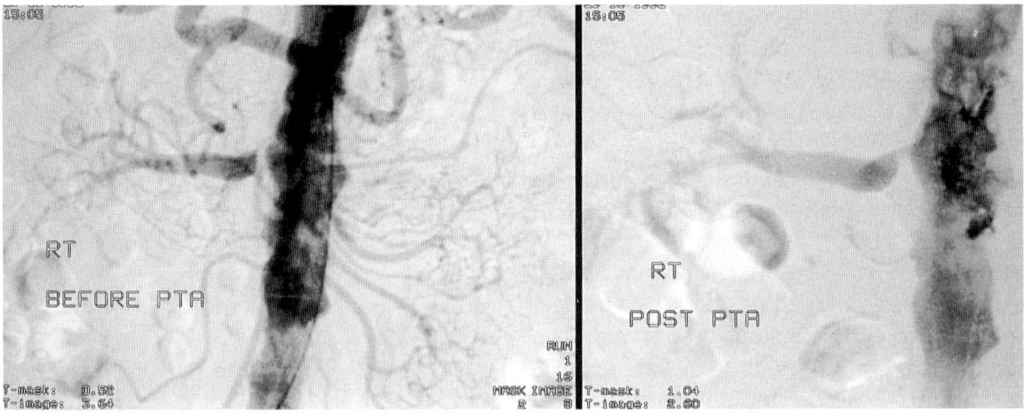

(a)

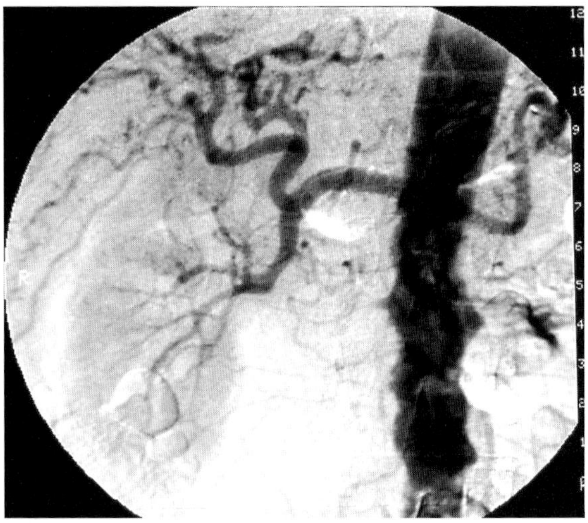

(b)

Figure 38.7 The angiograms (a) demonstrate a poor result from a second angioplasty to the ostial stenosis of the right renal artery. This patient underwent revascularization by direct anastomosis of the right renal artery to the common hepatic artery (b). In order to gain sufficient length of renal artery, dissection of the entire length was performed and despite the two previous angioplasties there was no technical difficulty or periarterial fibrosis encountered.

angiography is of extreme importance in order to exclude the quite high probability of significant stenosis of the celiac trunk.[32] Percutaneous angioplasty of a celiac artery stenosis in order to improve the inflow sufficiently to allow use of the hepatic or splenic artery for a renal revascularization is a possible solution to this problem.[33] There is little experience of visceral angioplasty reported in the literature. These are ostial lesions similar to those involving the renal artery and the probability of recurrence must be high. This approach, perhaps combined with stenting to optimize arterial inflow and thus allowing safe secondary renal revascularization by hepato or splenorenal bypass grafting merits further careful evaluation.

In the presence of significant celiac trunk stenosis, however, use of alternative inflow sites for bypass grafting is currently the preferred approach. The supraceliac or distal thoracic aorta is usually spared from significant disease, can be approached transabdominally and is ideal for secondary revacularization.[34] Other inflow sites include the superior mesenteric and iliac arteries although the high prevalence of aortoiliac arteriosclerosis in older patients makes the latter approach less attractive.[35, 36] Finally, where there is complex renal segmental arterial disease or extensive hilar fibrosis, the technique of extracorporeal reconstruction and autotransplantation is the method of choice. This elegant method allows safe and methodical reconstruction of the segmental vessels without concerns of warm ischemic damage to the kidney. The Cleveland Clinic reports the largest series of these procedures with excellent clinical results.

Saphenous vein aortorenal bypass grafts are susceptible to stenosis development which leads rapidly to complete thrombosis if not detected. Regular follow-up of a saphenous vein aortorenal bypass graft is vitally important for this reason with full angiography being performed at any sign of deteriorating renal function. Angioplasty of these lesions is usually successful. In the recently occluded saphenous aortorenal graft, an attempt at fibrinolysis is well worthwhile since the causative intrinsic lesion may be revealed and treated possibly by percutaneous angioplasty.[37] If the stenosis proves resistant to angioplasty or recurs, then in the presence of a patent graft a simpler technique such as an operative patch angioplasty may be all that is required. With the advent of rapid methods of intra-arterial fibrinolysis an attempt at clearance of a blocked graft might become a routine and acceptable approach to this problem.

For detailed descriptions of these techniques the reader is referred to Chapter 34 on renal artery endarterectomy; Chapter 35 on alternative renal artery bypass techniques; Chapter 37 on extracorporeal revascularization and autotransplantation; Chapter 39 on revascularization in the transplanted kidney; and Chapter 31 on fibrinolytic therapy.

Summary

The difficult problem of secondary renal revascularization is best managed by a conjoined approach of a nephrologist, vascular surgeon and interventional vascular radiologist. A flexible approach to achieving revascularization, including the more recent options of PTRA, stenting and fibrinolysis will yield the best clinical result with the lowest patient morbidity. Obviously such cases should be treated in centers that have extensive expertise and facilities in all three clinical disciplines.

References

1 Castaneda-Zuniga WR, Formanek A, Tradavarthy M *et al.* The mechanism of balloon angioplasty. *Radiology* 1980; **135:** 565–71.

2 Zollikofer CL, Salomonowitz E, Sibley *et al.* Transluminal angioplasty evaluated by electron microscopy. *Radiology* 1984; **153:** 369–74.

3 Cicuto KP, McLean GK, Oleaga JA *et al.* Renal artery stenosis: anatomic classification for percutaneous transluminal angioplasty. *Am J Radiol* 1981; **137:** 599–601.

4 Mills JL, Harris EJ, Taylor LM. The importance of routine surveillance of distal bypass grafts with duplex scanning: a study of 379 reversed vein grafts. 1990; *J Vasc Surg* **12:** 379–89.

5 Bandyk DF, Schmitt DD, Seabrook GR. Monitoring functional patency of *in situ* saphenous vein bypasses: the impact of a surveillance protocol and elective revision. *J Vasc Surg* 1989; **9:** 286–96.

6 Grondin CM, Campeau L, Lesperance J *et al.* Comparison of late changes in internal mammary artery and saphenous vein grafts in two consecutive series of patients 10 years after the operation. *Circulation* 1984; **70** (Supp.1)**:** 208–12.

7 Stanley JC, Ernst CB, Fry WJ. Fate of 100 aortorenal vein grafts: characteristics of late graft expansion, aneurysmal dilation and stenosis. *Surgery* 1973; **74:** 931–44.

8 Ekelund J, Gerlock J Jr, Goncharenko V. Angiographic findings following surgical treatment for renovascular hypertension. *Radiology* 1978; **126:** 345–9.

9 LoGerfo FW, Quist WC, Nowak MD *et al.* Downstream anastomotic hyperplasia: a mechanism of failure in Dacron arterial grafts. *Ann Surg* 1983, **197:** 479–83.

10 Berger K, Sauvage LR, Rao AM, Wood SJ. Healing of arterial prostheses in man: its incompleteness. *Ann Surg* 1972; **175:** 118–27.

11 Stanley JC, Fry WJ. Pediatric renal artery occlusive disease and renovascular hypertension. Etiology, diagnosis and operative treatment. *Arch Surg* 1981; **116:** 669–76.

12 Stanley JC, Whitehouse WM Jr, Zelenock GB *et al.* Reoperation for complications of renal artery reconstructive surgery undertaken for treatment of renovascular hypertension. *J Vasc Surg* 1985; **2:** 133–44.

13 Tegtmeyer CJ, Selby JB, Hartwell GD *et al.* Results and complications of angioplasty in fibromuscular disease. *Circulation* 1991; **83** (Supp.1)**:** 155–61.

14 Cluzel P, Raynaud A, Beyssen B *et al.* Stenoses of renal branch arteries in fibromuscular dysplasia: results of percutaneous transluminal angioplasty. *J Intervent Radiol* 1994; **193:** 227–32.

15 Weibull H, Bergquist D, Jendteg S *et al.* Clinical outcome and health care costs in renal revascularisation – percutaneous transluminal renal angioplasty versus reconstructive surgery. *Br J Surg* 1991; **78:** 620–4.

16 Baert AL, Wilms G, Amery A *et al.* Percutaneous transluminal renal angioplasty: initial results and long-term follow-up in 202 patients. *Cardiovasc Intervent Radiol* 1990; **13:** 22–8.

17 Plouin P-F, Darne B, Chatellier G *et al.*

Restenosis after a first percutaneous transluminal renal angioplasty. *Hypertension* 1993, **21:** 89–96.
18 Kremer-Hovinga TK, de Jong PE, de Zeeuw D *et al.* Restenosis prevalence and long-term effects on renal function after percutaneous transluminal renal angioplasty. *Nephron* 1986; **44** (Supp.1): 64–7.
19 Novick AC. Secondary renal vascular reconstruction for arterial disease in the native and transplant kidney. *Urol Clin North Am* 1994; **21:** 255–63.
20 Bergentz SE, Weibull H, Bergquist D. Long-term patency after reconstructive surgery and PTA for renal artery stenosis. In Greenhalgh RM, Hollier L (eds) *The Maintenance of Arterial Reconstruction*, pp. 384–96. London: WB Saunders, 1991.
21 Ernst CB, Stanley JC, Marshall FF, Fry WJ. Autogenous saphenous vein aortorenal grafts: a 10 year experience. *Arch Surg* 1972; **105:** 855–64.
22 van Bockel JH, van Schilfgaarde R, Felthuis W *et al.* The influence of surgical technique upon short-term and long-term anatomic results in reconstructive operation for renovascular hypertension. *Surg Gynecol Obstet* 1988; **166:** 402–8.
23 van Bockel JH, van Schilfgaarde R, van Brummelen P, Terpstra JL. Long-term results of renal artery reconstruction with autogenous artery in patients with renovascular hypertension. *Eur J Vasc Surg* 1984; **3:** 515–21.
24 Ramsay LE, Waller PC. Blood pressure response to percutaneous transluminal angioplasty for renovascular hypertension: an overview of published series. *Br Med J* 1990; **300:** 569–72.
25 Flechner SM. Percutaneous transluminal dilatation. A realistic appraisal in patients with stenosing lesions of the renal artery. *Urol Clin North Am* 1984; **11:** 515–27.
26 Weibull H, Bergquist D, Bergentz SE *et al.* Percutaneous transluminal renal angioplasty versus surgical reconstruction of atherosclerotic renal artery stenosis: a prospective randomised study. 1993; **18:** 841–52.
27 le Bird R, Warwick R, Hilson A *et al.* Renal artery angioplasty in severe atherosclerotic renovascular disease. *Br J Surg* 1995; **82:** 561.
28 Beebe HG, Chesebro K, Merchant F, Bush W. Results of renal artery balloon angioplasty limit its indications. *J Vas Surg* 1988; **8:** 300–6.
29 Dean RH, Callis JT, Smith BM, Meacham PW. Failed percutaneous transluminal renal angioplasty: experience with lesions requiring operative intervention. *J Vas Surg* 1987; **6:** 301.
30 McCann RL, Bollinger RR, Newman GE. Surgical renal artery reconstruction after percutaneous transluminal angioplasty. *J Vas Surg* 1988; **8:** 389–94.
31 Martinez AG, Novick AC, Hayes JM. Surgical treatment of renal artery stenosis after failed percutaneous transluminal angioplasty. *J Urol* 1990; **144:** 1094–6.
32 Valentine RJ, Martin JD, Myers SI. Asymptomatic celiac and superior mesenteric artery stenoses are more prevalent among patients with unsuspected renal artery stenosis. *J Vas Surg* 1991; **14:** 195.
33 Sniderman KW. Transluminal angioplasty in the management of chronic intestinal ischaemia. In Strandness DE, van Breda A (eds) *Vascular Diseases: Surgical and Interventional Therapy*. pp. 803–9. New York: Churchill Livingstone, 1994.
34 Novick AC, Stewart R. Use of the thoracic aorta for renal revascularisation. *J Uro* 1990; **143:** 77.
35 Khauli RB, Novick AC, Coseriu GU *et al.* Superior mesentero renal bypass for renal revascularisation with infrarenal aortic occlusion. *J Urol* 1985; **133:** 188–90.
36 Novick AC, Banowsky LH. Iliorenal saphenous vein bypass: an alternative for renal revascularisation in patients with a surgically difficult aorta. *J Urol* 1979; **122:** 243.
37 Libertino JA, Beckmann CF. Surgery and percutaneous angioplasty in the management of renovascular hypertension. *Urol Clin North Am* 1994; **21:** 235–43.

39

Revascularization for transplant renal artery stenosis

ZAKI SHAPIRA

Introduction

In principle there are two modalities for the treatment of hypertension caused by transplant renal artery stenosis (TRAS): the pharmacological (symptomatic) management and the revascularization of the stenotic lesion in the artery. Treatment is essential because untreated cases may lead to uncontrollable hypertension and deterioration of the renal graft function. Consequently, there is graft loss and serious danger to the patient due to cardiopulmonary complications.

Pharmacological management is usually reserved for patients found unsuitable for treatment by interventional revascularization. Those considered unsuitable are: (1) poor risk patients; (2) patients with complications relating to immunosuppressive therapy, i.e. malignancy, hepatic dysfunction and sepsis; (3) patients suffering from diffuse intraparenchymal stenoses which are inaccessible for the above procedures.[1]

Revascularization for TRAS should be offered to patients with documented stenosis who present with refractory hypertension and/or impaired graft function, with reasonable expectations of satisfactory results.

The accepted degree of lumen narrowing of the transplant artery for hemodynamics significance is 70–80% and above,[2,3] but 50% is also adequate if concommitant significant renal hypertension exists.[4–6]

Revascularization of the TRAS can be performed surgically or by utilizing techniques of invasive radiology, i.e. percutaneous transluminal angioplasty (PTA).

Surgical revascularization for TRAS

The techniques for TRAS repair have evolved in recent years from primarily surgical revascularization to the use of PTA as the first choice procedure.[4, 7] However, surgical intervention may be favored in:

1 Cases of anastomotic stenosis (Fig. 39.1). This type of stenosis is of short segment and attributed to technical errors in performing the anastomosis. This stenosis is typically dense and hence is often resistant to treatment with PTA.[8–11]
2 Stenosis due to twisting or kinking of the transplant artery. This stenosis is long and convoluted therefore not permitting safe accessibility to PTA.[4, 12, 13]

It also may be necessary in:

3 Failures of attempted revascularization by PTA.
4 Complications of PTA which might lead to impaired blood flow to the renal graft (i.e. intima dissection).

Contraindication for the use of surgical repair are:

1 In cases of chronic rejection (histologically confirmed).[14]
2 In cases where the stenosis is diffuse or extended into intrarenal arteries.[5]

The preferred surgical approach to the arteries is the intraperitoneal using a lower midline or paramedian incision.[4, 10, 14, 15] Approaching through the old transplant scar is extremely tedious and quite hazardous. Firstly, the iliac arteries should be exposed and isolated from the surrounding tissue and then the hypogastric and renal arteries. The renal artery should be traced distally and proximally to the stenotic segment controlled by vascular clamps (Fig. 39.2) The isolation could be difficult because of the dense scar formation surrounding the allograft and the likelihood of uretral and renal vein adherence to the renal artery.[2]

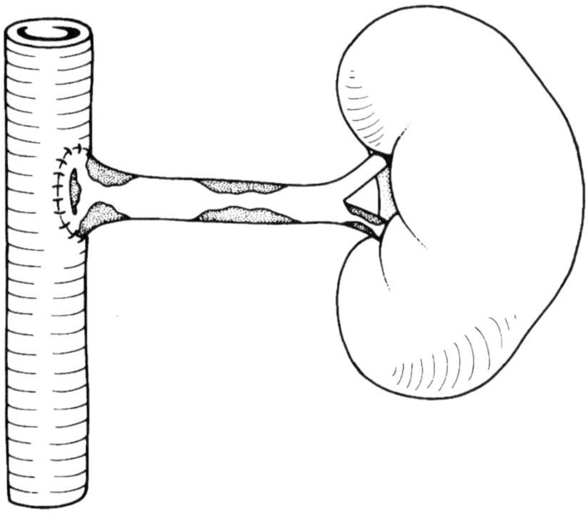

Figure 39.1. Typical localizations of TRAS: in the anastomotic line, along the main artery and in the secondary branch.

There is no need for cold perfusion of the graft during the revascularization repair because the graft usually resumes function soon after blood reperfusion has been initiated.[15]

Surgical techniques of revascularization of TRAS

Resection of the stenotic segment and direct arterial reanastomosis

Segmental arterial resection (Fig. 39.3) is an appropriate procedure for short segment stenosis like those which may occur in the anastomotic line of end renal artery to end hypogastric artery anastomosis. The artery, distal and proximal to

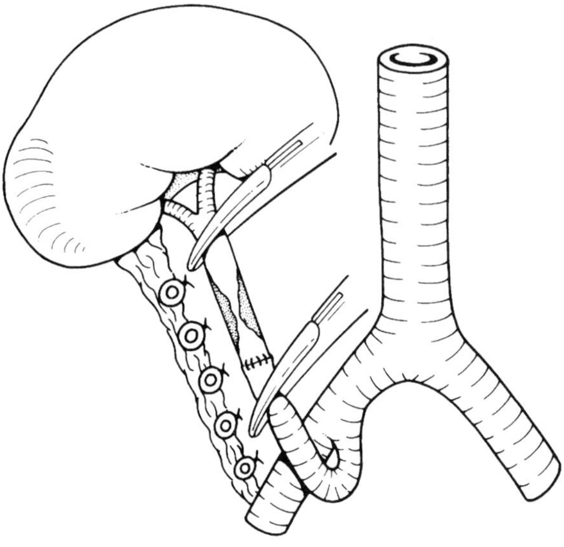

Figure 39.2. Isolation of the transplant renal artery distal and proximal to the stenosis site.

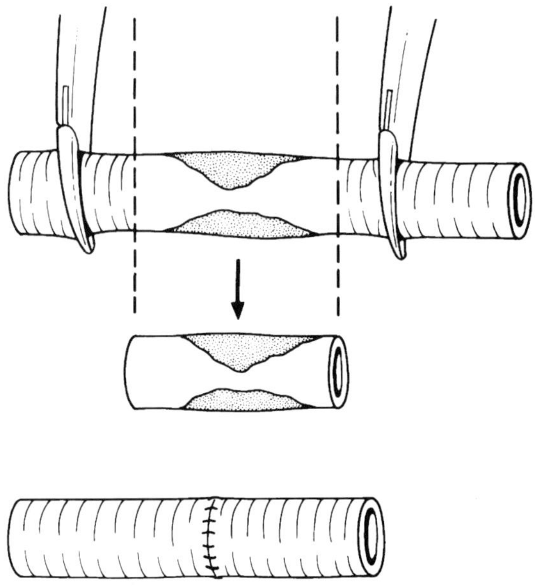

Figure 39.3. Segmental resection and reanastomosis.

the stenotic site, should be adequately isolated from surrounding tissues, to enable reanastomosis without tension.

We prefer to use interrupted monofilament sutures to anastomose arteries with a small diameter or continuous monofilament sutures between arteries with a larger diameter but leave large enough growth factors (Fig. 39.4). Taking these precautions into account might prevent restenosis of the new anastomosis.

Transection of the transplant artery distal to the anastomosis and end-to-side reimplantation

This technique is recommended for anastomotic stenosis of end renal artery to side common or external iliac artery anastomosis type. After isolation, the renal graft artery is transected distal to the stenosis. New end-to-side anastomosis is performed above or below the previous site of anastomosis to the appropriate iliac vessel (Fig. 39.5).

We prefer to use a vascular punch for adequate arteriotomy in the iliac vessel and to use interrupted monofilament sutures for the anastomosis in order to optimize the blood flow and prevention of stenosis.

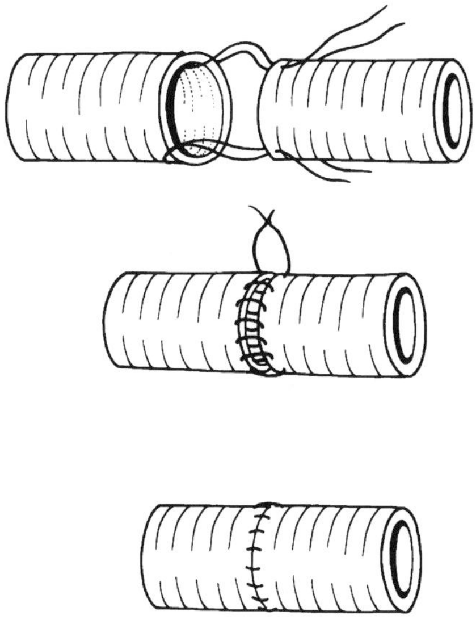

Figure 39.4. Continuous suture for end-to-end reanastomosis with growth factor to enable adequate widening after the resumption of blood flow.

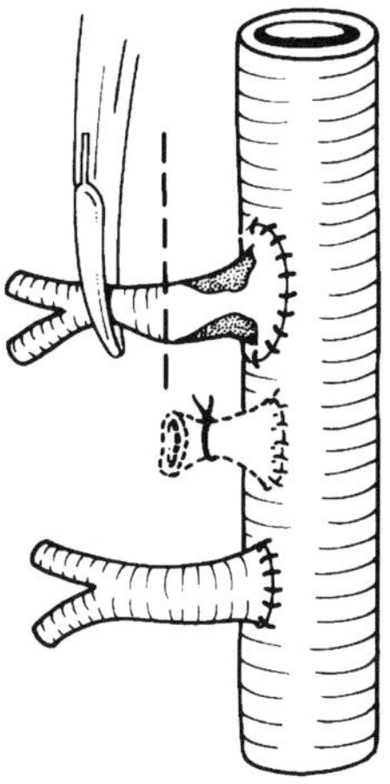

Figure 39.5. Transection of the artery distal to the stenosis and end-to-side reimplantation above or below the previous anastomosis.

The use of autologous saphenous vein grafts

Saphenous patch angioplasty

This is a popular repair procedure for stenosis, localized at any site along the transplant artery. This procedure might also be utilized in cases where the stenosis is localized or extended to the bifurcation of the main artery.[12]

The arteriotomy should be elongated enough, distally and proximally, along the edges of the stenosis. An eliptically shaped patch graft will permit dilatation of the artery at the stenotic site (Fig. 39.6).

Autogenous saphenous vein bypass graft

The use of autogenous saphenous vein conduit is a frequently employed procedure for bypassing native renal artery stenoses (Fig. 39.7).[16] This technique was readily adopted for the repair of TRAS.[12–15, 17] Utilizing this procedure enables the bridging of short or long segment stenoses where resection or transections and direct reanastomoses are not amenable.

The proximal anastomosis of the saphenous graft is firstly done end-to-side of the appropriate iliac artery in order to minimize the renal ischemic time. The distal anastomosis is then

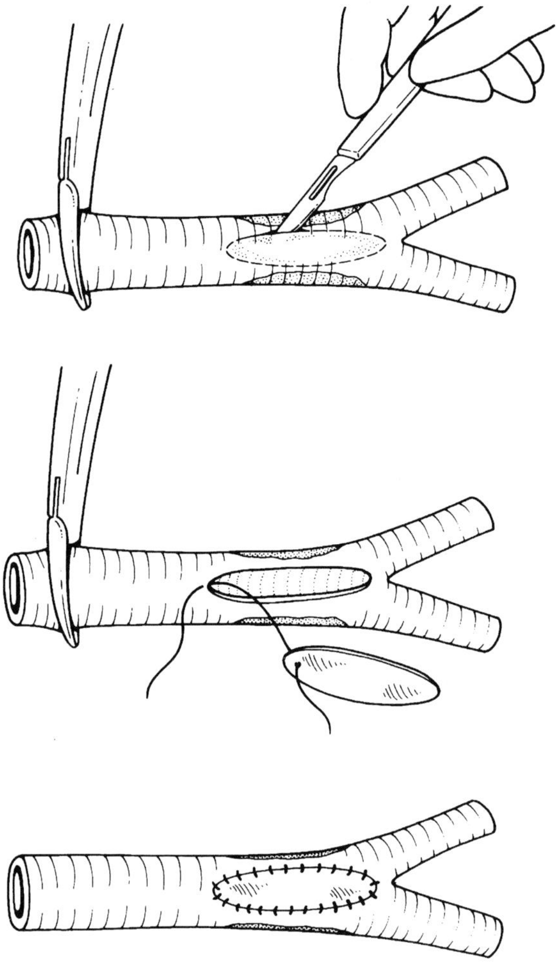

Figure 39.6. Arteriotomy extending proximally and distally to the stenotic segment and saphenous patch angioplasty.

performed end-to-side of the renal transplant artery. The arteriotomies of the the iliac artery and if possible of the transplant artery are preferably created with a vascular punch. Both edges of the saphenous graft should be spatulated in order to optimize blood flow and to prevent possible subsequent stenosis.

Autogenous saphenous vein interposition graft

This technique is similar to the previous one. The renal artery is transected at a level just distal to the stenosis and an end-to-end anastomosis is

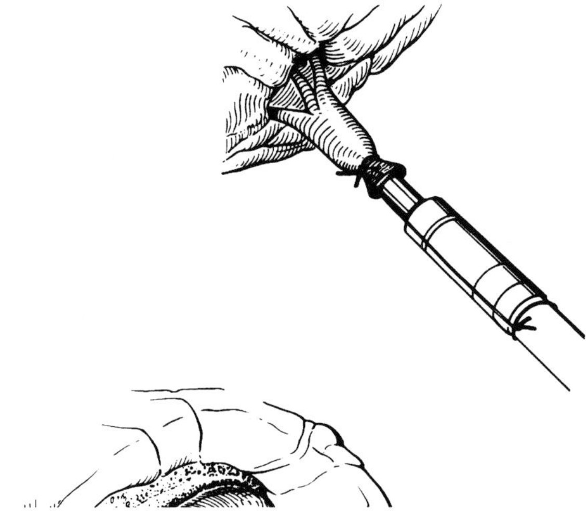

Figure 39.7. Saphenous vein bypassing the stenosis between the iliac artery and transplant renal artery.

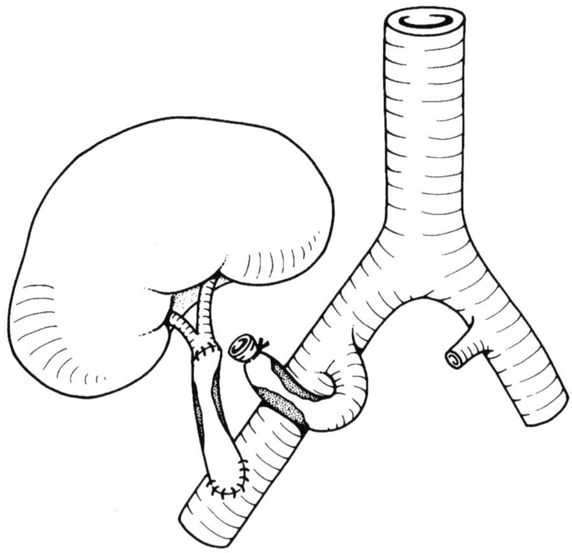

Figure 39.8. Transection of the transplant renal artery distal to the anastomosis and saphenous vein interposition between the renal artery (end-to-end) and iliac artery (end-to-side).

performed between the remnant of the renal artery and the saphenous graft. The proximal anastomosis is then created between the saphenous graft and the appropriate iliac artery end-to-side (Fig. 39.8), keeping the principles of vascular repair as mentioned before.

Postoperative management

In postoperative care and follow-up of patients who have undergone surgical revascularization, attention should be directed to the close monitoring of the renal graft perfusion and function. Deterioration of renal graft function which persists may indicate an impaired blood flow to the graft due to inadequate revascularization. Coincidental rejection or urine flow obstruction must be ruled out as a possible cause. Repeated isotope scans of the graft with 99 m-technetium and duplex ultrasonography of its artery are convenient tools in assessing the perfusion of the graft and the blood flow alterations.

The administration of short- or long-term anticoagulants after the procedure should be judged in respect to the size of the distal anastomosis, the revascularization type and the immediate technical results. In a situation where there is small-size anastomosis or long saphenous graft or unstable hemodynamic conditions during the operation, the administration of anticoagulants might prevent early thrombosis.

Results and complications of surgical revascularization of TRAS

The reported results and complication rates of surgical revascularization procedures for TRAS varies among studies. The immediate technical success rate has been known to range between 50 and 90%.[2, 4, 12, 14, 15, 19, 20] The reported improvement in renal graft function is between 38.8 and 44.4%[2, 10, 15] and the improvement in hypertension is between 44.4 and 100%.[2, 9, 13, 15] The complete cure rate is 22.2%.[2]

The occurence of restenosis is 9.3–12%[10, 13, 15, 20] and the rate of graft loss due to surgery varies between 2.38 and 20%.[2, 10, 13, 18] Reported mortality rates are between 1.6 and 5.5%.[2, 13, 15]

Data of 80 patients who underwent surgery for revascularization of TRAS collected from ten different publications by Grossman *et al.*[8] revealed a graft loss rate of 15%, reoperative rate of 13% and mortality rate of 5%.

Autogenous saphenous bypass graft revascularization procedure is the most frequently used surgery. The technical success with this procedure is reported to be between 50 and 94%.[12, 13, 17, 18] The rate of restenosis is between 4.7 and 6%.[13, 15] Improvement in blood pressure occurs in 60–100% of the cases.[12–15, 17]

Transection with end-to-side reimplantation and saphenous patch angioplasty are popular repair procedures. The technical success rates reported are: 80–100% [12, 18] and 70–100% [12, 14, 18] respectively.

In accordance with the experience gained in our center, improvement in blood pressure and renal function can be achieved in satisfactory rates by all the mentioned types of surgical repairs, providing that the procedures chosen have been adjusted to the requirements dictated by the localization length and etiology of the stenosis, and the principles for the prevention of restenosis or thrombosis have been strictly kept.

Interventional radiology for revascularization of TRAS

PTA

Utilizing PTA for the management of TRAS was first reported by Diamond and his collegues in 1979.[21] Since then PTA for revascularization of TRAS has rapidly replaced surgical interventions.[8, 22–26]

Percutaneous transluminal angioplasty became the treatment of choice for most types of TRAS because of its relative safety, simplicity and comparable clinical outcome to surgical corrections. The accepted *relative* contraindications for attempting PTA for revascularization of TRAS are:

1 In anticipation of inaccessibility of the artery, i.e. long convoluted stenosis resulting from twisting or kinking of the artery.
2 In diffuse stenosis involving several branches.
3 In anastomotic stenosis, which in most cases is resistant to this treatment.
4 The existence of significant coagulopathy should postpone the PTA procedure.

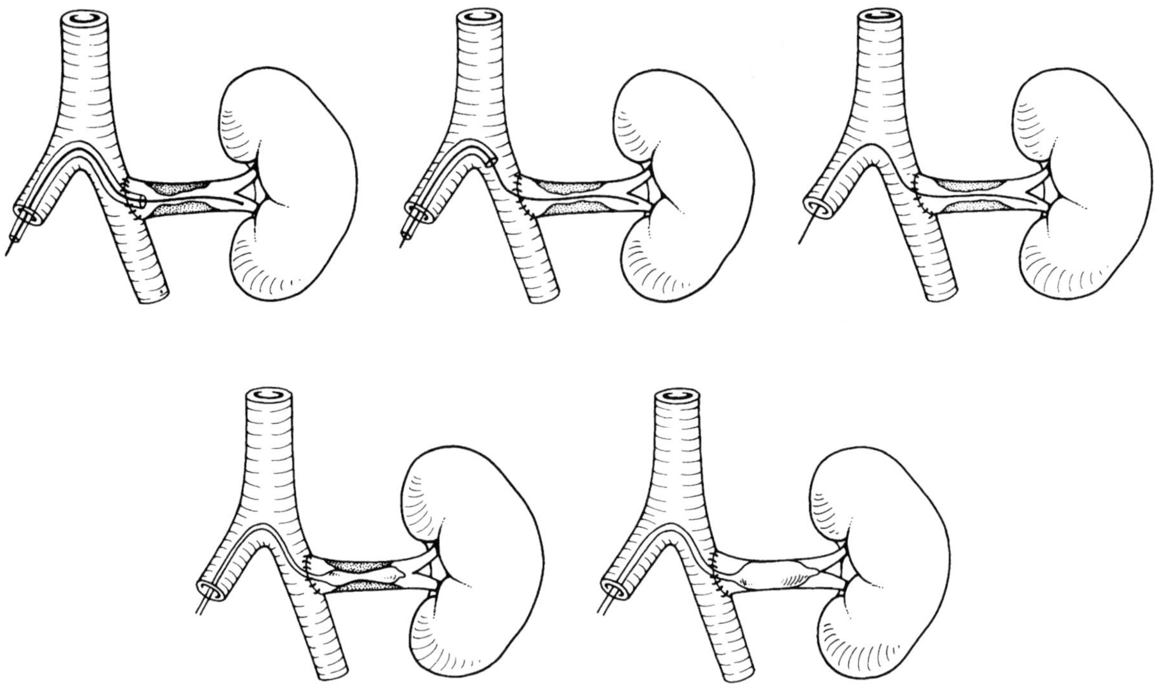

Figure 39.9. Contralateral insertion of selective arterial catheter toward the stenosis. Advancing of guidewire through the catheter and the stenosis. Replacement of the selective catheter with a balloon catheter and the inflating of the balloon until the 'waist' in the artery disappears.

Technique of PTA for TRAS

The performance of PTA for TRAS (Fig. 39.9) is based on the techniques described by Gruntzig.[27]

Preparations

Angioplasty as practised at our institution is in accordance with commonly accepted techniques.[5,6,11,28–31] Three days before the procedure, the patients are placed on short-acting antihypertensive drugs and 100 mg aspirin four times daily. The patient is told to fast during the 12 h preceding the procedure and is well hydrated in respect to his or her clinical condition. A normal coagulation profile and a patient's signed informed consent are mandatory prerequisites.

Techniques

The site of the femoral puncture is chosen according to the type of renal graft artery anastomosis. If the anastomosis is end-to-end, graft to hypogastric artery, then the ipsilateral femoral artery is the preferred catheter insertion site. In an end-to-side, graft to iliac artery anastomosis the contralateral femoral artery is chosen.

The patients are lightly sedated and the skin at the insertion site is locally anesthetized. Patients under 14 years of age often need general anesthesia for this procedure.

After percutaneous insertion of a selective catheter through the appropriate femoral artery, a small amount of non-ionic contrast medium is injected for a diagnostic image. The catheter tip is then directed fluoroscopically toward the lumen of the stenosis. A guidewire (usually 0.035 inch) is then advanced through the catheter and the stenosis. Then the selective catheter is advanced over the guidewire through the stenosis. The selective catheter is then exchanged for a short tip balloon catheter. Once the balloon is positioned in the lumen of the stenotic segment it is inflated with a pressure gauge syringe until the 'waist' in the balloon disappears. The balloon is kept inflated for 30 s but repeated inflation may be necessary in order to achieve satisfactory anatomical results, i.e. no more than 15% residual stenosis.

Anticoagulants (heparin 5000 units) are injected intra-arterially during the procedure. To prevent arterial spasms, intra-arterial nitroglycerine (100 μg) is injected per dilatation.

Post-procedural care

Patient care after completion of the procedure includes bed rest for 12–24 h and careful monitoring for possible complications, i.e. groin hematoma and impaired renal graft function. Anticoagulation is continued for 24 h and aspirin for 3 months is recommended, if not contraindicated.

Results and complications of PTA for TRAS

The initial technical success rate as reported by most of the recent studies is above 85%. However, recurrence of stenosis is reported to occur in between 11.1 and 20% of cases.[5, 6, 11, 28–30] Between 4 and 18% of the patients need secondary surgical intervention after failure of PTA as well as for graft salvage after severe complication of PTA, i.e. extensive artery dissection or perforation.[5, 6, 10, 11, 20, 30]

Graft loss rate as a result of PTA, reported in the majority of studies is approximately 5% with a range of between 0 and 18%. The common causes for graft loss are renal artery thrombosis and extensive renal artery or hypogastric artery dissection.[3, 10, 13, 17, 20, 25, 30, 32] There are almost no reports of mortality directly connected with PTA. Other less endangering complications of PTA are groin hematoma and arterial spasm.[5, 6, 11]

The choice of the revascularization procedure

The various publications on revascularization of TRAS show a disparity of success and complication rates (Table 39.1). In both procedures, the ranges of graft loss, restenosis, as well as technical success and blood pressure control are similar, but mortality is reported mainly in cases of surgical repair. For this reason it is well accepted by surgeons, radiologists and nephrologists that PTA should be the procedure of choice for revascularization of TRAS, providing no contraindication exists.

Further advantages of PTA are its relative simplicity and the acceptance of the procedure by the patients. Moreover failure of the PTA does not preclude the surgical intervention.

Primary surgical correction should be considered in cases of anastomotic or long convoluted stenoses and stenoses which respond poorly to treatment by PTA.

Successful revascularization of TRAS prolongs the renal graft and probably patient survival. One should however keep in mind that many TRAS could be prevented. The preventable stenoses are especially those whose etiology is concealed in the incorrect handling of the graft during preservation and implantation. Examples of such incorrect handling are: faulty suture technique; damage to the donor arterial intima by inaccurate cannulation for perfusion; improper apposition of the donor and recipient iliac vessels causing excessive length of the renal artery or renal artery–hypogastric artery conduit which may cause torsion and angulation.[33]

Table 39.1. Summary of success and complication rate ranges of surgical and PTA revascularization of TRAS

	Mortality (%)	Graft loss (%)	Restenosis (%)	Technical success (%)	Improvement in hypertension and/or graft function (%)
Surgical revascularization of TRAS	1.6–5.5	2.38–20	11.1–25	55–92.1	38.8–100
PTA for revascularization of TRAS	Almost no reports	5–18	11.1–20	58–93	63–93

References

1 Deglise-Favre, Hisse C, Lantz O *et al.* Long-term follow-up of 40 untreated cadaveric kidney transplant renal artery stenoses. *Transplant Proc* 1991; **23:** 1342–3.
2 Sagalowsky AI, Peters PS. Renovascular hypertension following renal transplantation. *Urol Clin North Am* 1984; **11:** 491–502.
3 Curtis JJ. Hypertension and kidney transplantation. *Am J Kidney Dis* 1986; **7:** 181–96.
4 Sutherland RS, Spees EK, Jones JW, Fink DW. Renal artery stenosis after renal transplantation: the impact of the hypogastric artery anastomosis. *J Urol* 1993; **149:** 980–5.
5 Bover J, Montana J, Castelao AM *et al.* Percutaneous transluminal angioplasty for treatment of allograft renal artery stenosis. *Transplant Proc* 1992; **24:** 94–5.
6 Thomas CP, Riad H, Johnson BF, Cumberland DC. Percutaneous transluminal angioplasty in transplant renal arterial stenoses: a long-term follow-up. *Transplant Int* 1992; **5:** 129–32.
7 Greenstein SM, Verstandig A, McLean GK *et al.* Percutaneous transluminal angioplasty. *Transplantation* 1987; **43:** 29–32.
8 Grossman RA, Dafoe DC, Shoenfeld RB *et al.* Percutaneous transluminal angioplasty treatment of renal transplant artery stenosis. *Transplantation* 1982; **34:** 339–43.
9 Chandrasoa P, Aberle AM. Anastomotic line renal artery stenosis after transplantation. *J Urol* 1986; **135:** 1159–62.
10 Roberts JP, Ascher NL, Fryd DS *et al.* Transplant renal artery stenosis. *Transplantation* 1989; **48:** 580–3.
11 Matalon TAS, Thompson MJ, Patel SK *et al.* Percutaneous transluminal angioplasty for transplant renal artery stenosis. *J Vasc Intervent Radiol* 1992; **3:** 55–8.
12 Dickerman RM, Pefers PC, Hull AR *et al.* Surgical correction of posttransplant renovascular hypertension. *Ann Surg* 1980; **192:** 639–44.
13 Benoit G, Hiesse C, Lcard P *et al.* Treatment of renal artery stenosis after renal transplantation. *Transplant Proc* 1987; **19:** 3600–1.
14 Tilney NL, Rocha A, Strom TB, Kirkman RL. Renal artery stenosis in transplant patients. *Ann Surg* 1984; **199:** 454–60.
15 Lacombe M. Renal artery stenosis after renal transplantation. *Ann Vasc Surg* 1988; **2:** 155–60.
16 Novick AC. Surgical correction of renovascular hypertension. *Surg Clin North Am* 1988; **68:** 1007–25.
17 DeMeyer M, Pirson Y, Dautrebande J *et al.* Treatment of renal graft artery stenosis comparison between surgical bypass and percutaneous transluminal angioplasty. *Transplantation* 1989, **47:** 784–8.
18 Merkus JWS, Huysmans FTM, Hoitsma AJ *et al.* Renal allograft artery stenosis: results of medical treatment and intervention. A retrospective analysis. *Transplant Int* 1993; **6:** 111–15.
19 Palleschi J, Novick AC, Braun WE, Magnusson MO. Vascular complications of renal transplantation. *Urology* 1980, **16:** 61–7.
20 Benoit G, Moukarazel M, Hisse L *et al.* Transplant renal artery stenosis: experience and comparative results between surgery and angioplasty. *Transplant Int* 1990; **3:** 137–40.
21 Diamond NG, Cassarella WJ, Hardy MA. Dilation of critical transplant renal artery stenosis by percutaneous transluminal angioplasty. *Am J Roentgenol* 1979; **133:** 1167–9.
22 Whiteside I, Cardella CJ, Yeung H *et al.* The role of percutaneous transluminal dilation in the treatment of transplant renal stenosis. *Clin Nephrol* 1982; **17:** 55–9.
23 Rankin RN, Illan RA, Keown PA. Percutaneous transluminal dilation of transplant renal artery stenosis. *Postgrad Med J* 1981; **57:** 300–3.
24 Lohr JW, MacDougal ML, Chonko AM *et al.* Percutaneous transluminal angioplasty in transplant renal artery stenosis: experience and review of the literature. *Am J Kidney Dis* 1986; **12:** 363–7.
25 Raynaud A, Bedrossian J, Remy P *et al.* Percutaneous transluminal angioplasty of renal transplant arterial stenoses. *Am J Roentgenol* 1986; **146:** 853–7.
26 Zajko AB, McLean GK, Grossman RA *et al.* Percutaneous transluminal angioplasty and fibrinolytic therapy for renal allograft arterial anastomosis and thromobosis. *Transplantation* 1982; **33:** 447–50.
27 Gruntzig A. Percutaneous transluminal recanalization (PTR) with the double-lumen dilatation catheter. In Zeitler E, Gruntzig A, Shoop W (eds) *Percutaneous Vascular Recanalization*, p. 17. Berlin: Springer-Verlag; 1978.
28 Spijkerboer M, Mali WP Th, Donckerwolcke RAMG. Renal transplant artery stenosis in children: treatment with percutaneous transluminal angioplasty. *Pediatr Radiol* 1992; **22:** 519–21.
29 McMullin ND, Reidy JF, Koppman CG *et al.* The management of renal transplant artery stenosis in children by percutaneous transluminal angioplasty. *Transplantation* 1992; **53:** 559–63.
30 Fauchald P, Vante K, Paulson D *et al.* Long-term clinical results of percutaneous transluminal angioplasty in transplant renal artery stenosis. *Nephrol Dial Transplant* 1992; **7:** 256–9.
31 Alaiabadi H, McLorie GA, Churchill M, Mcmullin N. Percutaneous transluminal angioplasty for transplant renal artery stenosis in children. *J Urol* 1990; **143:** 569–73.
32 Viron B, Lacomb M, Raynaud A *et al.* Delayed extensive arterial dissection after percutaneous transluminal angioplasty for transplant renal artery stenosis. *Nephron* 1991; **58:** 351–3.
33 Novick AC. Secondary renal vascular reconstruction for arterial disease in the native and transplant kidney. *Urol Clin North Am* 1994, **21:** 255–63.

Index

Abbreviations used in subheadings are: ARAS – Atherosclerotic renal artery stenosis; MRA – Magnetic resonance angiography; PTRA – Percutaneous transluminal renal angioplasty; RAS – Renal artery stenosis; RVH – Renovascular hypertension; TRAS – transplant renal artery stenosis